Medical Atlas of Cornea and External Diseases in Middle Eastern Populations

Anna Hovakimyan
Malayan Ophthalmologic Centre, Armenia

IGI Global
PUBLISHER of TIMELY KNOWLEDGE

A volume in the Advances in Medical Diagnosis, Treatment, and Care (AMDTC) Book Series

Published in the United States of America by
IGI Global
Medical Information Science Reference (an imprint of IGI Global)
701 E. Chocolate Avenue
Hershey PA, USA 17033
Tel: 717-533-8845
Fax: 717-533-8661
E-mail: cust@igi-global.com
Web site: http://www.igi-global.com

Library of Congress Cataloging-in-Publication Data

Names: Hovakimyan, Anna, 1970- author.
Title: Medical atlas of cornea and external diseases in Middle Eastern populations / by Anna Hovakimyan.
Description: Hershey, PA : Medical Information Science Reference, [2022] | Includes bibliographical references and index. | Summary: "This atlas presents around 700 pictures of different corneal pathologies and external diseases, of photo-documented cases by the author of over ten years of clinical practice"-- Provided by publisher.
Identifiers: LCCN 2021031288 (print) | LCCN 2021031289 (ebook) | ISBN 9781799869375 (hardcover) | ISBN 9781799869382 (ebook)
Subjects: MESH: Corneal Diseases--pathology | Conjunctival Diseases--pathology | Middle East | Atlas | Case Reports
Classification: LCC RE336 (print) | LCC RE336 (ebook) | NLM WW 17 | DDC 617.7/19--dc23
LC record available at https://lccn.loc.gov/2021031288
LC ebook record available at https://lccn.loc.gov/2021031289

This book is published in the IGI Global book series Advances in Medical Diagnosis, Treatment, and Care (AMDTC) (ISSN: 2475-6628; eISSN: 2475-6636)

British Cataloguing in Publication Data
A Cataloguing in Publication record for this book is available from the British Library.

All work contributed to this book is new, previously-unpublished material. The views expressed in this book are those of the authors, but not necessarily of the publisher.

For electronic access to this publication, please contact: eresources@igi-global.com.

Advances in Medical Diagnosis, Treatment, and Care (AMDTC) Book Series

ISSN:2475-6628
EISSN:2475-6636

Mission

Advancements in medicine have prolonged the life expectancy of individuals all over the world. Once life-threatening conditions have become significantly easier to treat and even cure in many cases. Continued research in the medical field will further improve the quality of life, longevity, and wellbeing of individuals.

The **Advances in Medical Diagnosis, Treatment, and Care (AMDTC)** book series seeks to highlight publications on innovative treatment methodologies, diagnosis tools and techniques, and best practices for patient care. Comprised of comprehensive resources aimed to assist professionals in the medical field apply the latest innovations in the identification and management of medical conditions as well as patient care and interaction, the books within the AMDTC series are relevant to the research and practical needs of medical practitioners, researchers, students, and hospital administrators.

Coverage

- Patient Interaction
- Critical Care
- Internal Medicine
- Patient-Centered Care
- Cancer Treatment
- Experimental Medicine
- Emergency Medicine
- Disease Management
- Alternative Medicine
- Medical Testing

IGI Global is currently accepting manuscripts for publication within this series. To submit a proposal for a volume in this series, please contact our Acquisition Editors at acquisitions@igi-global.com or visit: https://www.igi-global.com/publish/.

The Advances in Medical Diagnosis, Treatment, and Care (AMDTC) Book Series (ISSN 2475-6628) is published by IGI Global, 701 E. Chocolate Avenue, Hershey, PA 17033-1240, USA, www.igi-global.com. This series is composed of titles available for purchase individually; each title is edited to be contextually exclusive from any other title within the series. For pricing and ordering information please visit https://www.igi-global.com/book-series/advances-medical-diagnosis-treatment-care/129618. Postmaster: Send all address changes to above address.

Titles in this Series

For a list of additional titles in this series, please visit: www.igi-global.com/book-series/advances-medical-diagnosis-treatment-care/129618

Using Narrative Writing to Enhance Healing During and After Global HealthCrises
Jennifer Lynne Bird (Oxbridge Academy, USA)
Medical Information Science Reference • © 2022 • 241pp • H/C (ISBN: 9781799890515) • US $295.00

Handbook of Research on Pathophysiology and Strategies for the Management of COVID-19
Omar El Hiba (Chouaib Doukkali University, Morocco) Jayakumar Radhakrishnan (Veterans Affairs Medical Center, USA) Tiziano Balzano (University Hospital HM Puerta del Sur, Spain) and Faical Isbaine (Emory University, USA)
Medical Information Science Reference • © 2022 • 352pp • H/C (ISBN: 9781799882251) • US $425.00

Strategies to Overcome Superbug Invasions Emerging Research and Opportunities
Dimple Sethi Chopra (Punjabi University, India) and Ankur Kaul (Institute of Nuclear Medicine and Allied Sciences, India)
Medical Information Science Reference • © 2021 • 319pp • H/C (ISBN: 9781799803072) • US $225.00

Integrated Care and Fall Prevention in Active and Healthy Aging
Patrik Eklund (Umea University, Sweden)
Medical Information Science Reference • © 2021 • 348pp • H/C (ISBN: 9781799844112) • US $345.00

Cases on Applied and Therapeutic Humor
Michael K. Cundall Jr. (North Carolina A&T State University, USA) and Stephanie Kelly (North Carolina A&T State University, USA)
Medical Information Science Reference • © 2021 • 267pp • H/C (ISBN: 9781799845287) • US $255.00

Artificial Intelligence for Accurate Analysis and Detection of Autism Spectrum Disorder
Sandeep Kautish (Lord Buddha Education Foundation, Nepal & Asia Pacific University of Technology & Innovation, Malaysia) and Gaurav Dhiman (Government Bikram College of Commerce, India)
Medical Information Science Reference • © 2021 • 224pp • H/C (ISBN: 9781799874607) • US $295.00

Diagnostic and Treatment Methods for Ulcerative Colitis and Colitis-Associated Cancer
Ashok Kumar Pandurangan (B. S. Abdur Rahman Crescent Institute of Science and Technology, India)
Medical Information Science Reference • © 2021 • 309pp • H/C (ISBN: 9781799835806) • US $295.00

IGI Global
PUBLISHER of TIMELY KNOWLEDGE

701 East Chocolate Avenue, Hershey, PA 17033, USA
Tel: 717-533-8845 x100 • Fax: 717-533-8661
E-Mail: cust@igi-global.com • www.igi-global.com

To my family and my mentors, without whose continuous support over the years, this atlas would not have come through, and who make it all these efforts worthwhile. To Malayan Eye Center, where I work as head of the Cornea-Uveitis Department since 2005, and to Dr. Alexander Malayan, who has played a pivotal role in my professional career.

Table of Contents

Preface

This atlas presents over 800 pictures of different corneal pathologies and external diseases, narrowed down from 13000 photo-documented cases over ten years of clinical practice. This book contains unique cases that are very rare in other countries, and even a few cases that are not included in other similar books. These individual cases could be related to the specific geographic area, as well as to the social conditions of life. The photos regarding corneal ulcers/keratitis caused by specific and isolated microorganisms, with before and after treatment photos, will give a general idea to any clinician on how the appearance of the eye will end up. It is important to emphasize that corneal ulcers present a vision-threatening condition and that's why they have been prioritized in this atlas. A few of the patients that traveled remotely and were successfully treated did not return to our hospital for follow up, which is why in these few cases, the book misses after-treatment photos.

I would like to mention several diseases that are exceptionally common in Middle Eastern populations, especially in Armenia; We see many vernal disease cases starting from early Spring till late Fall. We have described an atypical case of inferiorly localized shield ulcer with before and after-treatment photos that have been described only in India (2 cases so far to our knowledge). Atopic conjunctivitis though, is extremely rare in this region. We see about 400-450 new keratoconus cases per year at our hospital. Within 1 year around 350 cases undergo collagen cross-lining, 25-30 cases get Ferrara Ring implants, and about 30-50 cases undergo transplant surgery. Fuchs uveitis syndrome is very common, accounting to 7.8 – 8% of all uveitis cases referrals, whereas Fuchs endothelial dystrophy is very rare. Herpetic keratitis is also extremely common in Armenia; we see about 40-50 new cases per year at our hospital with different presentations (the treatment options we offer are covered in Ch. 5).

This atlas can be an ideal handbook for junior practitioners, including residents and students. This comprehensive collection of Middle Eastern patients can be an excellent supplement to the existing literature in this field. All the cases were exclusively diagnosed and treated by me at Malayan Eye Center in Yerevan, Armenia. All surgeries have been performed by me with the exception of initial cases of KPro surgeries that were performed with Dr. Aldave and Dr. Hovhanesian. In several PK cases, a few sutures have been done by young doctors in my department under my supervision. Due credits are given under the few photos taken from other practitioners.

Acknowledgment

I would like to express my profound gratitude to my junior colleagues Araks Davtyan and Artak Kirakosyan. Araks Davtyan helped with the editing of the volume. Her attention to detail and the level of depth with descriptions of pathologies, often borrowed from BCSC Cornea volume and the 2017 4th Edition of Cornea (edited by M.J. Mannis and E. J. Holland), made an invaluable contribution towards finalizing this atlas. Artak Kirakosyan was always standing by with his smartphone, taking high-quality pictures, and organizing them into suitable folders to facilitate the writing of this atlas. It is important to mention at this point that some earlier images, taken with a different device before the smartphone (iPhone X), have been discarded due to quality issues. In case of interest, these pictures of prior years can be shared through private messages. Ani Hambardzumyan was my main collaborator 15 years ago, with whom I started thinking about generating such an atlas and used the photo camera attached to the Haag-Streit slit lamp for taking photos. A few rare cases from these times that never appeared again in practice have been included in the book for completeness.

I am incredibly grateful to all my mentors, who have made enormous contributions to the development of my career, including Alexander Malayan, Roger Ohanesian, John Hovanesyan, Emmett Cunningham, Todd Margolis, Ed Holland, Anthony Aldave, Lee Shahinian, and many other colleagues, learning from whom has been a great privilege.

I would also like to express my sincere thankfulness to all my colleagues throughout the country for referring the most challenging cases, especially corneal ulcers, to my department.

Chapter 1
Eyelid Diseases

ABSTRACT

This chapter reviews eyelid malpositions, benign and malignant tumors, infections, and inflammatory diseases of the eyelid. Eyelid lesions can originate in any layer or structure within the eyelid and eyelid adnexa. Benign tumors of the eyelid can often be diagnosed based on their characteristic appearance. A biopsy should be performed if an eyelid lesion is not easily diagnosed based on clinical appearance. Blepharitis and meibomitis are very common disorders. Despite their prevalence, these diseases are often overlooked and misdiagnosed. Meibomian gland dysfunction is a major cause of evaporative dry eye and can occur along with aqueous deficient dry eye. Bacteria, fungi, viruses, and parasites can cause infection of the eyelids in different locations, anterior, posterior, angular, which can have different courses, acute, intermediate, or chronic. This chapter also contains photos with a rare disorder, Urbach-Wiethe disease, demonstrating the lesions of lipoid proteinosis at the lower and upper eyelids.

DISORDERS OF EYELIDS

Malposition of Eyelids

Normal eyelid apposition, blinking, and closure are necessary for maintenance of a healthy ocular surface. Eyelid malpositions more frequently involve the lower eyelid. Malposition of eyelids includes ectropion, entropion, trichiasis, distichiasis, floppy eyelid syndrome (discussed in chapter 3 - Conjunctivitis), lid imbrication syndrome, lagophthalmos, and eyelid retraction.

Ectropion can be congenital, involutional, cicatricial, paralytic, mechanical or inflammatory. Involutional ectropion is caused by laxity of retractors and/or canthal tendons (Stefanyszy, 1985). It is almost always seen in the lower lids in elderly patients (Fig 1). The treatment involves surgical repair with control of inflammation.

DOI: 10.4018/978-1-7998-6937-5.ch001

Figure 1. Involutional ectropion. The everted lower lid is seen

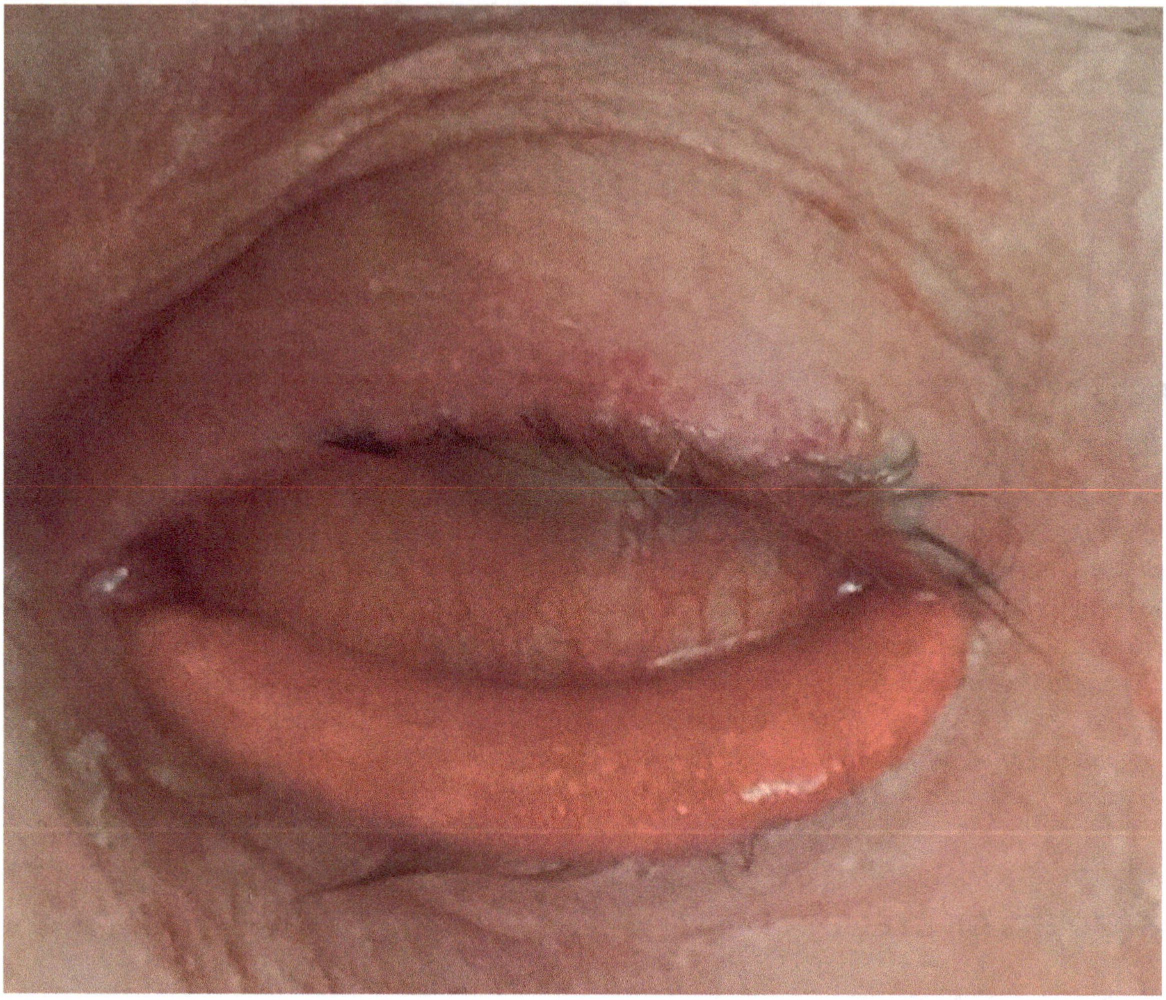

Entropion is an eversion of eyelids inward. It can be congenital, involutional, cicatricial, and acute spastic. Involutional entropion is the most common form of entropion, usually seen in elderly patients, mainly involving the lower eyelids (Nowinski et al, 1985) (Fig 2). In spastic entropion, therapeutic management with lubrication, bandage contact lens may be helpful. Other types of entropion require surgical interventions with different techniques.

Trichiasis is a condition where the lashes are misdirected backward toward the cornea, but the tarsal plate maintains normal apposition to the globe (Lyon et al, 1994). Trichiasis is usually secondary to chronic inflammatory diseases, including: blepharitis, trachoma, ocular cicatricial pemphigoid, Stevens-Johnson syndrome, or chemical burns, but can be idiopathic as well (Fig 3). Trichiasis may occur diffusely across the entire eyelid margin, or in small segments. There are several ways to treat Trichiasis, including Epilation, Electrolysis, Cryotherapy, and Blue-green argon laser ablation. Epilation is appropriate for a few misdirected lashes, although the lashes can grow back within 4–6 weeks. Electrolysis can treat individual eyelashes for more permanent results (Lyon et al, 1994). Cryotherapy is effective for groups of eyelashes (Sullivan et al, 1976). Blue-green argon laser ablation can be used to treat trichiasis, with variable results (Bartley et al, 1992).

Figure 2. Involutional entropion. The insight everted lower eyelid is seen

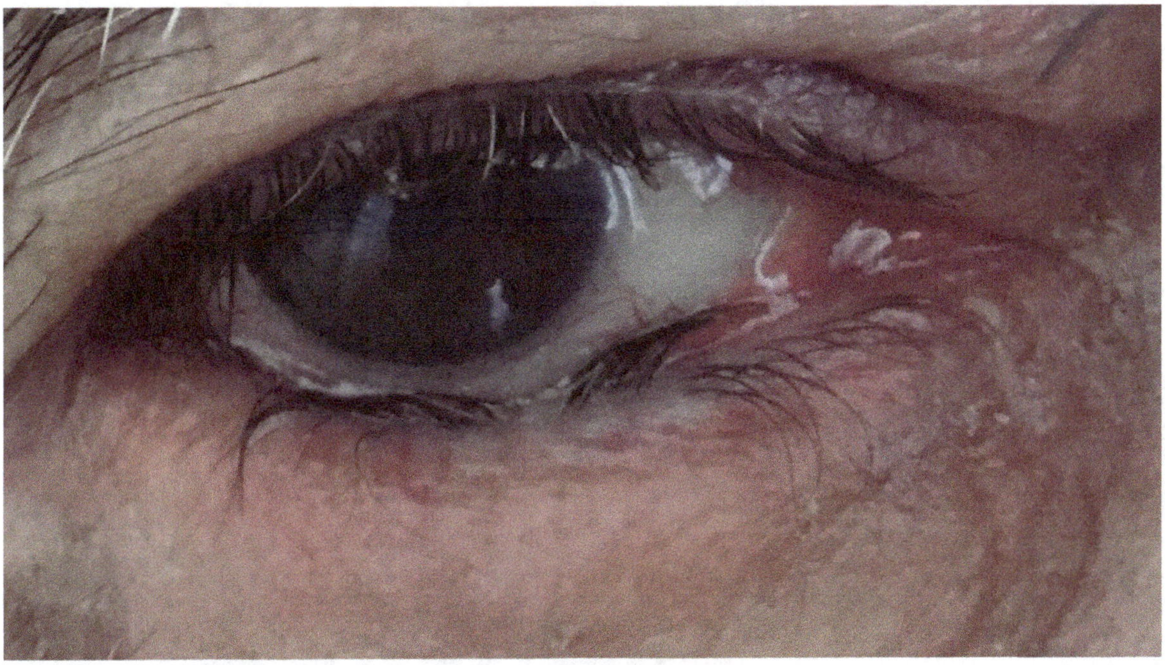

Figure 3. Trichiasis, eyelashes growing backward and misdirected

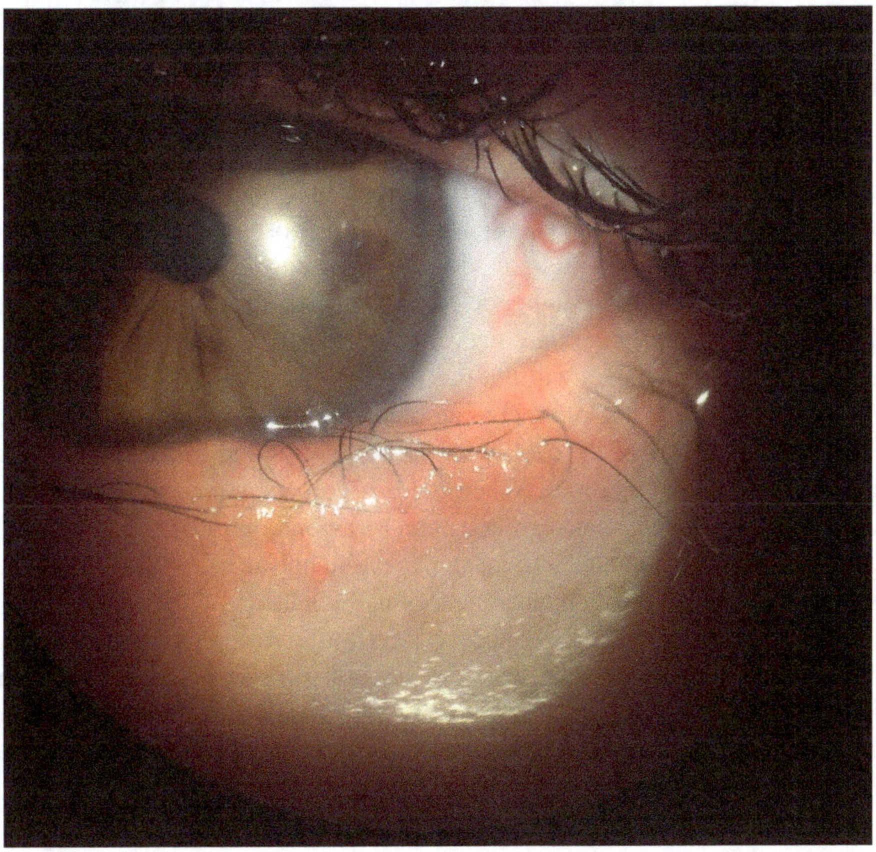

Distichiasis is a congenital or acquired condition when an extra row of eyelashes emerges from the meibomian gland orifices. Acquired distichiasis can occur due to trauma and chronic inflammatory diseases of the eyelids and conjunctiva (Fig 4). Focal areas may be treated by epilation or electrolysis. Cryotherapy applied to the posterior lamella can also be used for a few lashes. In the case of more extensive distichiasis, the eyelid can be split along the gray line and the posterior lamella can be treated with cryotherapy or focal hyfrecation. The posterior lid margin and tarsal plate containing the distichiatic hair follicles can be excised directly (Lyon et al, 1994).

Figure 4. Distichiasis. An additional fine row of eyelashes is seen

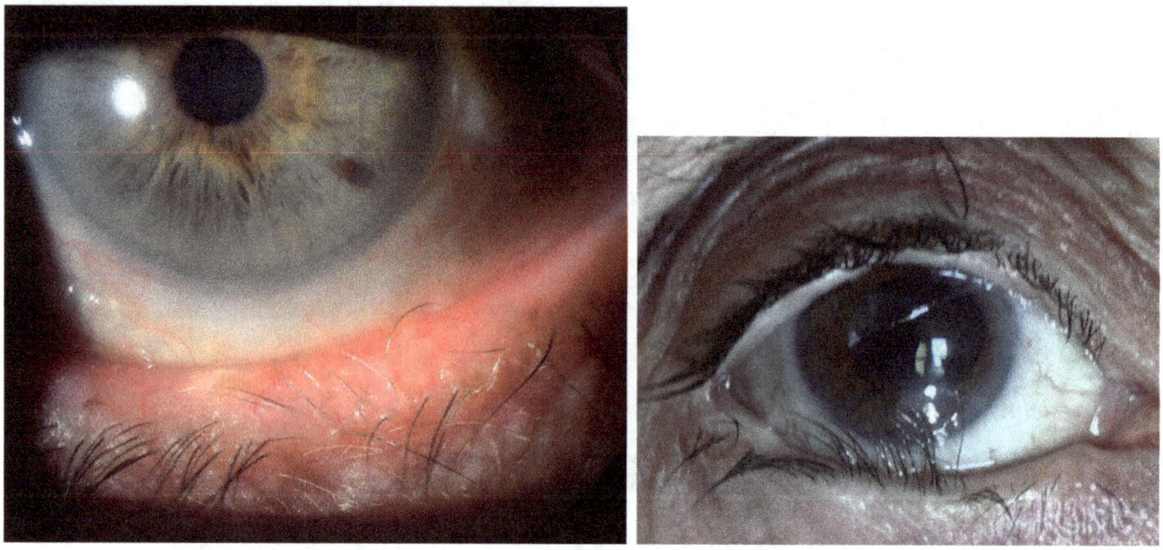

Lagophthalmos is the inability to close the eyelids properly. Thus, a portion of the eye remains open when blinking, as well as during sleep, and gets damaged from exposure (Hall, 1936; Howitt, 1966; Fuchs et al, n.d.). Lagophthalmos can develop due to several factors such as a forward projection of the eye within the orbit, vertical shortening of the upper or lower eyelids, dysfunction of the protractor orbicularis oculi muscle (Fig 6; 7), or its seventh cranial nerve motor innervation (Fig 5), adhesions between the globe and upper lid, etc. Artificial tears without preservatives can be administered frequently in order to improve the patient's tear film. The ointment can be applied at nighttime or during the day if there is severe corneal exposure. Taping of the eyelids at night can offer additional ocular surface protection without resorting to surgery (Lemp, 2009). When there is corneal exposure and recovery is expected within a matter of weeks, a temporary tarsorrhaphy can be a good option. If there is no full lid closure, gold or platinum weight can be implanted into the upper eyelid in patients with paralytic lagophthalmos. This will result in a gravity-dependent enhancement of eyelid closure (Siah et al, 2018). Patients with lagophthalmos secondary to upper eyelid retraction (i.e. from thyroid eye disease) can have recession surgery of the upper eyelid retractor muscles (levator palpebrae superioris and Müller's muscles). Lower eyelid laxity occurs in facial nerve paralysis and floppy eyelid syndrome. Lid tightening procedures such as lateral tarsal strip will lead **to improved apposition of the lower eyelid to the globe and decrease scleral exposure and epiphora symptoms (Kwon, 2015).**

Figure 5. Lagophthalmos caused by seventh nerve dysfunction. Bell's palsy is seen

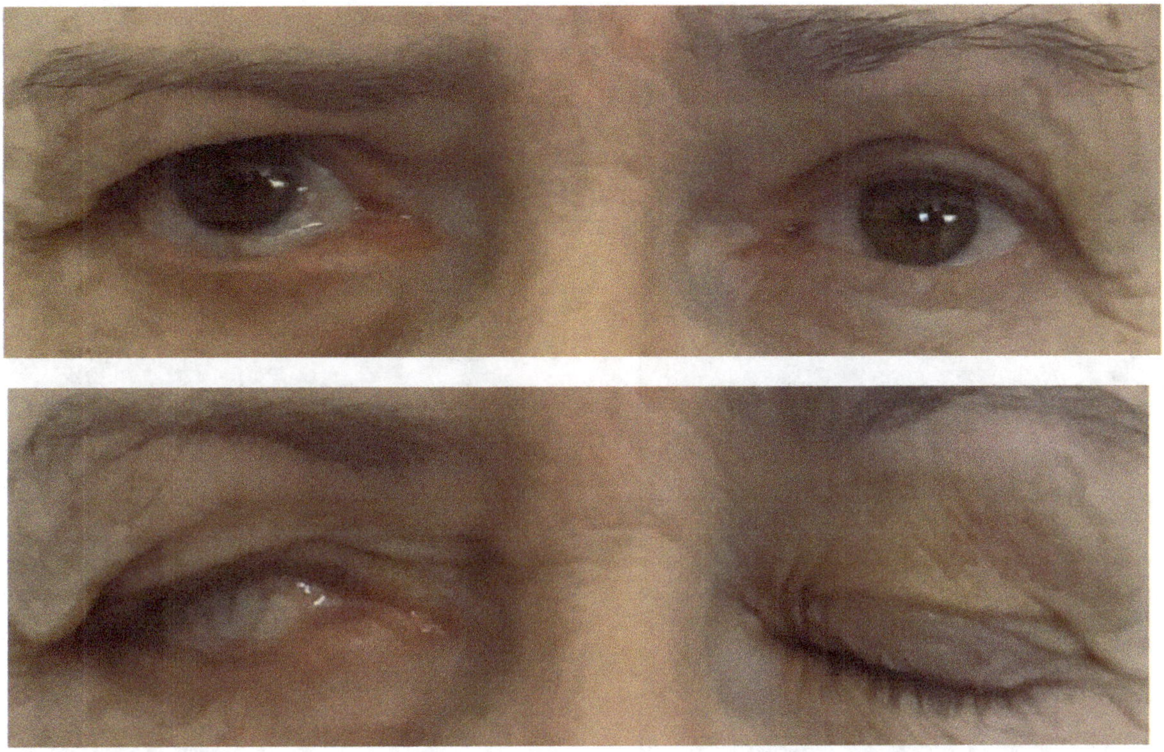

Figure 6. Lagophthalmos caused by ectropion with exposure keratopathy. Hypopyon is noted

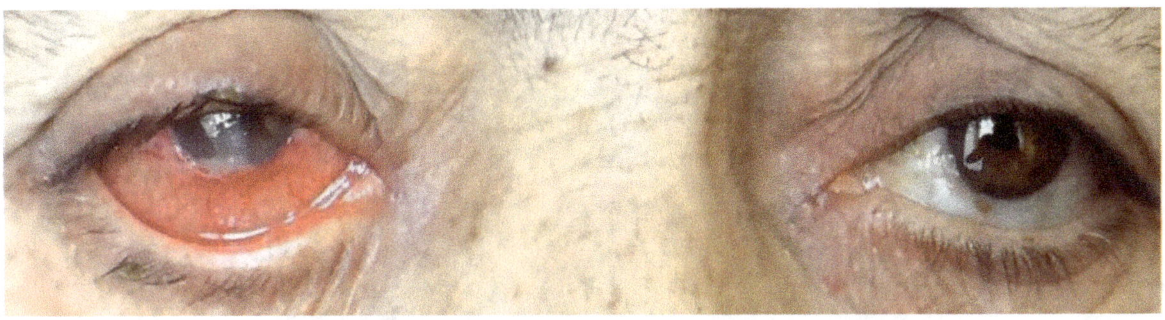

Figure 7. The same eye. Incomplete eyelids closure is noted

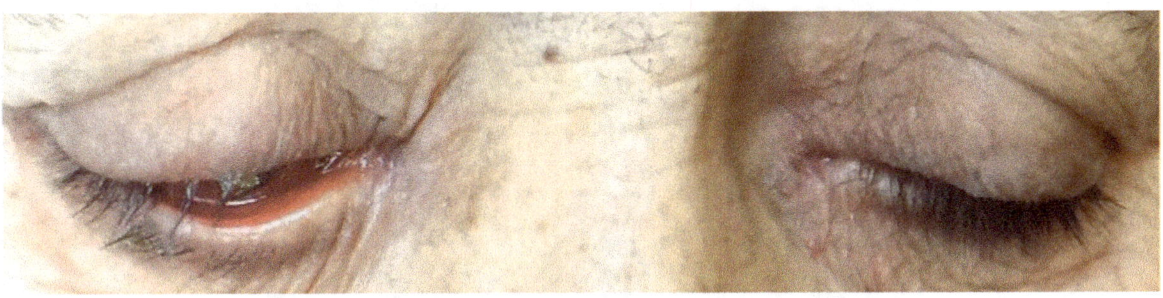

Orbital fat prolapse is a movable yellowish mass, usually located in the superotemporal quadrant beneath the conjunctiva (Glover, 1987). Localized weakness or thinning of Tenon's capsule due to aging or surgical trauma is its main cause. Typically, males are more likely to get affected than females (Fig 8, 9). Surgical repair of orbital fat prolapse is indicated for discomfort or for cosmetic complaints. Standard surgical method involves resection of herniated fat through conjunctival incision.

Figure 8. Orbital flat prolapse is seen in inferotemporal quadrant (unusual location)

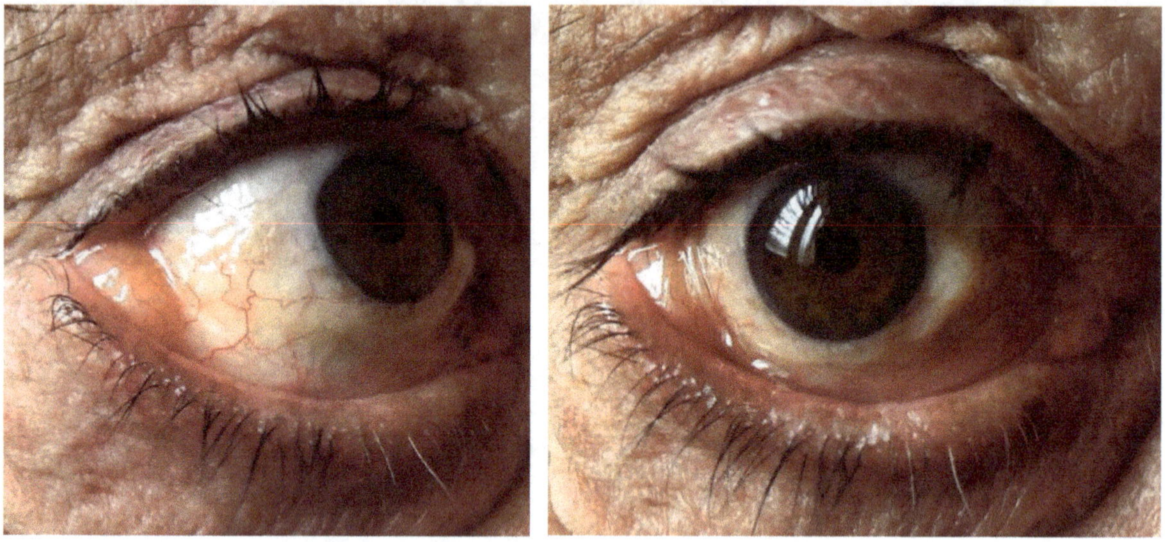

Figure 9. The same eye under slit lamp. Yellowish mass is seen under conjunctiva

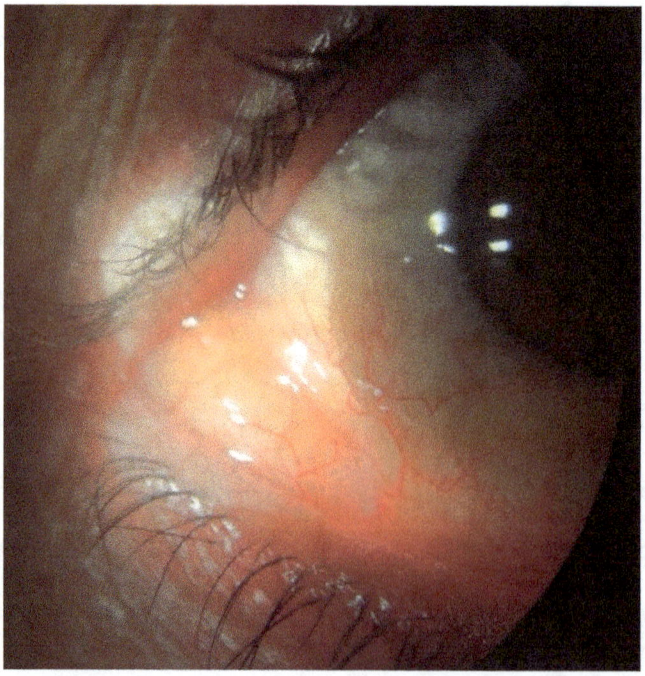

Benign Lid Tumors

Numerous benign tumors can originate in any layer or structure within the eyelid and eyelid adnexa. Benign tumors of the eyelid are usually diagnosed based on their characteristic appearance.

Acrochordon (skin tags) is considered a common benign eyelid tumor (Domonkos, 1982). Clinically, they are small, multiple, flesh-colored lesions attached to the eyelid margin or skin by a thin pedicle. Rarely they can be large and pedunculated (Fig 10). Treatment is surgical: cryotherapy or shave excision.

Figure 10. Acrochordon as a small pedunculated lesion is seen

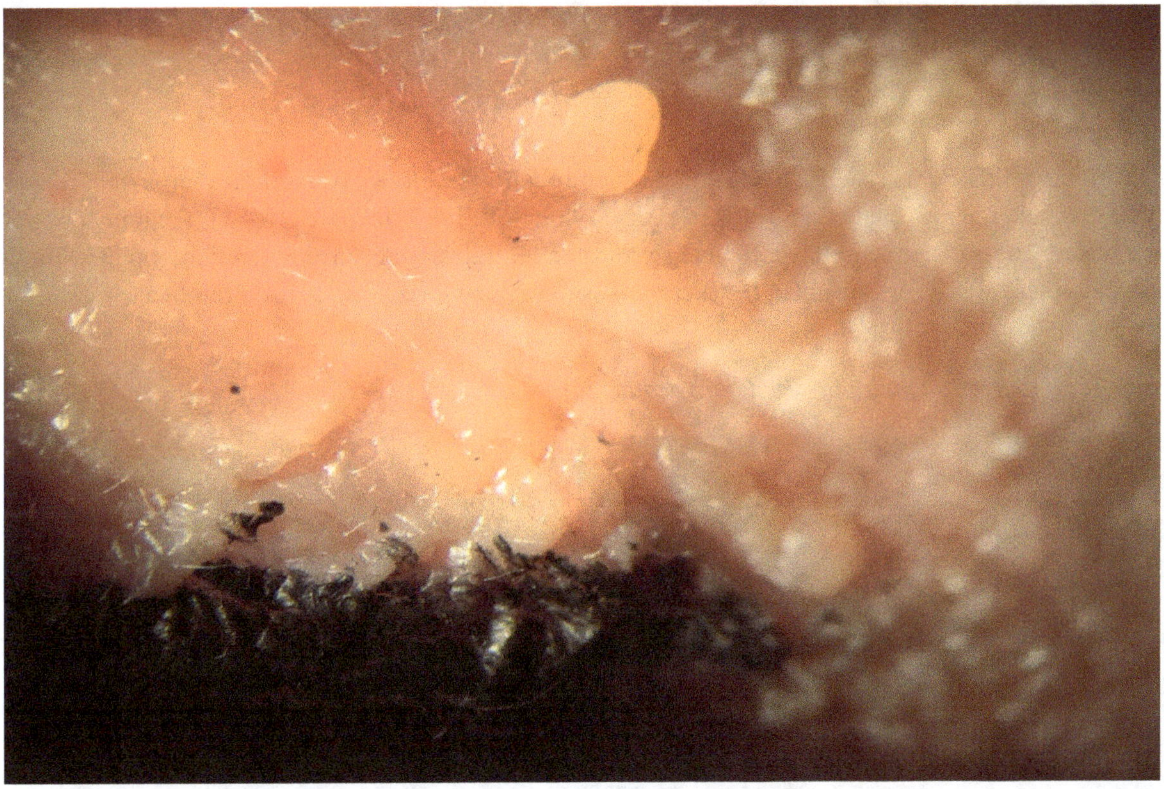

Cavernous hemangioma is considered to be the most common benign primary orbital tumor of adults. Eyelid involvement is rare (Jakobiec et al, 1991). Eyelid lesions, usually multiple, are compressible, can present as deep dermal and subcutaneous nodules. (Fig 11). Treatment indications include threatened or manifest amblyopia due to induced astigmatic refractive error or occlusion amblyopia, optic neuropathy due to tumor compression, exposure keratopathy due to massive proptosis. Surgical excision is the recommended treatment when indicated.

Pyogenic granuloma is not an accurate term, as this lesion is not pyogenic or granulomatous. Previously, it was thought that this lesion was caused by a pyogenic infection of a small wound. According to histological appearance, "eruptive hemangioma" or "hemangioma of granulation tissue" are more correct terms. It is the most commonly acquired vascular lesion of the eyelid and can be considered an inflammatory lesion. Clinically, a pedunculated, reddish lesion with frequent superficial ulcerations of

Figure 11. Cavernous hemangioma. The same eye under slit lamp (left)

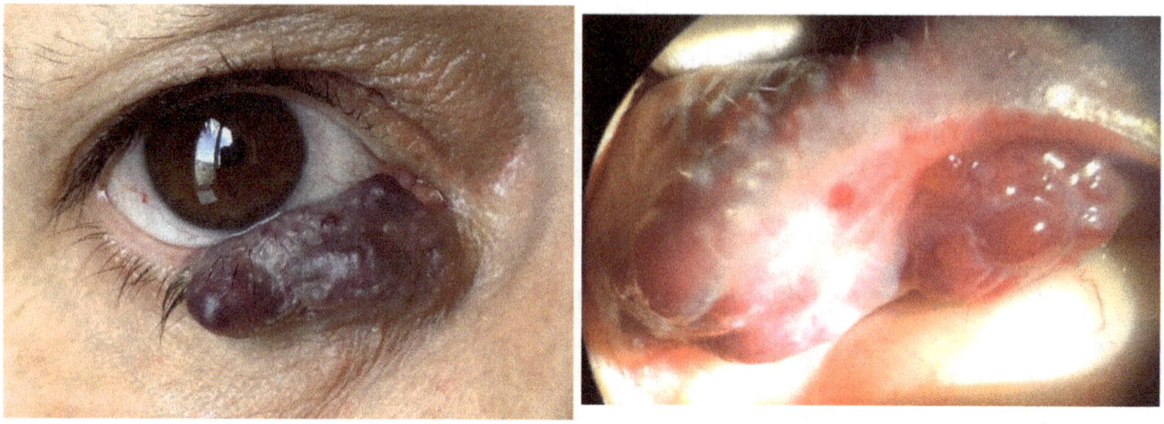

the overlying epithelium is seen. This lesion most commonly develops after minor trauma or surgery or may be associated with a chalazion (Fig 12) (Ferry, 1989; Soll, 1993; Jakobiec, 1988). Treatment options include: surgical excision, curettage, topical steroids and intralesional steroid injection, topical Timolol 0.5% and other topical (or oral) beta-blockers, cryosurgery, cauterization or laser removal.

Figure 12. Pyogenic granulomas. Reddish, pedunculated lesions are seen

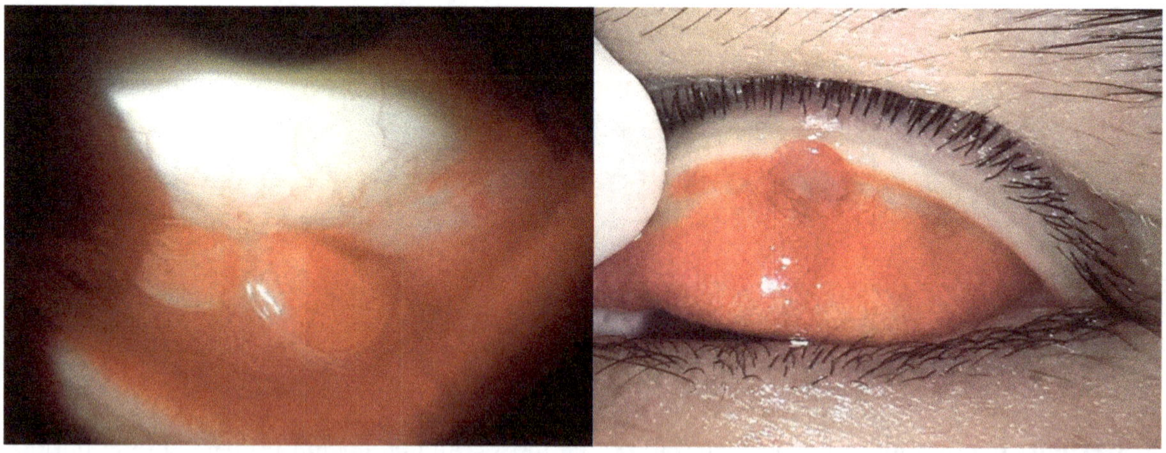

Apocrine hidrocystoma (cyst of Moll) represents a true adenoma of the secretory cells of the glands of Moll, rather than a retention cyst (Alessi, 1997). Clinically, apocrine hidrocystomas represents as translucent or bluish, and is usually seen as solitary lesions near the eyelid margin (Fig 13). Treatment is surgical excision.

Xanthelasmas are common dermal lesions located at medial aspects of the upper and lower eyelids, usually seen in middle-aged to elderly patients (female preponderance). Xanthelasmas are usually bilateral, plaque-like, yellow, flat, or slightly raised lesions derived from histiocytes (Fig 14, 15). Although the lesions can be found in association with diabetes and other hyperlipidemic conditions, most patients have no underlying systemic disease (Amrith, 1999). The recommended treatment is surgical excision for cosmetic concerns. Recurrences are common (Rohrich, 2002).

Figure 13. Cyst of Moll. The translucent cyst located at lid margin is seen

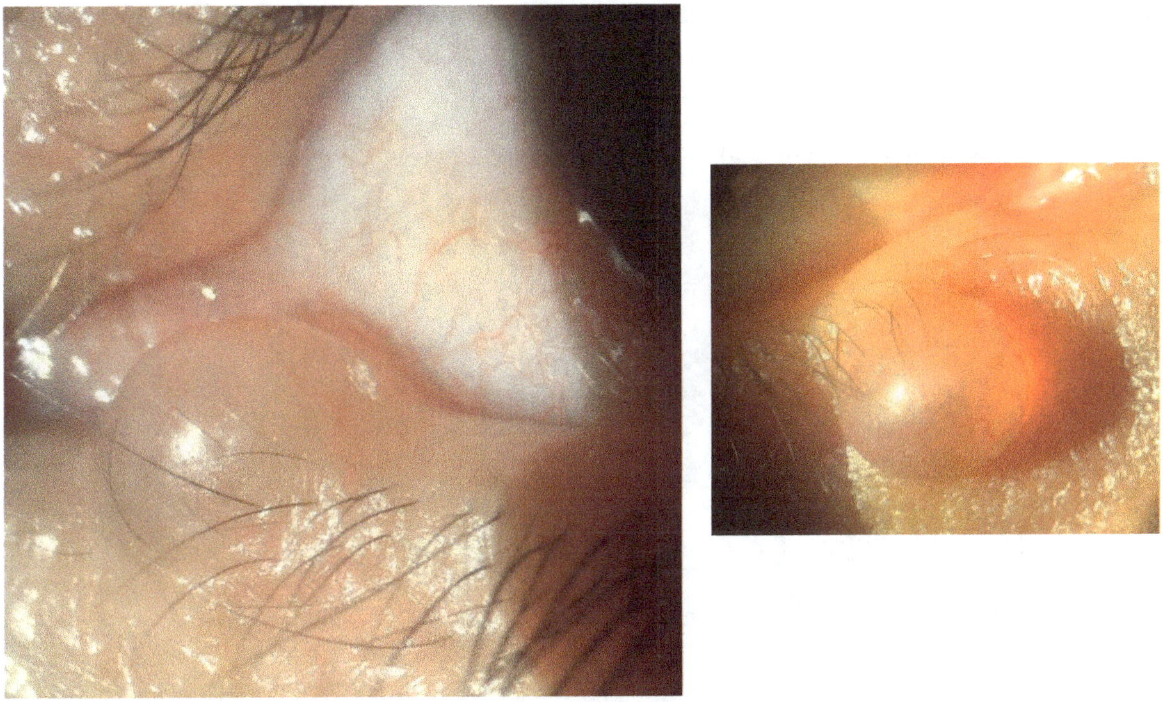

Figure 14. Bilateral Xanthelasma of upper eyelid. The yellow, flat small lesions are seen

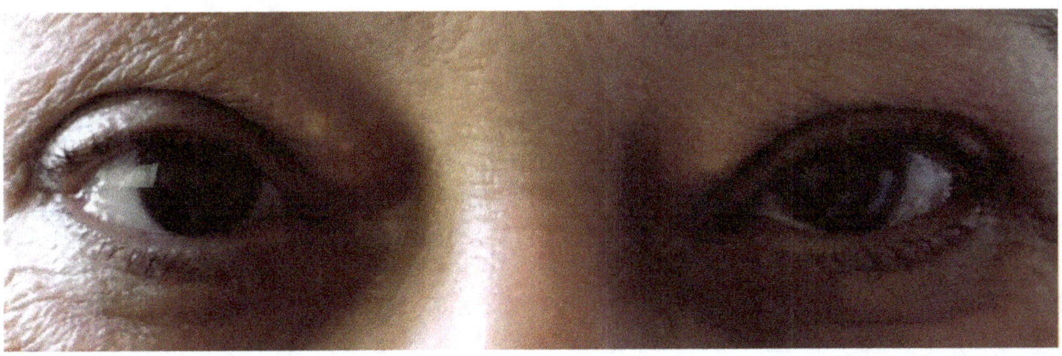

Figure 15. Bilateral xanthelasma of upper eyelid associated with trichofolliculoma of the lower left eyelid

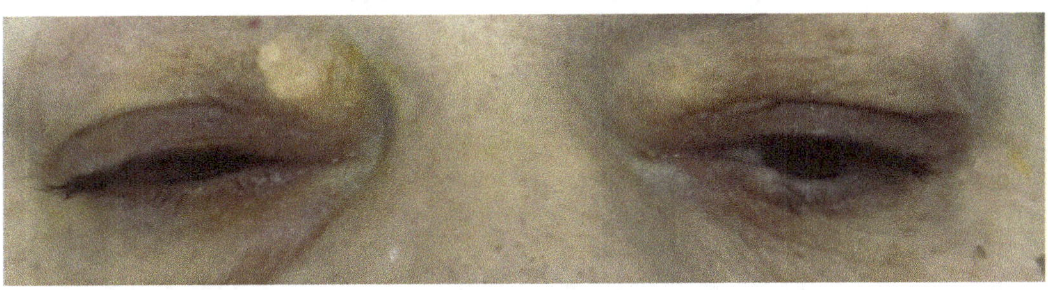

Trichofolliculoma is a solitary, slightly elevated, dome-shaped, flesh-colored nodule (Pinkus, 1965). A central umbilicated area representing the opening of a dilated follicle is considered a diagnostic feature (Fig 16). Treatment is surgical excision for cosmetic purposes.

Figure 16. Trichofolliculoma of lower eyelid is seen (Figure 15 close-up)

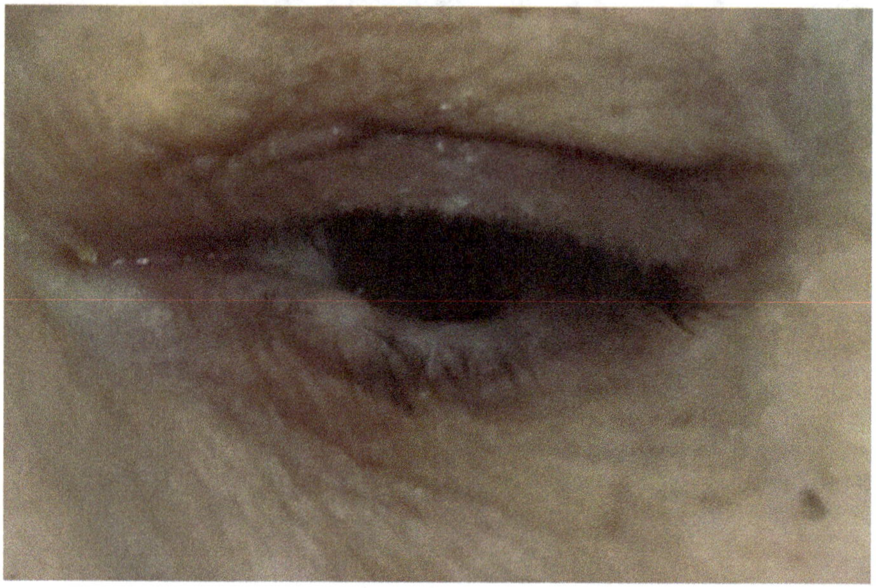

Urbach–Wiethe disease (lipoid proteinosis) is a rare, recessively inherited disorder characterized by the accumulation of hyaline-like material in the skin, mucous membranes, brain, and other organs (Fig 17). The first symptom is often a weak cry with a hoarse voice. Dermatological changes are the most apparent symptoms of Urbach–Wiethe disease; patients may also have neurological symptoms. There is currently no known effective treatment. D-penicillamine, oral dimethyl sulfoxide, acitretin, topical corticosteroids, and carbon dioxide laser have been used with varying degrees of success. Treatment with acitretin has shown some efficacy for hoarseness after use over a long period, but there has been variable success in treating the skin lesions (Hamada, 2002).

Epidermal inclusion cyst arises from the infundibulum of the hair follicle. It can occur spontaneously or after surgery or trauma (McGavran, 1966). Clinically, it represents a slow-growing, elevated, round, smooth, firm, keratin-filled lesion (Fig 19). Recommended treatment is marsupialization or, if possible, complete excision of the cyst without violation of the cyst wall.

The nevus of Ota, known as oculodermal melanocytosis, represents a bluish discoloration of the eyelids and periorbital skin. It usually has a unilateral involvement. Uveal melanomas are frequently associated with this condition (Dutton, 1984). The temple, forehead and malar region can be involved (Fig 20). In the early phase, cryosurgery, surgical excision, skin grafting, and dermabrasion are typically employed (Ono et al, 1998). Since the development of laser technology, several lasers have been introduced into the treatment of benign pigmentary lesions (Seo, 2015).

Figure 17. Urbach-Wiethe disease. The lesions of lipoid proteinosis are seen at the lower and upper eyelid

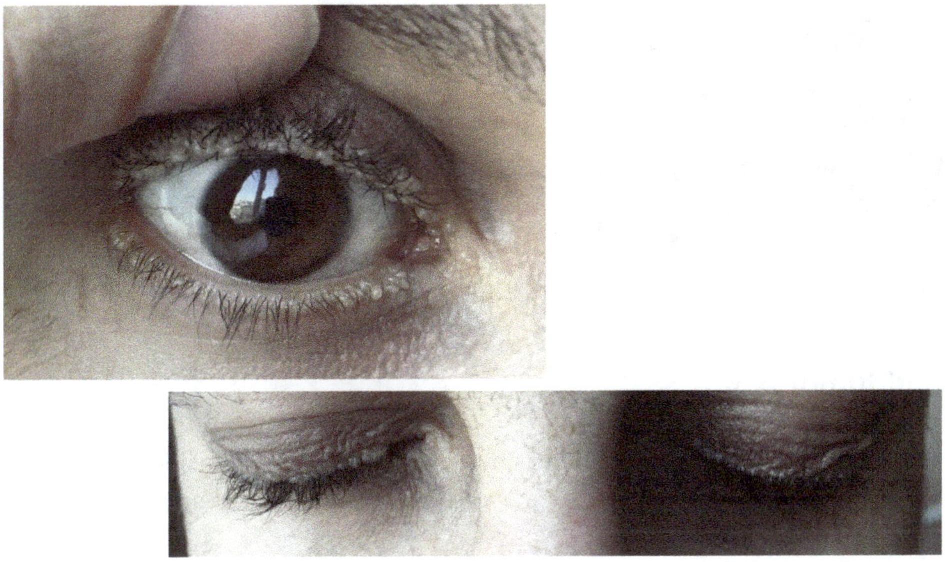

Figure 18. The same patient. Lesions are seen under slit lamp

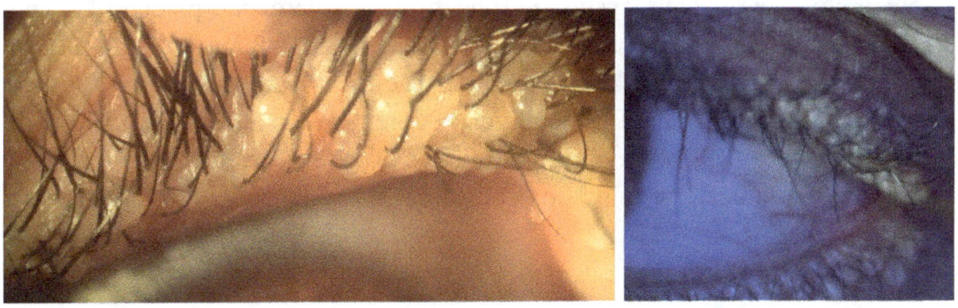

Figure 19. Epidermal inclusion cyst is seen

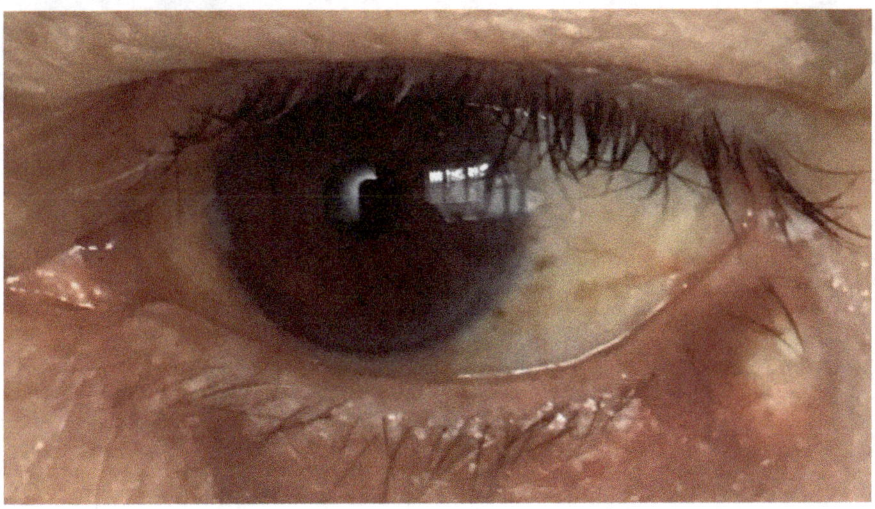

Figure 20. Nevus Ota (bilateral, more expressed in the left eye)

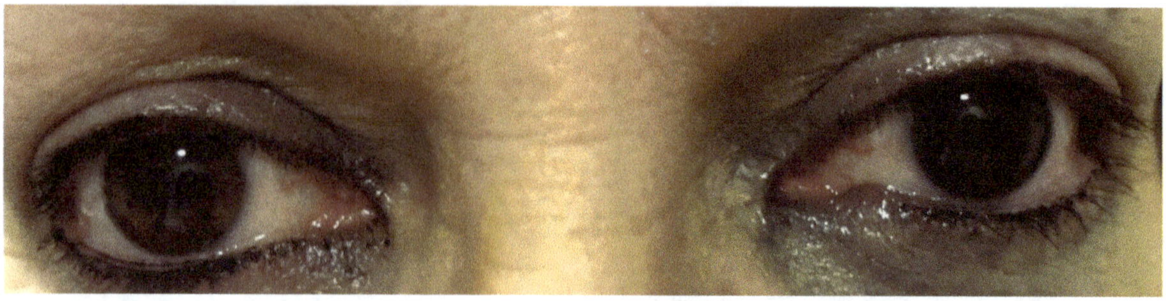

Malignant lid tumors

The eyelids are affected by skin cancer and are often overlooked when considering suspicious skin lesions. Eyelid skin cancer treatment includes removal of the offending lesion, while preserving as much normal tissue as possible.

Basal cell carcinoma (BCC) is the most common skin cancer among all eyelid malignancies. Basal cell carcinoma is a tumor with many clinical and histologic manifestations and develops from the basal layer and epidermal appendages (Rubin, 2005). Clinical representations occur in different varieties, including nodular, noduloulcerative, pigmented, cystic, morpheaform or sclerosing, plaque-like, and superficial (Fig 21, 22, 23). If a lesion is small, excisional biopsy with at least 2–3 mm of margin of normal tissue should be considered. In simple surgical excisions, the specimen should be examined histologically to confirm the margins are clear. Surgical excision, cryosurgery, radiotherapy, and Mohs micrographic surgery have been reported to achieve five-year cure rates of 90%. Currently, the best available option is surgical excision with standard frozen section control or Mohs micrographic surgery (Lane, 2005).

Figure 21. CC in early stage

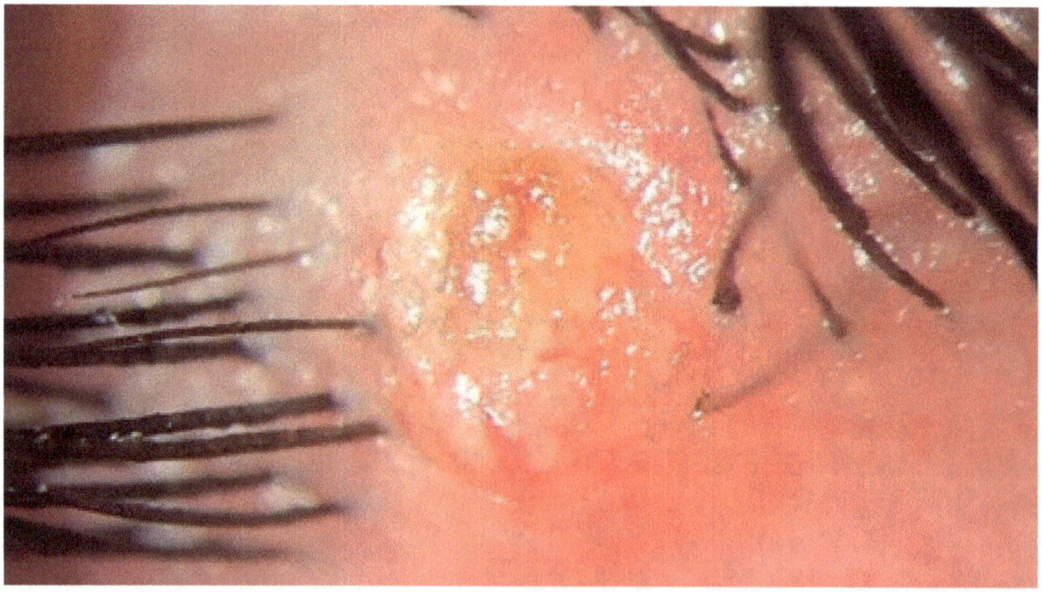

Figure 22. The nodular basal cell carcinoma. Exophytic growth and sharp delineation from normal skin are seen

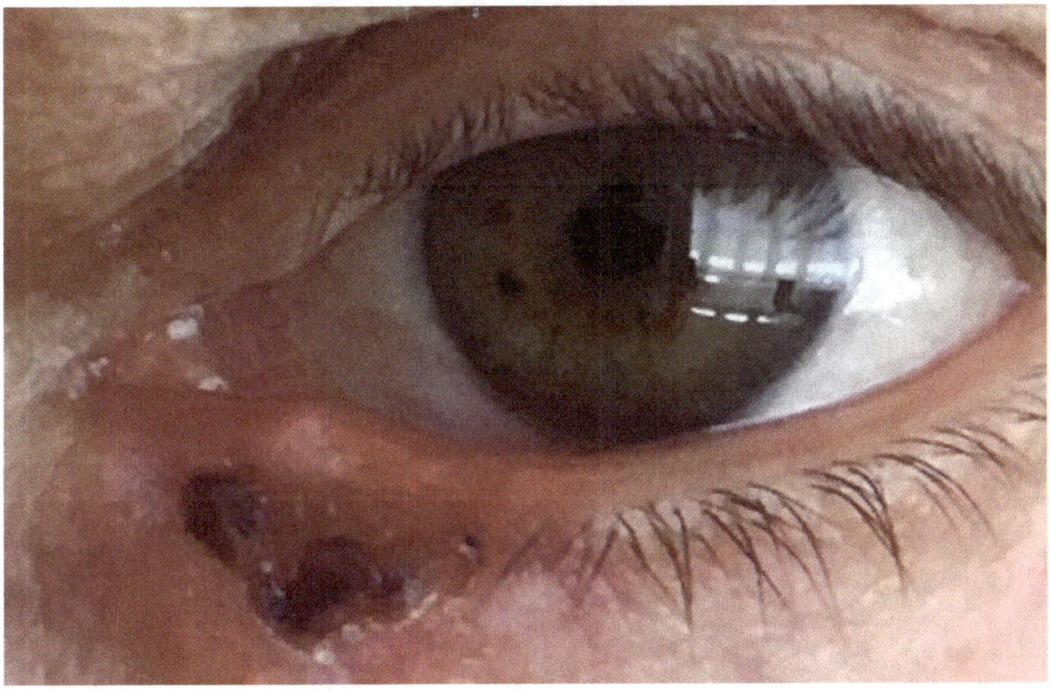

Figure 23. Basal cell carcinoma (through the courtesy of Dr. Gharakeshishyan)

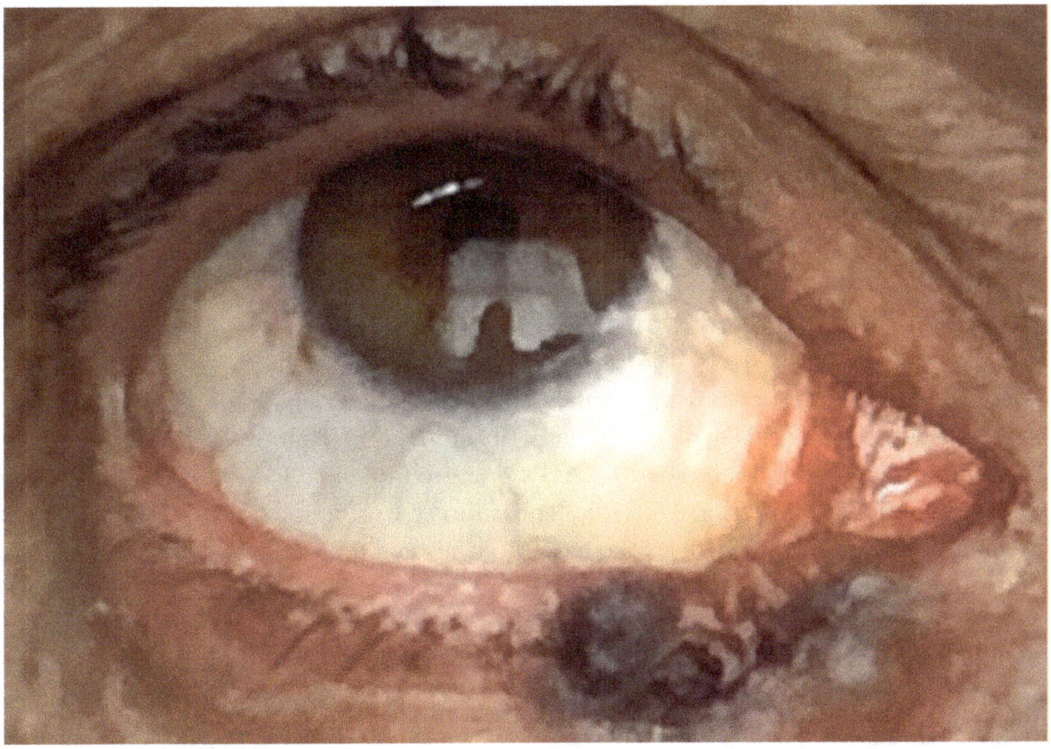

Figure 24. Sebaceous cell carcinoma (biopsy proven) through the courtesy of Dr. Gharakeshishyan

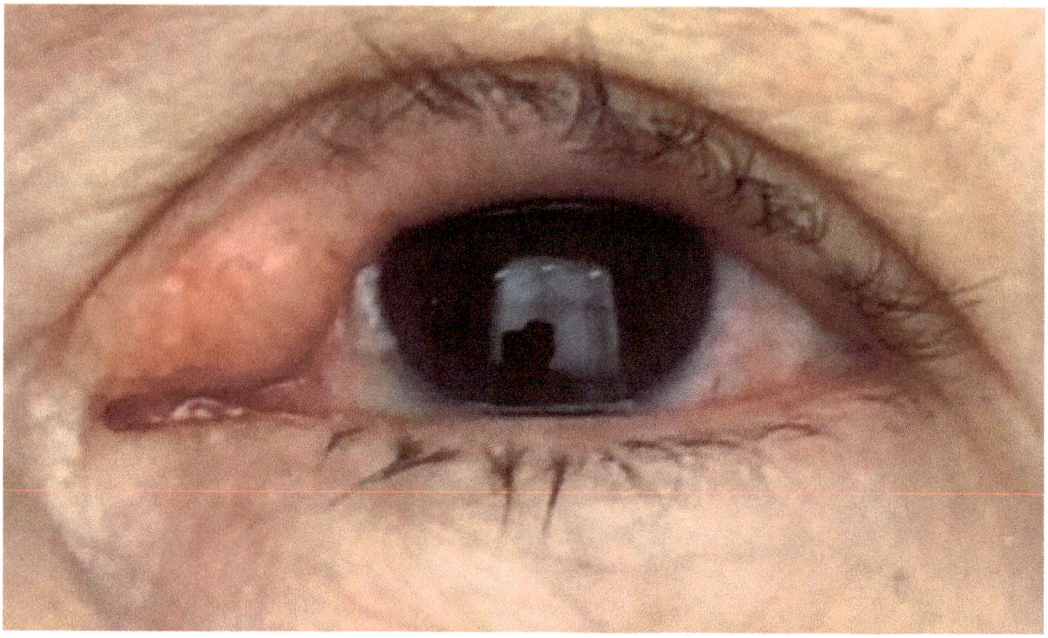

Sebaceous cell carcinoma is the third most common eyelid malignancy. It is a potentially lethal tumor because the morbidity and mortality rates are quite high. It usually originates from meibomian glands, rarely from other sebaceous glands (Doxanas, 1984). The sebaceous carcinoma can be mistaken for a chalazion. Clinically, it represents a firm and immobile nodule, with yellowish coloration. Loss of eyelashes can occur (Fig 24). With histologic confirmation of sebaceous cell carcinoma, the surgeon must consider the extent of possible pagetoid involvement of the bulbar conjunctiva.

Squamous cell carcinoma (SCC) is a malignant neoplasm of the epidermal keratinizing cells. SCC of the eyelids is a potentially lethal tumor due to possible invasion into the orbit.[32] It can spread to regional lymph nodes and metastasize to distal sites (Fig 25). After an incisional biopsy with confirmation of the diagnosis, the preferred method of management for primary periocular SCC is surgical excision with microscopic monitoring of tissue margins (Faustina, 2004).

Eyelid Inflammation and Infections

Blepharitis is one of the most common disorders encountered in ophthalmology. It is estimated that eye care specialists see blepharitis in 47% of their patients[1]. Despite its prevalence, the disease is often overlooked and misdiagnosed. According to AAO's preferred Practice Pattern (2013), blepharitis can have two forms: anterior and posterior. Anterior blepharitis is the inflammation of the lid margin anterior to the gray line. It predominately involves the base of lashes and their follicles. Posterior blepharitis is the inflammation posterior to the gray line, with predominate involvement of the meibomian glands and their orifices. Recent literature has used the terms posterior blepharitis and meibomian gland dysfunction (MGD) synonymously, but they don't have the same meaning. Posterior blepharitis is used to describe inflammatory conditions of the posterior lid margin, whereas MGD is only one of the possible causes of inflammatory disease.

Figure 25. Squamous cell carcinoma is seen on the inferior eyelid through the courtesy of Dr. Gharakeshishyan

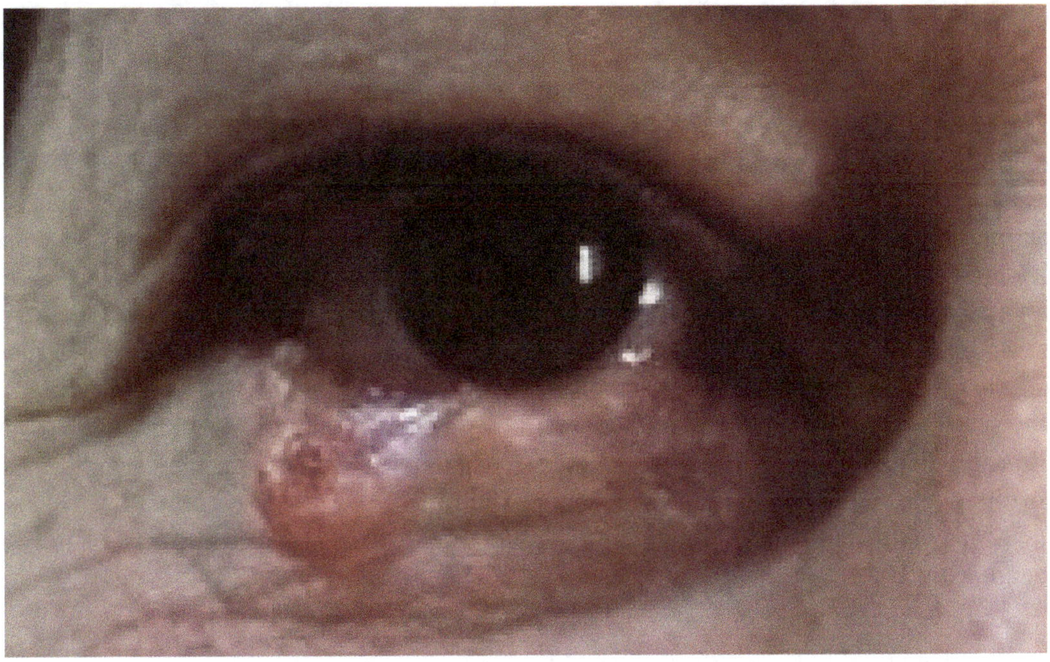

Meibomian gland dysfunction is the major cause of evaporative dry eye and can occur along with aqueous deficient dry eye. Recent clinical studies identified MGD either alone or in combination with aqueous tear deficiency as the most commonly occurring form of dry eye, suggesting that MGD be considered as a part of dry eye disease (Lemp, 2012).

According to McCulley's classification, blepharitis and meibomian gland dysfunction are categorized as follows:

1. Staphylococcal: anterior lid inflammation with collarettes and madarosis.
2. Seborrheic: anterior lid disease with greasy scales with minimal inflammation.
3. Mixed seborrheic and staphylococcal: findings of seborrheic with increased inflammation
4. Seborrheic with secondary meibomitis: spotty distributing of meibomian obstruction.
5. Seborrheic with secondary meibomitis: with occluded and inflamed meibomian glands
6. Primary meibomitis: diffuse obstruction and inflammation of meibomian glands in association with seborrheic dermatitis or acne rosacea.

International Workshop on Meibomian Gland Dysfunction /The International Workshop on Meibomian Gland Dysfunction: Executive Summary. *Invest Ophthalmol Vis Sci.* 52:1922 2011/ has more detailed classification of MGD based on delivery speed and primary/secondary causes respectively.

Treatment options include warm compresses, eyelid cleansing, including eyelid massage in cases of MGD to express the meibomian glands, antibiotics (topical and/or systemic), topical anti-inflammatory agents (e.g., corticosteroids, cyclosporine). Eyelid cleansing is especially useful for anterior blepharitis, while warm compresses are especially helpful for posterior blepharitis and MGD. A topical antibiotic ointment such as bacitracin or erythromycin can be prescribed and applied on the eyelid margins one or more times daily or at bedtime for a few weeks. Doxycycline, minocycline, or tetracycline can be given daily, and tapered after clinical improvement is noted. Alternatively, oral erythromycin or azithromycin can be used especially in women of childbearing age and children. A brief course of topical corticosteroids may be helpful for eyelid or ocular surface inflammation such as marginal keratitis, or phlyctenules. Corticosteroid eye drops or ointments are typically applied several times daily to the eyelids or ocular surface. Once the inflammation is controlled, the corticosteroid can be tapered and discontinued and then used intermittently to maintain patient comfort. Because many blepharitis patients have tear film instability, artificial tears may improve symptoms when used as an adjunct to eyelid cleansing and medications. If artificial tears are used more than four times per day, non-preserved tears should be used to avoid preservative toxicity, Topical cyclosporine and/or punctal plugs may also be helpful in managing coexisting aqueous tear deficiency (American Academy of Ophthalmology, 2018).

Staphylococcal blepharitis is seen more commonly in younger individuals with female preponderance. Clinically, staphylococcal blepharitis represents as hard, brittle fibrinous scales and hard, matted crusts surrounding individual cilia on the anterior eyelid margin (Dougherty et al, 1985; Dougherty et al, 1985; McCulley et al, 1982). The removal of hard crusts may reveal small ulcers of the anterior eyelid margin (Fig 26, 27).

Figure 26. Staphylococcal blepharitis. Crusts within eyelashes are seen

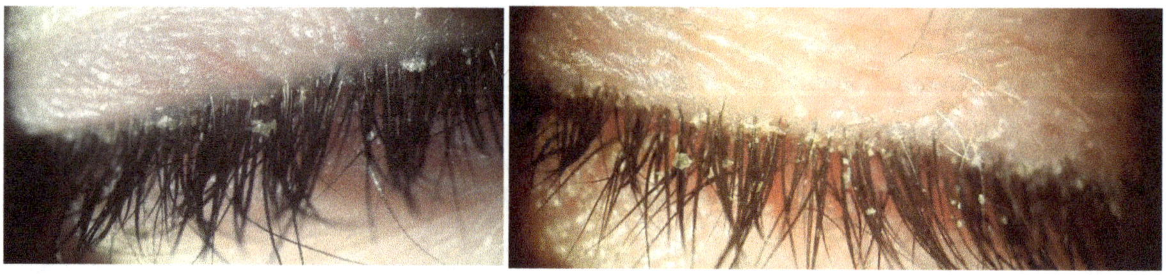

Figure 27. Bilateral staphylococcal blepharitis in a child

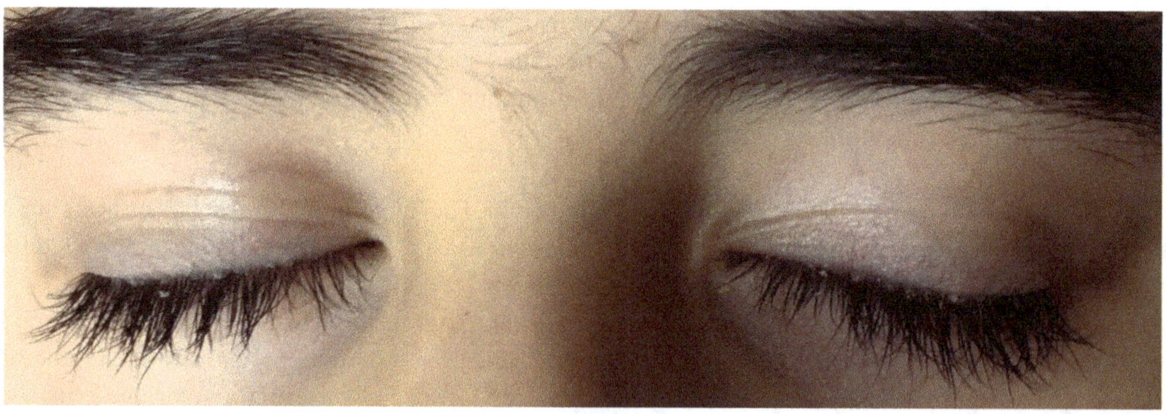

Seborrheic blepharitis can develop alone or in combination with staphylococcal blepharitis or meibomian gland dysfunction. Inflammation is located mainly at the anterior eyelid margin (McCulley, 1982; Shine, 1993). Clinically, usually oily, and greasy crusting is seen on the eyelids, eyelashes, and eyebrows (Fig 28).

Figure 28. Seborrheic blepharitis. Oily and greasy crusts are seen

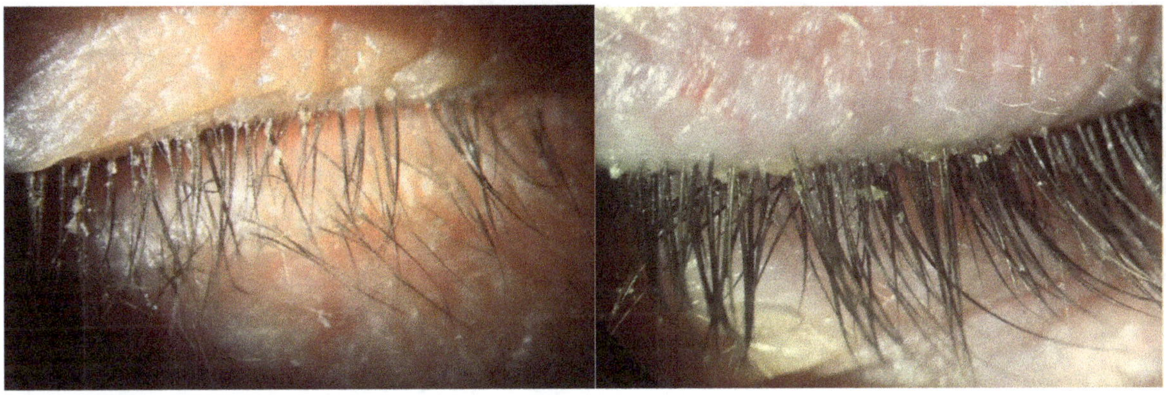

Meibomian seborrhea is characterized by dilated meibomian ductules, which are easily expressed. Clinically, foamy secretion accumulated at lid margin can be observed (Fig 29) (McCulley, 1982; Foulks et al, 2003).

Figure 29. Meibomian seborrhea. Foamy secretion is seen at lid margin with debris in tear film (left photo)

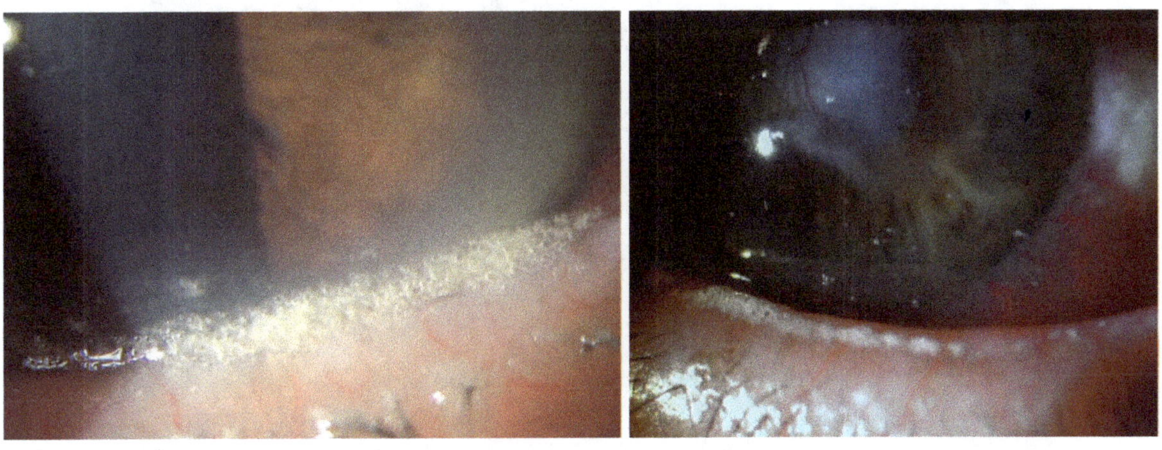

Seborrheic blepharitis with secondary meibomitis clinically represents with a thick, toothpaste-like secretion. The glands are plugged, and the secretions can be expressed with moderate pressure on the lid margin (Fig 30) (Foulks et al, 2003).

Figure 30. Obstructed meibomian glands are seen. The toothpaste-like secretion is seen

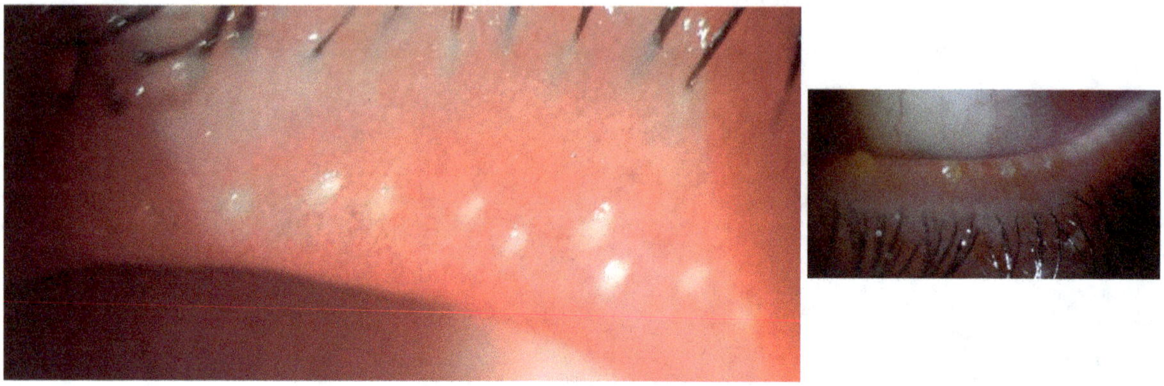

Rosacea is an oculodermatologic condition commonly presenting along with meibomian gland dysfunction. This condition's pathogenesis is not well-known, but it seems to be mainly a disorder of vasodilation. Sebaceous glands of the skin are also affected in these patients (Fig 31, 32). Severe or prolonged MGD in advanced rosacea is often associated with inflammation in the cornea, which results in vascularization

Figure 31. Rosacea. Dilated superficial vessels are seen on face skin

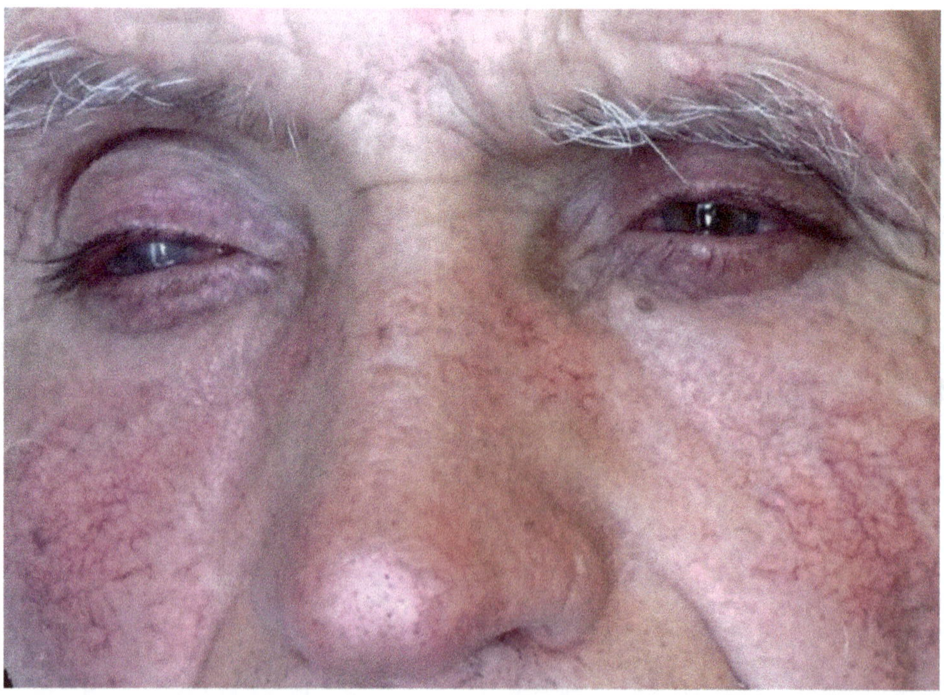

Figure 32. The same patient under slit lamp. The thickened lid margin (thylosis) with telangiectasia and obstructed meibomian glands are seen

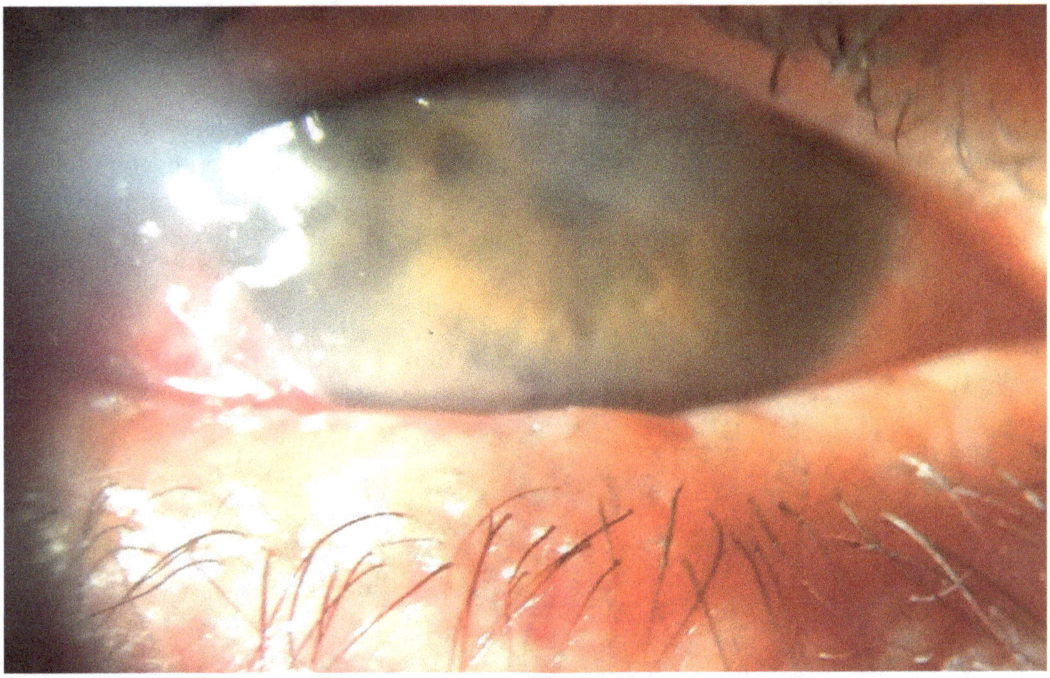

or scarring of the cornea (Starr et al, 1969; Steinhoff et al, 2013; Hoang-Xuan et al, 1991). It is named rosacea keratitis (rosacea keratitis is discussed more detailed in Noninfectious corneal disease, chapter 6). Oral azithromycin (off-label) has been used successfully in the management of acne rosacea as an alternative to oral tetracyclines, particularly in combination with 0.1% topical tacrolimus. FDA issued a warning that oral azithromycin may lead to abnormalities in the electrical activity of the heart, with the potential to create serious irregularities in heart rhythm (American Academy of Ophthalmology, 2018). Frequent preservative-free artificial tears, punctual occlusion, and topical cyclosporine help in patients with dryness. Eyelid hygiene, topical antibiotics, and oral omega-3 fatty acid supplementation may help to control blepharitis (Macsai, 2008).

Angular blepharitis is an inflammation of the lateral lid margins and canthal region, mainly caused by Moraxella or Staphylococcus species (Din, 2012). Clinically, angular blepharitis is characterized by redness of skin and dried crusts, usually with bilateral involvement (Fig 33).

Figure 33. Angular blepharitis. The erythematous, scaly skin

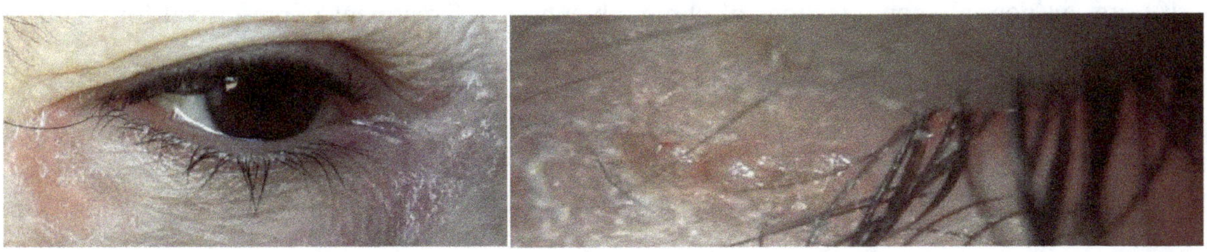

Hordeolum is an acute, painful, suppurative, nodular infectious lesion of the eyelid, usually caused by Staphylococcus species (Fig 34). The infection may affect the glands of Zeis, Moll, or hair follicles (Fig 36). In this case, the lesion is called external hordeolum (Duderstadt, 2013). In contrast, when the meibomian glands are infected, the condition is referred to as internal hordeolum (Fig 37). Hordeolum may be associated with both blepharitis and MGD (Fig 35). The natural history of acute internal hordeolum generally spans one to two weeks, beginning with the appearance of an abscess and concluding with spontaneous draining of the abscess. Warm compress, lid massage and scrubs may accelerate the healing process. A topical antibiotic is usually not effective. If the condition is severe, systemic antibiotics or surgical incision and drainage may be implemented (Lindsley et al, 2013).

Figure 34. Hordeolum. Nodular lesion with overlying skin redness is seen

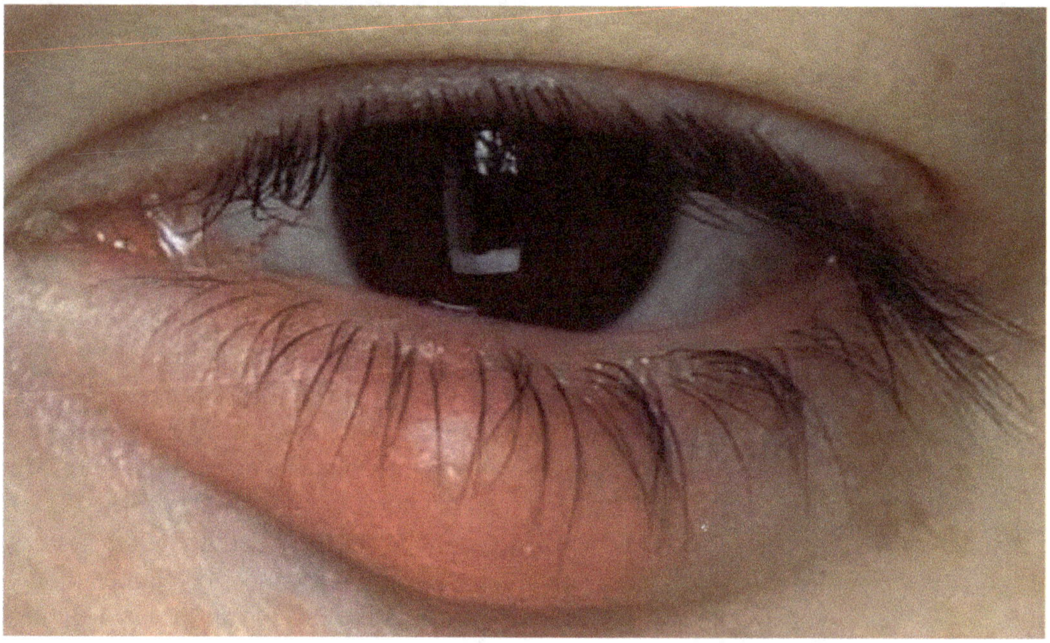

Chalazion represents a chronic granuloma that occurs after obstruction of Zeis or meibomian glands. The nodules frequently arise in and around the meibomian glands and may be more prominent on either the skin or the conjunctiva (Fig 38). Warm compresses can soften and drain the gland ducts, steroid intralesional injections may help to resolve. If medical treatment is not helpful, surgical removal is advocated (Lindsley et al, 2013).

Thylosis (Fig 32), **poliosis** (whitening of eyelashes, Fig 39) and **madarosis** (absence of eyelashes, Fig 40) present possible complications of chronic blepharitis. Treatment is prescribed for control of blepharitis.

Preseptal and orbital cellulitis are two acute infectious diseases that have potential morbidity and mortality. Preseptal cellulitis usually refers to infections localized anterior to the orbital septum; in orbital cellulitis, infectious process is located in the orbital septum with involvement of the globe. Preseptal cellulitis occurs mostly in the pediatric population (Lee et al, 2011). Cellulitis has an acute unilateral

Figure 35. The same patient under slit lamp. Associated blepharitis is seen

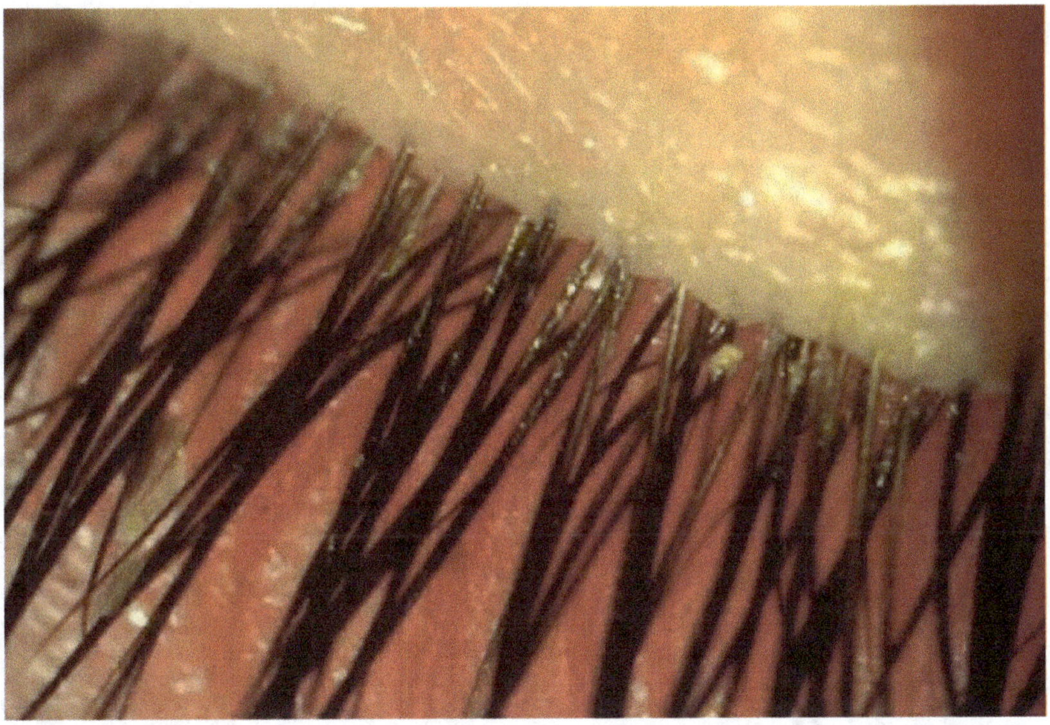

Figure 36. Zeis gland abscess

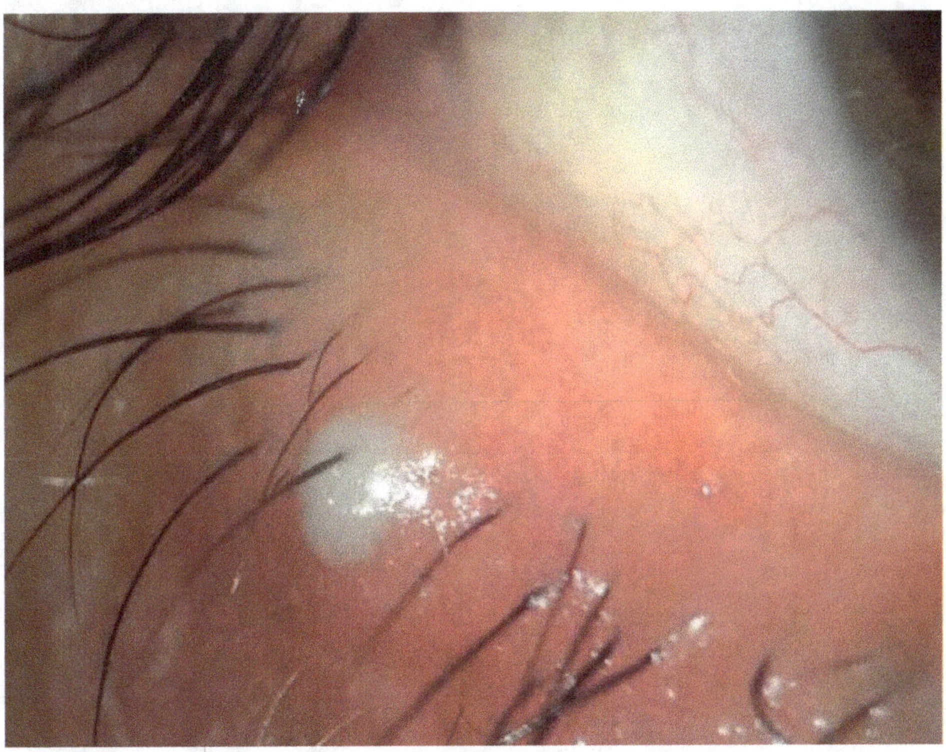

Figure 37. Internal hordeolum. Purulent nodular lesion is seen

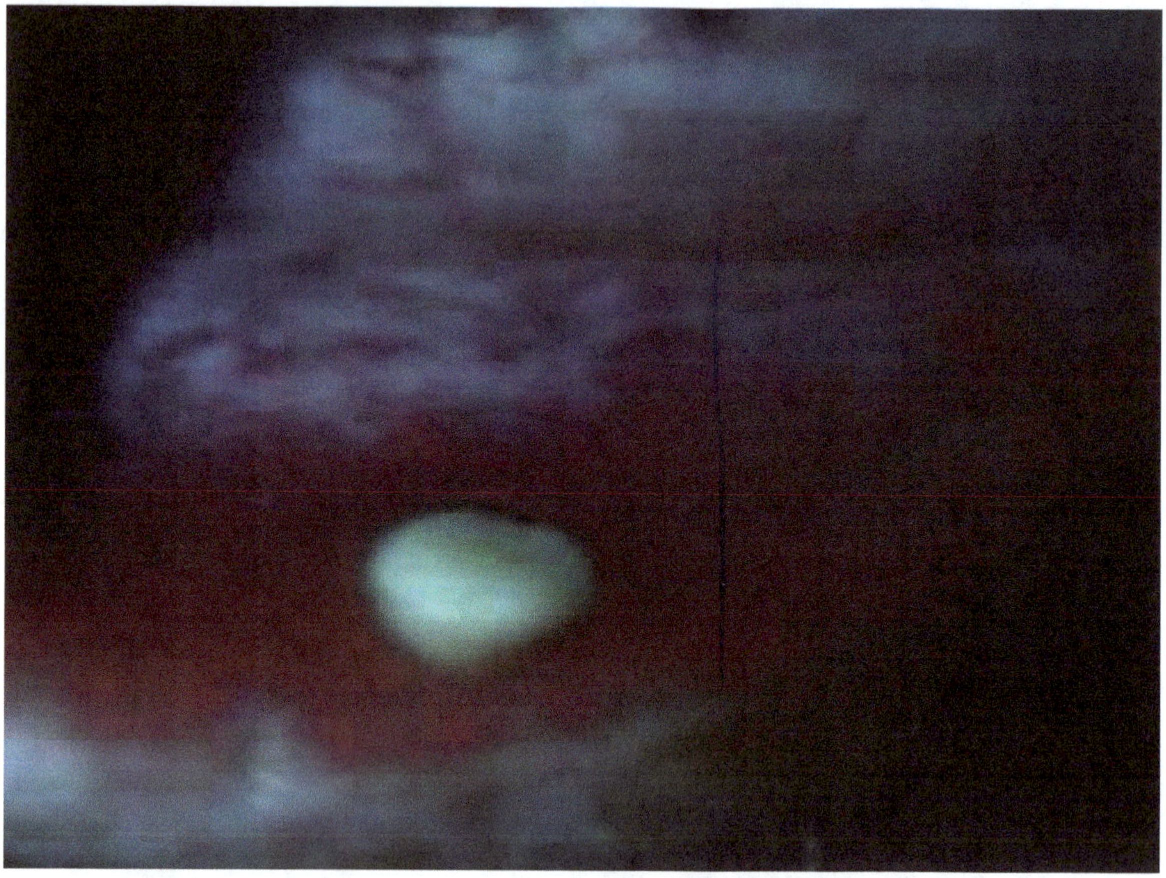

Figure 38. Chalazions of the upper eyelid. The elevated nodular lesions, central and far temporal (circled) without redness are seen

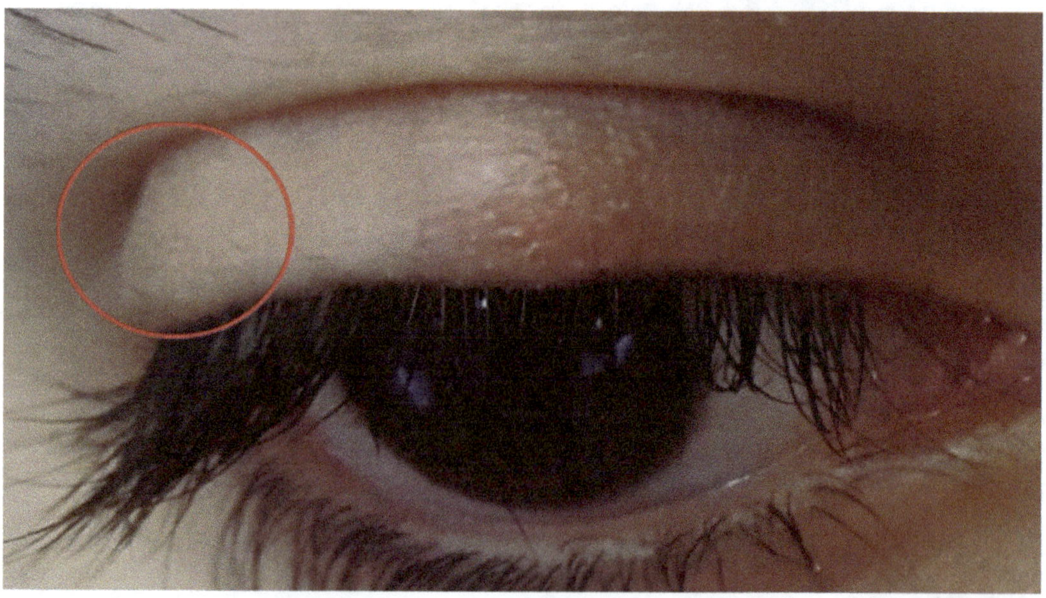

Figure 39. Poliosis of eyelashes are seen

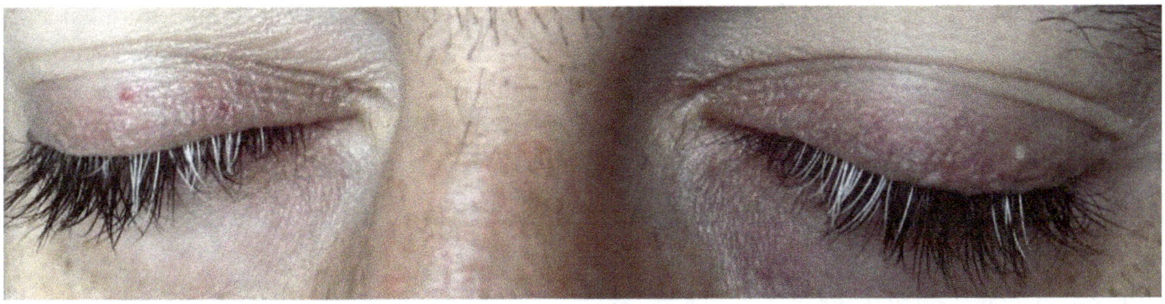

Figure 40. Madarosis associated with blepharitis

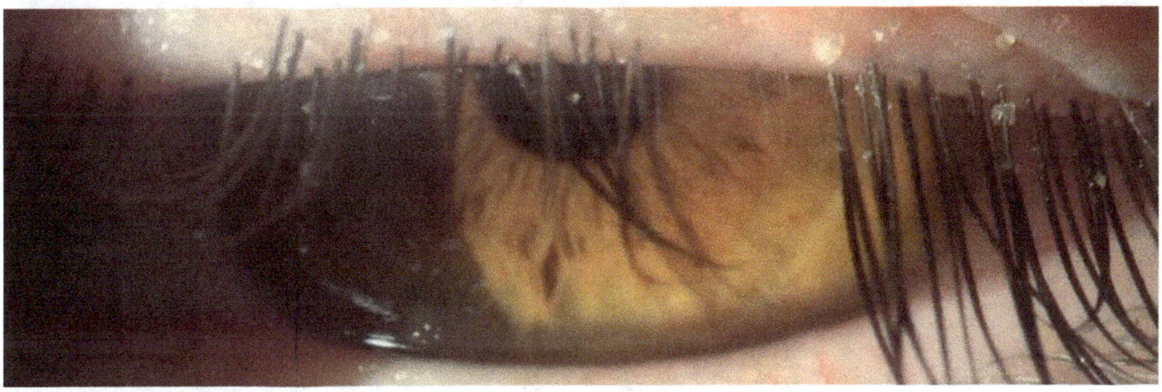

Figure 41. Preseptal cellulitis. The swollen, edematous, eyelids are seen

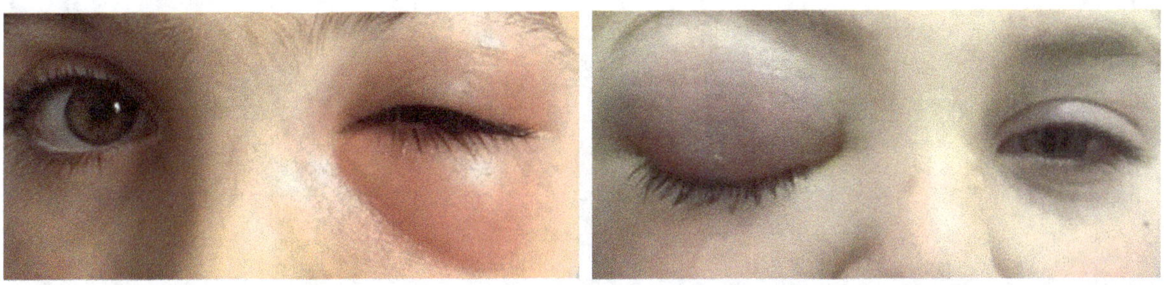

onset accompanied by pain, redness, swelling, and warmth erythema that can be associated with fever and malaise (Fig 41). The main infectious causes are Staph. Aureus, Streptococcus pyogenes Haemophilus influenzae and Streptococcus pneumoniae. Majority of children with non-severe preseptal cellulitis can be managed as outpatients with oral antibiotics. Highly febrile children with toxic appearing and/or having neutrophilic leukocytosis should have parenteral antibiotics (Block, 2013).

Demodex blepharitis (Fig 42) is the most common parasitic eyelid infection, which is caused by Demodex mites; Demodex folliculorum, and Demodex brevis. Demodex mites inhabit follicles with or without hair in areas of high sebum production. They can be observed in the skin of almost the entire body, such as the face, scalp, etc (Kosik-Bogack, 2013; Zhao, 2012) Demodex blepharitis is associated with reactive hyperkeratosis, which refers to the classic clinical finding of semitransparent "sleeves" around the eyelashes, termed as cylindrical dandruff (Fig 43). Demodicosis is currently considered to be commonly associated with rosacea. Improvement in symptoms and signs was recently reported in a small case series, in which a group of patients used 50% tea tree oil eyelid scrubs weekly, and tea- tree-oil shampoo scrubs daily for a minimum of 6 weeks. Oral Ivermectin has also been reported to be of benefit in some cases of recalcitrant Demodex blepharitis (Bravo, 2015).

Figure 42. Demodex blepharitis

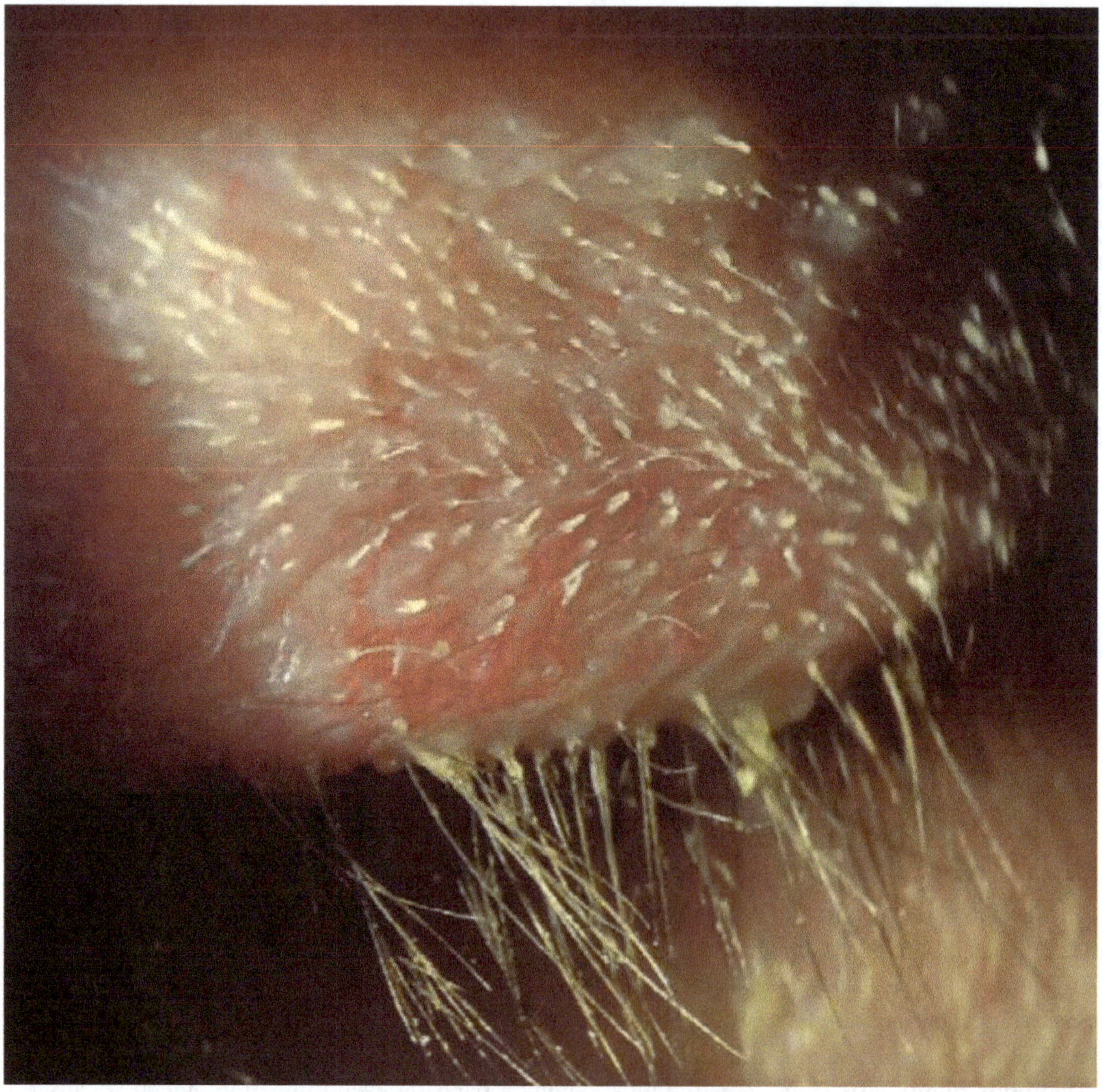

Figure 43. Microscopic picture of Demodex on the eyelash

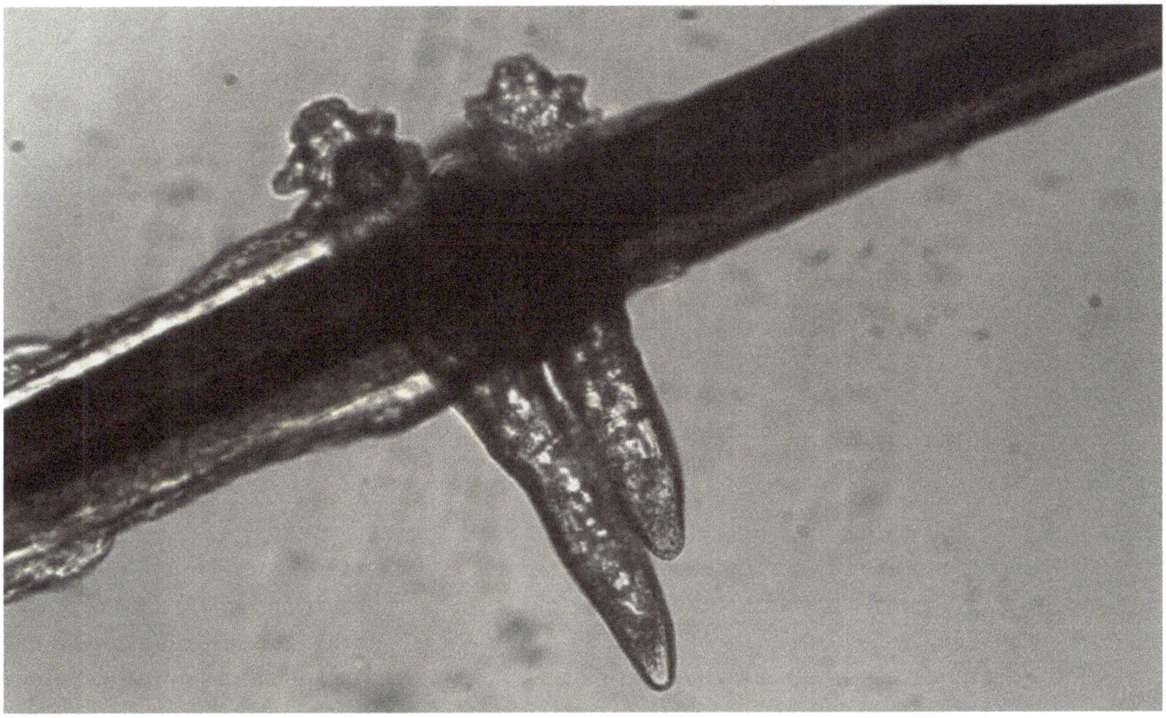

Viral infections of eyelids are usually caused by herpes simplex, varicella zoster viruses, molluscum contagiosum (discussed in chapter 3, Conjunctivitis), human papilloma viruses (HPV), etc.

HSV Blepharitis is an eyelid infection caused by the herpes simplex virus, either with HSV-1 or HSV-2 (rarely). Eyelids involvement with HSV-1 can be a primary or recurrent infection. Clinically,

Figure 44. Herpetic vesicles are seen on the upper eyelid

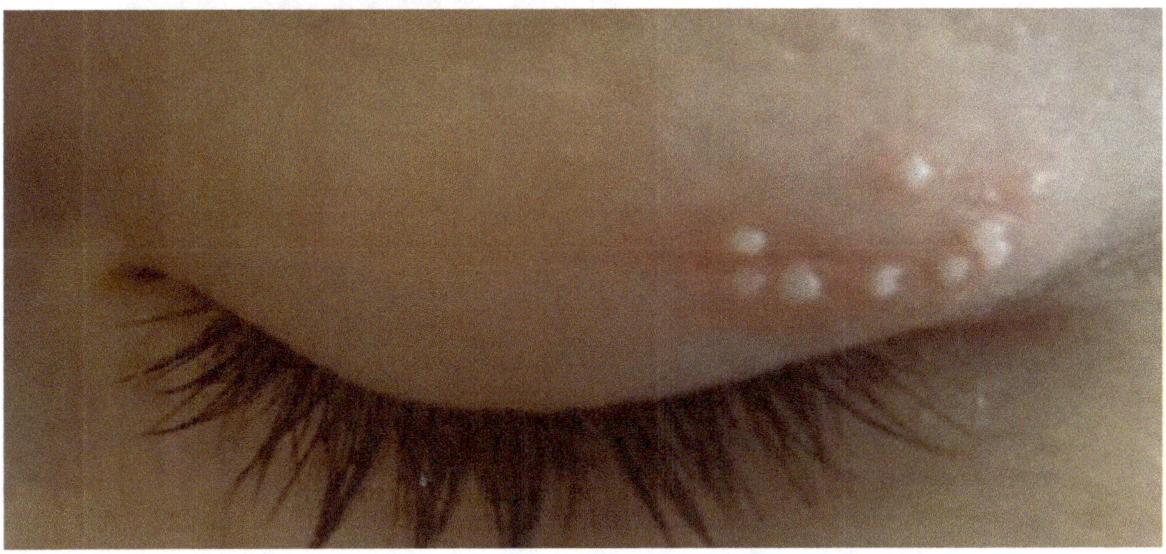

Figure 45. Herpetic blepharitis of lower eyelid. Multiple vesicles are seen

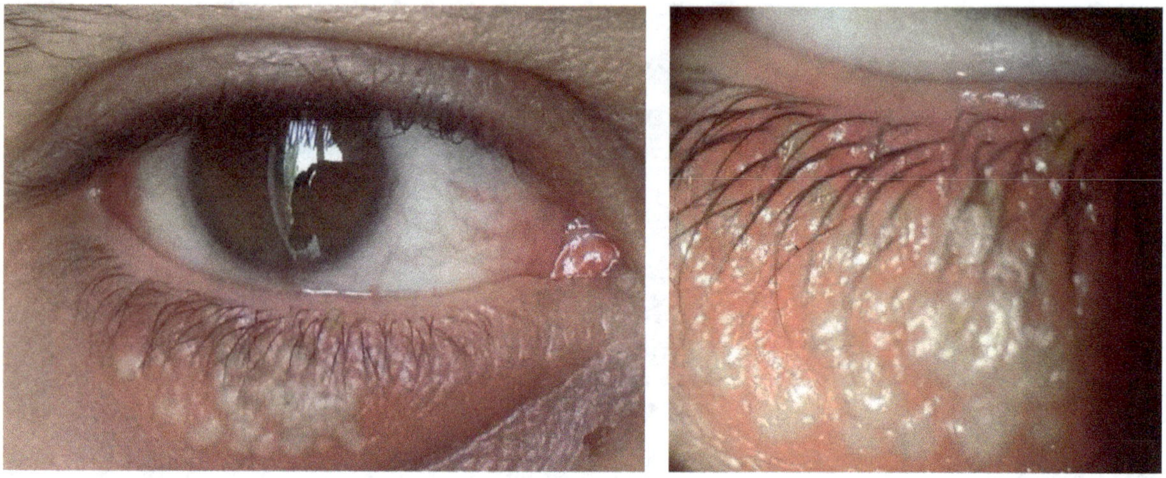

it is presented with multiple vesicles on a raised, edematous, erythematous base, similar to lesions on mouth and nose. In a primary infection, lesions may be more severe, diffuse, and involve the periorbital skin (Fig 44, 45) (Liu, 2012). Primary ocular HSV infection is a self-limited disease, and when limited to the eyelid skin, it does not necessarily require any specific therapy. Patients with significant primary

Figure 46. Papilloma of upper eyelid

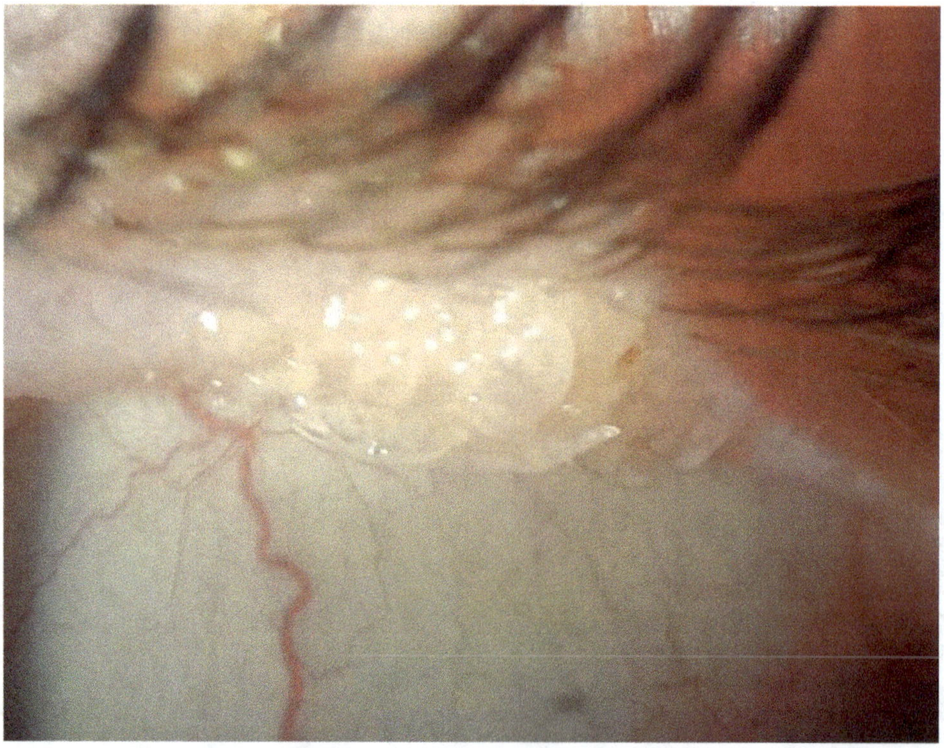

Figure 47. Presumed papilloma of lower eyelid

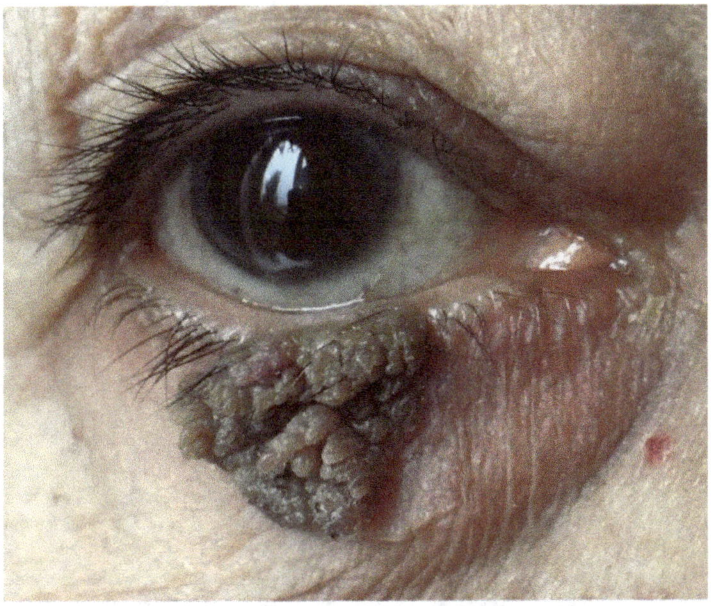

eyelid HSV infection may benefit from oral acyclovir that may shorten the course of the disease, reduce the chance of corneal involvement, and decrease patient morbidity.

Eyelid papilloma is a common eyelid tumor usually caused by papillomavirus.

Eyelid involvement may have different ways of presentation, including a skin tag, and can be solitary or multiple, rough or smooth (Fig 46, 47). It is benign, painless, and has very little to no risk for cancer growth (Bravo, 2015). Oral cimetidine, topical interferon or mitomycin, excision and intraoperative application of MMC have been reported as alternative therapies for recurrent lesions (Ma'luf, 2010).

Contact dermatitis of the eyelids is a common condition and can be associated with other ocular allergies.[57] Usually, a history of lotions, creams (Fig 48), or topical medications (Fig 49) is present. The periocular skin is erythematous, edematous, and may show scaling and crusting. The management of eyelid dermatitis involves ongoing avoidance of exposure to irritants and allergens, along with the use of topical anti-inflammatory agents including topical corticosteroids and topical calcineurin inhibitors. There are no randomized trials assessing the efficacy and safety of these agents for eyelid eczema, and their use is based on limited evidence from small observational studies, indirect evidence based on their use in other types of eczema, and clinical experience (Fonacier et al, 2004).

Atopic dermatitis is an inflammation which results in itchy, red, swollen, and cracked skin. Ocular involvement usually refers to atopic keratoconjunctivitis, but atopic dermatitis may present with thickened, scaly, erythematous, and fissured periocular skin (Fig 50, 51) (Fonacier, 2004).The topical application of a vasoconstrictor-antihistamine combination may bring transient relief of symptoms but is unlikely to alter the immunopathologic process or its sequelae. Nonsteroidal medications have been shown to be effective in reducing itching, tearing, and photophobia. Topical mast cell stabilizers one to four times a day are recommended for the whole year to patients with perennial symptoms. Cyclosporine A and tacrolimus, both orally and topically have been shown to be effective at treating AKC, as well as reducing the amount of topical steroid use. In rare cases of uncontrolled dermatitis, with vision-threatening complications, oral steroids are indicated (Stumpf, 2006).

Figure 48. Contact dermatitis caused by face cream

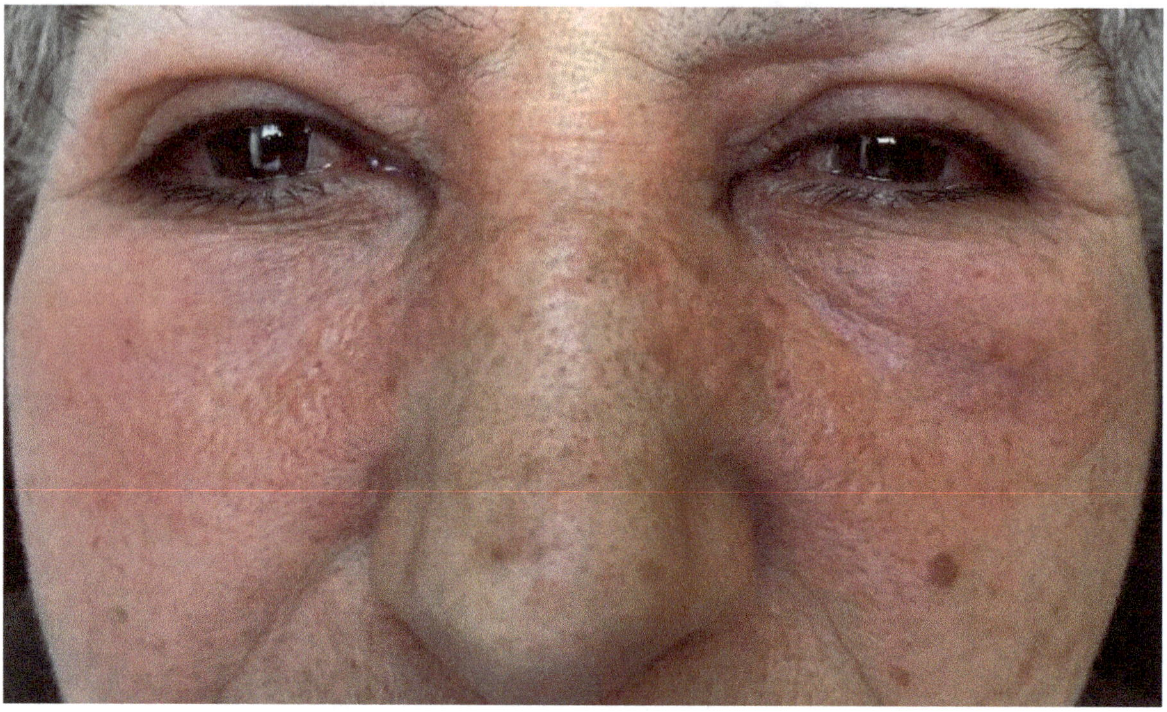

Figure 49. Contact dermatitis associated with allergic conjunctivitis due to topical Maxitrol drops. Edematous eyelids with redness and crusts are seen

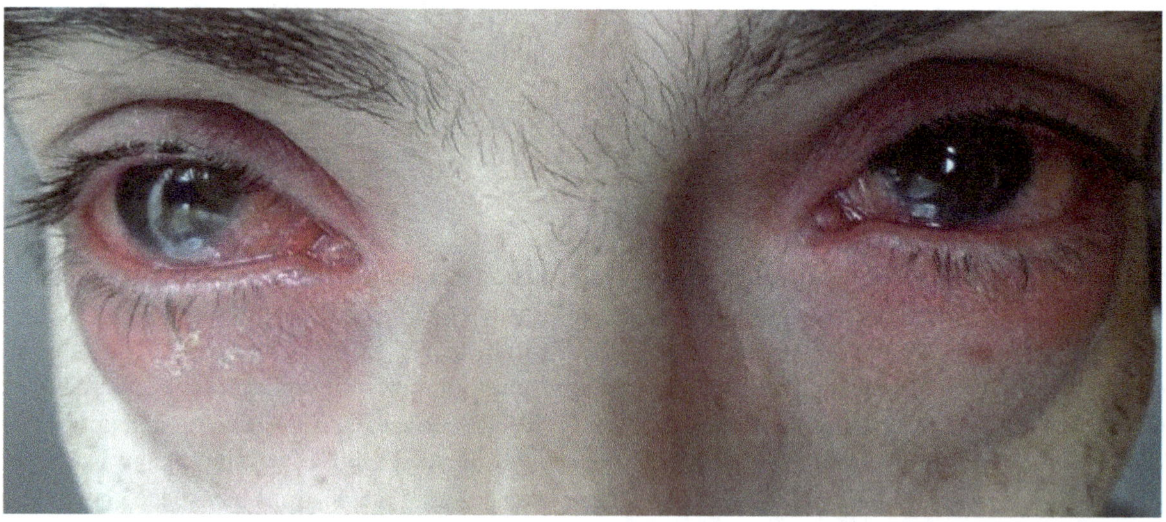

Figure 50. Atopic dermatitis. The thickened periocular skin and crusts are seen

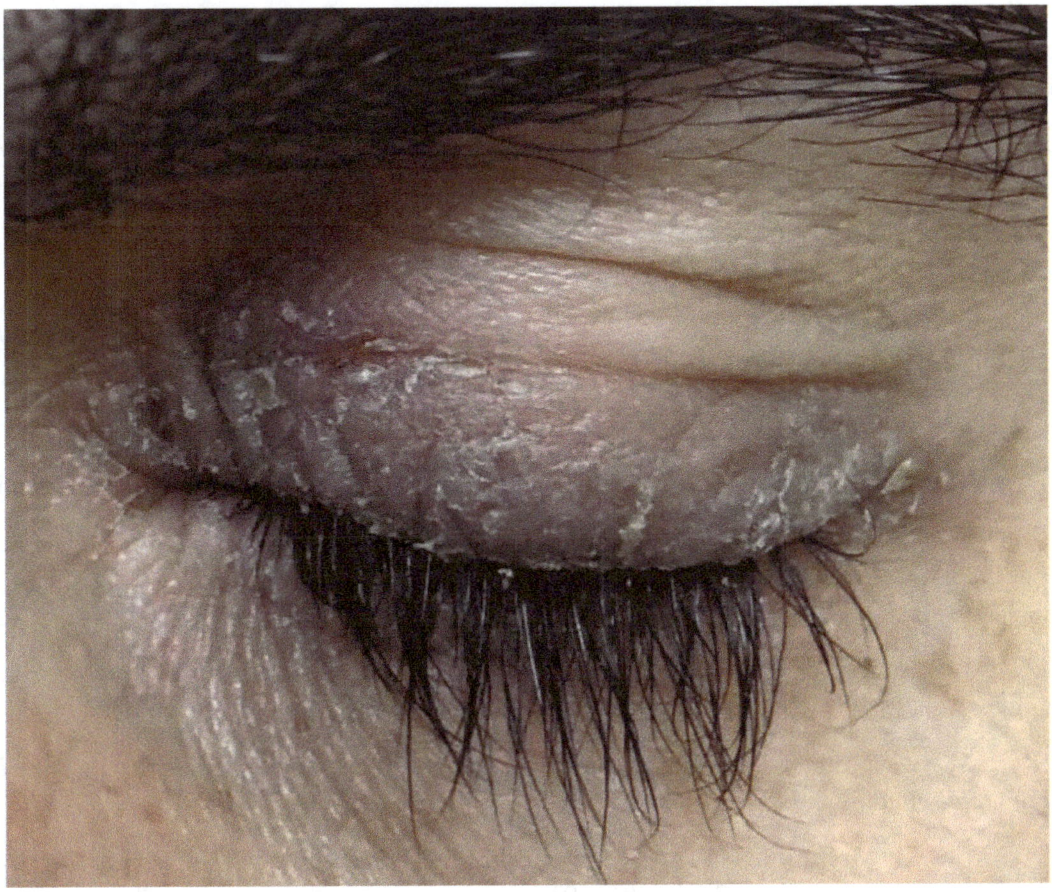

Figure 51. The same patient under slit lamp

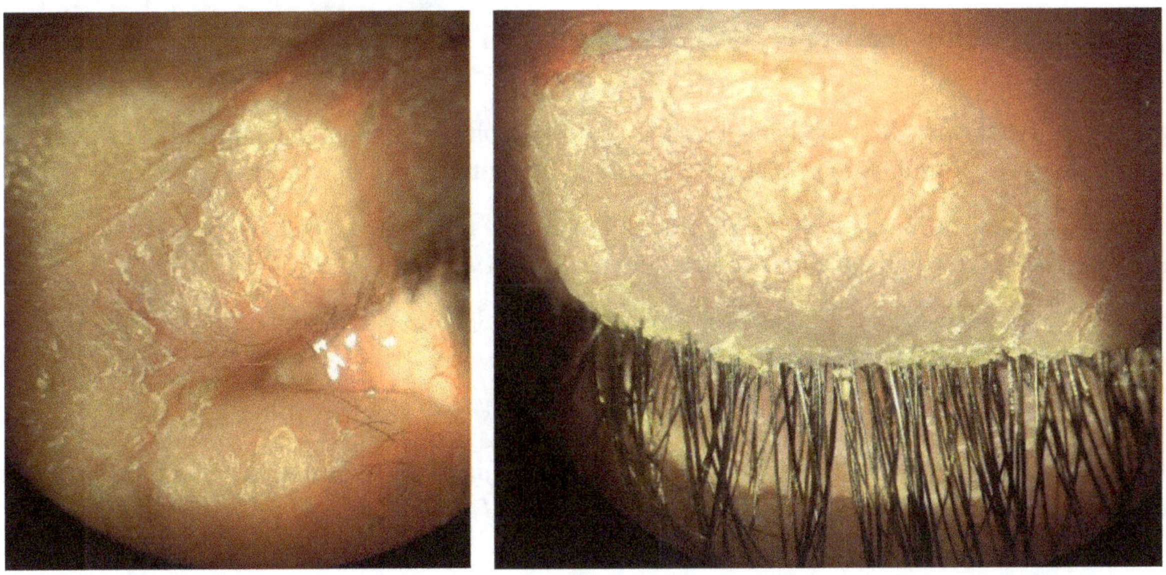

REFERENCES

Alessi, E., Gianotti, R., & Coggi, A. (1997). Multiple apocrine hidrocystomas of the eyelids. *British Journal of Dermatology*, *137*, 642–645.

American Academy of Ophthalmology Cornea/External Disease Panel. (2018). *Preferred Practice Pattern®. Blepharitis*. San Francisco, CA: American Academy of Ophthalmology. www.aao.org/ppp

Amrith, S., Hong Low, C., & Cheah, E. (1999). Erdheim–Chester disease: A bilateral orbital mass as an indication of systemic disease. *Orbit (Amsterdam, Netherlands)*, *18*, 99–104.

Bartley, G. B., & Lowry, J. C. (1992). Argon laser treatment of trichiasis. *American Journal of Ophthalmology*, *113*, 71–74.

Block, S. L. (2013). Getting an eyeful of preseptal cellulitis. *Pediatric Annals*, *42*(3), 99–102.

Bravo, I. G., & Félez-Sánchez, M. (2015). Papillomaviruses: Viral evolution, cancer and evolutionary medicine. *Evolution, Medicine, and Public Health*, *2015*(1), 32–51.

Din, N., & Patel, N. N. (2012). Blepharitis – a review of diagnosis and management. *Int J Ophthalmol Prac.*, *3*(4), 150–155.

Domonkos, A. N., Arnold, H. L., & Odom, R. B. (1982). *Andrew's diseases of the skin*. WB Saunders Philadelphia.

Dougherty, J. M., & McCulley, J. P. (1984). Comparative bacteriology of chronic blepharitis. *The British Journal of Ophthalmology*, *68*(8), 524–528.

Dougherty, J. M., & McCulley, J. P. (1986). Bacterial lipases and chronic blepharitis. *Investigative Ophthalmology & Visual Science*, *27*(4), 486–491.

Doxanas, M. T., & Green, W. R. (1984). Sebaceous gland carcinoma. Review of 40 cases. *Archives of Ophthalmology*, *102*(2), 245–249.

Duderstadt, K. (2013). Pediatric Physical Examination: An Illustrated Handbook (2nd ed.). Elsevier Health Sciences.

Dutton, J. J., Anderson, R. L., & Schelper, R. L. (1984). Orbital malignant melanoma and oculodermal melanocytosis: Report of two cases and review of the literature. *Ophthalmology*, *91*, 497–506.

Faustina, M., Diba, R., & Ahmadi, M. A. (2004). Patterns of regional and distant metastasis in patients with eyelid and periocular squamous cell carcinoma. *Ophthalmology*, *111*(10), 1930–1932.

Ferry, A. P. (1989). Pyogenic granulomas of the eye and ocular adnexa: A study of 100 cases. *Transactions of the American Ophthalmological Society*, *87*, 327.

Fonacier, J. (2001). Ocular allergies. *Current Allergy and Asthma Reports*, *1*(4), 389–396.

Foulks, G. N., & Bron, A. J. (2003). Meibomian gland dysfunction: A clinical scheme for description, diagnosis, classification, and grading. *The Ocular Surface*, *1*, 107–126.

Freeman, A. K., Serle, J., VanVeldhuisen, P., Lind, L., Clarke, J., Singer, G., & Lebwohl, M. (2004). Tacrolimus ointment in the treatment of eyelid dermatitis. *Cutis*, *73*(4), 267.

Fuchs, A., & Wu, F. C. (n.d.). Sleep with half open eyes (physiological lagophthalmos). *American Journal of Ophthalmology*, *1*, 717.

Glover, A. T., & Grove, A. S. (1987). Jr Subconjunctival orbital fat prolapse. *Ophthalmic Plastic and Reconstructive Surgery*, *3*(2), 83–86.

Groden, L. R., Murphy, B., & Rodnite, J. (1991). Lid flora in blepharitis. *Cornea*, *10*(1), 50–53.

Hall, A. J. (1936). Some observations on the active opening and closing of the eyes. *The British Journal of Ophthalmology*, *20*, 257–295.

Hamada, T. (2002). Lipoid proteinosis. *Clinical and Experimental Dermatology*, *27*(8), 624–629.

Hoang-Xuan, T., Rodriguez, A., & Zaltas, M. M. (1990). Ocular rosacea. *Ophthalmology*, *97*, 1468–1475.

Howitt, D. A., & Goldstein, J. H. (1969). Physiological lagophthalmos. *American Journal of Ophthalmology*, *68*, 355.

Jakobiec. (1988). Cornealtumors. In *The cornea*. Churchill Livingstone.

Jakobiec, F. A., & Jones, I. S. (1991). *Vascular tumors, malformations, and degenerations. In Clinical ophthalmology* (Vol. 2). JB Lippincott.

Kosik-Bogacka. (2013). Demodex folliculorum and Demodex brevis in healthy and immunocompromised patients. *Ophthalmic Epidemiology*, *20*(3), 159–163.

Kwon, Jang, & Yoon. (2015). Long-Term Outcome of Combined Lateral Tarsal Strip With Temporal Permanent Tarsorrhaphy for Correction of Paralytic Ectropion Caused By Facial Nerve Palsy. *J Craniofac Surg.*, *26*(5), 409-12.

Lane, J. E., & Kent, D. E. (2005). Surgical margins in the treatment of nonmelanoma skin cancer and Mohs micrographic surgery. *Current Surgery*, *62*(5), 518–526.

Lee, S., & Yen, M. T. (2011). Management of preseptal and orbital cellulitis. *Saudi Journal of Ophthalmology*, *25*(1), 21–29.

Lemp, Crews, & Bron. (2012). Distribution of aqueous-deficient and evaporative dry eye in a clinic-based patient population. *Cornea, 31*(472).

Lemp, M. A., & Nichols, K. K. (2009). Blepharitis in the United States 2009: A survey based perspective on prevalence and treatment. *Ocul Suft.*, *7*(Suppl. 2), S1–S14. doi:10.1016/S1542-0124(12)70620-1 PMID:19383269

Lindsley, J. J. (2013). Interventions for acute internal hordeolum. *Cochrane Database of Systematic Reviews*, (4), CD007742.

Liu, S., Pavan-Langston, D., & Colby, K. A. (2012). Pediatric herpes simplex of the anterior segment: Characteristics, treatment, and outcomes. *Ophthalmology*, *119*(10), 2003–2008.

Luz Fonacier, M. D., & David, I. (2015, May-June). Contact Dermatitis: A Practice Parametere Update 2015. *The Journal of Allergy and Clinical Immunology. In Practice*, *3*(3), S1–S39.

Lyon, D. B., & Dortzbach, R. K. (1994). *Entropion, trichiasis, and distichiasis. In Ophthalmic plastic surgery: Prevention and management of complications*. Raven Press New York.

Ma'luf, R. N. (2010). Treatment of recurrent eyelid margin verruca vulgaris with mitomycin C. *Ophthalmic Plastic and Reconstructive Surgery*, *26*(3), 214–215.

Macsai, M. S. (2008). The role of omega-3 dietary supplementation in blepharitis and meibomian gland dysfunction (AOS thesis). *Trans Am Ophthalmol Soc.*, *106*(336).

McCulley, J. P., Dougherty, J. M., & Deneau, D. G. (1982). Classification of chronic blepharitis. *Ophthalmology*, *89*, 1173–1180.

McCulley, J. P., Dougherty, J. M., & Deneau, D. G. (1982). Classification of chronic blepharitis. *Ophthalmology*, *89*, 1173–1180.

McGavran, M. H., & Binnington, B. (1966). Keratinous cysts of the skin. *Archives of Dermatology*, *94*, 499–508.

Nowinski, T. S., & Anderson, R. L. (1985). The medial spindle procedure for involutional medial ectropion. *Archives of Ophthalmology*, *103*(11), 1750–1753. doi:10.1001/archopht.1985.01050110146045 PMID:3904688

Ono, I., & Tateshita, T. (1998). Efficacy of the ruby laser in the treatment of Ota's nevus previously treated using other therapeutic modalities. *Plastic and Reconstructive Surgery*, *102*, 2352–2357.

Pinkus, H., & Sutton, R. (1965). Trichofolliculoma. *Archives of Dermatology*, *91*, 46–49.

Rohrich, R. J., Janis, J. E., & Pownell, P. H. (2002). Xanthelasma palpebrarum: A review and current management principles. *Plastic and Reconstructive Surgery*, *110*, 1310–1314.

Rubin, A. I., Chen, E. H., & Ratner, D. (2005). Basal-cell carcinoma. *The New England Journal of Medicine*, *353*(21), 2262–2269.

Seo, H. M., Choi, C. W., & Kim, W. S. (2015). Beneficial effects of early treatment of nevus of Ota with low-fluence 1,064-nm Q-switched Nd:YAG laser. *Dermatologic Surgery*, *41*, 142–148.

Shields, C. L., & Shields, J. A. (2004). Tumors of the conjunctiva and cornea. *Survey of Ophthalmology*, *49*(1), 3–24.

Shine, W. E., & McCulley, J. P. (1993). Role of wax ester fatty alcohols in chronic blepharitis. *Investigative Ophthalmology & Visual Science*, *34*, 3515–3521.

Siah, W. F., Nagendran, S., Tan, P., Ali Ahmad, S. M., Litwin, A. S., & Malhotra, R. (2018, February). Late outcomes of gold weights and platinum chains for upper eyelid loading. *The British Journal of Ophthalmology*, *102*(2), 164–168.

Soll, S. M., Lisman, R. D., & Charles, N. C. (1993). Pyogenic granuloma after transconjunctival blepharoplasty: A case report. *Ophthalmic Plastic and Reconstructive Surgery*, *9*, 298–301.

Starr, P. A. J., & McDonald, A. (1969). Oculocutaneous aspects of rosacea. *Proceedings of the Royal Society of Medicine*, *62*, 9.

Stefanyszyn, M. A., Hidayat, A. A., & Flanagan, J. C. (1985). The histopathology of involutional ectropion. *Ophthalmology*, *92*(1), 120–127. doi:10.1016/S0161-6420(85)34061-7 PMID:4038795

Steinhoff, M., Schauber, J., & Leyden, J. J. (2013). New insights into rosacea pathophysiology: A review of recent findings. *Journal of the American Academy of Dermatology*, *69*, 515.

Stumpf, T., Luqmani, N., & Sumich, P. (2006). Systemic tacrolimus in the treatment of severe atopic keratoconjunctivitis. *Cornea*, *25*(10), 1147–1149.

Sullivan, H., Beard, C., & Bullock, J. D. (1976). Cryosurgery for treatment of trichiasis. *American Journal of Ophthalmology*, *82*, 117–121.

Zhao, Y. E., Wu, L. P., & Hu, L. (2012). Association of blepharitis with Demodex: A meta-analysis. *Ophthalmic Epidemiology*, *19*(2), 95–102.

Chapter 2
Dry Eye Disease

ABSTRACT

Dry eye disease, also known as dry eye syndrome and keratoconjunctivitis sicca (KCS), is a disorder of the tear film that develops due to reduced tear production or tear film excessive evaporation, associated with ocular discomfort and an inflammatory disease of the ocular surface. Dry eye is a common cause of ocular irritation necessitating ophthalmic care. Systemic medications like diuretics, antihistamines, anticholinergics, antidepressants, and retinoids can also cause symptoms of dry eye. Environmental factors such as reduced humidity, increased wind, air conditioning, and heating may increase the ocular discomfort of patients. The definition, causes, and classification of dry eye syndrome are discussed in this chapter. A rare manifestation of the disease presenting a severe consequence like corneal perforation is included to highlight the importance of early recognition and treatment and to highlight the possible severities of the disease. Post treatment photos are included to show the appearance of the sequela.

DRY EYE SYNDROME

According to the International Dry Eye Workshop (DEWS 2017), dry eye is defined as a "multifactorial disease of the tears and ocular surface that results in symptoms of discomfort, visual disturbance, and tear film instability with potential damage to the ocular surface." It is accompanied by increased osmolarity of the tear film and inflammation of the ocular surface. Classically, DED has been divided into two subtypes: aqueous tear-deficient dry eye (ADDE) and evaporative dry eye (EDE). Clinically, the borders between the two are less clear, and both are leading to dysfunctional tear syndrome with hyperosmolarity, inflammation, and tear instability.

Epidemiological studies on dry eye syndrome have controversial findings regarding their prevalence. Approximately 1 out of 7 individuals aged 65 to 84 years reports symptoms of dry eye often or all of the time. Men's Health Study revealed that the prevalence of dry eye in men increased from 3.9% to 7.7% when men aged 50 to 54 were compared with men over 80. In a similar Women's Health Study of over 39,000 women, the prevalence of dry eye was 5.7% among women younger than 50 and increased to

DOI: 10.4018/978-1-7998-6937-5.ch002

9.8% among women over 75. Many risk factors for dry eye have been proposed. Older age and female gender have been identified as major risk factors.Use of glaucoma medication containing benzalkonium chloride (BAK) is another risk factor. Smoking and multivitamin use is shown to be associated with an increased risk of dry eye, whereas caffeine use is associated with a decreased risk. More recent reports have suggested a relationship between botulinum toxin injection and dry eye.. Rheumatoid arthritis, among systemic diseases, is one of the most common that can lead to dry eye disease.

Table 1. Etiologic classification of dry eye from the definition and classification of dry eye disease

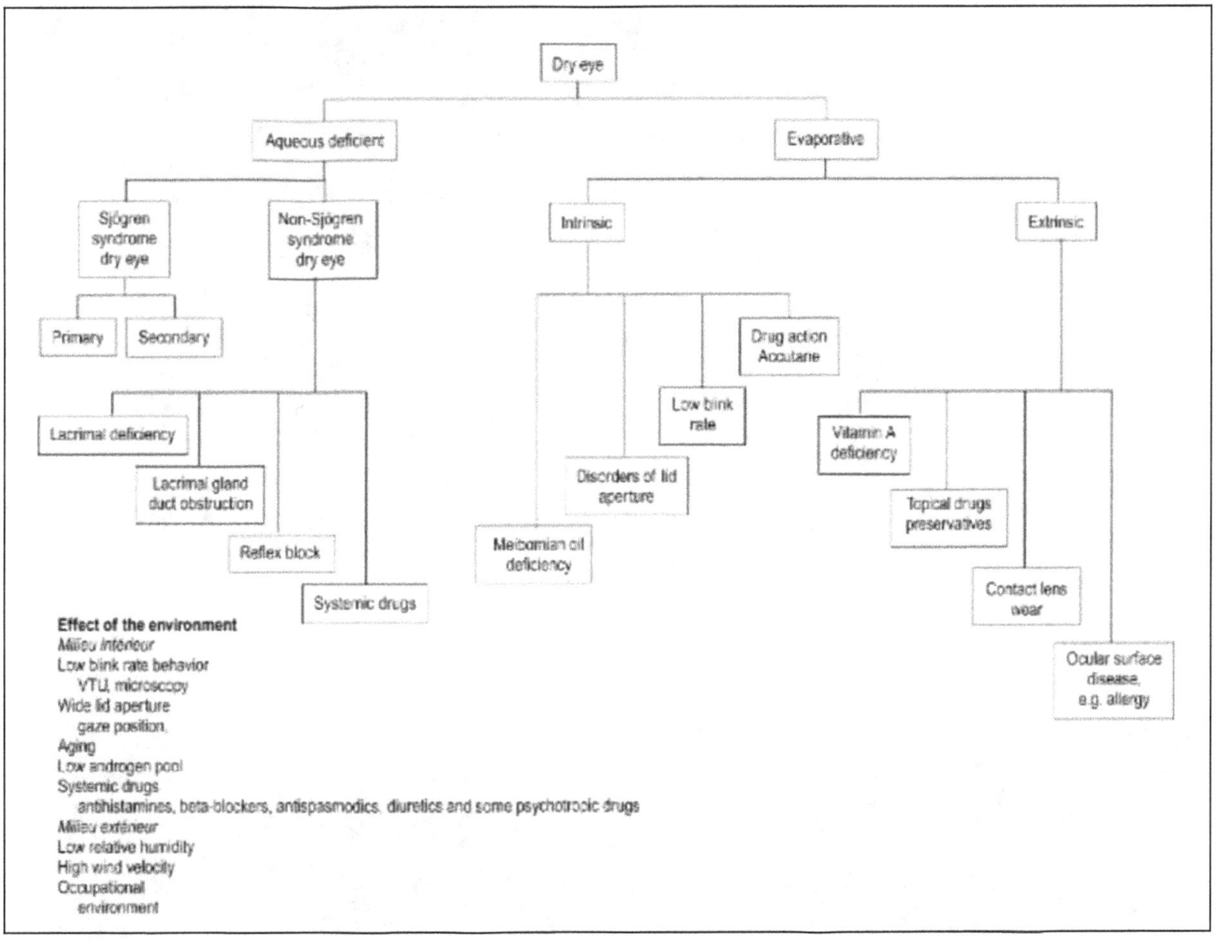

Oculus Surf (2017;5:75–92)

The most common diagnostic tests are the measurement of tear break-up time (TBUT), ocular surface staining, Schirmer strips (Fig 5), and measurement of corneal sensation (Wolffsohn et al, 2017; Belmonte et al, 2017). Ocular surface damage can be assessed by staining with one or more dyes, including fluorescein (Fig 2), Rose Bengal, or Lissamine green (Fig 6).

Figure 1. Schirmer test. A Schirmer strip is placed in the lateral one-third of the lower lid. The distance of wetting (counted by mm) shows lacrimal production

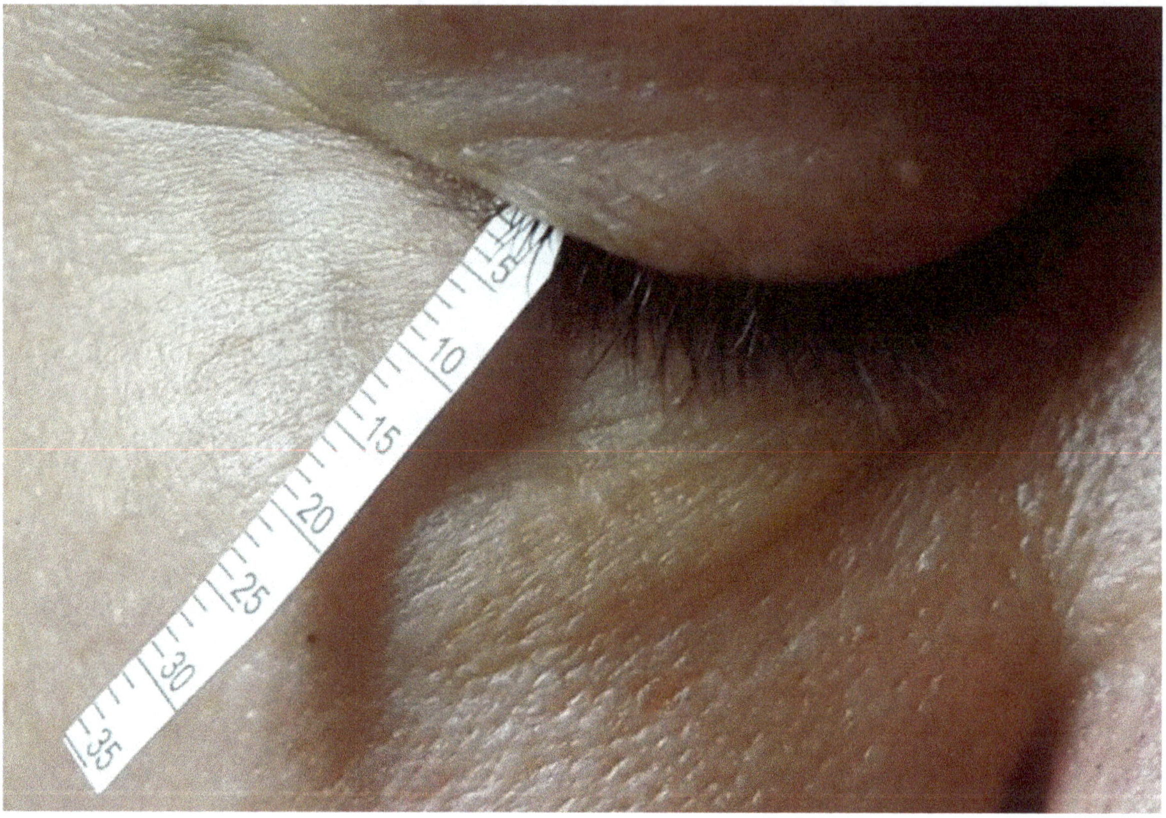

Figure 2. Sjögren syndrome. The right and left eyes of the same patient. Severe dryness is seen. The cornea is stained with Fluorescein; the photo is taken under Cobalt-blue illumination with the yellow-blue filter

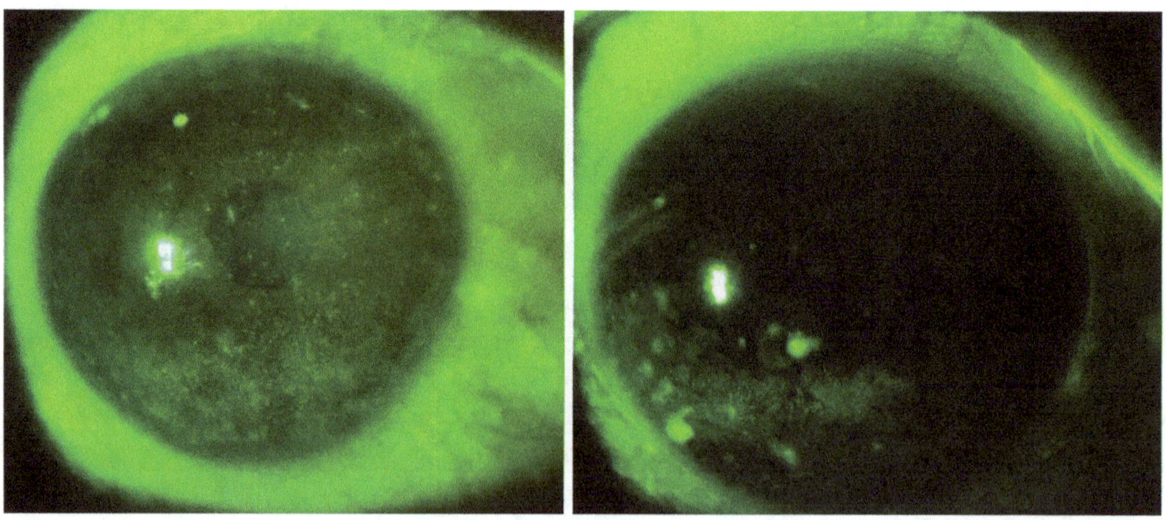

Figure 3. Dry eye syndrome. Rose-Bengal staining of interpalpebral conjunctiva (left photo) and the same eye under a slit-lamp (right photo)

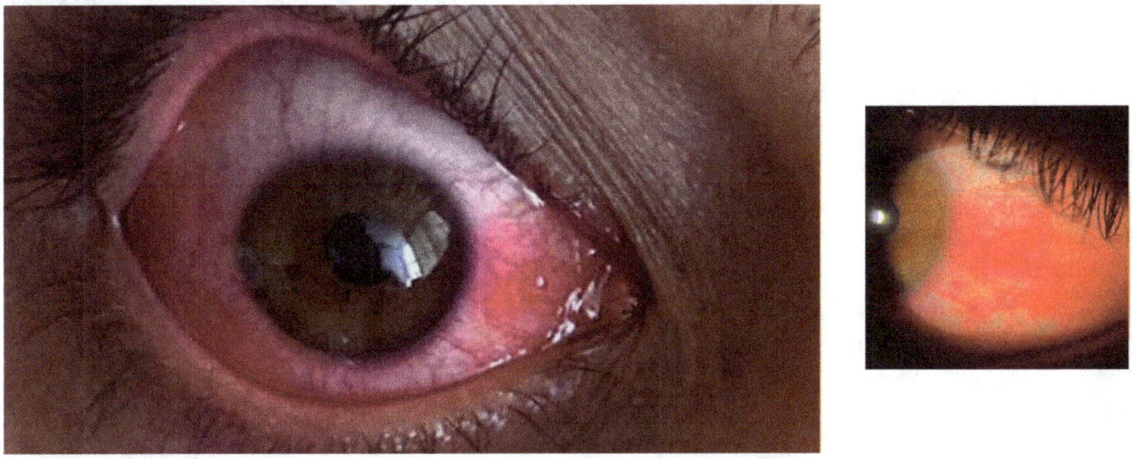

Assessment of tear film composition is an additional method to diagnose dry eye disease, which includes osmolarity testing and tear protein analysis (lysozyme, lactoferrin).

TBUT refers to measuring the time between the last blink and the appearance of the first break (randomly distributed dry spot or hole) in the precorneal fluorescent tear film after application of fluorescein dye. It is a clinical test used to assess for evaporative dry eye disease. A TBUT under 10 seconds is considered abnormal.

Schirmer test is the most commonly used technique for measuring tear secretion. A Schirmer strip is usually placed in the lateral one-third of the lower lid. The distance of strip wetting after five minutes shows aqueous tear production. More than 10 mm of moisture on the paper after 5 minutes without topical anesthesia and 5 mm with anesthesia is a sign of normal tear production (Fig 1).

Reduced corneal sensation is another sign of dry eye. The simplest technique for measuring corneal sensitivity is to gently touch the surface of the cornea and conjunctiva with a few strands from a cotton swab or dental floss and grade the patient's response. Another method of assessment is using a Cochet–Bonnet esthesiometer.

Ocular surface damage is commonly assessed by staining with fluorescein, Rose Bengal, or Lissamine green. Fluorescein sodium is considered to be the most commonly used dye in ophthalmology. Fluorescein generally stains the cornea to a greater degree than the conjunctiva (Fig 2), whereas Rose Bengal and Lissamine green have greater sensitivity of staining the conjunctiva (Fig 3). The classical location for conjunctival staining in dry eye syndrome is the interpalpebral conjunctival zone.

ADDE (aqueous tear-deficient dry eye) has 2 subtypes: Sjögren syndrome dry eye (SSDE) and non-Sjögren syndrome dry eye.

Sjögren syndrome is an autoimmune exocrinopathy with the involvement of lacrimal and salivary glands, as well as other organs (Fig 3, 4, 5). The glands become infiltrated by activated T cells, which cause acinar and ductal epithelial cell death and hyposecretion of the tears or saliva (Hayashi et al, 2003). Many autoimmune diseases especially rheumatoid arthritis can affect lacrimal gland causing secondary Sjögren syndrome and lead to dry eye disease (Fig 6-9) (Generali et al, 2015).

Figure 4. Sjögren syndrome. The enlarged salivary gland is seen

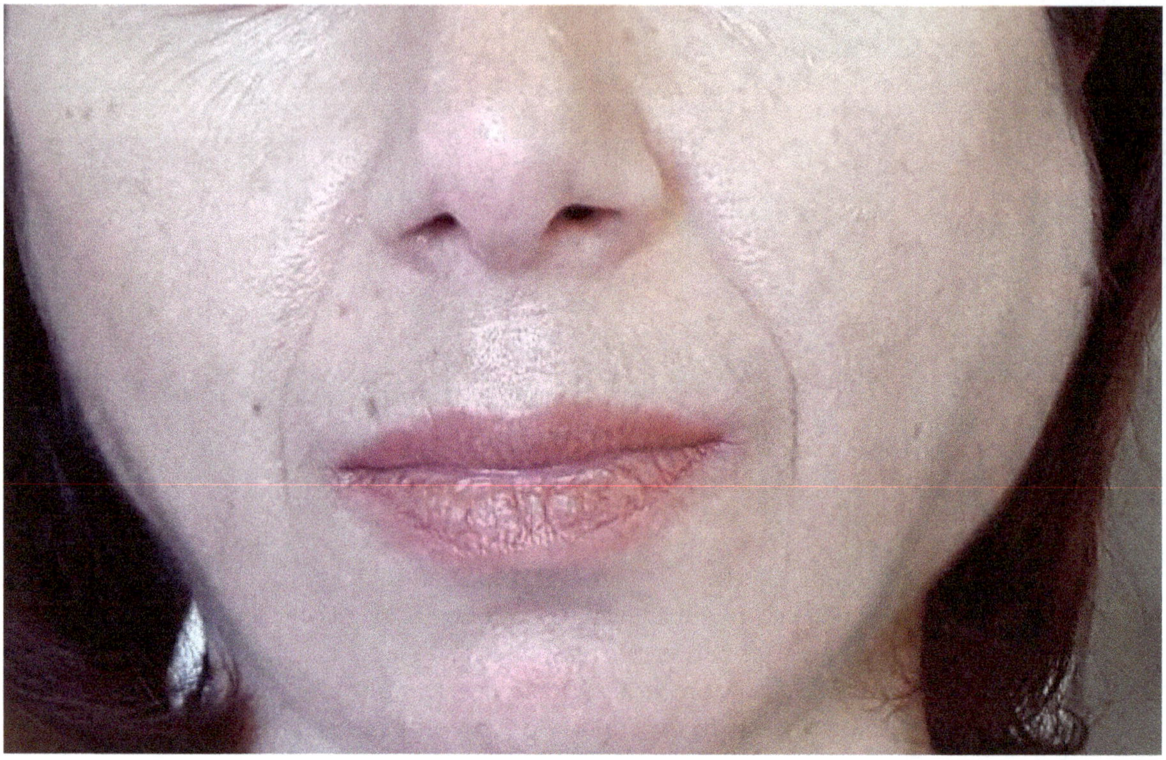

Figure 5. Sjögren syndrome. The enlarged lacrimal glands are seen

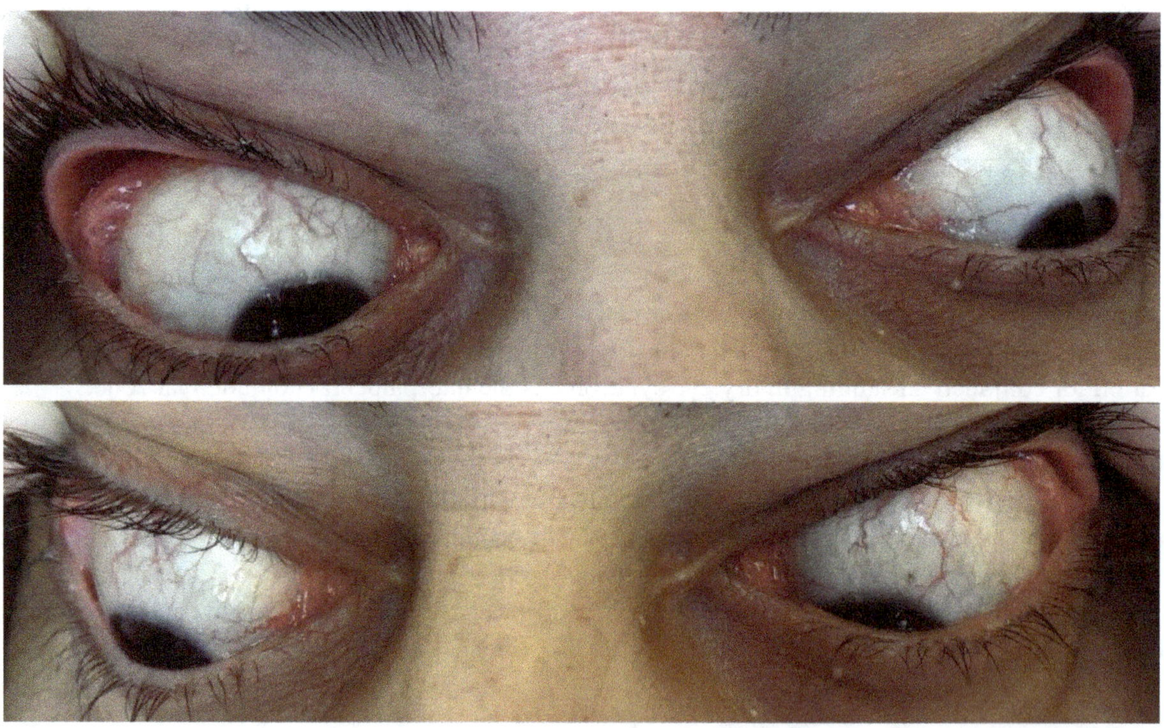

Figure 6. The enlarged lacrimal glands of the same patient under a slit lamp

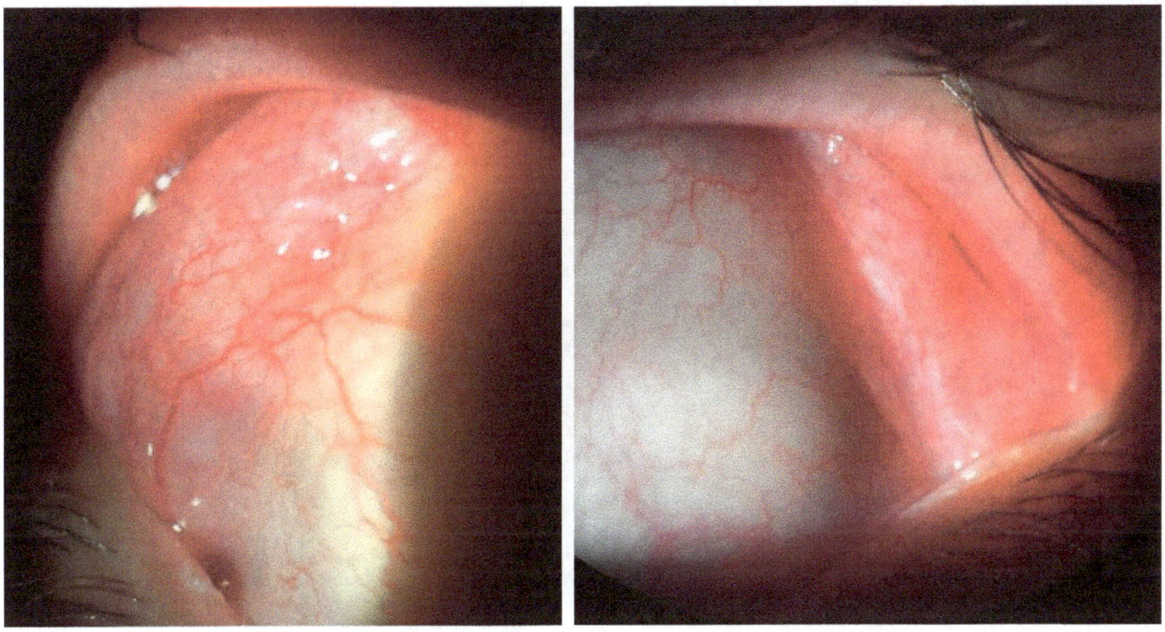

Figure 7. Corneal perforation due to severe dry eye associated with RA

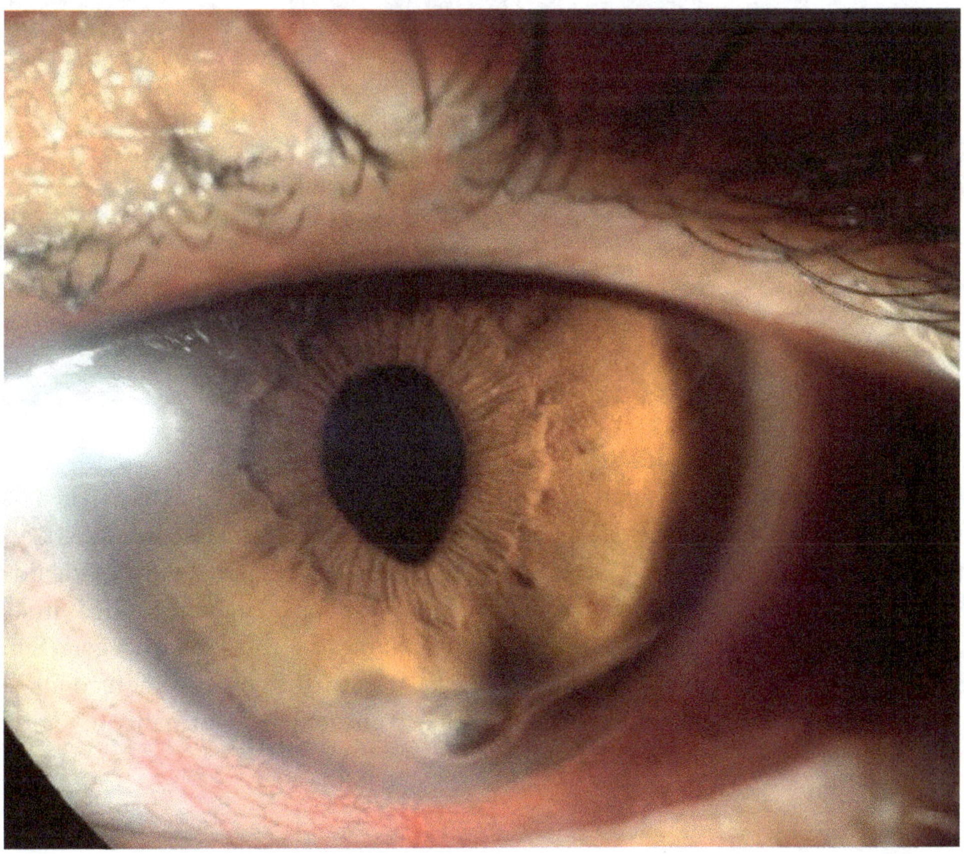

Figure 8. Severe dry eye due to rheumatoid arthritis (RA). Corneal perforation is seen, note the very shallow anterior chamber (right photo)

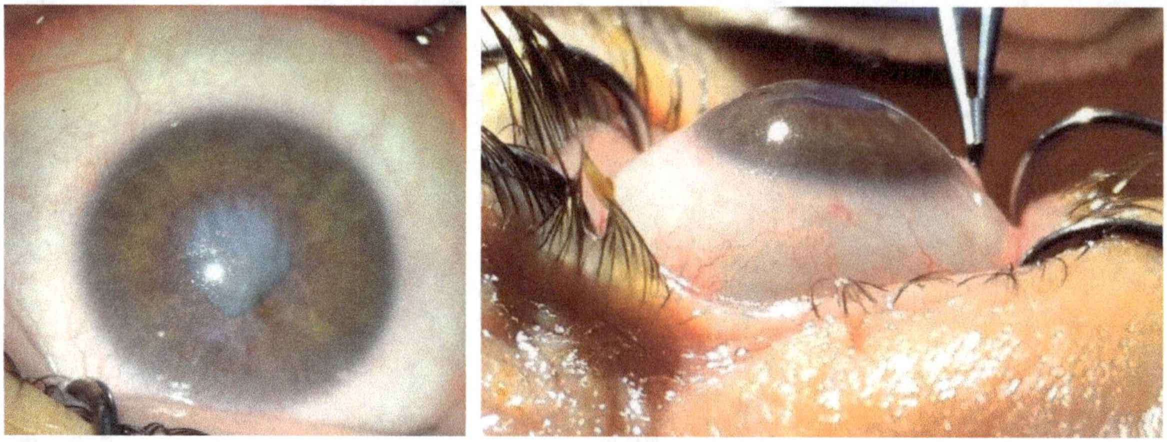

Figure 9. The same eye covered with amniotic membrane (left photo) and the next day after surgery (right photo). The anterior chamber is deep

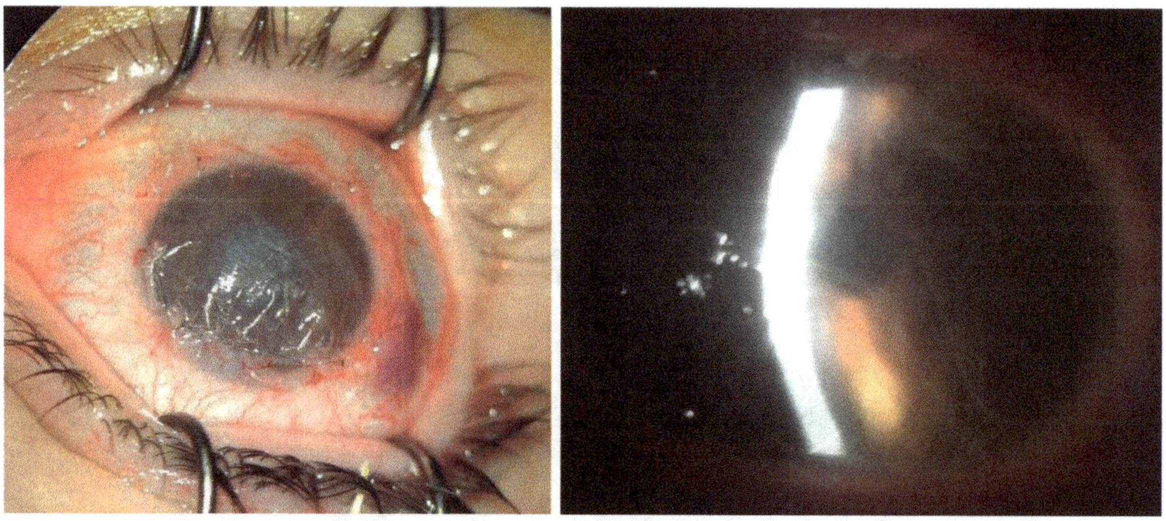

Non-Sjögren syndrome dry eye is a form of ADDE due to lacrimal dysfunction, when the systemic autoimmune features of SSDE have been excluded. The most common form is age-related dry eye, which represents primary ductal obstruction of lacrimal gland leading to lacrimal gland dysfunction (Obata et al, 1995). The effecting factors to these age-related symptoms are considered the changes in sex hormone levels, specifically a physiologic decrease in androgens and/or an increase in estrogen (Sullivan et al, 2002). (Fig 10). Congenital alacrima is also a possible cause, and the most common condition is Riley-Day syndrome, where the tear production is decreased due to congenital abnormality of parasympathetic innervation of lacrimal gland (Simson, 2006).

Figure 10. The same eye after 20 days of treatment. Mild anterior stromal scar is formed

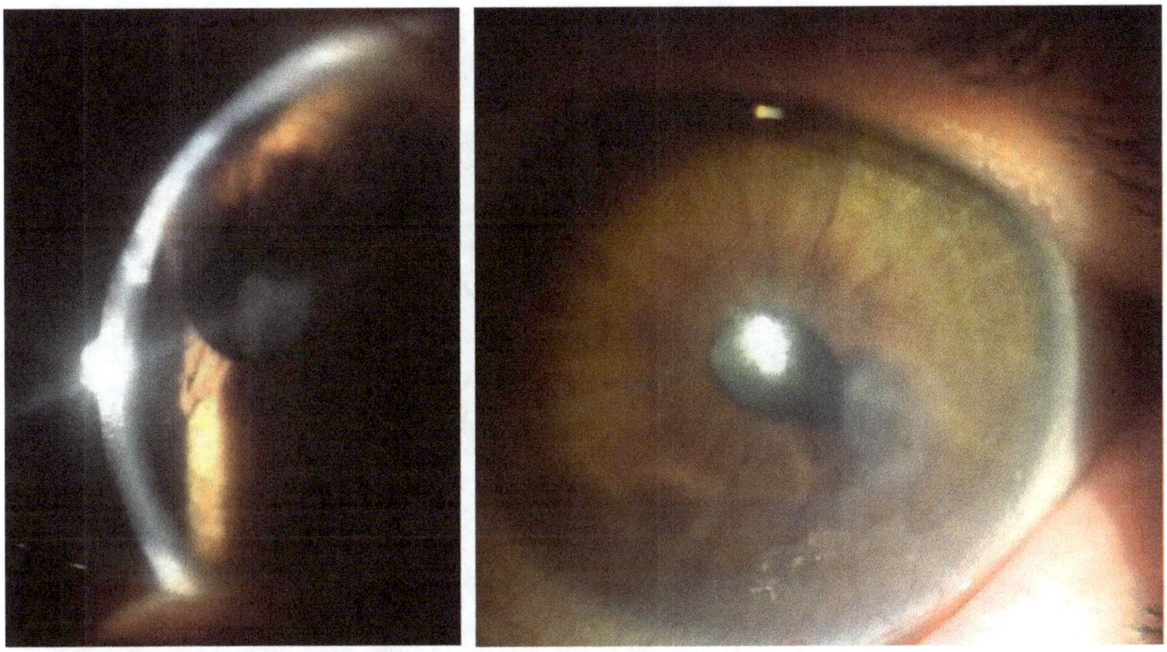

Figure 11. Bilateral epitheliopathy due to dry eye syndrome, patient in menopause

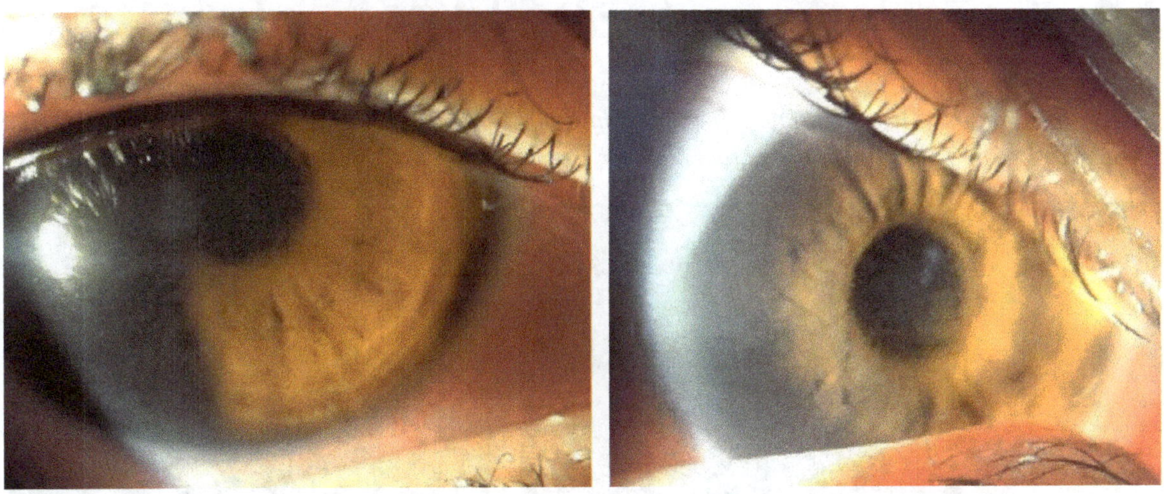

Lacrimal gland can be secondarily affected in sarcoidosis (Fig 11, 12), lymphoma, hemochromatosis, and amyloidosis (Fox, 1994). Some systemic infections can also cause tear production failure, including EBV, HTLV-1, and HIV-1 (Itescu, 1991).

Reflex hyposecretion could lead to dry eye disease due to either sensory block including diabetes mellitus (Kaiserman, 2005) neurotrophic keratitis (Cavanagh et al, 1989) or motor block as a side effects of systemic drug use, especially with anticholinergic effects (Moss et al, 2004).

Figure 12. Lacrimal gland enlargement and infiltration in sarcoidosis

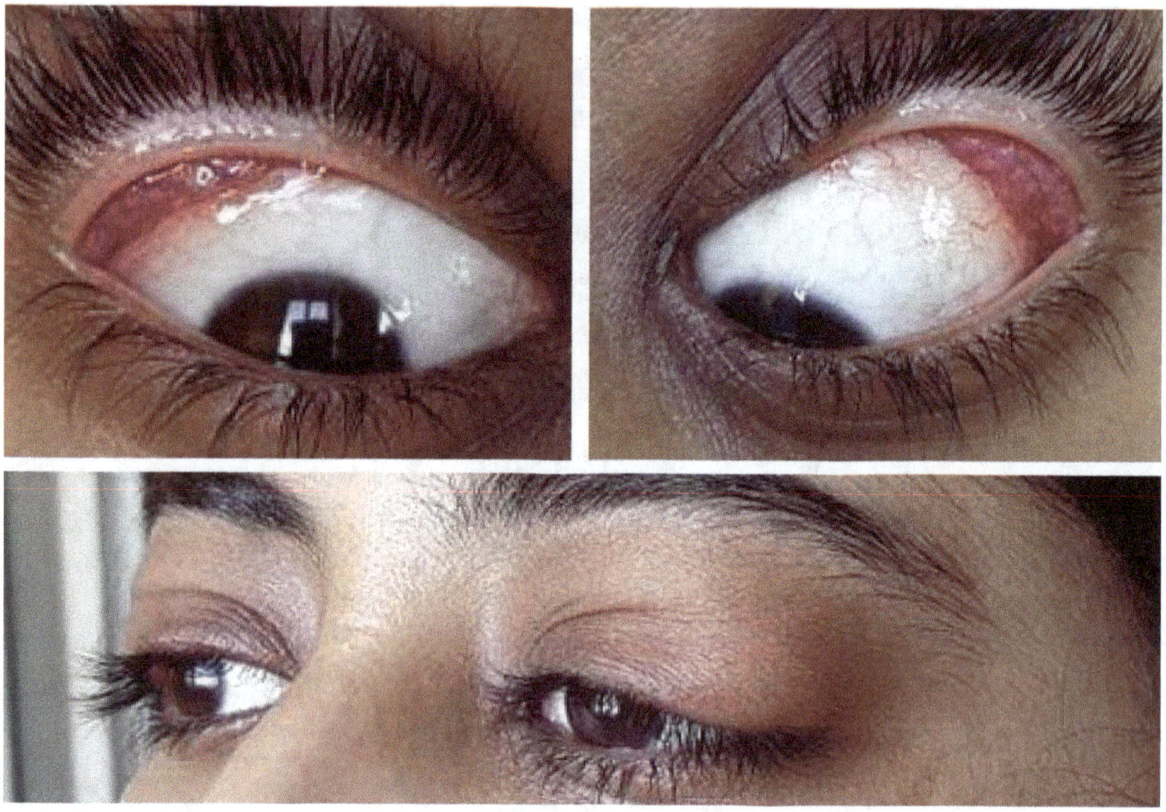

Figure 13. Sarcoidosis. The right and left eyes of the same patient. Severe dryness is seen. The cornea is stained with Fluorescein; the photo is taken under Cobalt-blue illumination with the yellow-blue filter

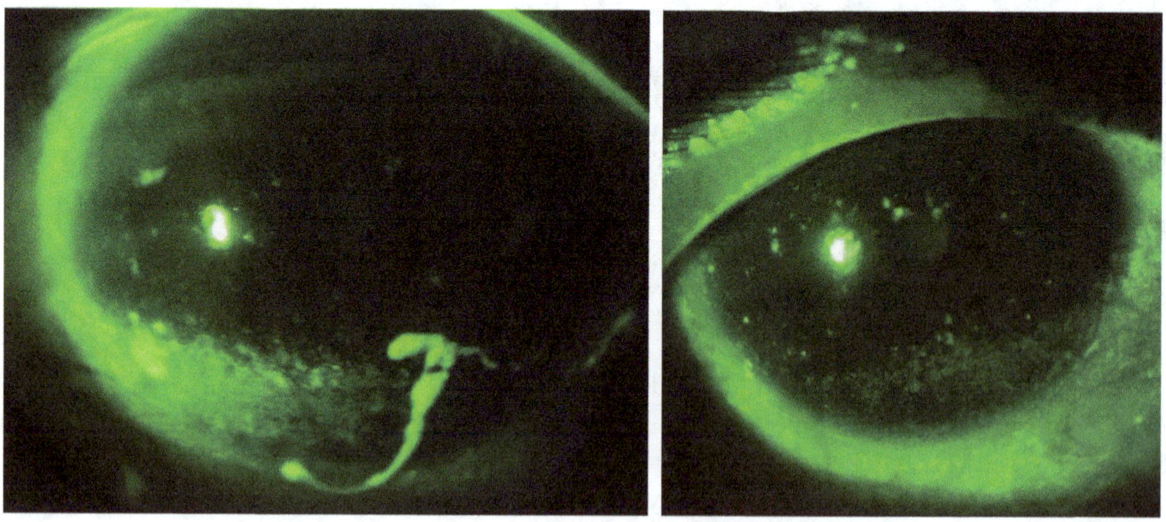

Evaporative dry eye classically has intrinsic causes (conditions affecting lid structure or dynamics) and extrinsic causes (external cause of ocular surface exposure) but the boundaries are very blurred within them.

Intrinsic causes include meibomian gland dysfunction that results in tear instability and faster evaporation from ocular surface (discussed more detailed in Chapter 1) (Nichols, 2011). This is considered the most common cause of evaporative dry eye syndrome (Fig 13) (Bron, 2004). Meibography is a relatively new technique to assess and visualize meibomian glands (Fig 14). An increasingly exposed evaporative surface is another reason of intrinsic causes and occurs in patients with proptosis[26], especially with thyroid disease, as well as due to increased interblink duration (Nakamori, 1997).

Extrinsic causes include ocular surface diseases (chronic ocular surface disease, vit A deficiency) (Hori, 2004) that lead to imperfect surface wetting and contact lens wear (Nichols, 2006). (Fig 15). The use of topical drops containing preservatives, especially BAK, are one of the most common causes of dry eye (Pisella, 2002).

Lubricants, artificial tears, ointments, and gels continue to be the mainstay of treatment for dry eye syndrome. Punctal occlusion/plugs are one of the most useful therapies for patients with aqueous-deficient DED. In severe cases of dry eye contact lenses can help and hydrate the corneal surface, especially when filamentary keratopathy is associated. Cyclosporine 0.05% or 0.1%, and Xiidra are considered tear stimulation agents. Autologous serum tears are effective in severe DED. Corticosteroids nonspecifically inhibit many aspects of the inflammatory response. Several studies show that short-term topical corticosteroid use (at least four weeks) alleviate the signs and symptoms of DED.

Figure 14. Occlusive meibomitis is seen

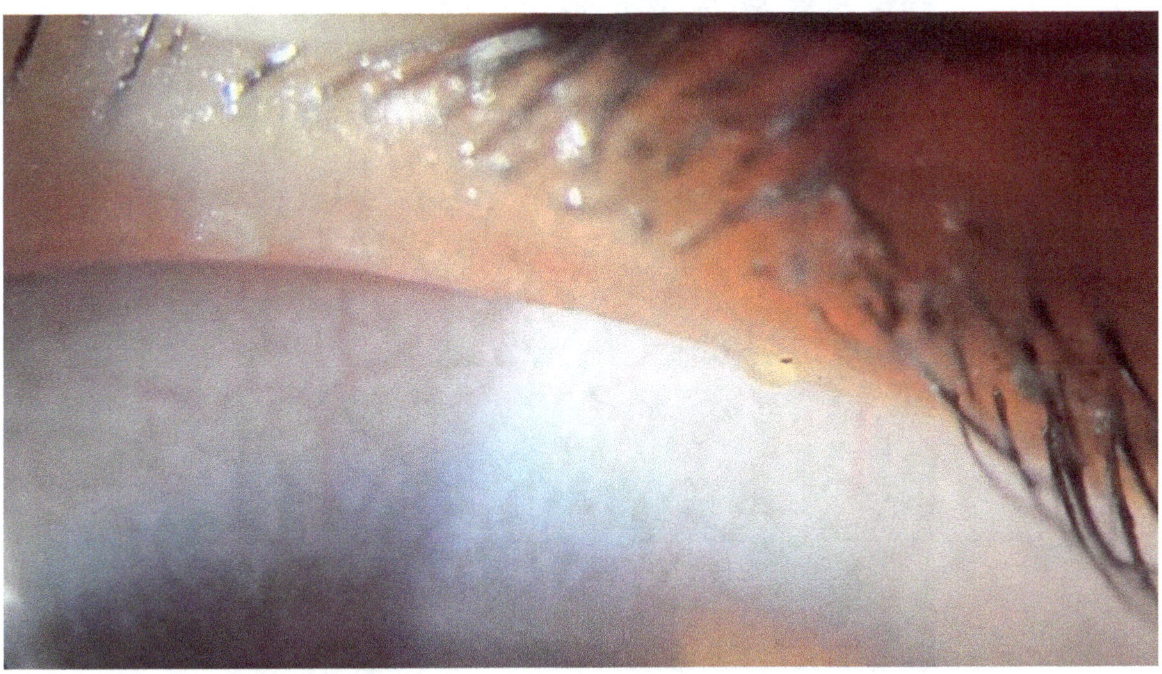

Figure 15. Lacry-Diag Mentonierre system meibography. The damaged meibomean glands are visualized. Lower and upper lids of the same patient

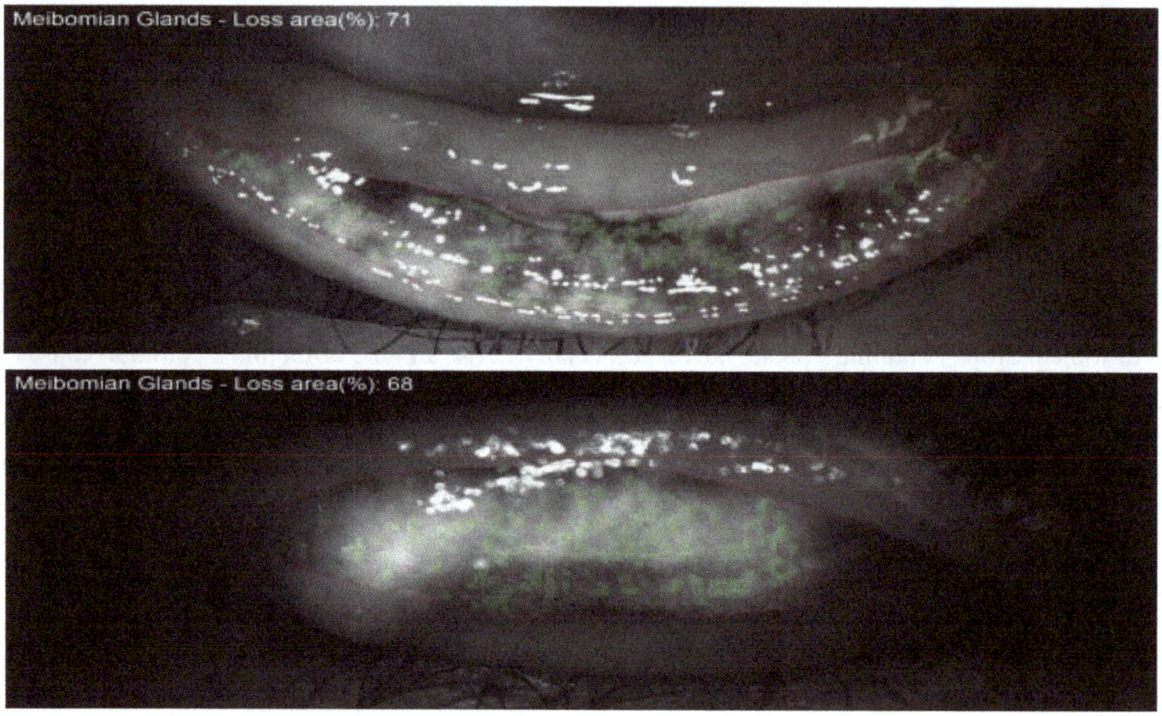

Figure 16. Mild epitheliopathy due to dry eye associated with contact lens wear

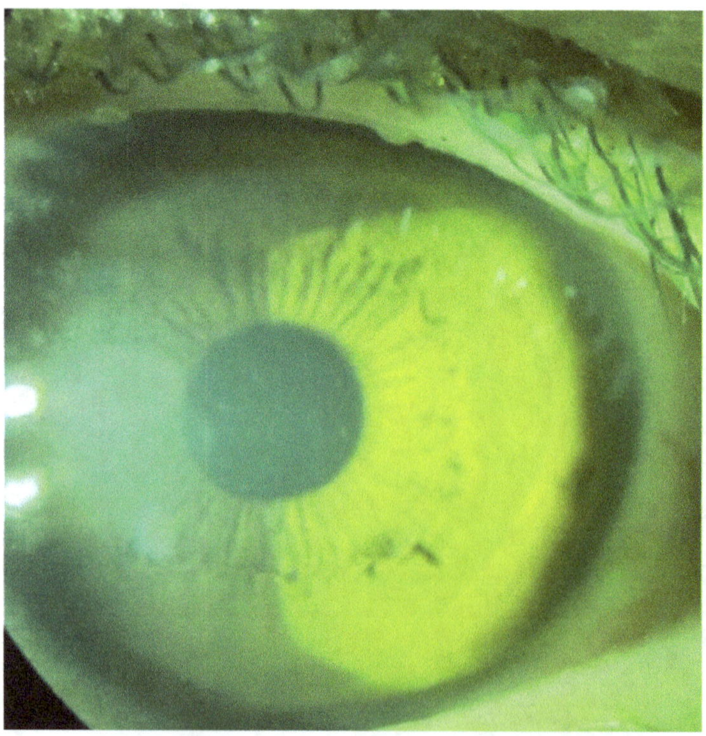

REFERENCES

Asbell, P. A. (2006). Increasing importance of dry eye syndrome and the ideal artificial tear: Consensus views from a roundtable discussion. *Current Medical Research and Opinion*, *22*(11), 2149–2157. doi:10.1185/030079906X132640 PMID:17076975

Belmonte, C., Nichols, J. J., Cox, S. M., Brock, J. A., Begley, C. G., Bereiter, D. A., Dartt, D. A., Galor, A., Hamrah, P., Ivanusic, J. J., Jacobs, D. S., McNamara, N. A., Rosenblatt, M. I., Stapleton, F., & Wolffsohn, J. S. (2017). TFOS DEWS II pain and sensation report. *The Ocular Surface*, *15*(3), 404–437. doi:10.1016/j.jtos.2017.05.002 PMID:28736339

Bron, A. J., & Tiffany, J. M. (2004). The contribution of Meibomian disease to dry eye. *Cornea*, *2*, 149–164. PMID:17216085

Cavanagh, H. D., & Colley, A. M. (1989). The molecular basis of neurotrophic keratitis. *Acta Ophthalmologica. Supplementum*, *192*, 115–134. PMID:2554641

Craig, J. P., Nichols, K. K., Akpek, E. K., Caffery, B., Dua, H. S., Joo, C.-K., Liu, Z., Nelson, J. D., Nichols, J. J., Tsubota, K., & Stapleton, F. (2017). TFOS DEWS II definition and classification report. *The Ocular Surface*, *15*(3), 276–283. doi:10.1016/j.jtos.2017.05.008 PMID:28736335

Fox, R. I. (1994). Systemic diseases associated with dry eye. *International Ophthalmology Clinics*, *34*(1), 71–87. doi:10.1097/00004397-199403410-00008 PMID:8169074

Generali, E., Cantarini, L., & Selmi, C. (2015). Ocular involvement in systemic autoimmune diseases. *Clinical Reviews in Allergy & Immunology*, *49*(3), 263–270. doi:10.100712016-015-8518-3 PMID:26494481

Gold-von Simson, F. B., & Axelrod, F. B. (2006). Axelrod: Familial dysautonomia: update and recent advances. *Current Problems in Pediatric and Adolescent Health Care*, *36*(6), 218–237. doi:10.1016/j.cppeds.2005.12.001 PMID:16777588

Hayashi, Y., Arakaki, R., & Ishimaru, N. (2003). The role of caspase cascade on the development of primary Sjögren's syndrome. *The Journal of Medical Investigation*, *50*, 32–38. PMID:12630566

Hori, Y., Spurr-Michaud, S., Russo, C. L., Argu¨eso, P., & Gipson, I. K. (2004). Differential regulation of membrane-associated mucins in the human ocular surface epithelium. *Investigative Ophthalmology & Visual Science*, *45*(1), 114–122. doi:10.1167/iovs.03-0903 PMID:14691162

Itescu, S. (1991). Itescu: Diffuse infiltrative lymphocytosis syndrome in human immunodeficiency virus infection – a Sjögren's-like disease. *Rheumatic Diseases Clinics of North America*, *17*(1), 99–115. doi:10.1016/S0889-857X(21)00091-0 PMID:2041892

Jones, L., & Laura, E. (2017, July). TFOS DEWS II Management and Therapy Report. *The Ocular Surface*, *15*(3), 575–628. doi:10.1016/j.jtos.2017.05.006 PMID:28736343

Kaiserman, I., Kaiserman, N., Nakar, S., & Vinker, S. (2005). Dry eye in diabetic patients. *American Journal of Ophthalmology*, *139*(3), 498–503. doi:10.1016/j.ajo.2004.10.022 PMID:15767060

Lemp, M. A., Crews, L. A., Bron, A. J., Foulks, G. N., & Sullivan, B. D. (2012). Distribution of aqueous-deficient and evaporative dry eye in a clinic-based patient cohort: A retrospective study. *Cornea*, *31*(5), 472–478. doi:10.1097/ICO.0b013e318225415a PMID:22378109

Leung, E. W., Medeiros, F. A., & Weinreb, R. N. (2008). Prevalence of ocular surface disease in glaucoma patients. *Journal of Glaucoma*, *17*(5), 350–355. doi:10.1097/IJG.0b013e31815c5f4f PMID:18703943

McCarty, C. A., Bansal, A. K., Livingston, P. M., Stanislavsky, Y. L., & Taylor, H. R. (1998). The epidemiology of dry eye in Melbourne, Australia. *Ophthalmology*, *105*(6), 1114–1119. doi:10.1016/S0161-6420(98)96016-X PMID:9627665

Moss, S. E., Klein, R., & Klein, B. E. (2000). Prevalence of and risk factors for dry eye syndrome. *Archives of Ophthalmology*, *118*(9), 1264–1268. doi:10.1001/archopht.118.9.1264 PMID:10980773

Moss, S. E., Klein, R., & Klein, B. E. (2004). Incidence of dry eye in an older population. *Archives of Ophthalmology*, *122*(3), 369–373. doi:10.1001/archopht.122.3.369 PMID:15006852

Nakamori, K., Odawara, M., Nakajima, T., Mizutani, T., & Tsubota, K. (1997). Blinking is controlled primarily by ocular surface conditions. *American Journal of Ophthalmology*, *124*(1), 24–30. doi:10.1016/S0002-9394(14)71639-3 PMID:9222228

Nichols, J., & Sinnott, L. T. (2006). Tear film, contact lens, and patient-related factors associated with contact lens-related dry eye. *Investigative Ophthalmology & Visual Science*, *47*(4), 1319–1328. doi:10.1167/iovs.05-1392 PMID:16565363

Nichols, K. K., Foulks, G. N., Bron, A. J., Glasgow, B. J., Dogru, M., Tsubota, K., Lemp, M. A., & Sullivan, D. A. (2011). The International Workshop on Meibomian Gland Dysfunction: Executive Summary. *Investigative Ophthalmology & Visual Science*, *52*(4), 1922–1929. doi:10.1167/iovs.10-6997a PMID:21450913

Nowak, M., Marek, B., & Kos-Kudla, B. (2005). Tear film profile in patients with active thyroid orbitopathy. *Klinika Oczna*, *107*, 479–482. PMID:16417002

Obata, S., Yamamoto, S., Horiuchi, H., & Machinami, R. (1995). Histopathologic study of human lacrimal gland. Statistical analysis with special reference to aging. *Ophthalmology*, *102*(4), 678–686. doi:10.1016/S0161-6420(95)30971-2 PMID:7724184

Ozgur, O. K., Murariu, D., Parsa, A. A., & Parsa, F. D. (2012). Dry eye syndrome due to botulinum toxin type-A injection:guideline for prevention. *Hawai'i Journal of Medicine & Public Health: a Journal of Asia Pacific Medicine & Public Health*, *71*(5), 120–123. PMID:22737648

Pisella, P. J., Pouliquen, P., & Baudouin, C. (2002). Prevalence of ocular symptoms and signs with preserved and preservative free glaucoma medication. *The British Journal of Ophthalmology*, *86*(4), 418–423. doi:10.1136/bjo.86.4.418 PMID:11914211

Rossi, G. C., Tinelli, C., Pasinetti, G. M., Milano, G., & Bianchi, P. E. (2009). Dry eye syndrome-related quality of life inglaucoma patients. *European Journal of Ophthalmology*, *19*(4), 572–579. doi:10.1177/112067210901900409 PMID:19551671

Schaumberg, D. A., Sullivan, D. A., Buring, J. E., & Dana, M. R. (2003). Prevalence of dry eye syndrome among US women. *American Journal of Ophthalmology, 136*(2), 318–326. doi:10.1016/S0002-9394(03)00218-6 PMID:12888056

Schaumberg, Dana, Buring, & Sullivan. (2009). Prevalence of dry eye disease among US men: estimates from the Physicians' Health Studies. *Arch Ophthalmol., 127*(6), 763-768.

Schein, O. D., Muñoz, B., Tielsch, J. M., Bandeen-Roche, K., & West, S. (1997). Prevalence of dry eye among the elderly. *American Journal of Ophthalmology, 124*(6), 723–728. doi:10.1016/S0002-9394(14)71688-5 PMID:9402817

Sullivan, D. A., Sullivan, B. D., Evans, J. E., Schirra, F., Yamagami, H., Liu, M., Richards, S. M., Suzuki, T., Schaumberg, D. A., Sullivan, R. M., & Dana, M. R. (2002). Androgen deficiency, Meibomian gland dysfunction, and evaporative dry eye. *Annals of the New York Academy of Sciences, 966*(1), 211–222. doi:10.1111/j.1749-6632.2002.tb04217.x PMID:12114274

Wolffsohn, J. S., Arita, R., Chalmers, R., Djalilian, A., Dogru, M., Dumbleton, K., Gupta, P. K., Karpecki, P., Lazreg, S., Pult, H., Sullivan, B. D., Tomlinson, A., Tong, L., Villani, E., Yoon, K. C., Jones, L., & Craig, J. P. (2017). TFOS DEWS II diagnostic methodology report. *The Ocular Surface, 15*(3), 539–574. doi:10.1016/j.jtos.2017.05.001 PMID:28736342

Yazdani, C., McLaughlin, T., Smeeding, J. E., & Walt, J. (2001). Prevalence of treated dry eye disease in a managed carepopulation. *Clinical Therapeutics, 23*(10), 1672–1682. doi:10.1016/S0149-2918(01)80136-3 PMID:11726003

Chapter 3
Conjunctivitis

ABSTRACT

Conjunctivitis represents an inflammation of conjunctiva with cellular infiltration, exudation, and vascular dilation. According to the course of the disease, conjunctivitis can be acute, hyperacute, and chronic. Morphologically, conjunctivitis can appear with papillary reaction, follicular reaction, cicatrizing, granulomatous and membranous changes. This chapter discusses all types of conjunctivitis, their clinical signs and symptoms, and basic approaches of treatment. This chapter includes before and after treatment photos of atypical inferiorly localized shield ulcer, Tularemia-associated Parinaud oculoglandular syndrome, and Stevens-Johnson disease. Pictures are included In the ligneous conjunctivitis patient's case taken at diagnosis as well as 10 years later, demonstrating stable condition with appropriate treatment throughout the period.

INTRODUCTION

Morphologic Responses

Papillary response is a nonspecific sign of conjunctival inflammation. Papillae are characterized by folds or projections of hypertrophic epithelium, which contain a fibrovascular core (Duke-Elder et al, 1961). Giant papillae are greater than 1mm in diameter and are usually found in the upper eyelid (Fig 1).

Follicles are yellowish-white, round elevations of conjunctiva caused by lymphocytic response. The central part of the follicle is avascular. Follicles can be seen in the upper tarsal conjunctiva, lower cul-de-sac, as well as at the limbus (Fig 2) (Arffa, 1991).

Membranes are composed mainly of fibrin attached to the epithelial conjunctival surface. True membranes cause bleeding while removing, which differentiates them from pseudomembranes (Fig 3).

Cicatrization presents as a foreshortening of conjunctival fornix and as a symblepharon formation in its early stage. Cicatrizing conjunctivitis can lead to an ankyloblepharon formation if left untreated (Fig 4).

Granulomas affect the conjunctival stroma. Conjunctival granuloma can be observed in Sarcoidosis and Parinaud Oculoglandular Syndrome. It can also occur because of a retained foreign body (Fig 5) (Chin, 1994).

DOI: 10.4018/978-1-7998-6937-5.ch003

Conjunctivitis

Table 1. Algorithm for diagnosing acute conjunctivitis

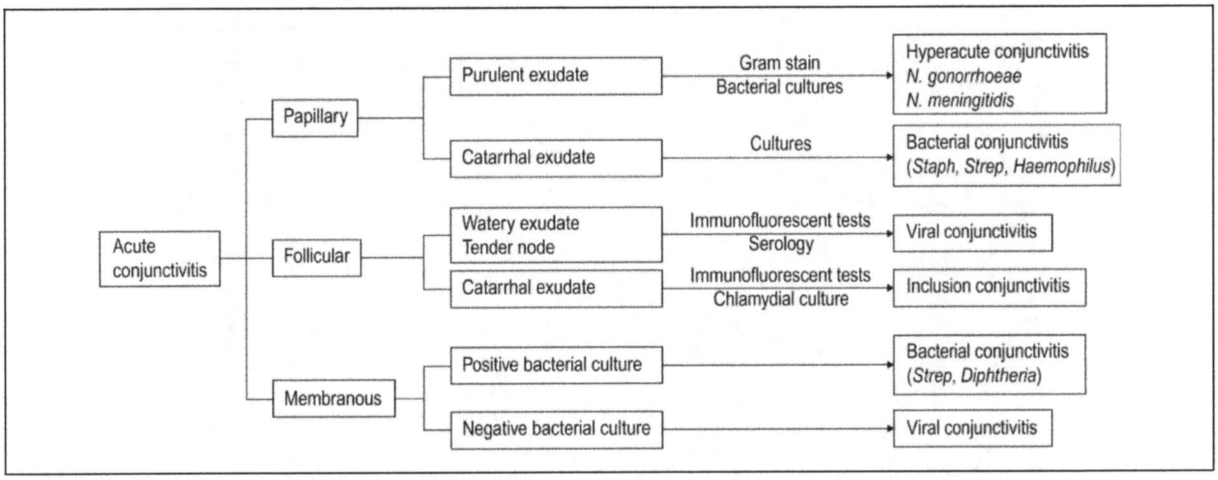

(Adapted from Buttross M, Stern GA: Acute conjunctivitis. In: Margo C, Hamed LM, Mames RN, editors: *Diagnostic problems in clinical ophthalmology.*Philadelphia: WB Saunders; 1994.)

Table 2. Algorithm for diagnosing chronic conjunctivitis

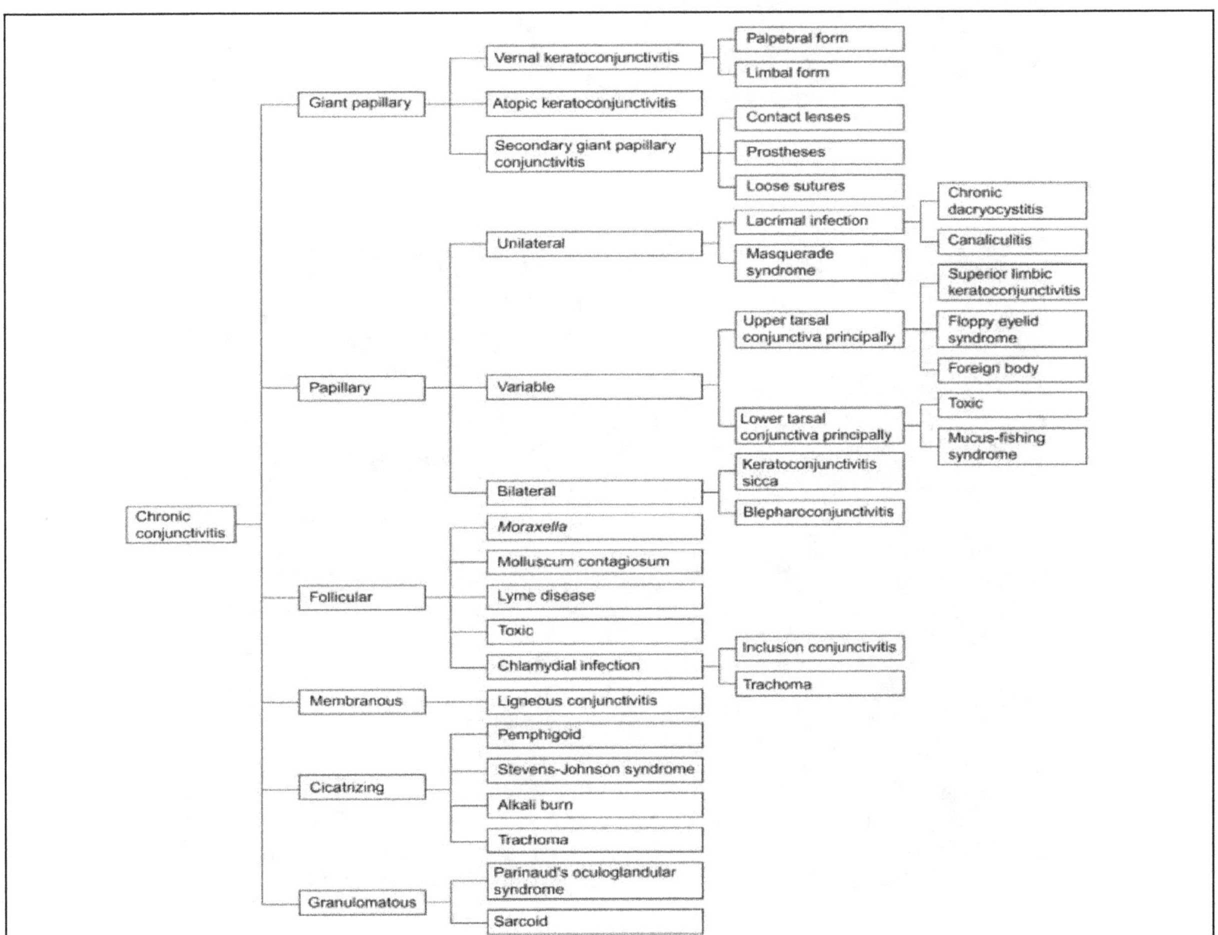

(Adapted from Buttross M, Stern GA: Acute conjunctivitis. In: Margo C, Hamed LM, Mames RN, editors: *Diagnostic problems in clinical ophthalmology.*Philadelphia: WB Saunders; 1994.)

Figure 1. Papillary reaction

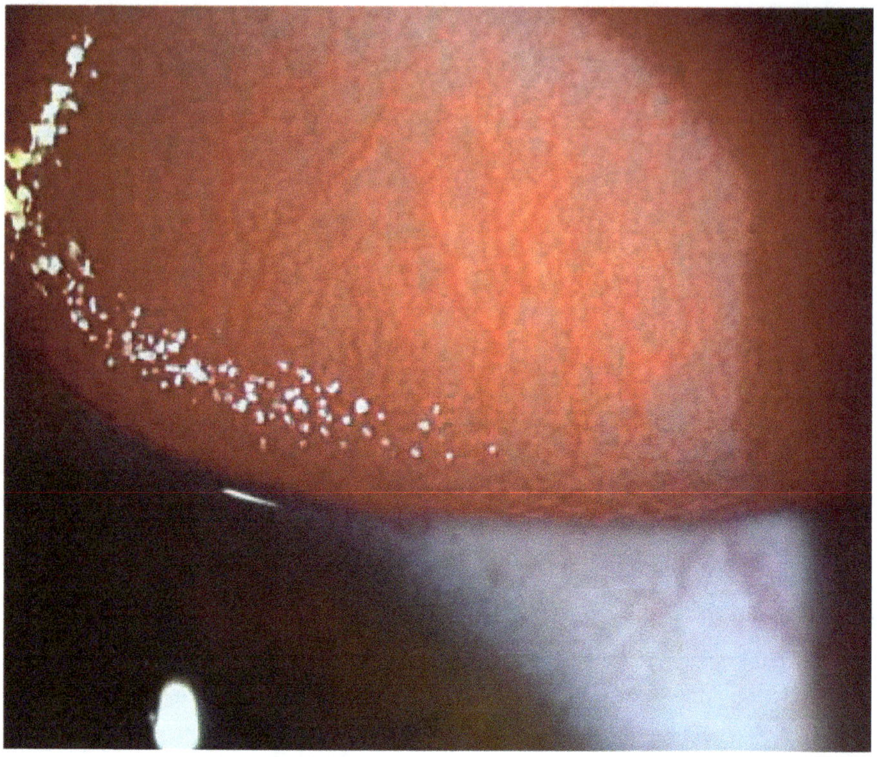

Figure 2. Follicular reaction

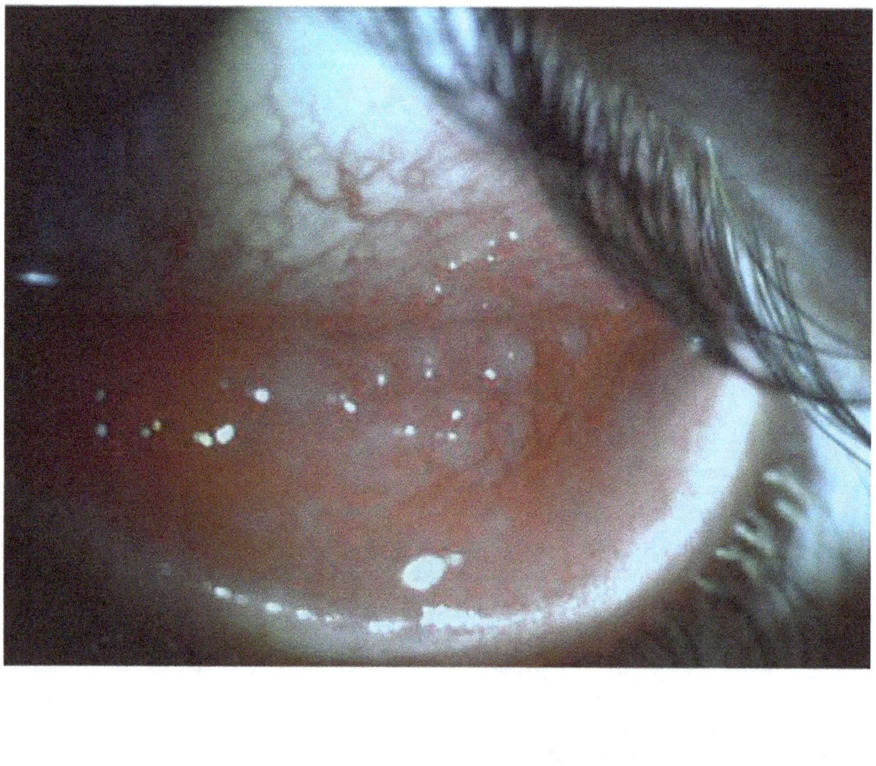

Figure 3. Membranous conjunctivitis

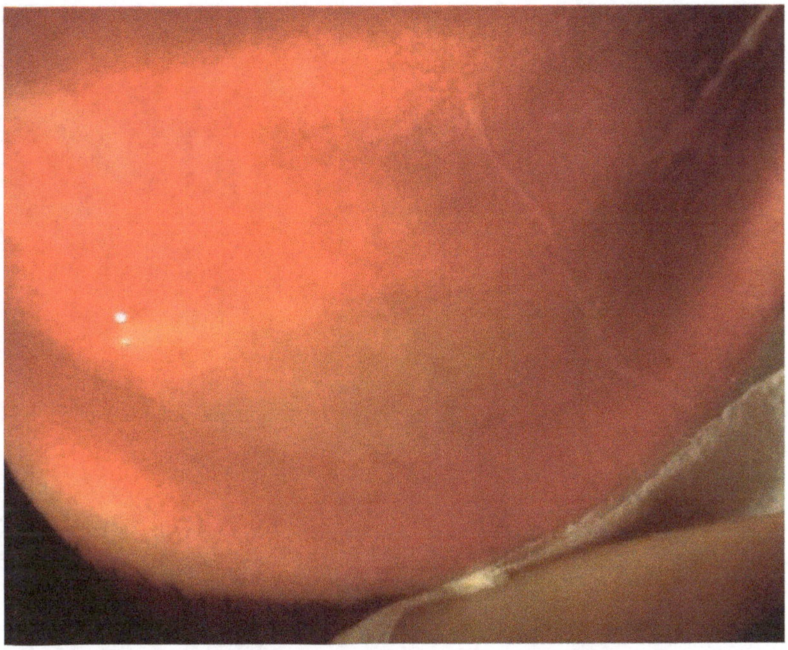

Figure 4. Symblepharon in cicatrizing conjunctivitis

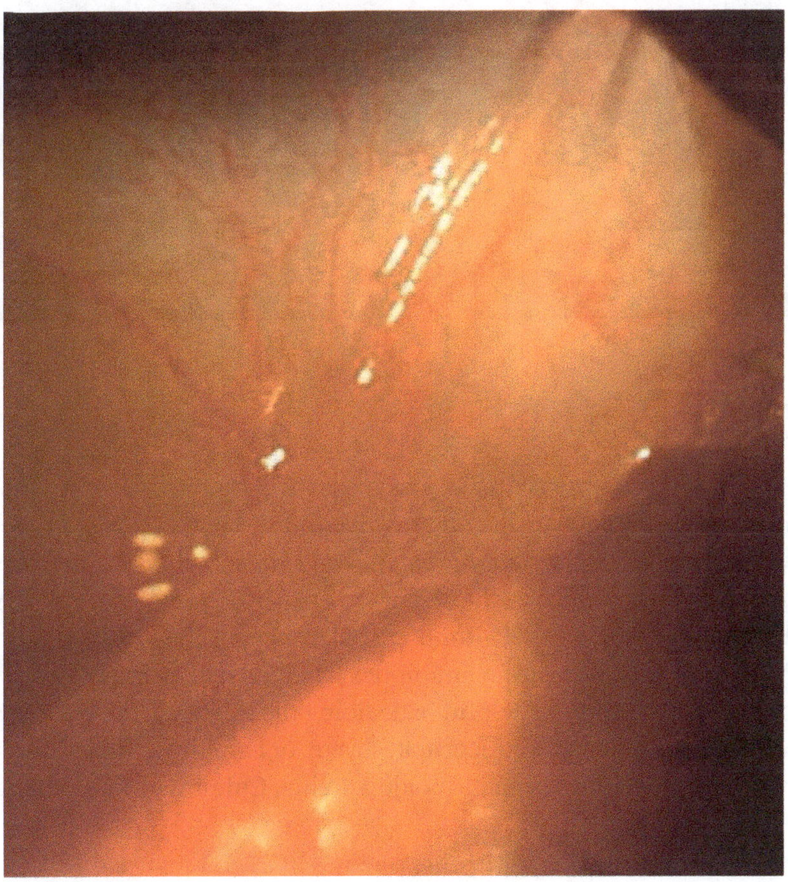

Figure 5. Granulomatous conjunctivitis

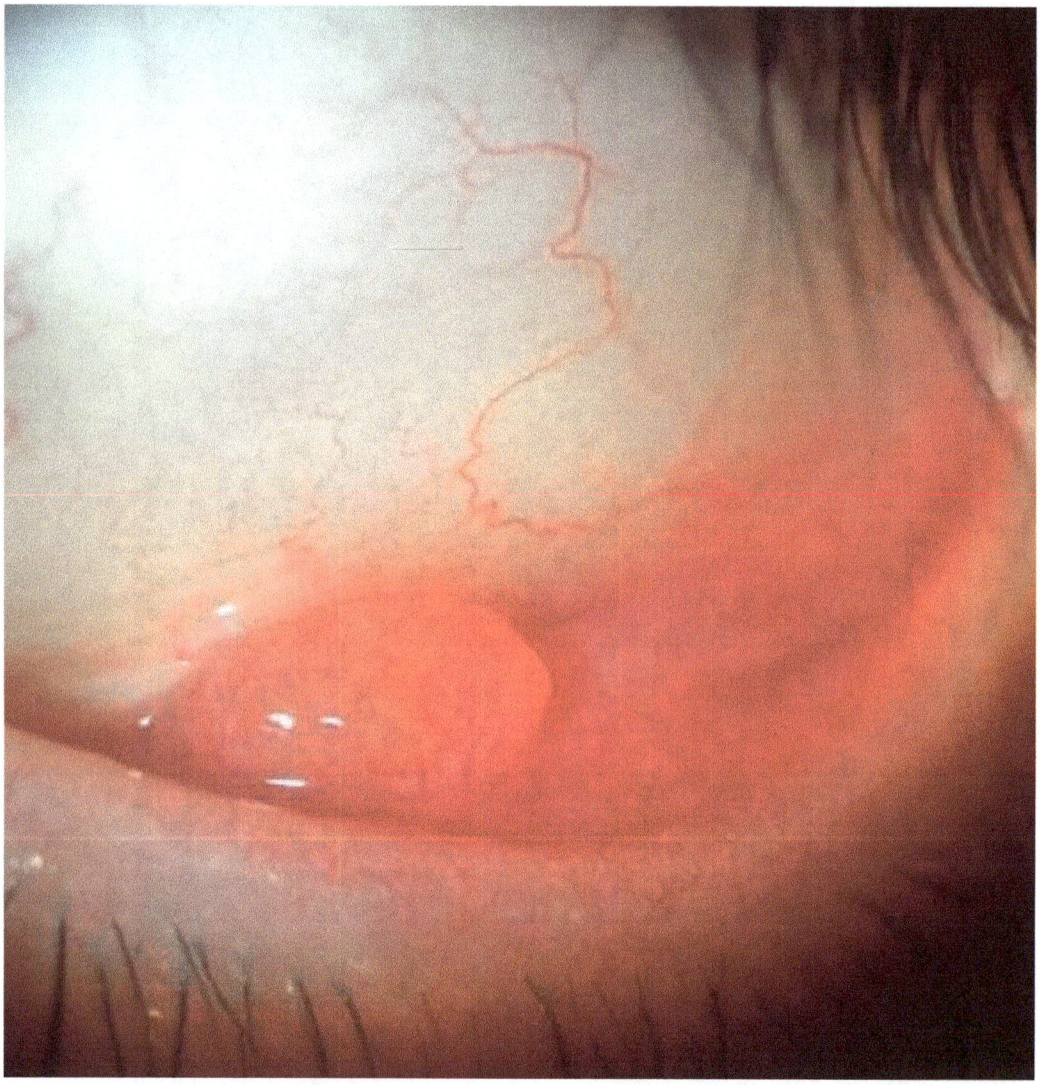

Acute Conjunctivitis

The cause of **acute papillary conjunctivitis** in most cases is bacterial conjunctivitis with catarrhal or mucopurulent exudate. One or two eyes may be involved in the process (Fig 8). Secondary punctate epitheliopathy may be developed. Staphylococcus aureus and Haemophilus influenzae are the most commonly isolated organisms (Fig 6, 7) (Locatcher-Khorazo et al, 1972; Perkins et al, 1995). Studies show that bacteria are eliminated in 7 days in self-limiting adult mucopurulent acute bacterial conjunctivitis. The use of a 7-day course of broad-spectrum antibiotics has shown to clear bacteria within 5 days. Cultures for routine conjunctivitis are rarely helpful in deciding the treatment course and are cost-effective. Bacterial cultures though, are indicated for recurrent, severe, or chronic purulent conjunctivitis (Rapoza, 1996). In cases of suspected infectious neonatal conjunctivitis, Cultures of the conjunctiva are indicated almost always.

Figure 6. Bacterial conjunctivitis. Purulent discharge, conjunctival swelling and mild injection are seen

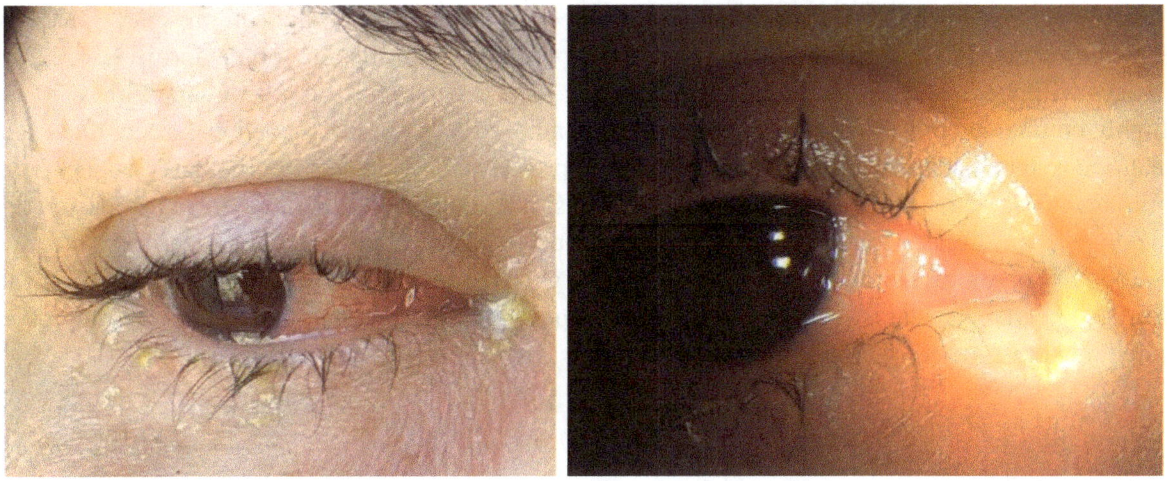

Figure 7. Bacterial conjunctivitis. Catarrhal discharge and conjunctival injection are seen

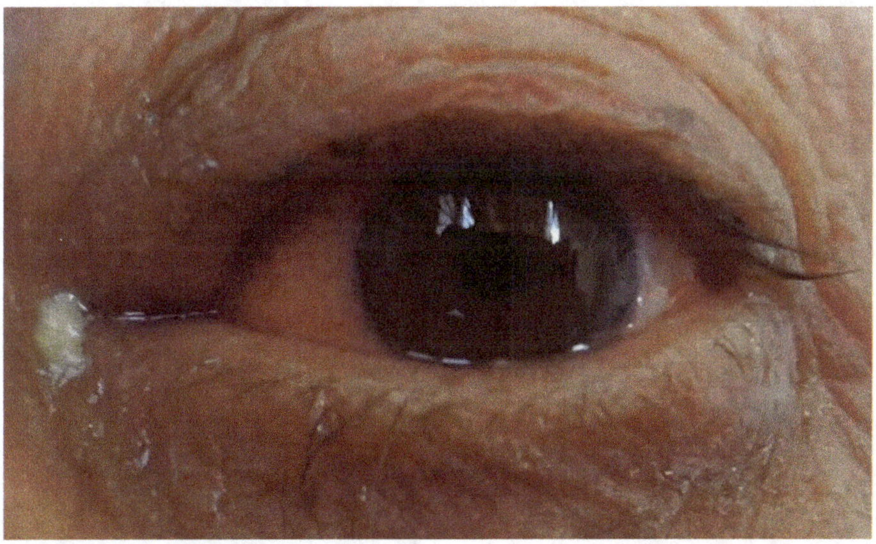

Figure 8. Severe bacterial conjunctivitis

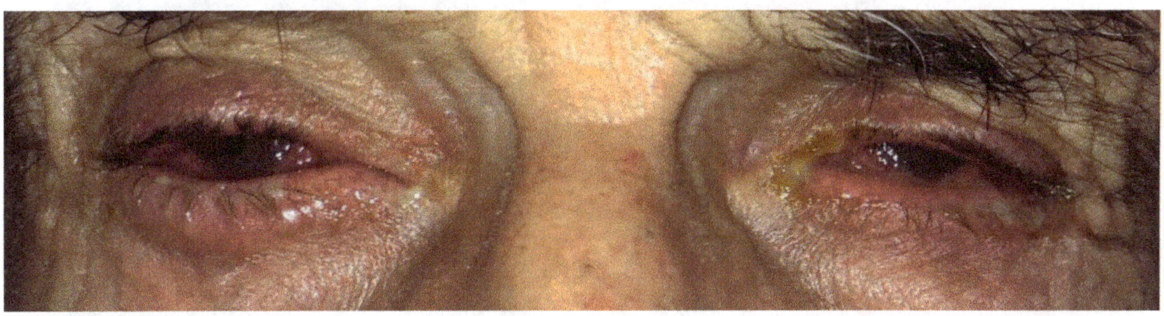

Acute follicular conjunctivitis includes viral infections and chlamydial inclusion conjunctivitis. Adenovirus is responsible for most of the acute viral conjunctivitis cases and can present as epidemic keratoconjunctivitis, pharyngeal conjunctival fever or nonspecific follicular conjunctivitis. Small hemorrhages within conjunctiva may be observed (Fig 9, 10, 11). Epidemic keratoconjunctivitis (EKC) is a highly contagious infection and generally affects one eye and then the second eye a few days later. Preauricular lymphadenopathy is usually present. Approximately 2 weeks after the onset, subepithelial infiltrates can appear, representing a delayed hypersensitivity response and can interfere with vision (Fig 12) (Centers for Disease Control, 1990). There is no proven effective treatment for adenoviral infection, however, use of topical ganciclovir 0.15% ophthalmic gel has been quite effective in treating EKC (Tabbara, 2001). Artificial tears, topical antihistamines, topical steroids, oral analgesics, or cold compresses, diluted povidone iodine 2% may be used to minimize symptoms.

Figure 9. Adenoviral conjunctivitis. Marked palpebral edema, conjunctival injection and mucopurulent discharge are seen

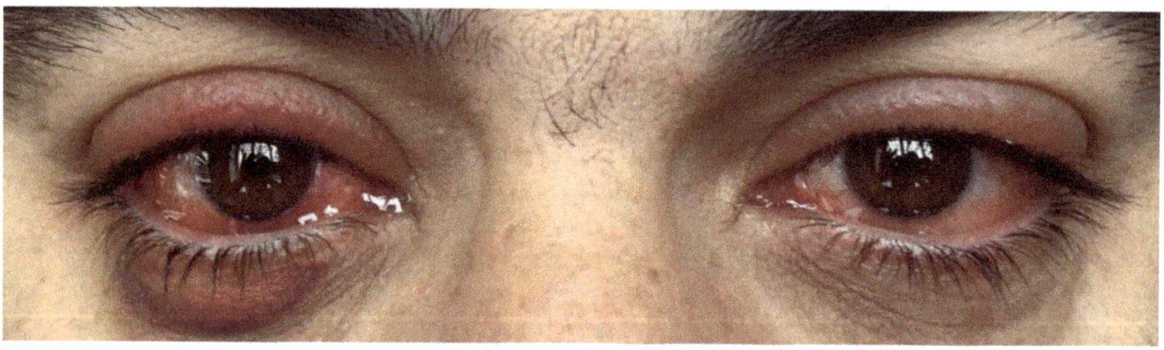

Figure 10. Adenoviral conjunctivitis. Follicles with mucous discharge are seen on the lower eyelid

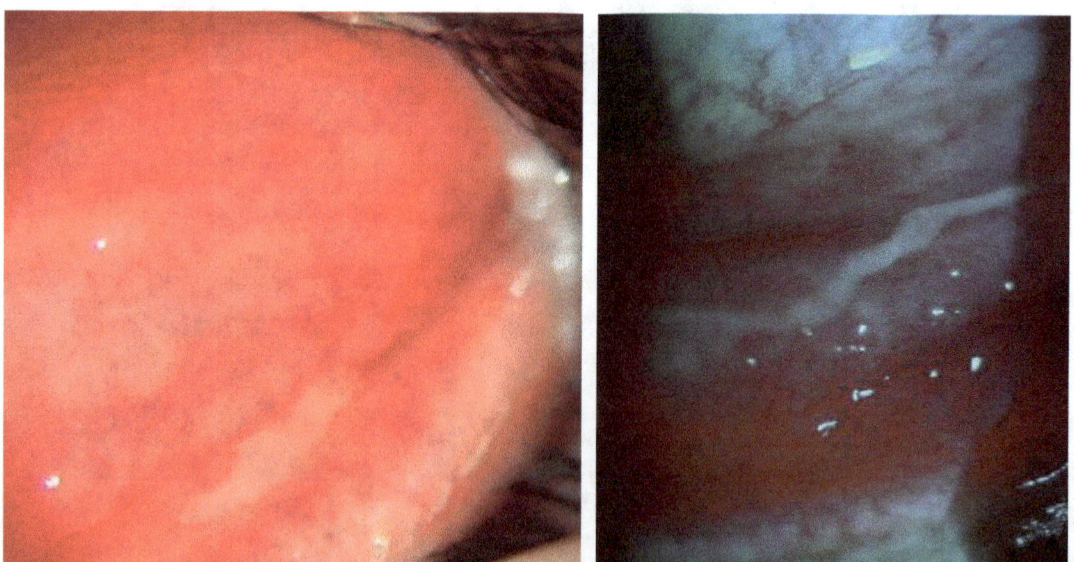

Figure 11. Adenoviral conjunctivitis. Small hemorrhages are seen on the upper eyelid

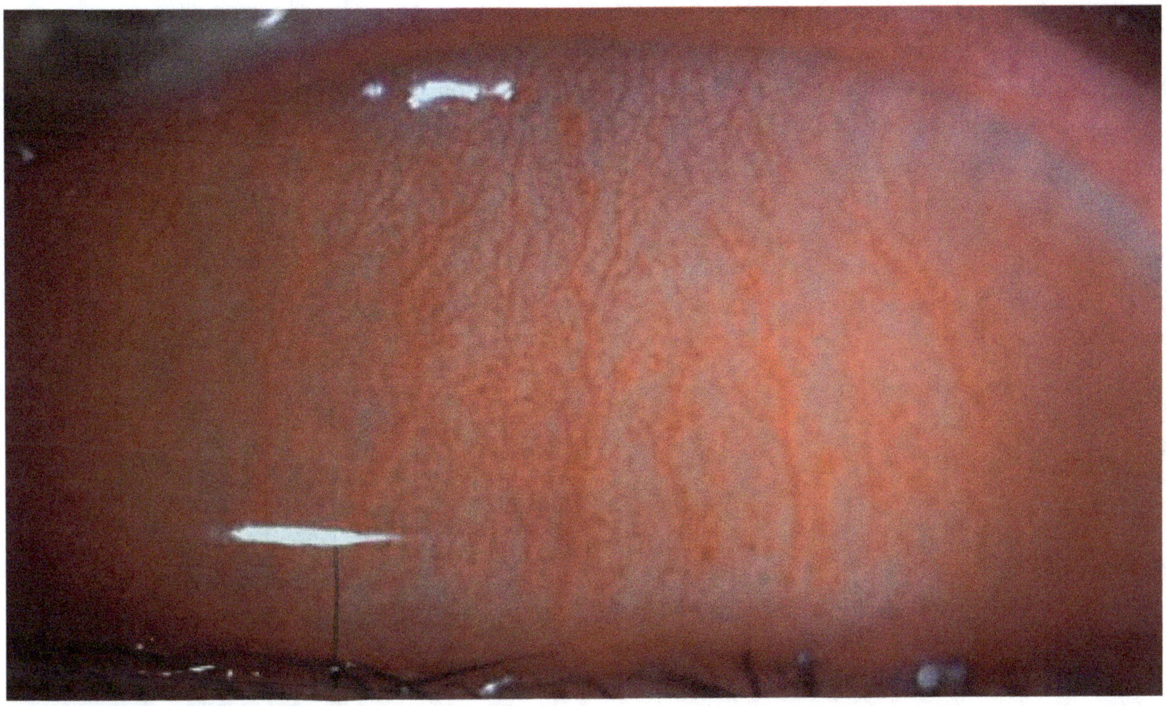

Figure 12. Adenoviral keratoconjunctivitis (EKC), corneal subepithelial infiltrates

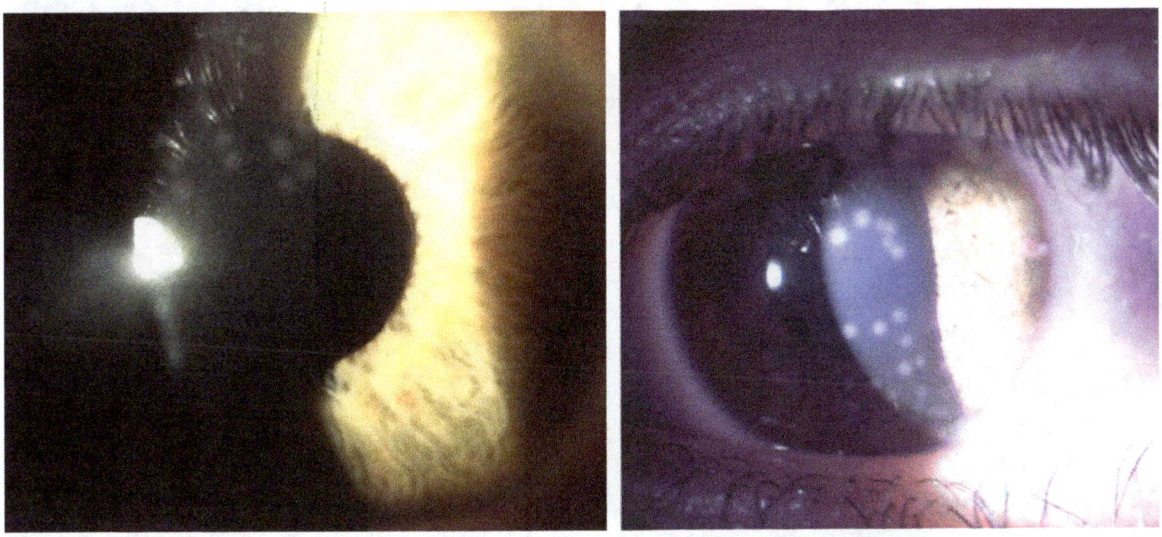

Chlamydia trachomatis is a Gram-negative obligate intracellular bacterium and is considered the cause of trachoma (A-C serotypes) and inclusion conjunctivitis (D-K serotypes). Inclusion conjunctivitis is an oculogenital disease that most commonly affects sexually active young adults (Fig 13) (Schachte, 1990). Inclusion conjunctivitis is generally a unilateral condition. Bulbar follicles are common and represent a pathognomonic sign of chlamydial infection (Fig 14). Treatment of adult inclusion conjunctivitis includes either a single oral dose of azithromycin, 1 g, or a 7-day course of twice daily oral doxycycline, 100 mg (Hammerschlag, 1989).

Figure 13. Inclusion conjunctivitis. Follicles with mucous discharge and injection are seen on the upper tarsal conjunctiva

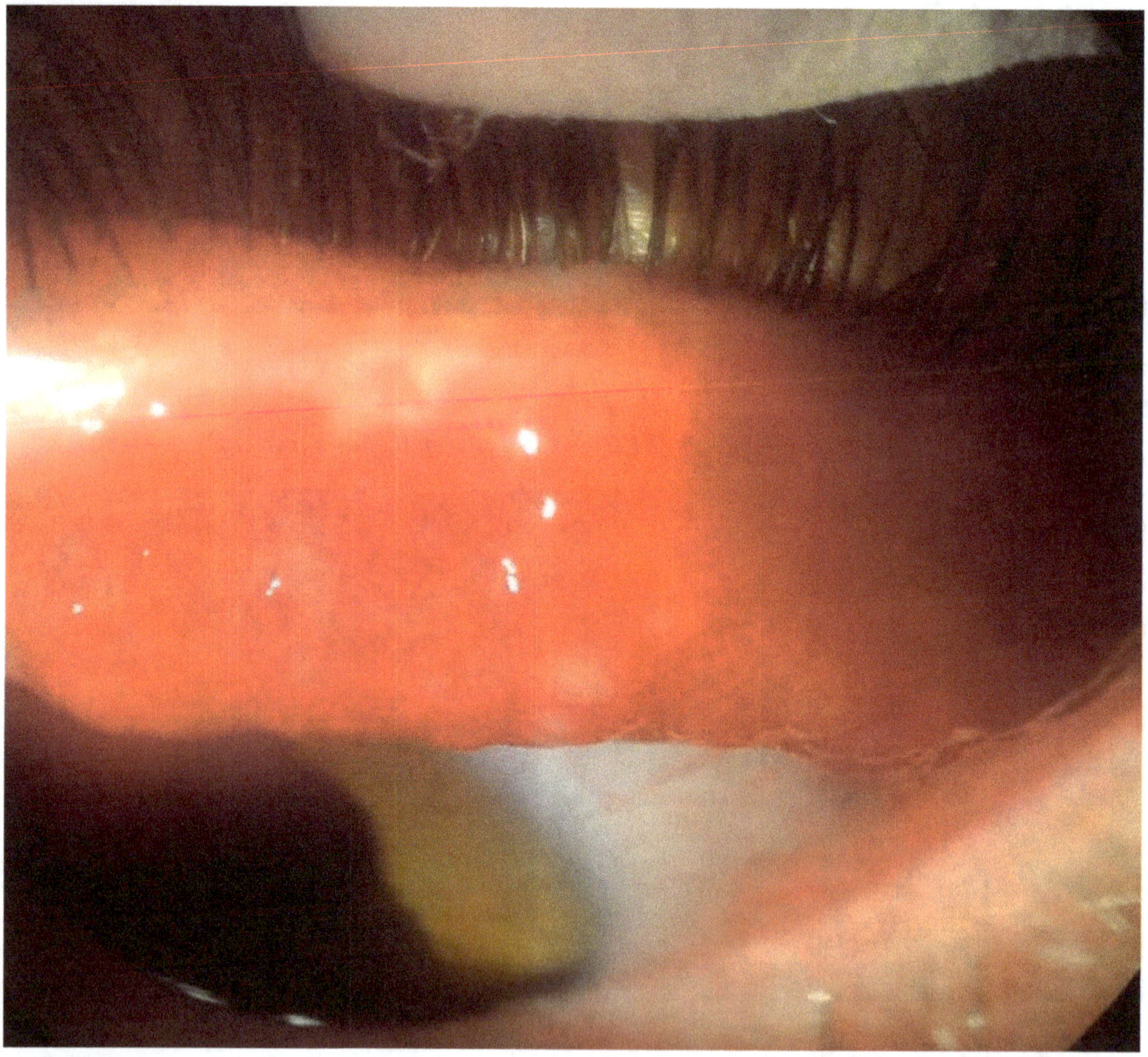

Figure 14. Inclusion conjunctivitis. Bulbar follicles are seen

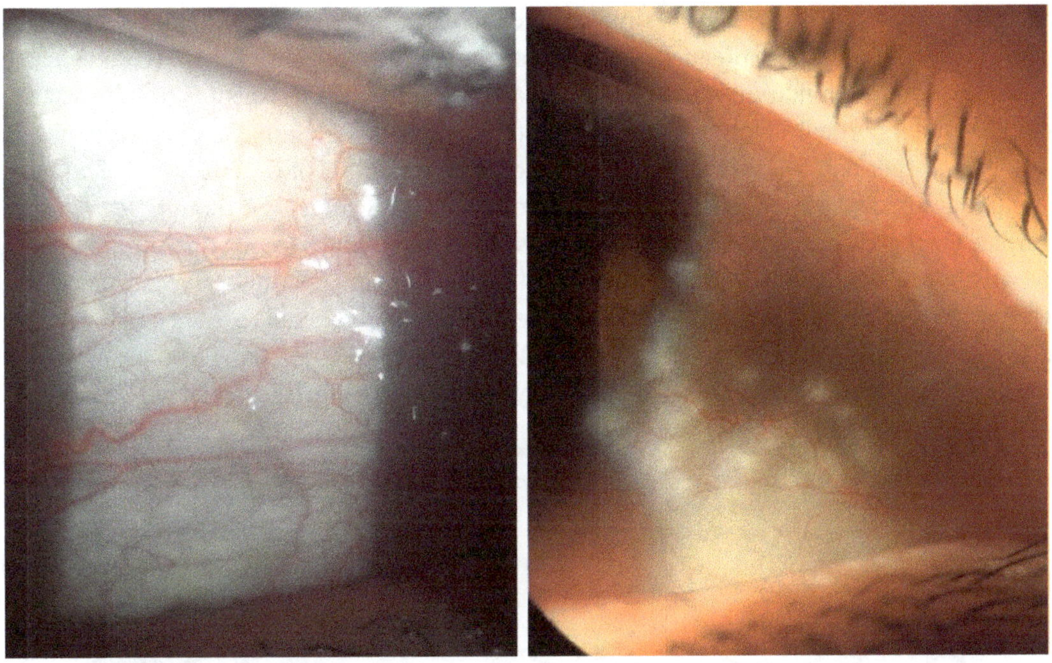

Figure 15. Herpes simplex blepharoconjunctivitis associated with herpes nasalis. Multiple herpetic vesicles on upper and lower eyelids

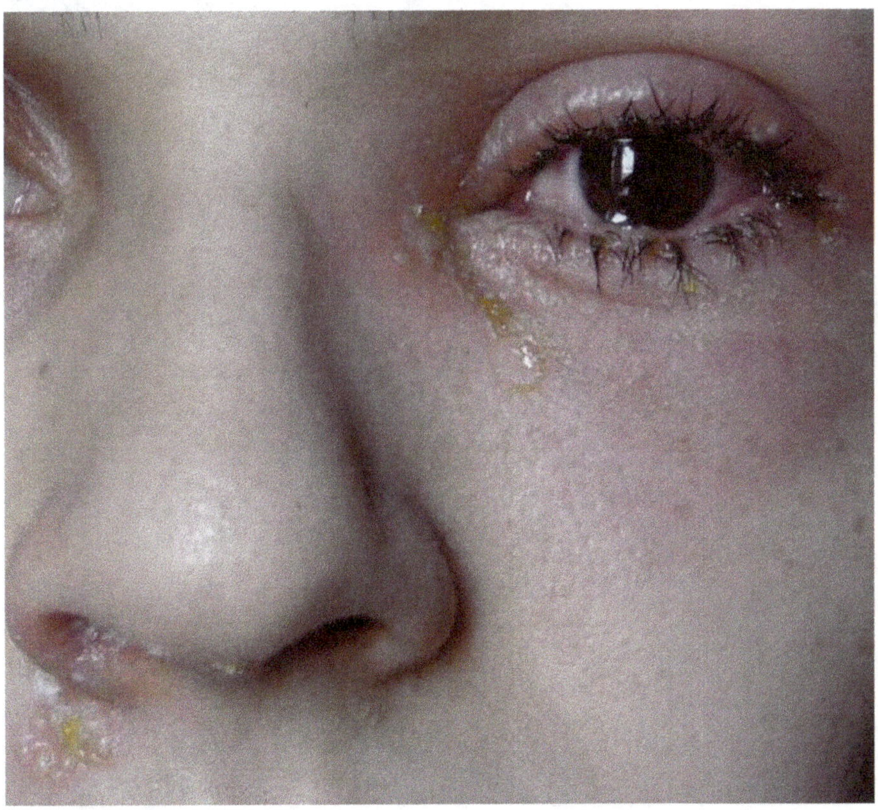

Primary herpes simplex, varicella zoster (VZV) and Epstein-Barr viruses (EBV) can cause acute follicular conjunctivitis. Primary herpes simplex infection is usually associated with lesions on the lid. Clinically, watery discharge with preauricular lymphadenopathy is seen (Fig 15, 16) (Glasser et al, 1986). Herpes simplex virus conjunctivitis is a self-limited acute condition. Treatment is usually advised when there is concomitant corneal involvement. Possible topical options include ganciclovir 0.15% gel used three to five times per day or trifluridine 1% solution five to eight times per day. Topical trifluridine causes epithelial toxicity if used for more than 2 weeks. Topical ganciclovir though, is less toxic to the ocular surface (Duke-Elder, 1961). Topical antivirals alone have shown to be unhelpful in treating VZV conjunctivitis but may be used as additive treatment in unresponsive patients (Wilhelmus et al, 2015). With persistent or recalcitrant acute/subacute disease in immunocompetent patients, oral antivirals may be of help at a dose of 800 mg five times daily for 7 days for acyclovir, 1000 mg every 8 hours for 7 days for valacyclovir, or 500 mg three times daily for 7 days for famciclovir (Li et al, 2018; Szeto et al, 2017).

Figure 16. Zoster skin rash associated with blepharoconjunctivitis

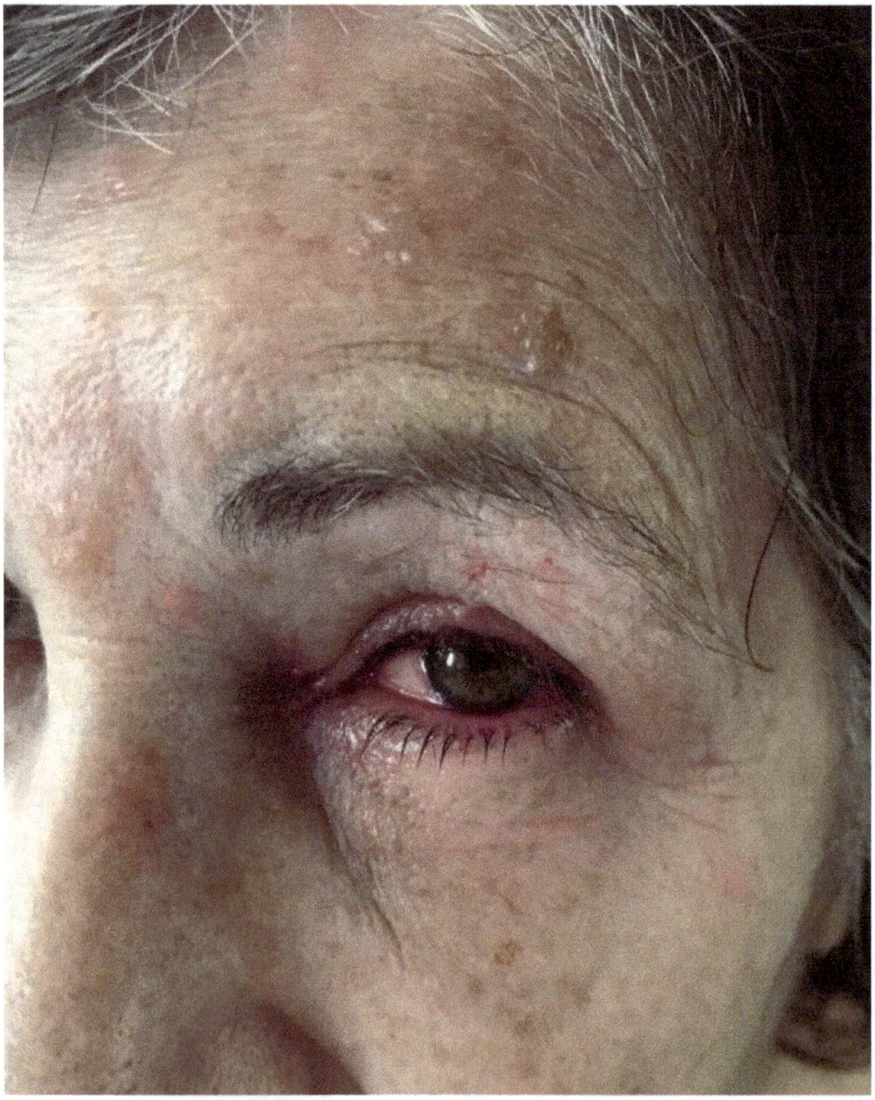

Acute membranous and pseudomembranous conjunctivitis may be caused by viral and bacterial infections. Adenoviral conjunctivitis, particularly EKC, is the most common cause of membranous/pseudomembranous conjunctivitis (Fig 17, 20, 21, 22) (Vastine et al, 1987). Debridement of the membrane can be considered to prevent corneal epithelial abrasions or permanent cicatricial changes (e.g., foreshortening of the conjunctival fornix) for patients with adenoviral membranous conjunctivitis (Boralkar, 1989). Staph aureus and β-hemolytic streptococci are the most common causes of bacterial membranous conjunctivitis. C. diphtheriae was previously considered to be the most common bacterial cause of membranous conjunctivitis; however, it is very rare nowadays (Fig 18, 19). Diphtheritic conjunctivitis is usually associated with systemic disease, thus, systemic antibiotic therapy with erythromycin and antitoxin therapy is required. Pseudomembranous/membranous conjunctivitis can be observed in ocular GVHD as well.

Figure 17. Adenovirus-associated pseudomembrane

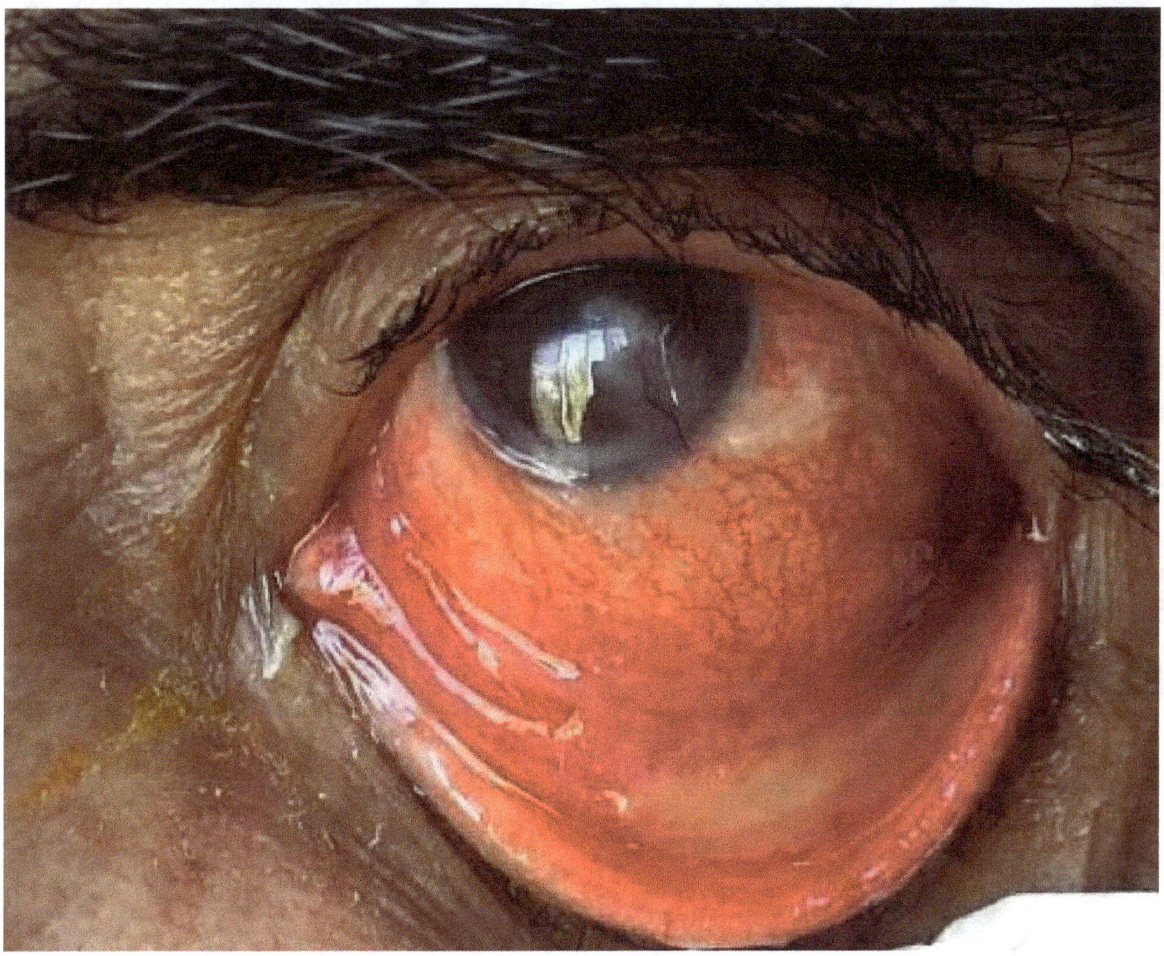

Figure 18. Membranous conjunctivitis caused by C. diphtheriae. Conjunctival membrane is seen (Photo is blurred because it was taken 22 years ago, and this was the only case during the 25 years of our practice)

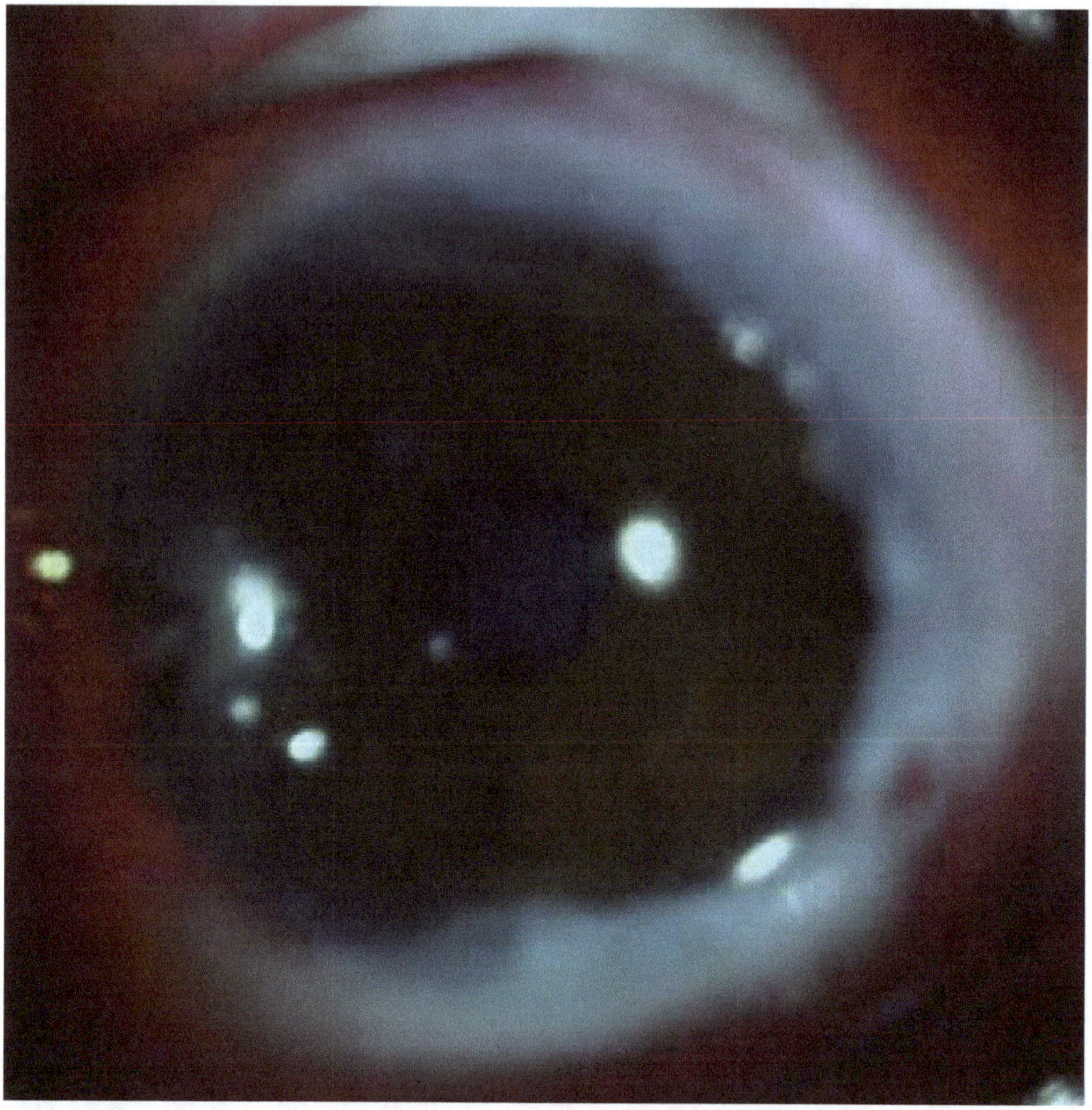

Figure 19. Pseudomembrane caused by Corynebacterium striatum

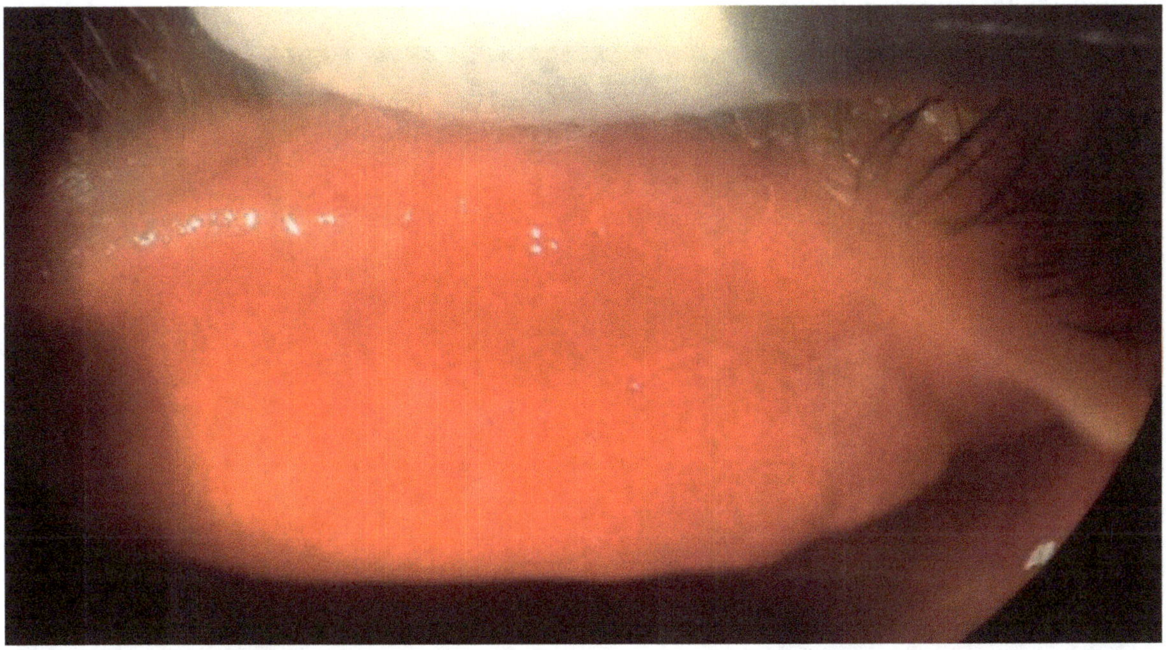

Figure 20. Dense Adenoviral pseudomembrane

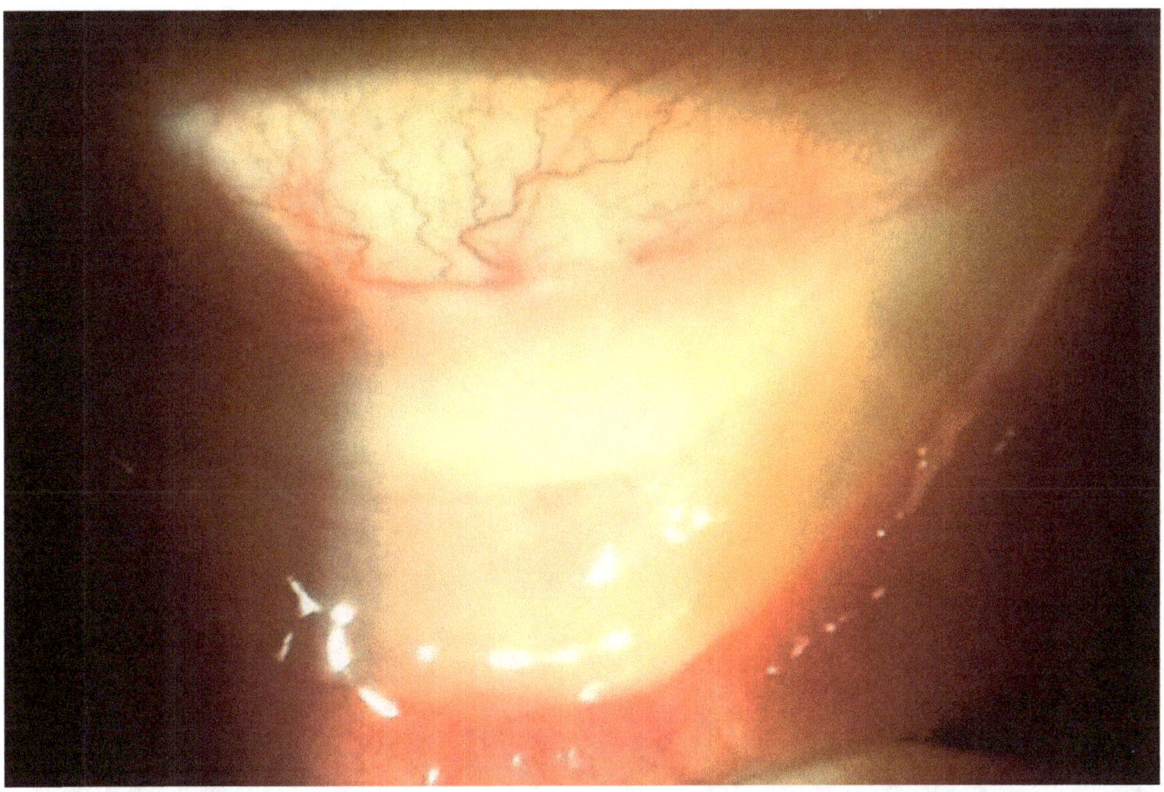

Figure 21. The same patient. Adenoviral pseudomembrane removal under a slit lamp. The white peeled membrane on forceps is visible

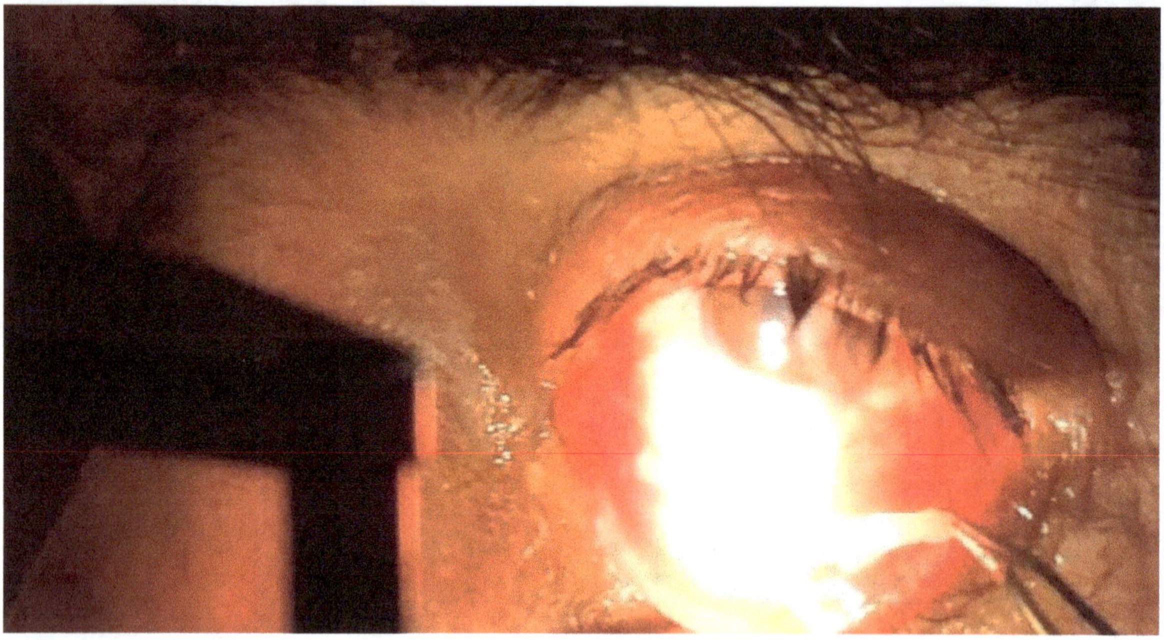

Figure 22. The same patient 1 week after pseudomembrane removal. Treatment included topical ganciclovir, mild steroids and artificial tears

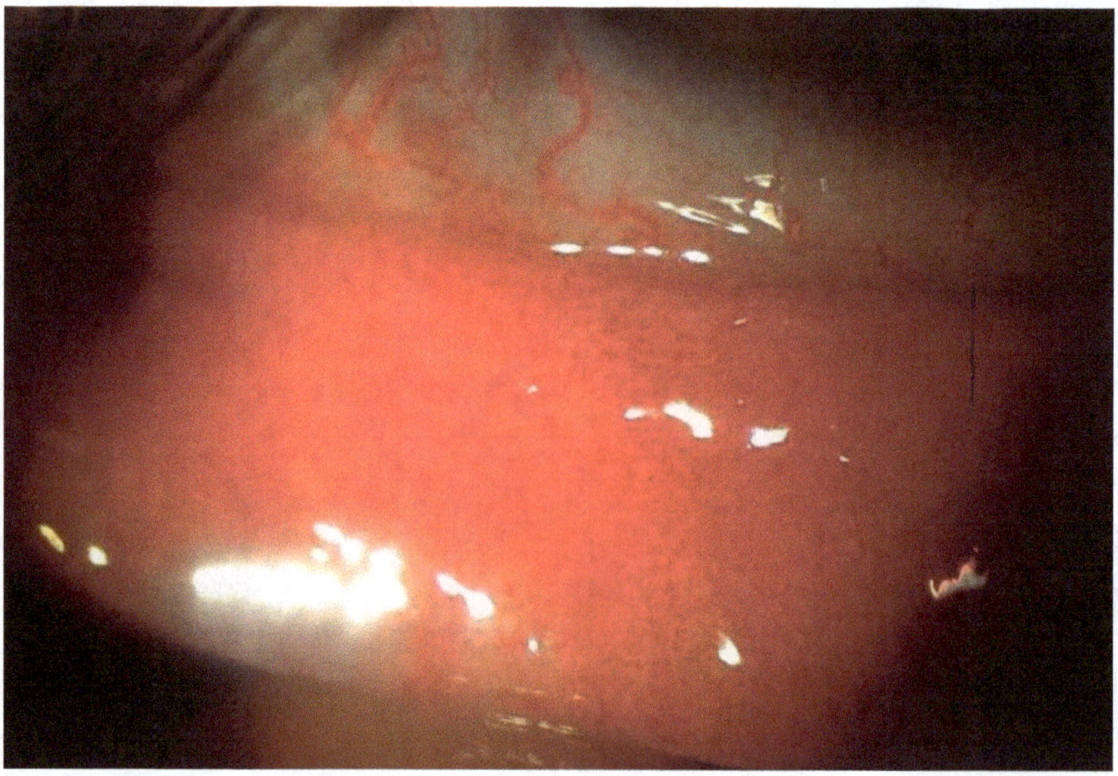

Chronic Conjunctivitis

Giant papillary conjunctivitis, according to definition, is a conjunctivitis when papillae are greater than 1mm in diameter. Vernal and atopic keratoconjunctivitis are two primary forms of giant papillary conjunctivitis (GPC). Secondary forms of GPC are related to chronic contact lens use (Fig 30), ocular prosthesis, or exposed sutures.

Vernal keratoconjunctivitis (VKC) is a bilateral, allergic, seasonal, recurrent disease that affects mainly children and young adults. Clinically, VKC has 2 forms; palpebral and limbal. The characterized feature of palpebral VKC is giant papillae on the upper tarsal conjunctiva (Fig 23). In limbal VKC, both tarsal conjunctivae reveal diffuse papillary reaction (Abelson, 1987). The thickened, gelatinous opacification of the upper limbus is seen in limbal VKC with whitish excrescences (Trantas dots) within thickened limbus (Fig 24, 25, 26). Corneal involvement may represent sterile shield-shaped epithelial defect (vernal ulcer) localized superiorly, although extremely rare presentation of inferiorly localized ulcers have been reported as well (Fig 27, 28, 29) (Hovakimyan et al, 2020). Topical corticosteroids are usually necessary to control severe symptoms and signs for acute exacerbations of vernal/atopic conjunctivitis (Naderan et al, 2017). Topical cyclosporine 2% has demonstrated an alleviation in signs and symptoms compared with placebo after two weeks of use in patients with VKC (Kiliç, 2006). Commercially available 0.05% topical cyclosporine has also been shown to be effective in more frequent dosing for the treatment of severe vernal/atopic conjunctivitis. It has been shown to be effective in preventing seasonal recurrences too[2] Use of cyclosporine may allow for reduced use of topical steroids. Randomized clinical trials have demonstrated the efficacy of 0.1% topical tacrolimus in patients who had failed conjunctivitis therapy with topical corticosteroids, cyclosporine, and/or antiallergy medications (Pucci, 2015).

Figure 23. Palpebral form of VKC. Giant papillae are seen on upper tarsal conjunctiva

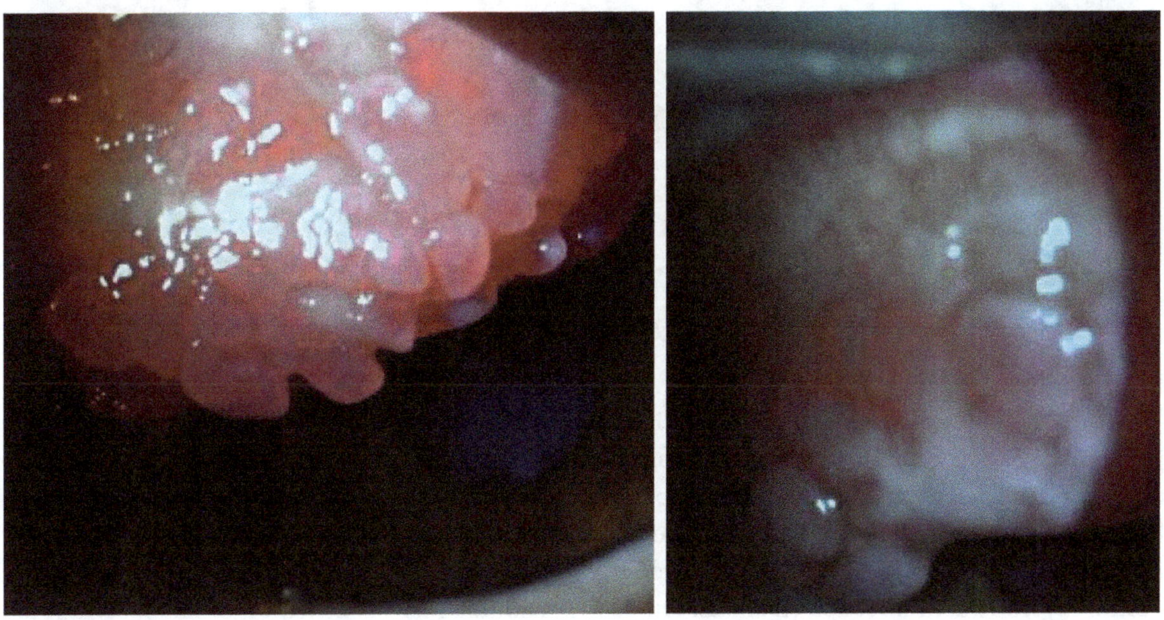

Figure 24. limbal form of VKC without magnification (left photo) and under slit lamp (right photo)

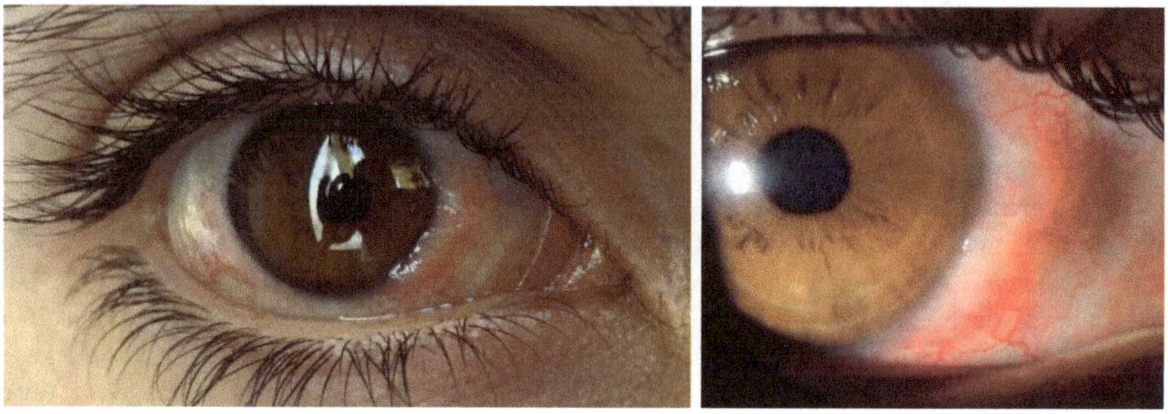

Figure 25. VKC, limbal form

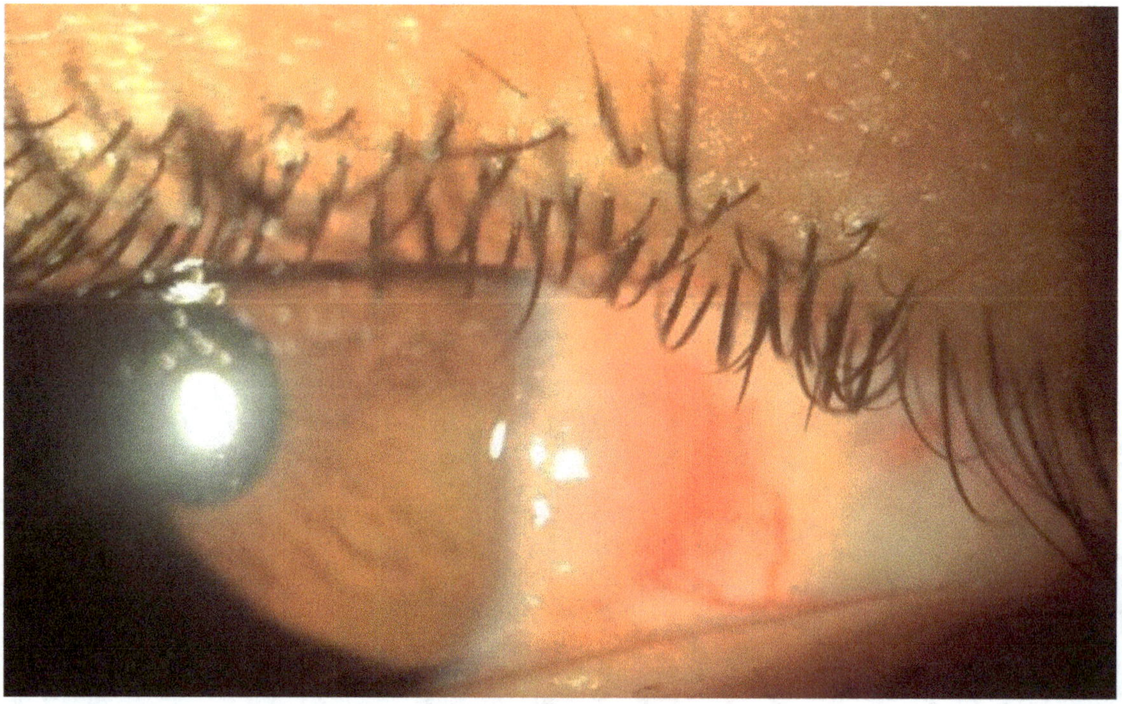

Lacrimal drainage system infection, particularly chronic dacryocystitis (Fig 31) and chronic canaliculitis (Fig 32) may be associated with **chronic papillary conjunctivitis**. Slit lamp exam may reveal diffuse, unilateral papillary conjunctivitis, and mucopurulent discharge (Jones, 1966). The lower canaliculus is affected more frequently. The main difference between chronic dacryocystitis and chronic canaliculitis is epiphora, which is present in chronic dacryocystitis. The most common cause of chronic canaliculitis is Actinomyces israelii infection (Duke-Elder, 1974). The treatment is based on broad-spectrum topical antibiotics. Doxycycline 100mg one or two times daily can be effective. Chronic dacryocystitis is treated surgically.

Figure 26. Limbal form of VKC. Trantas dots are seen on superior thickened limbus

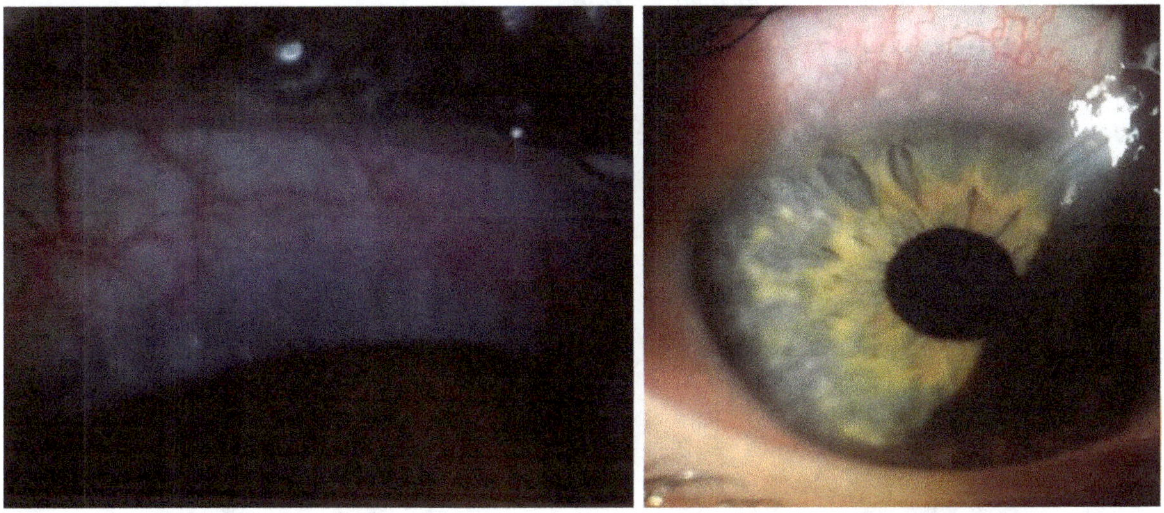

Figure 27. Shield ulcer caused by VKC. Oval epithelial defect with edematous edges

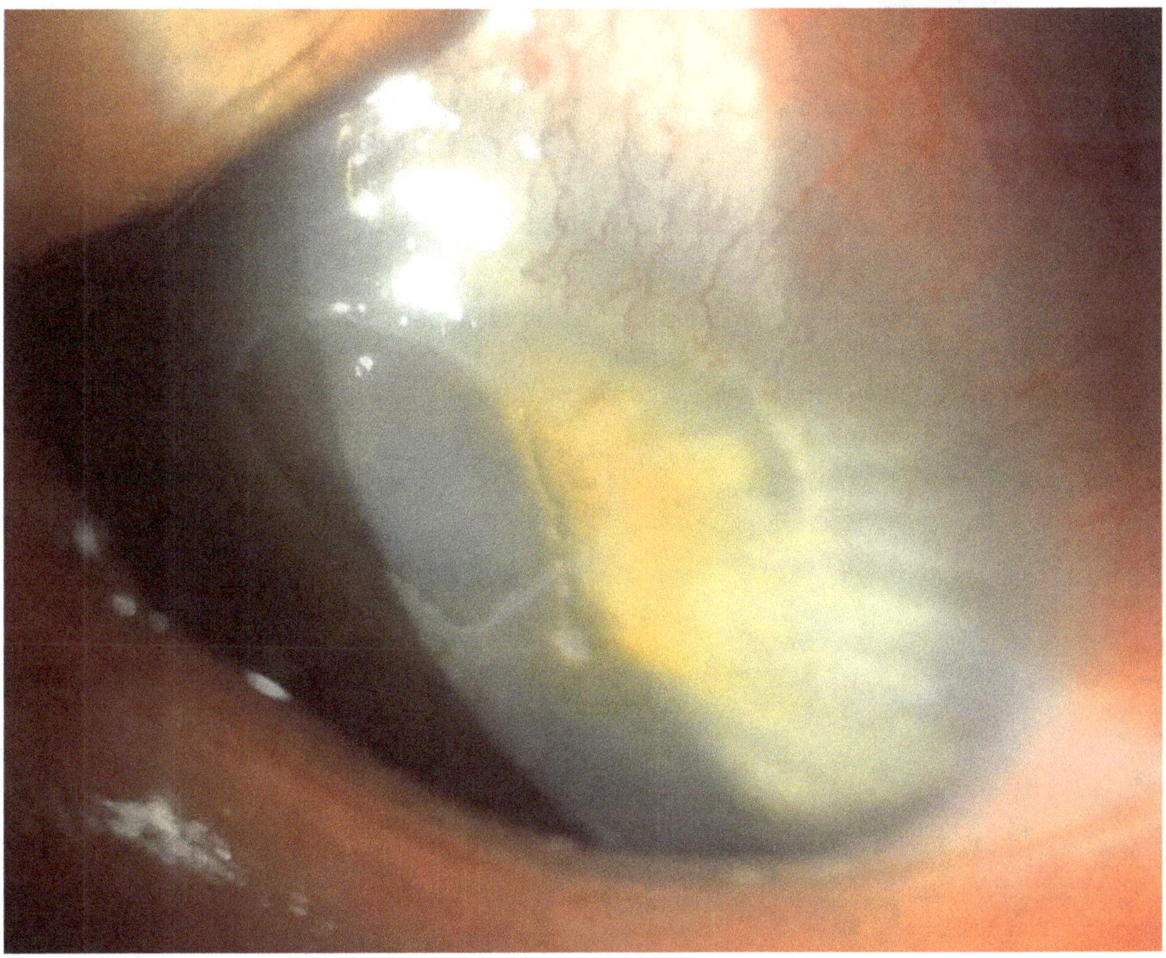

Figure 28. The fellow right eye of the same patient with two (typically and atypically localized) shield ulcers. Second atypical shield-ulcer located inferiorly

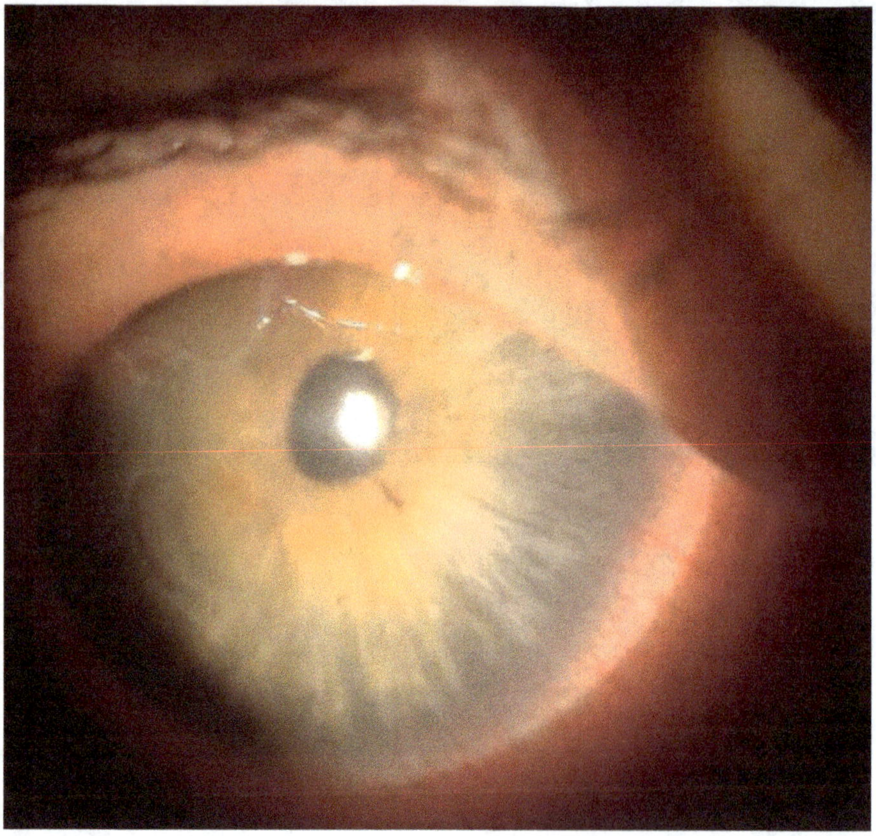

Figure 29. The same patient after treatment with topical mild steroids, bandage contact lens, antiallergic drops, and Doxycycline orally. Inferior ulcer totally healed, superior ulcer full epithelized with fibrotic changes. Note the giant papillae on superior tarsal conjunctiva

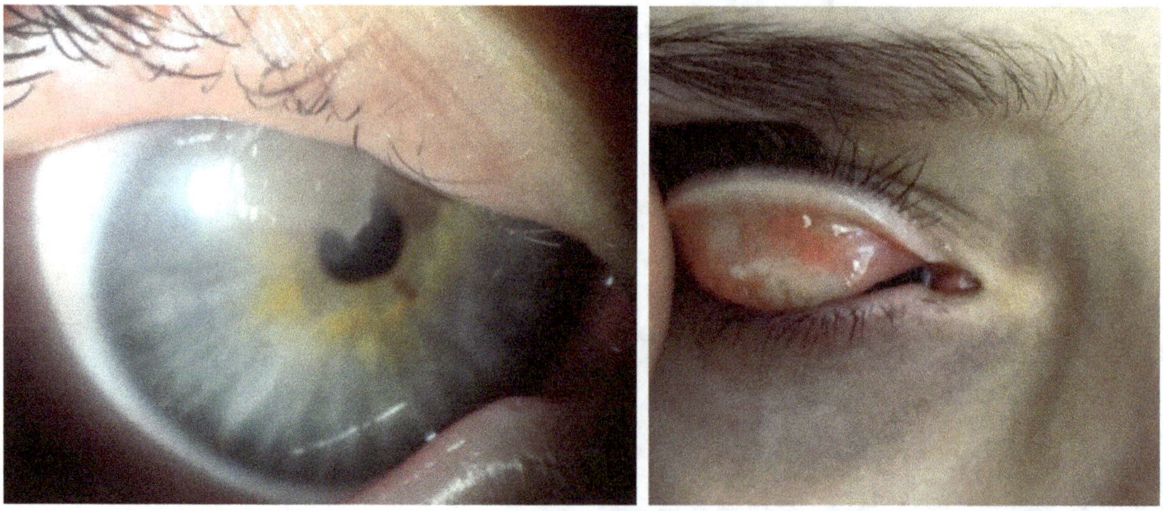

Figure 30. Secondary giant papillary conj-is associated with chronic contact lens wear

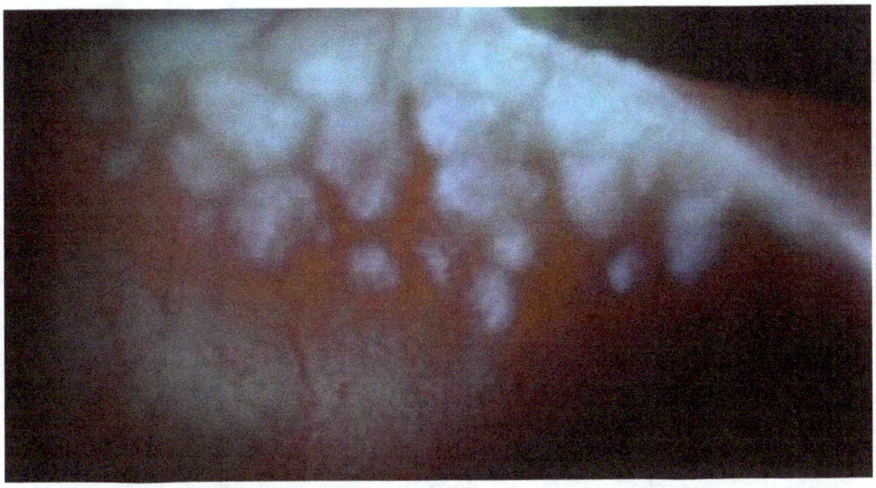

Figure 31. Chronic canaliculitis. Mucopurulent discharge from inferior punctum

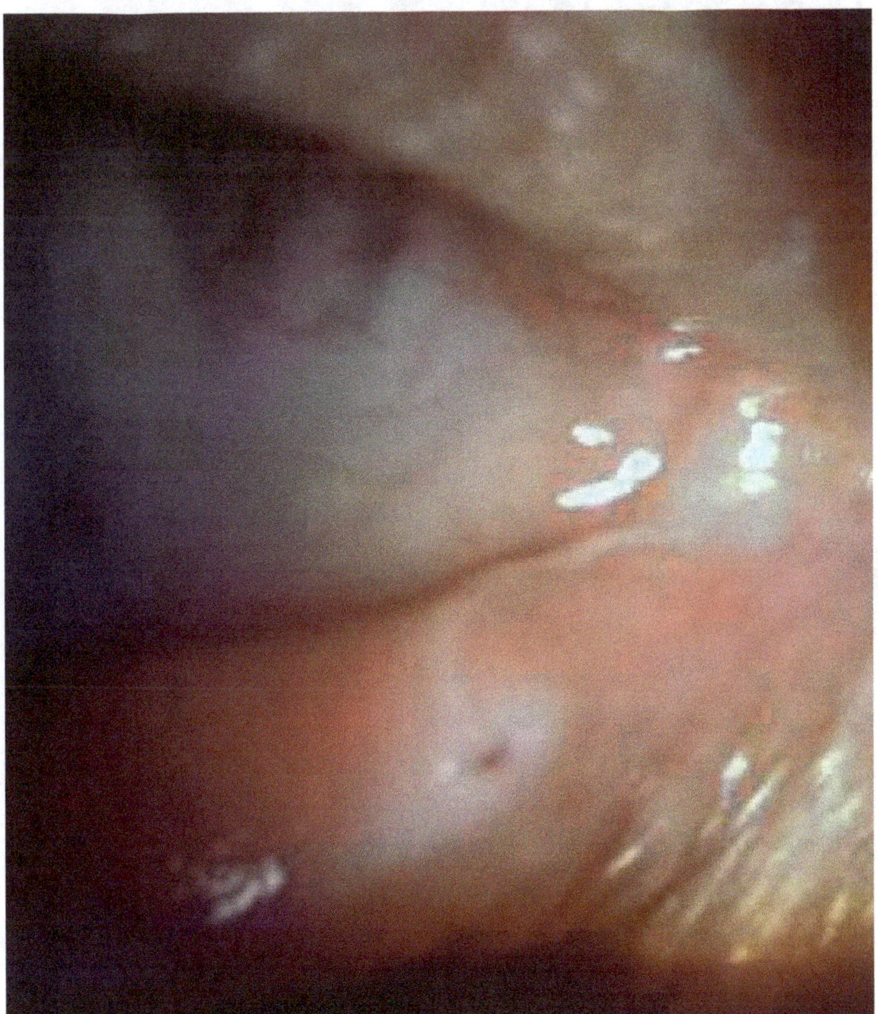

Figure 32. Chronic dacryocystitis. Mucopurulent discharge is seen with hyperemic and edematous dacryocyst-overlying skin

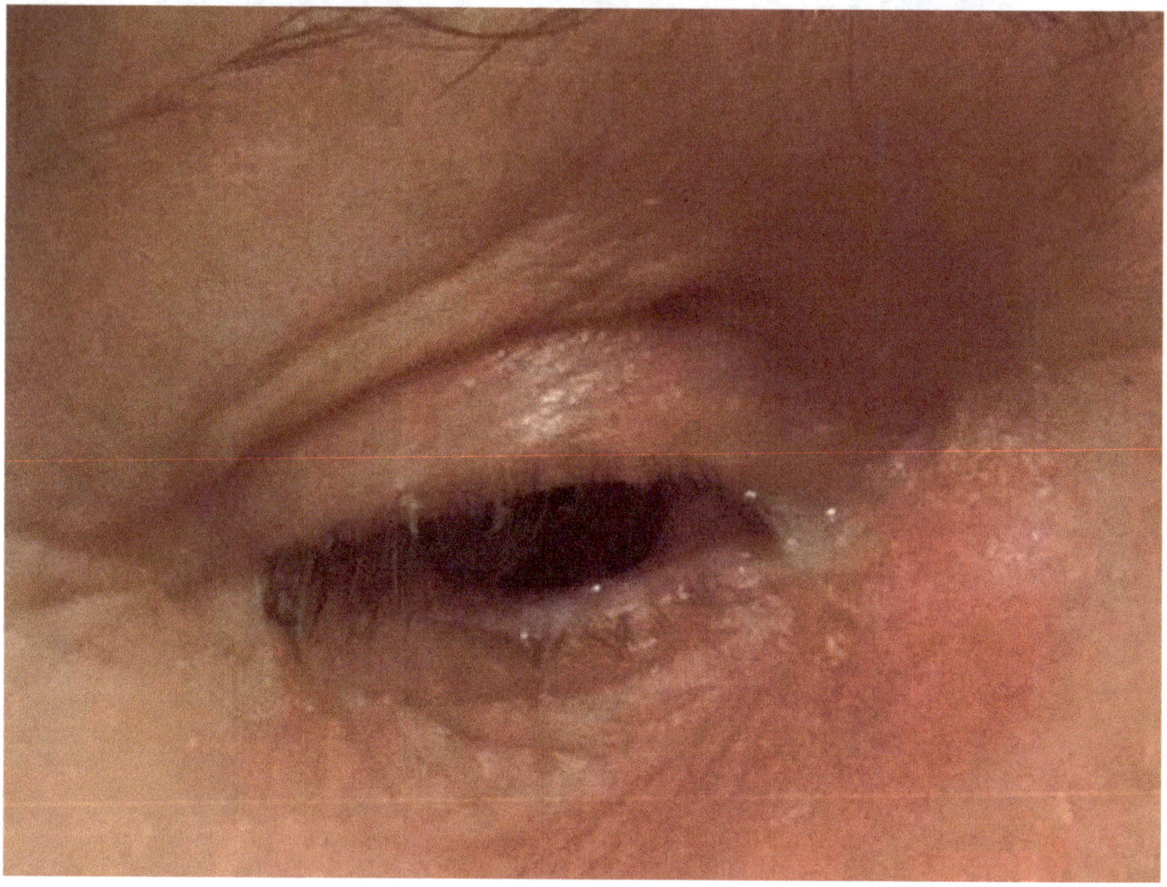

Figure 33. Superior limbic keratoconjunctivitis, hyperemic upper bulbar conjunctiva

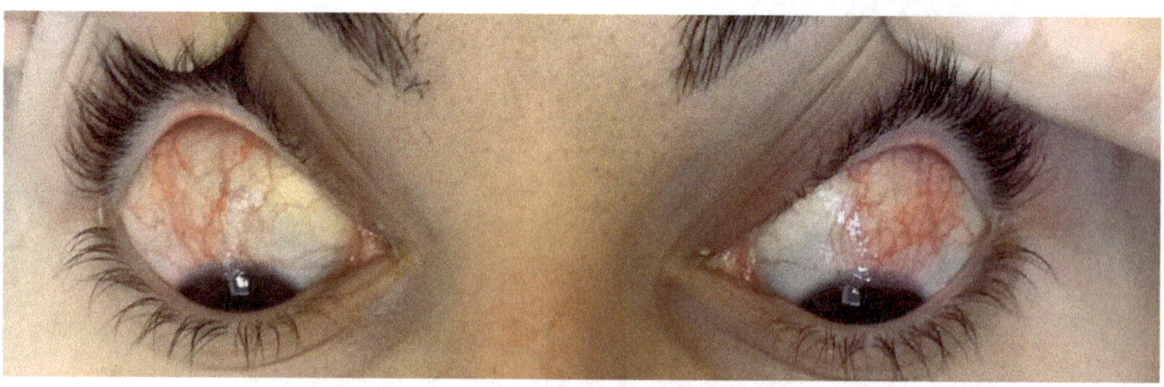

Superior limbic keratoconjunctivitis is a noninfectious disease, typically presenting with a thickened upper eyelid, a velvet papillary hypertrophy of upper tarsal conjunctiva (Fig 34), and a hyperemic upper bulbar conjunctiva, which is redundant and moveable (Fig 33). Keratinization of the superior limbal and bulbar conjunctiva is present and can be stained with rose Bengal (Fig 35). Often, filamentary keratopathy and punctate epithelial keratopathy are observed. Superior limbic keratoconjunctivitis can be associated with thyroid diseases (Bainbridge, 1998; Culbertson et al, 1994). Mild cases of SLK may respond to treatment of concomitant dry eye syndrome with lubricants, mast-cell stabilizers, cyclosporin (Perry, 2003). Associated filamentary keratitis may occasionally respond to topical 10% acetylcysteine (Albietz, 2003)or hypertonic (5%) saline Persistent symptoms may necessitate surgical intervention such as cautery (chemical or thermal) to tighten redundant conjunctiva or conjunctival resection·

Figure 34. The upper tarsal papillary conjunctivitis (velvet hypertrophy) and rose Bengal stained bulbar conjunctiva

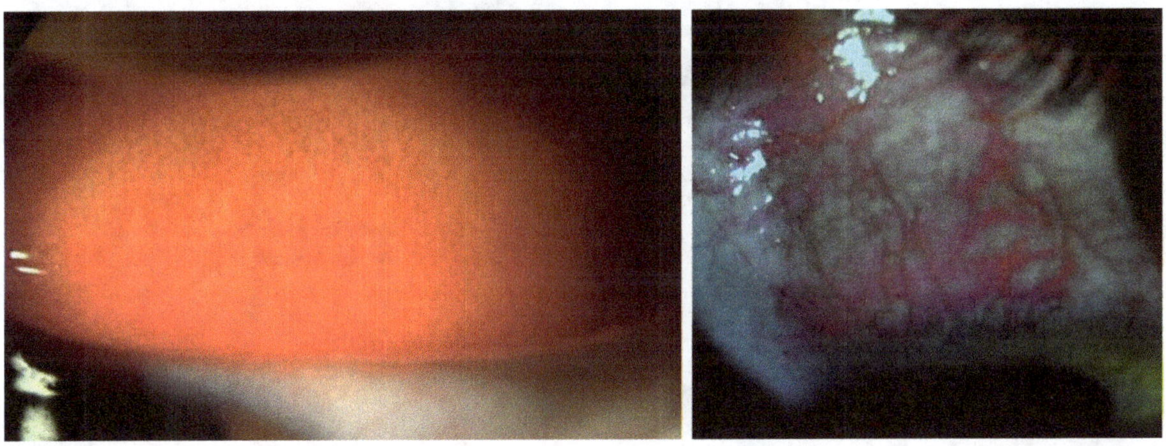

Figure 35. Superior limbic keratoconjunctivitis. The keratinized bulbar conjunctiva stained with rose Bengal

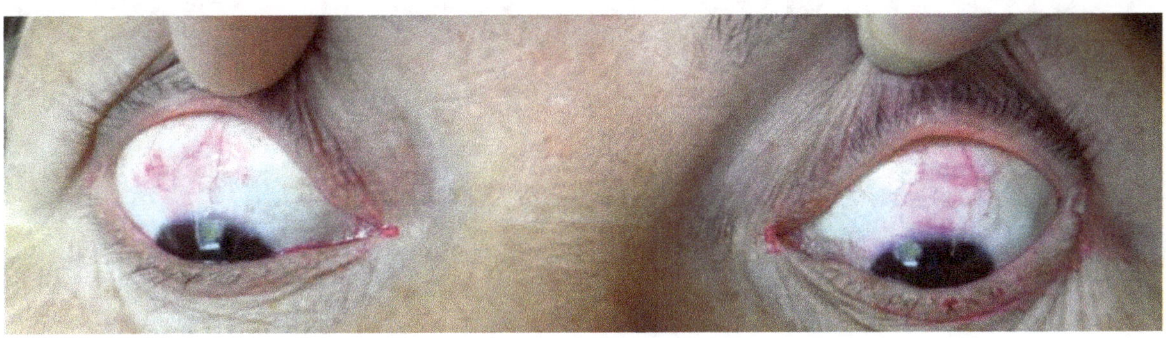

Floppy eyelid syndrome occurs predominantly in obese males who are used to sleeping face down. It is characterized by floppy, rubbery, easily everted upper tarsal plates and by papillary reaction of the upper tarsal conjunctiva (Fig 36,37,38). Floppy eyelid syndrome can be associated with obstructive sleep apnea, keratoconus and obesity (Compton et al, 2016). Temporary relief of floppy eyelid syndrome can be managed by taping the patient's eyelids shut or by having the patient wear a protective shield while sleeping. Lubricants may help in managing mild cases. Definitive therapy involves surgical procedures such as lateral canthus repair horizontal shortening of the upper eyelid, or excision of the medial upper lid (Periman, 2002).

Figure 36. Floppy eyelid syndrome. Rubbery, floppy, easily everted eyelid with severe papillary reaction

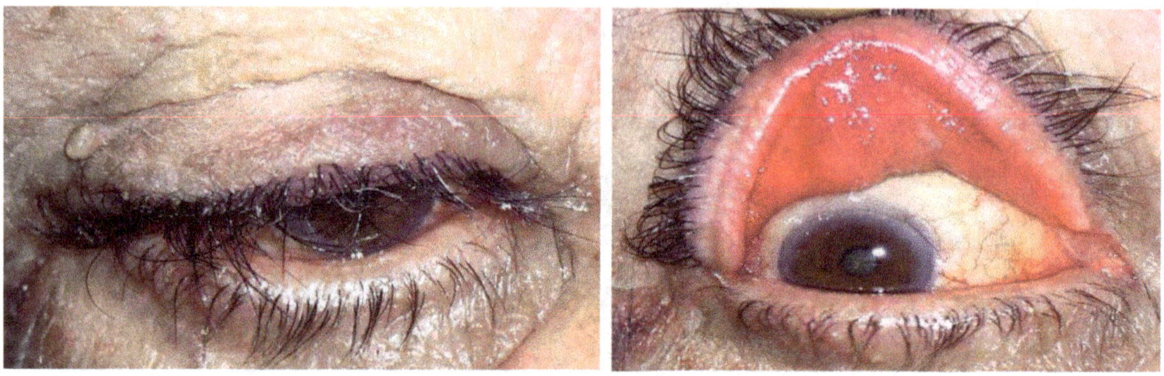

Figure 37. Papillary reaction of upper tarsal conjunctiva under slit lamp

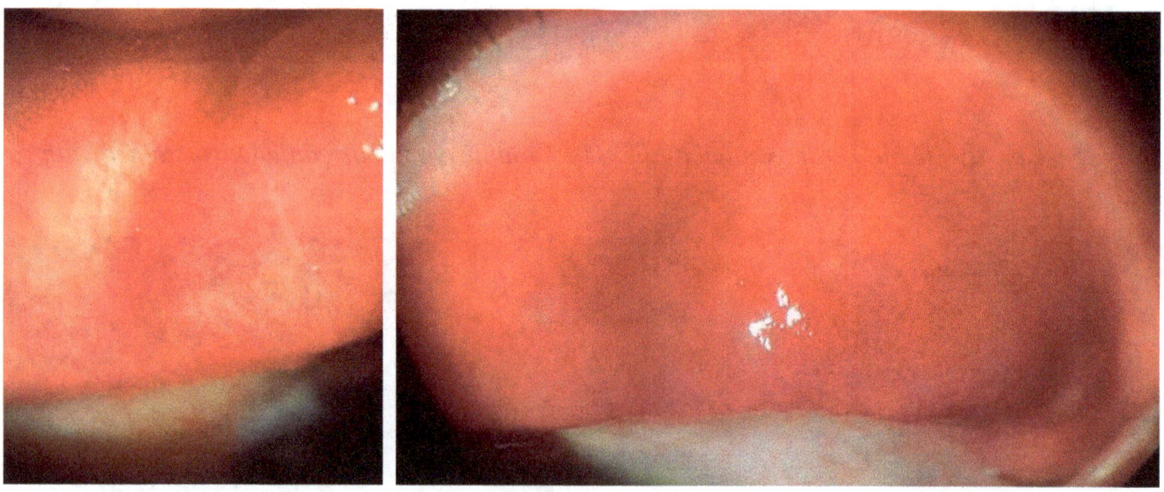

Figure 38. The same patient. Easily everted upper eyelid is shown

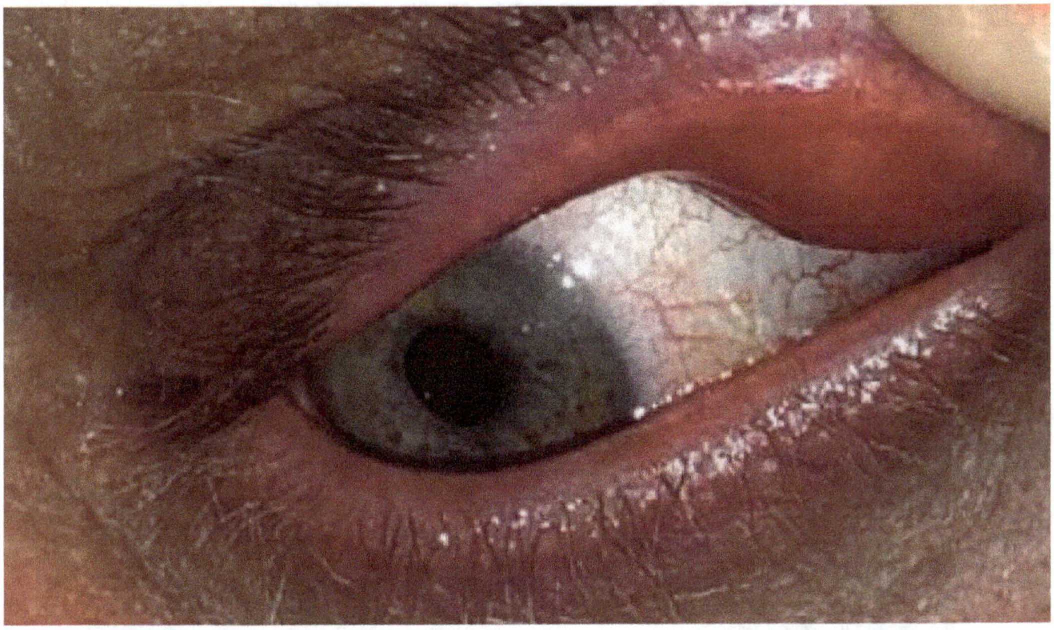

Keratoconjunctivitis sicca is another cause of chronic papillary conjunctivitis, which is usually observed bilaterally. This disorder represents the insufficiency of the quantity and quality of precorneal tear film (Behrens, 2006). Clinical signs include a decreased tear lake, debris in the tear film, and interpalpebral rose Bengal and lissamine green staining of the corneal and conjunctival keratinized epithelium (Discussed more detailed in chapter 2) (Fig 39,40).

Mucus-fishing syndrome is a mechanically induced, chronic papillary conjunctivitis. These patients exacerbate their conjunctival irritation by frequent removal of excess mucus discharge (Fig 41) (O'Brien, 2013). The patients admitted to mechanical removal of the mucus strands. The epithelial injury created by mucus fishing generates the ocular surface irritation, resulting in more mucus production, creating a vicious cycle. The nasal and inferior bulbar conjunctiva are the most frequently involved, as they are the most accessible areas. Treatment consists of eliminating the digital manipulation (if possible), increase lubrication and using mucolytic agents, such as acetylcysteine 10% topically, for reducing mucus production.

Allergic conjunctivitis is an inflammatory response of the conjunctiva to an allergen. It is usually seasonal and is associated with upper respiratory tract symptoms. Presence of rhinitis often terms this condition as allergic rhinoconjunctivitis (McCulley et al, 1985). Allergic conjunctivitis is almost always bilateral with watery or mucus discharge. Clinically, the eyelids and conjunctiva are edematous. Diffuse conjunctival injection is seen with papillary reaction of conjunctiva (Fig 42). Mild allergic conjunctivitis can be treated with a topical antihistamine/vasoconstrictor agent or with the more effective second-generation topical histamine H1-receptor antagonists (Owen et al, 2004). Many topical medications can be stored in the refrigerator, as the cooling sensation upon instillation of the eye drop may provide symptomatic relief. If the symptoms are not adequately controlled, a brief course (1 to 2 weeks) of topical corticosteroids with a low side effect profile can be added to the regimen. In severe cases, topical cyclosporine or tacrolimus can be considered (Erdinest et al, 2014).

Figure 39. Keratoconjunctivitis sicca. Mucous debris in tear film

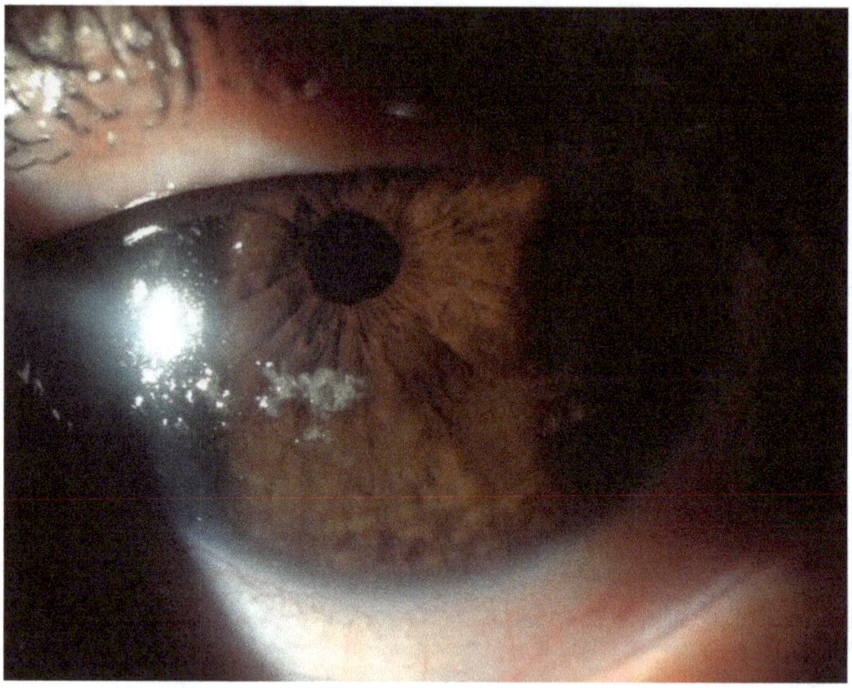

Figure 40. Keratoconjunctivitis sicca associated with Sjogren syndrome. The keratinized epithelium stained with Fluorescein is seen. The photo is taken under Cobalt-blue illumination with a yellow-blue filter

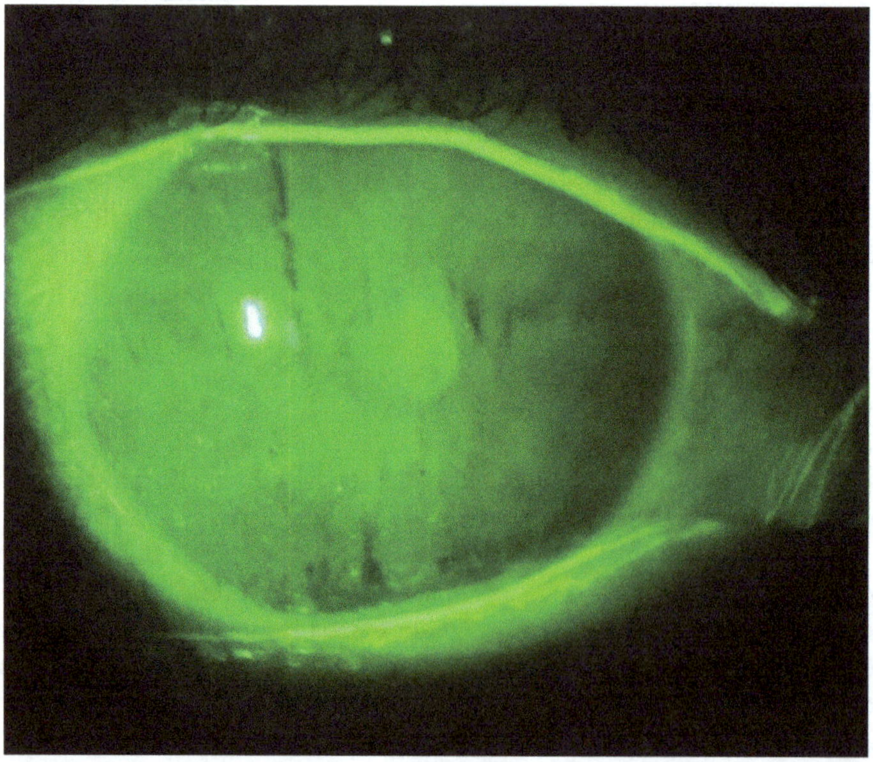

Figure 41. Mucus discharge between two eyelids in mucus-fishing syndrome

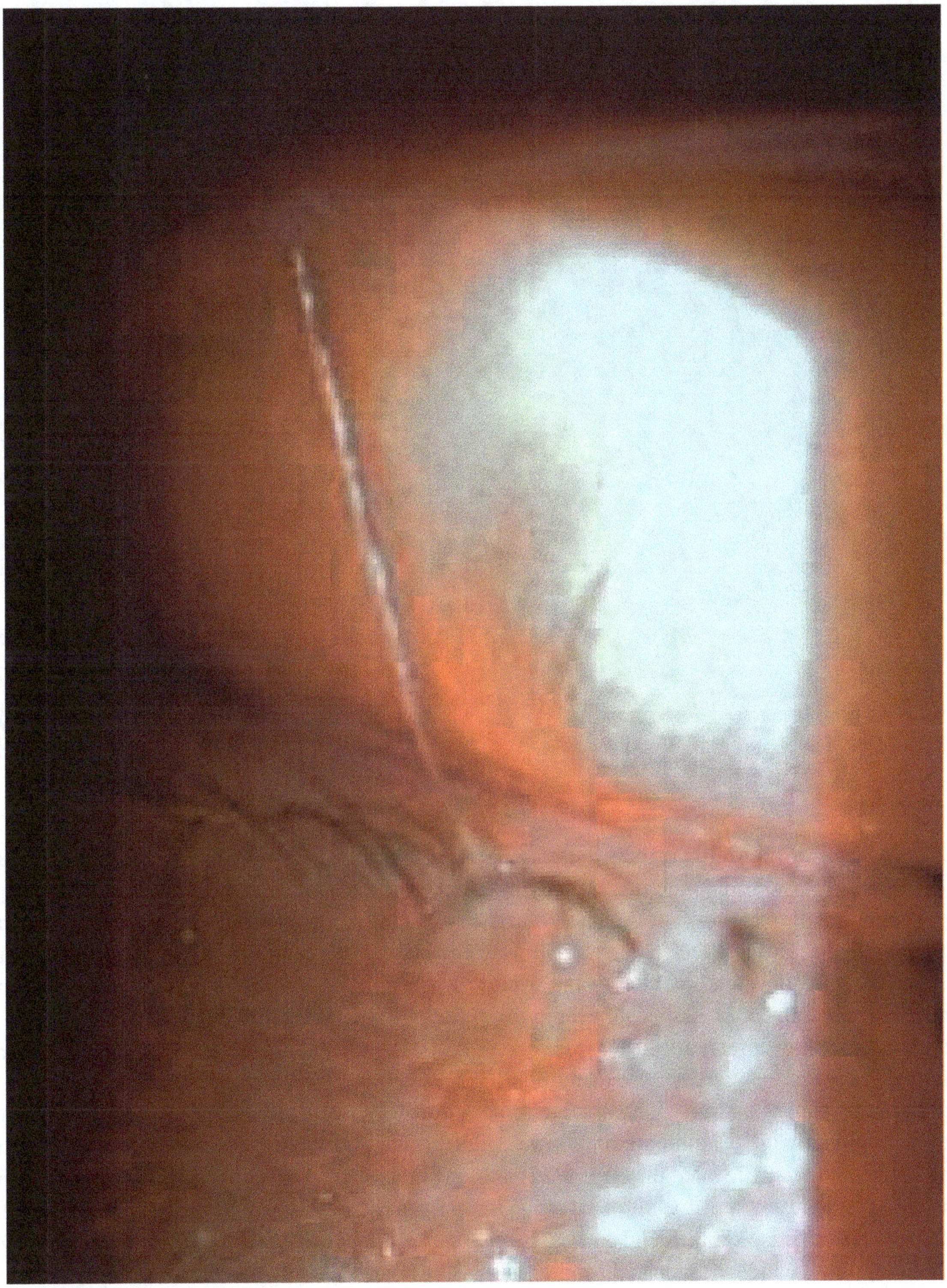

Figure 42. Allergic conjunctivitis. Palpebral edema, diffuse conjunctival injection and watery discharge are seen

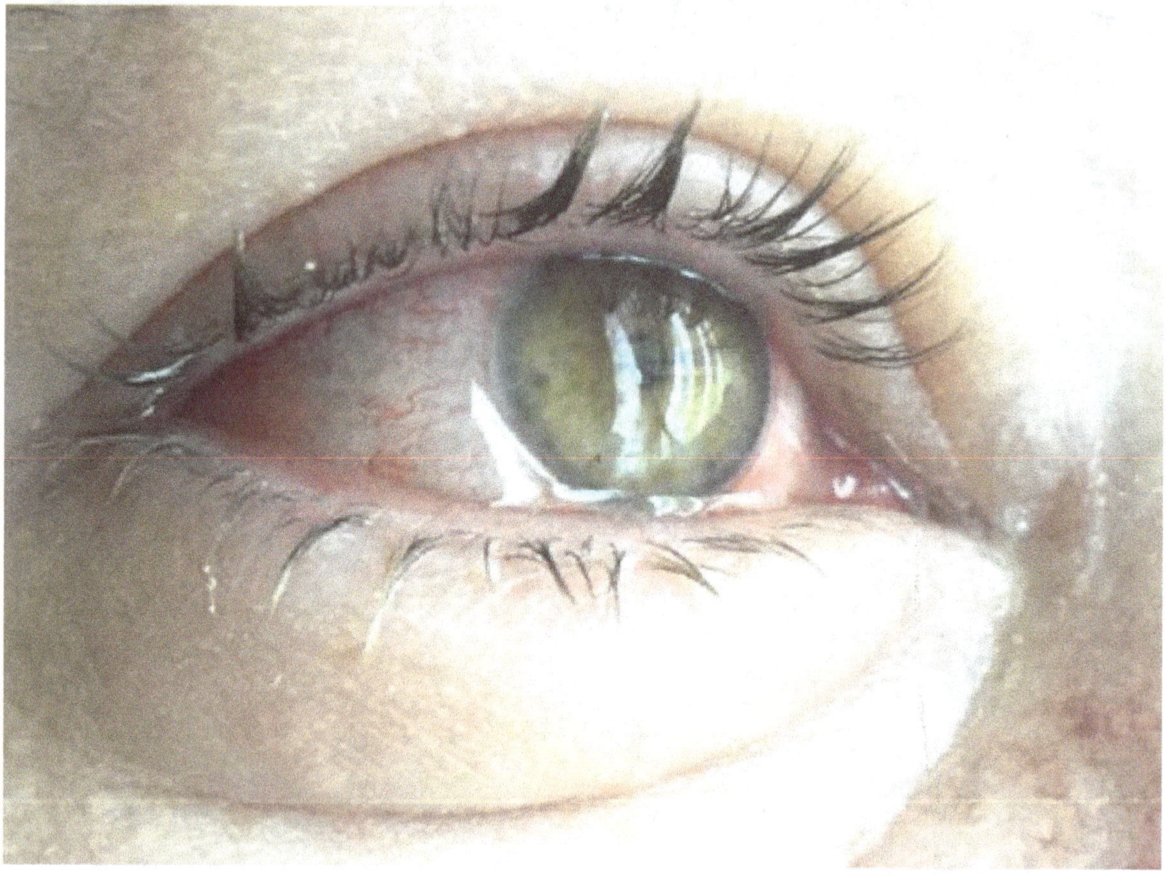

Chlamydial conjunctivitis is the most common chronic follicular conjunctivitis and may manifest as trachoma or inclusion conjunctivitis. Trachoma in endemic developing countries is the most common cause of blindness. Trachoma is a bilateral, chronic follicular conjunctivitis, which can cause corneal and conjunctival scarring (MacCallan et al, 1931). The classic scar sign of trachoma is considered the Arlt's line located above and parallel to the eyelid margin of the tarsal conjunctiva (Fig 43). Topical tetracycline 1% ointment or suspension three times a day for a minimum of six weeks is the current recommended treatment for active disease (West et al, 2004). Oral azithromycin shows great efficacy in treating trachoma as a single 1 g dose (Solomon, 2004).

Molluscum contagiosum belongs to DNA poxviruses and can cause chronic, follicular, mainly unilateral conjunctivitis. It is more common in children and adults. The typical lesions are pink, umbilicated and are usually located on the eyelid margin (Fig 44,45,46). Conjunctivitis and keratitis from molluscum contagiosum are a result of viral shedding from the eyelid lesion(s) onto the surface of the eye. Superficial punctate keratitis and corneal pannus can occur (Charteris et al, 1995; Chen et al, 2013). Treatment options include incision and curettage (aggressive enough to cause bleeding), simple excision, excision and cautery, and cryotherapy. In adults, large and multiple molluscum lesions with relatively little conjunctival inflammation may indicate an immunocompromised state (Gonnering et al, 1988).

Figure 43. Trachoma. Presumed Arlt's line. Patient claims to have had trachoma in childhood

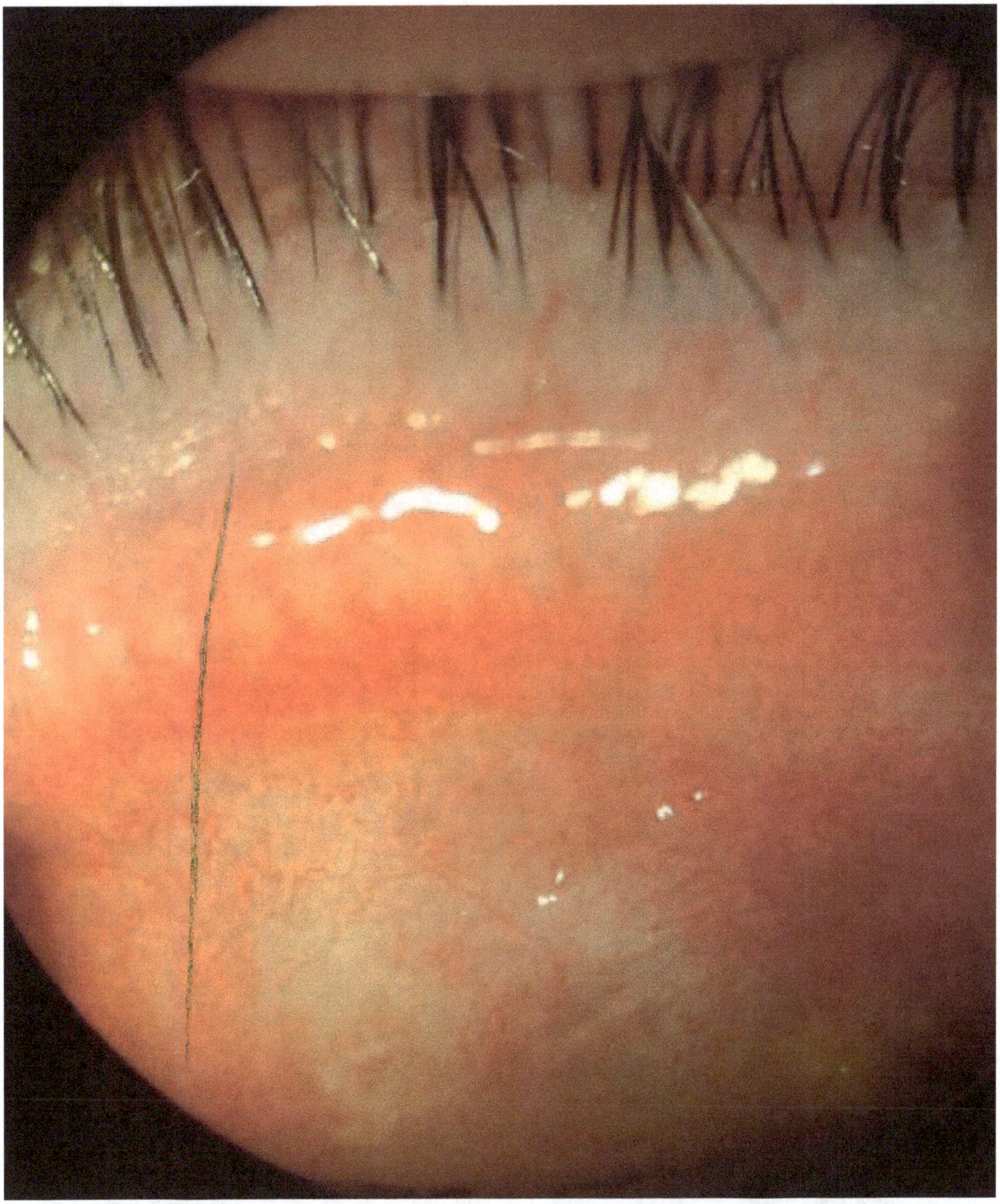

Figure 44. Umbilicated lesion of molluscum contagiosum is seen on the lower eyelid margin

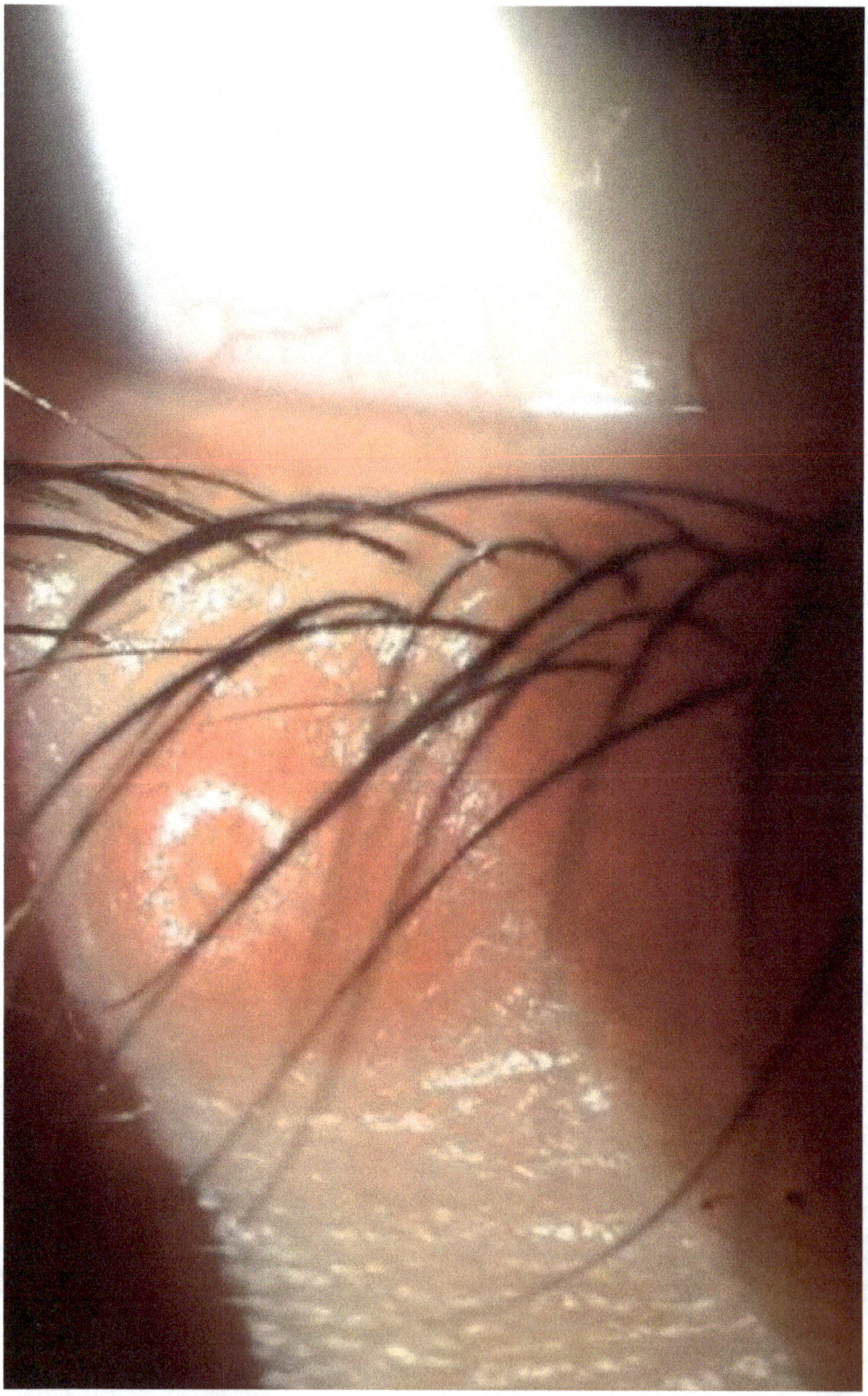

Figure 45. Two nasally located molluscum contagiosum lesions and associated follicular conjunctivitis (right photo)

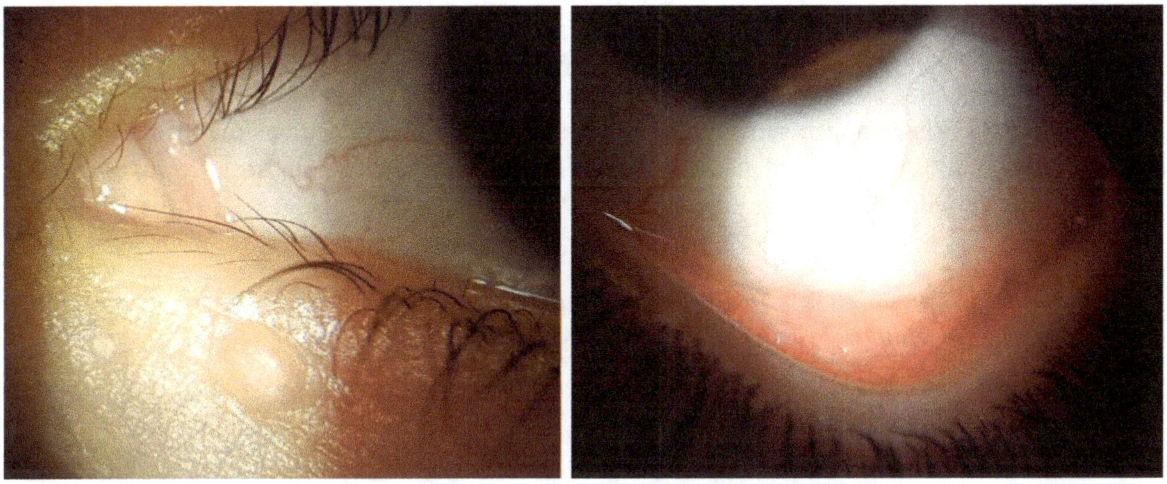

Figure 46. Multiple lesions of molluscum contagiosum on the upper lid margin

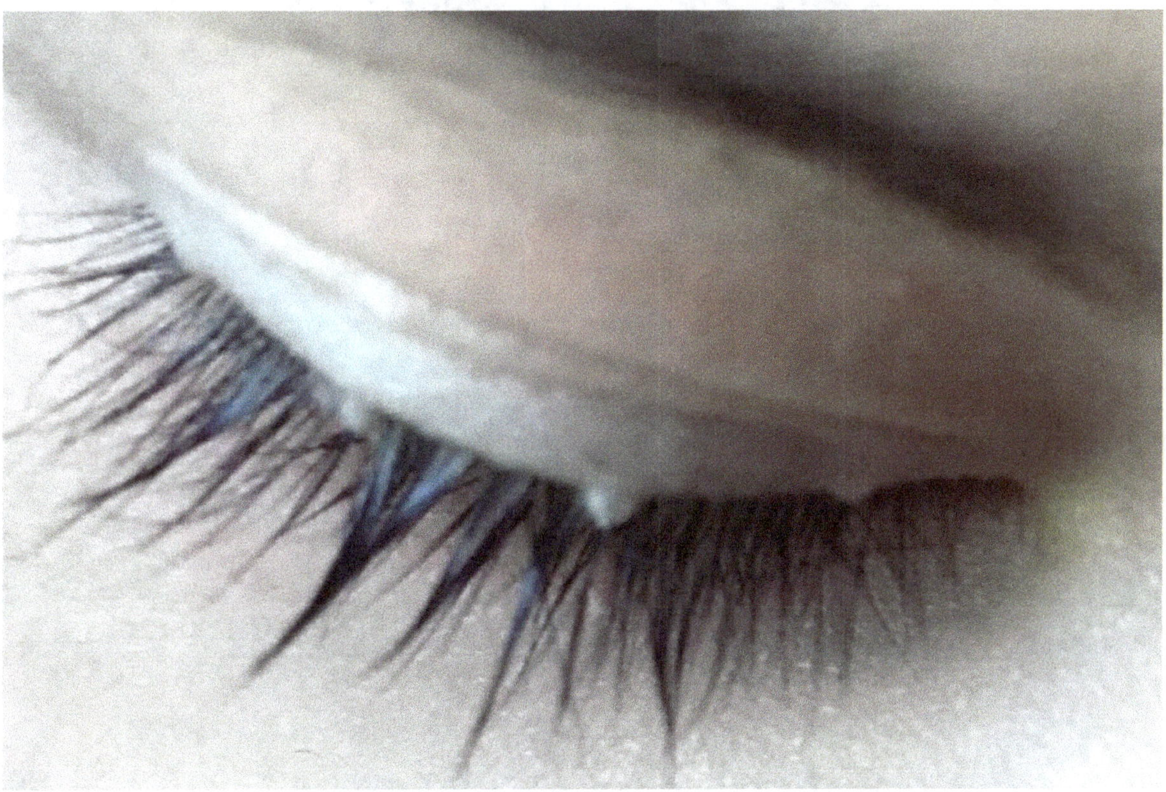

Ligneous conjunctivitis (LC) is the only chronic membranous conjunctivitis and is associated with type 1 plasminogen deficiency (Mingers et al, 1999). (Fig 47,48, 49). The true ligneous lesion represents a highly vascularized, raised, friable lesion, which can be easily removed, although it tends to bleed while removing. These lesions are usually located on the upper and lower tarsal conjunctiva but may be seen on the bulbar conjunctiva as well. After removal without appropriate therapy, the recurrence of lesions is seen within days. Plasminogen substitution is presently being investigated as the primary treatment for LC (Mingers et al, 1997). Topical plasminogen preparations extracted from fresh frozen plasma have successfully been employed in the treatment of LC (Watts et al, 2002).

Figure 47. Ligneous conjunctivitis. The ligneous membranous lesions are seen on the lower and upper palpebral region. The child is 25 months old

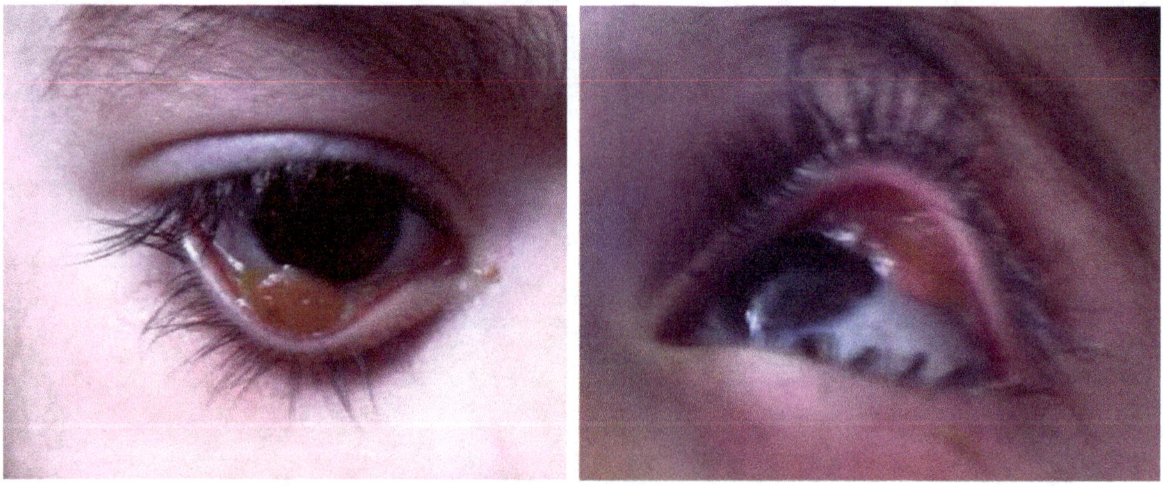

Figure 48. Ligneous conjunctivitis. The same patient: picture was taken over an old photo provided by parents

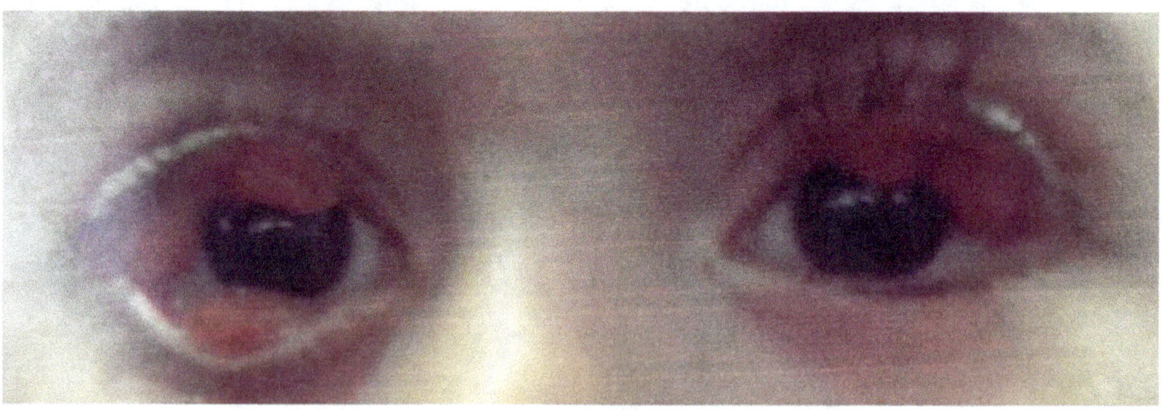

Figure 49. Ligneous conjunctivitis. The same patient (12 years old) after 10 years of monthly treatment with topical plasminogen and systemic plasminogen

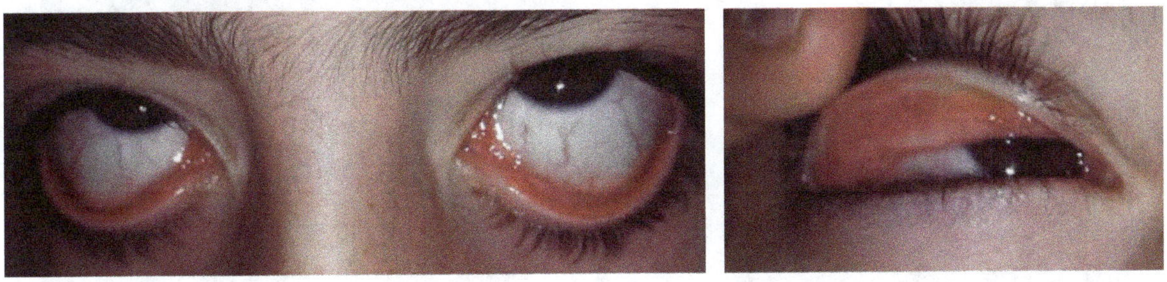

Ocular mucous membrane pemphigoid, also known as ocular cicatricial pemphigoid (OCP), is a cicatrizing conjunctivitis characterized by a slow progression from chronic conjunctivitis to subepithelial scarring, leading to fornix foreshortening, symblepharon (Fig 50), and even ankyloblepharon formation (Fig 51) (Chan et al, 2002). Ocular mucous membrane pemphigoid is found more commonly in elderly women. Mild and slowly progressive disease may be treated using mycophenolate mofetil, dapsone, azathioprine, or methotrexate (Saw et al, 2008). For severe inflammation or for inflammation unresponsive to treatment with other agents, cyclophosphamide should be considered (Wilkins, 2008).

Figure 50. OCP. Symblephara are seen

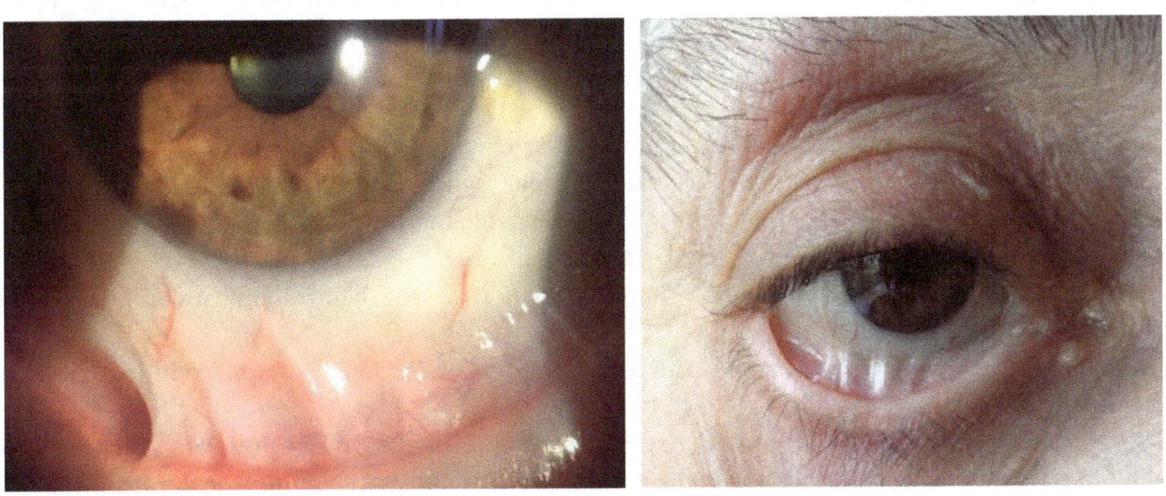

Stevens-Johnson syndrome (SJS), and its severe variant, toxic epidermal necrolysis (TEN), are severe disorders that can affect the skin and mucous membranes. Historically, erythema multiforme (erythema multiforme major) has been a part of SJS and TEN but is now considered a distinct entity that usually does not cause long-term ophthalmological sequelae. Erythema multiforme and SJS/TEN were thought to be immune-mediated responses to certain drugs (Carbamazepine, Sulfasalazine, Phenobarbital, etc.) and infections (mostly Mycoplasma pneumoniae). The ocular findings in SJS have 2 phases: acute and chronic. In the acute phase, many conditions starting from simple conjunctival hyperemia up to very

Figure 51. Ankyloblepharon due to OCP

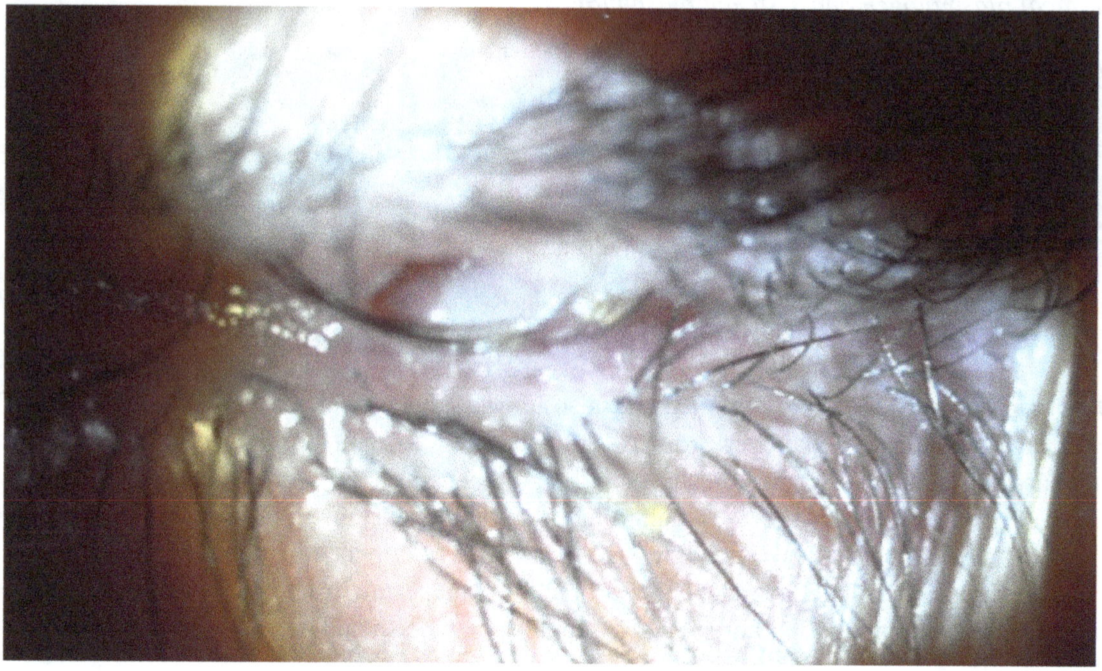

extensive sloughing of the ocular surface, tarsal conjunctiva and lid margins can be seen (Fig 52, 53). Uncommonly, corneal ulceration may occur. In chronic phase scarring, symblepharon and cicatrization are formed (Fig 54, 55) (Chang et al, 2007). Acute systemic management by a multidisciplinary medical team often involves immunosuppressive and immunomodulatory therapies. Medical management with topical lubricants, antibiotics, and anti-inflammatories is recommended (Jain et al, 2016). Lid hygiene and periodic sweeping of the conjunctival fornices prevents synechiae formation. Early amniotic membrane transplantation is a useful adjunct to stabilize the ocular surface, impede and treat cicatrization and conjunctival and corneal defects (Gregory et al, 2016).

Membranous conjunctivitis with symblepharon formation due to Chemical injuries are discussed in Chapter 11 "Corneal trauma".

Granulomatous conjunctivitis can be caused by sarcoidosis, retained foreign body (Fig 56), and Parinaud oculoglandular syndrome.

Sarcoidosis is a systemic chronic inflammatory disease characterized by the presence of noncaseating granulomas (Brownstein et al, 1990; Jabs et al, 1986). Uveitis is the most common ocular manifestation. Involvement of the lids, the lacrimal glands, the orbit, and the cornea can occur as well. Conjunctival granulomas are small, round, or oval nodules and have yellow-brown or red color. They can be surrounded by erythema or edema (Fig 57). Methotrexate has proven effective and relatively safe in the treatment of both system and ocular (Baughman et al, 1987; Dev et al, 1999) disease, allowing for reduction or even discontinuation of systemic steroids in many patients. Azathioprine, chlorambucil, and cyclophosphamide have also been effective in some patients with refractory disease· The tumor necrosis factor blockers infliximab and adalimumab have been shown to be effective in treating sarcoid ocular inflammation, while etanercept has not been shown to be helpful and, actually, has been associated with onset of sarcoidosis in rare cases (Baughman et al, 2012).

Figure 52. Steven-Johnson syndrome caused by Mycoplasma pneumonitis, acute phase. Mucus membranes inflammation of the eyes and mouth noted

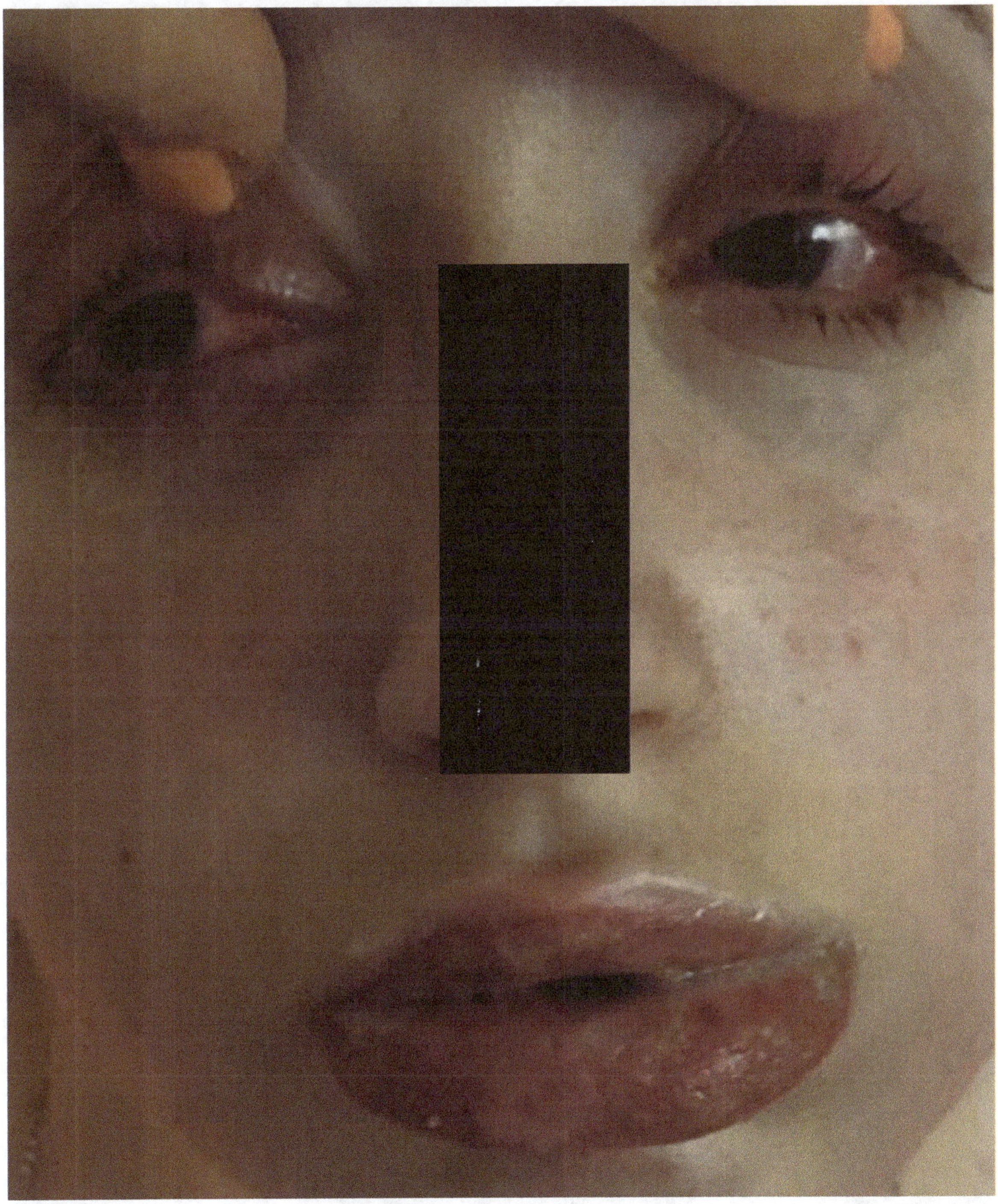

Figure 53. The same patient. Severe dryness associated with filamentary keratopathy is noted

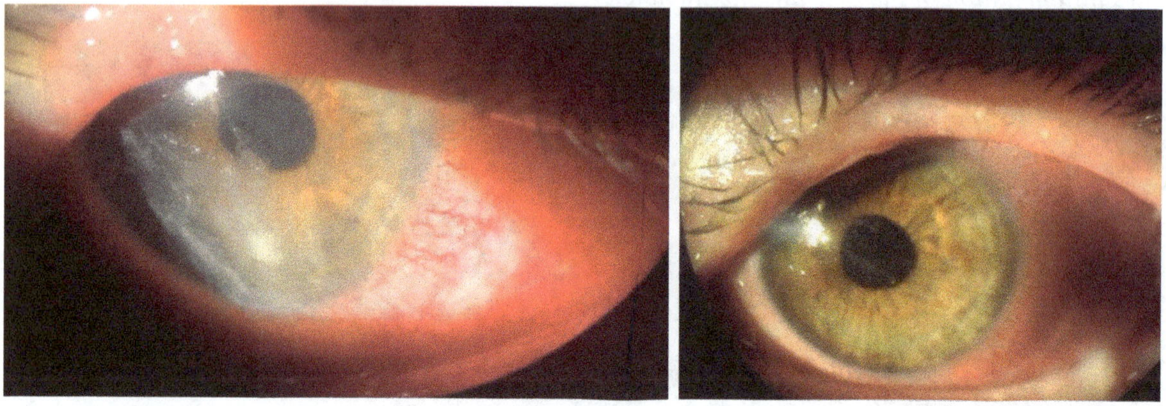

Figure 54. SJS, the same patient after the acute phase

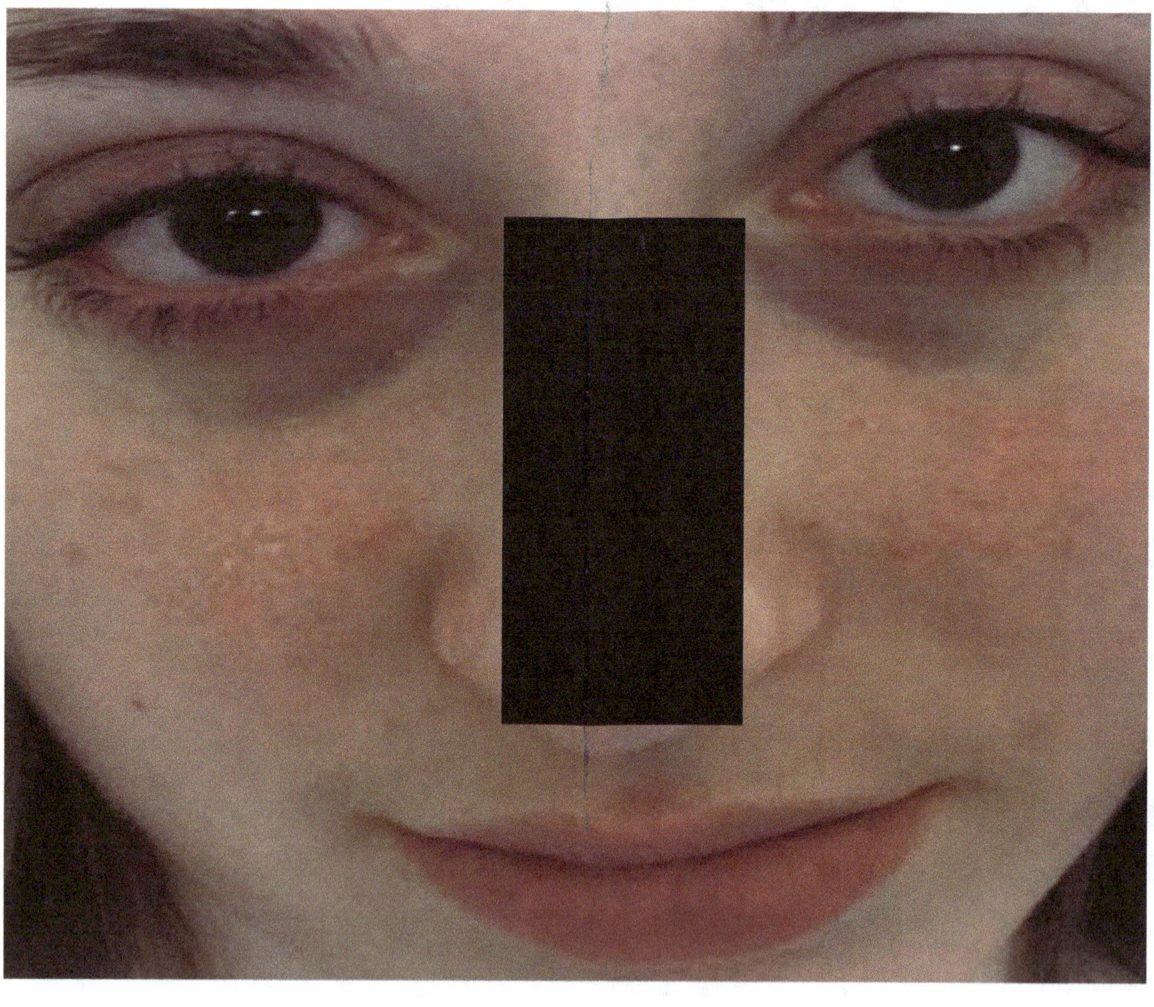

Figure 55. SJS, the same patient, in the chronic phase. Symblephara are formed

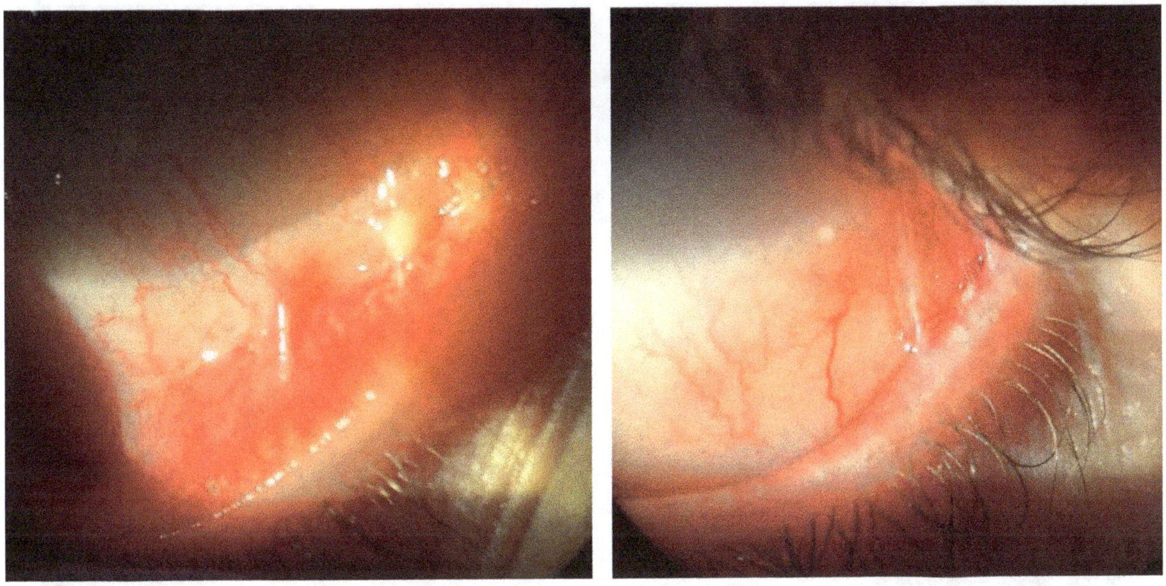

Figure 56. lower tarsal conjunctival granuloma associated with retained foreign body

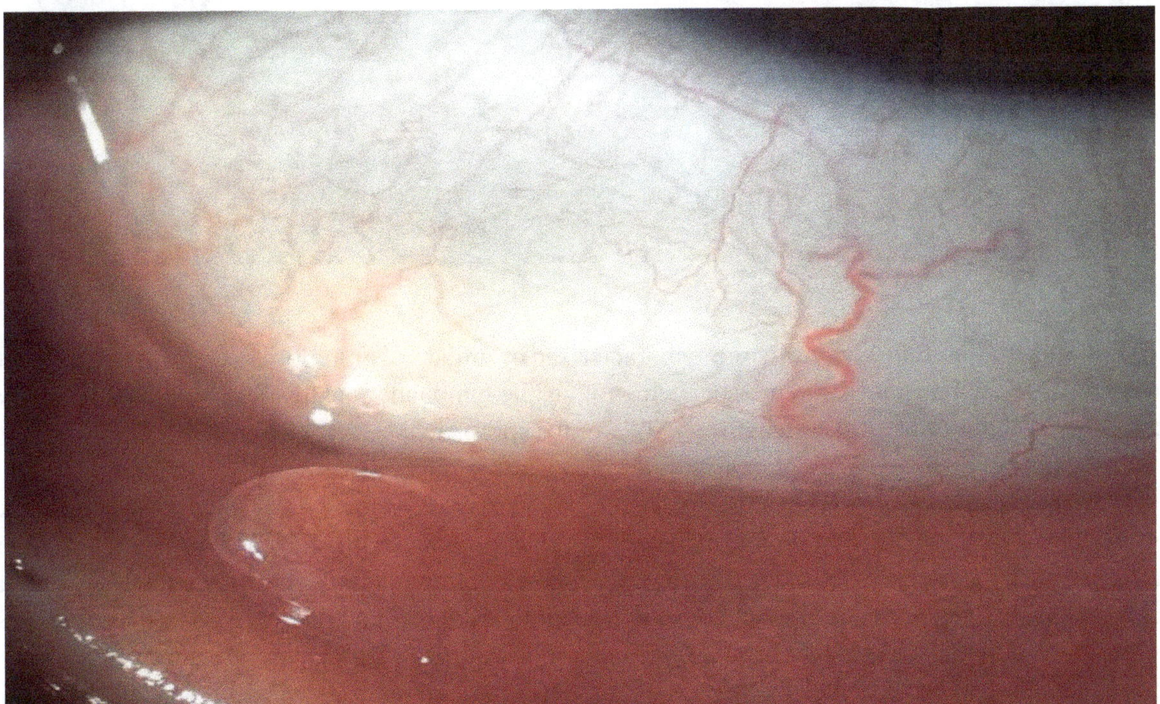

Figure 57. Conjunctival granulomata associated with sarcoidosis (biopsy proven)

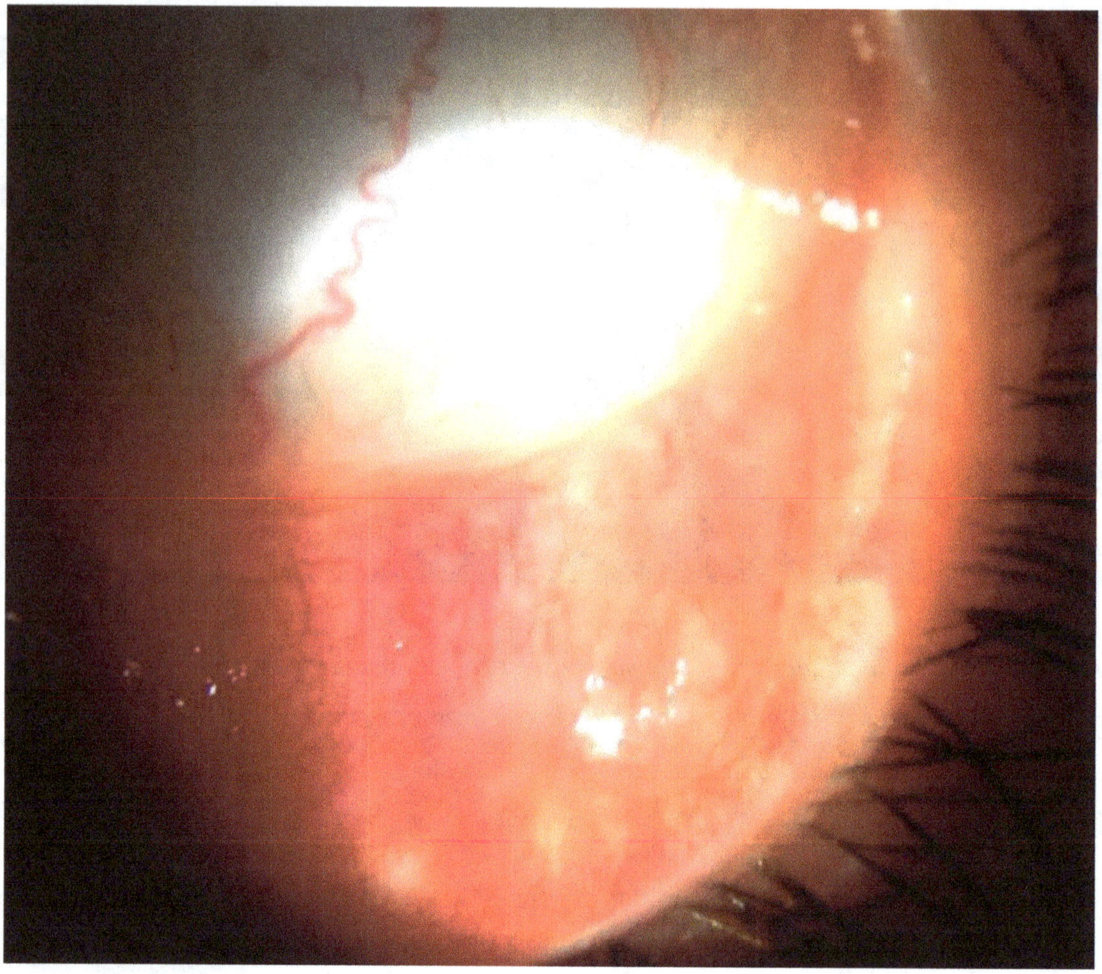

Parinaud oculoglandular syndrome is characterized by unilateral granulomatous conjunctivitis with a localized follicular response, often associated with visible lymphadenopathy. Parinaud oculoglandular syndrome may develop in cat-scratch disease, tularemia, sporotrichosis, etc (Chin et al, 1993). The most common cause of Parinaud oculoglandular syndrome is cat-scratch disease, and Bartonella henselae is the causative organize (Cassady et al, 1953). The infection may gain entry to the eye via the conjunctiva from facial cat scratches, but cat bite/scratch may not always be present (Fig 59). No specific treatment trials address the issue of antibiotic treatment in Parinaud oculoglandular syndrome. However, a meta-analysis of available randomized and nonrandomized clinical trials found no evidence to support the use of antibiotics in uncomplicated CSD. Cure rates and time course of the disease are unaffected by antibiotic treatment compared to placebo (Prutsky et al, 1967). Tularemia, caused by Francisella tularensis, is the second common cause of Parinaud syndrome, usually associated with severe systemic symptoms. Patients mention contact with ticks, rabbits, squirrels (Fig 60,61,62) (Steinemann et al, 1999). Topical broad-spectrum antibiotics should be combined with systemic antibiotic therapy. Medications such as Moxifloxacin, ciprofloxacin, levofloxacin, doxycycline, and systemic gentamicin are attractive alternatives to traditional seven days IM streptomycin injections (Tarnvik et al, 2003).

Figure 58. Parinaud oculoglandular syndrome associated with cat-scratch disease. The granuloma of lower tarsal conjunctiva with surrounded follicular reaction is seen

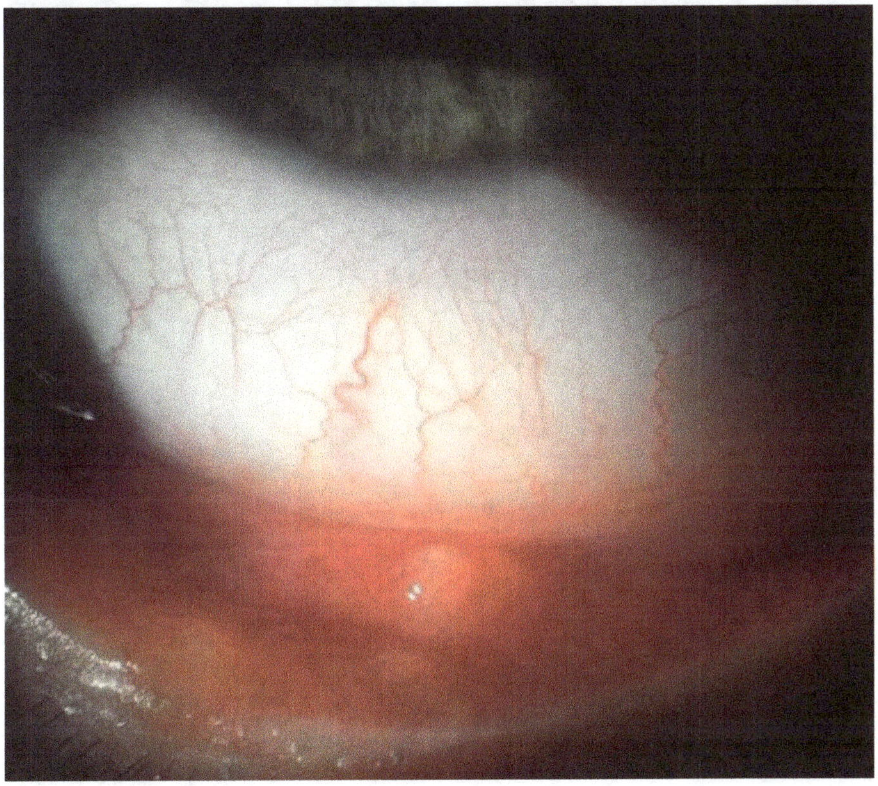

Figure 59. Parinaud oculoglandular syndrome associated with tularemia. Marked discharge and ulceration are seen over granuloma and follicular reaction

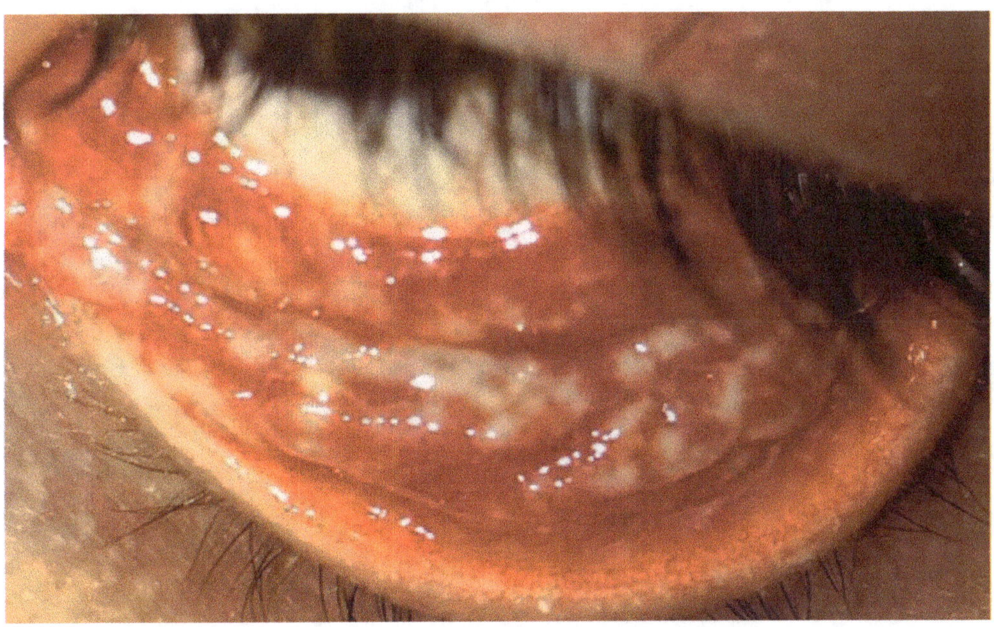

Figure 60. The same patient. Ipsilateral lymphadenopathy is noted

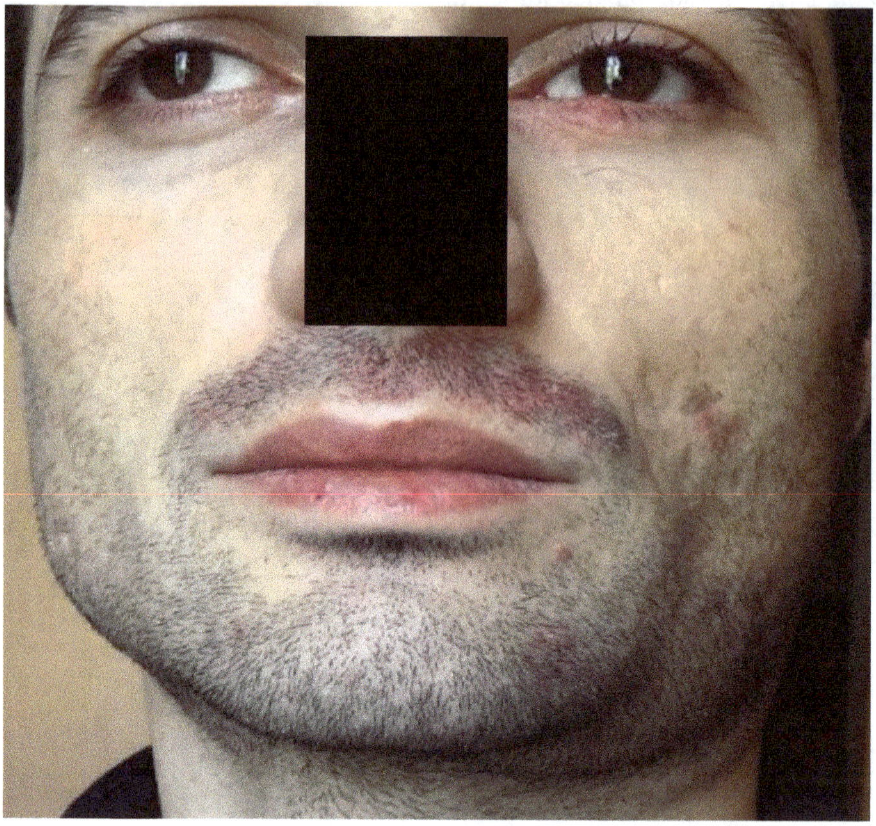

Figure 61. The same patient after a 3-week treatment with oral Doxycycline, topical mild steroids, lubricants and topical antibiotics

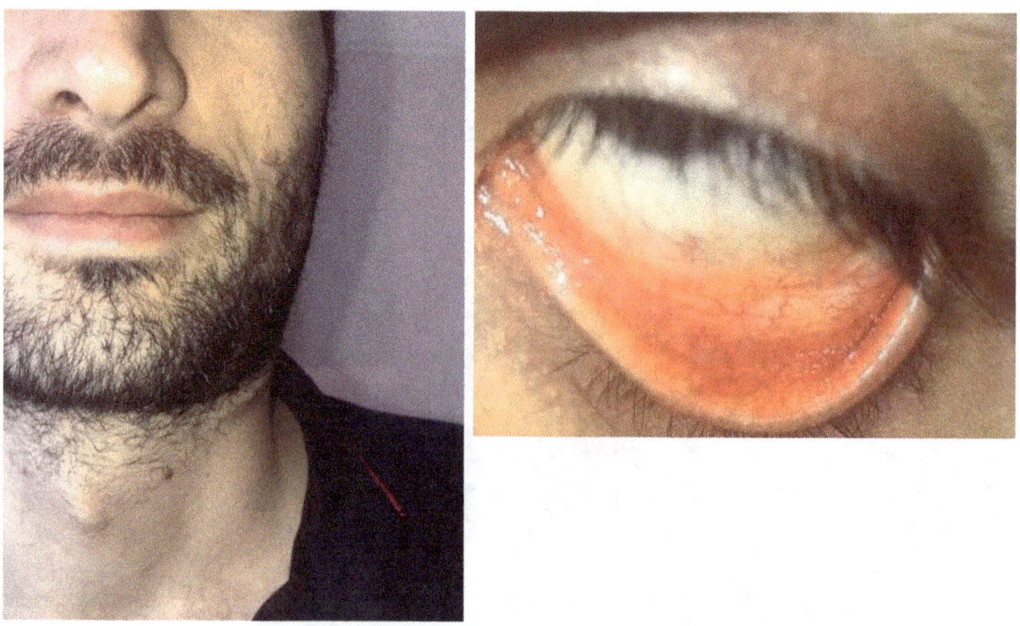

REFERENCES

Arffa, R. C. (1991). *Conjunctivitis. I. Follicular, neonatal, and bacterial. In diseases of the cornea* (3rd ed.). Mosby St Louis.

Duke-Elder, A. G. (1961). *Leigh: Inflammations of the conjunctiva and associated inflammations of the cornea. S Duke-Elder System of ophthalmology. In Diseases of the outer eye* (Vol. 8). Mosby.

Chin. (1994). Parinaud's oculoglandular conjunctivitis. In *Clinical ophthalmology*. JB Lippincott.

Locatcher-Khorazo & Seegal. (1972). *Microbiology of the eye*. Mosby.

Abelson, M. B., & Allansmith, M. R. (1987). *Ocular allergies. G Smolin RA Thoft The cornea*. Little Brown Boston.

Albietz, Sanfilippo, Troutbeck, & Lenton. (2003). Management of filamentary keratitis associated with aqueous-deficient dry eye. *Optom Vis Sci., 80*(6), 420-430.

Arffa, R. C. (1991). *Chlamydial infections. RC Arffa Grayson's diseases of the cornea* (3rd ed.). Mosby St Louis.

Bainbridge, J. W., Mackie, I. A., & Mackie, I. (1998). Diagnosis of Theodore's superior limbic keratoconjunctivitis. *Eye, 12*, 748–749.

Baughman, R. P., Costabel, U., & du Bois, R. M. (2008). Treatment of sarcoidosis. *Clinics in Chest Medicine, 29*, 533–548.

Baughman, R. P., & Lower, E. E. (1997). Alternatives to corticosteroids in the treatment of sarcoidosis. *Sarcoidosis, Vasculitis, and Diffuse Lung Diseases, 14*, 121–130.

Baughman, R. P., Lower, E. E., & Ingledue, R. (2012). Management of ocular sarcoidosis. *Sarcoidosis, Vasculitis, and Diffuse Lung Diseases, 29*, 26–33.

Behrens, A., Doyle, J. J., & Stern, L. (2006). Dysfunctional tear syndrome: A Delphi approach to treatment and recommendations. *Cornea, 25*, 900–907.

Boralkar, A. N. (1989). Diphtheritic conjunctivitis: A rare case report in Indian literature. *Indian Journal of Ophthalmology, 101*, 437.

Brownstein, S., Liszauer, A. D., Carey, W. D., & Nicolle, D. A. (1990). Sarcoidosis of the eyelid skin. *Canadian Journal of Ophthalmology, 25*, 256–259.

Cassady, J. V., & Culbertson, C. S. (1953). Cat-scratch disease and Parinaud's oculoglandular syndrome. *Archives of Ophthalmology, 50*, 68–74.

Centers for Disease Control. (1990). Epidemic keratoconjunctivitis in an ophthalmology clinic – California. *MMWR, 39*, 598. PMID:2166898

Chan, L., Ahmed, A. R., & Anhalt, G. (2002). The first international consensus on mucous membrane pemphigoid: Definition, diagnostic criteria, pathogenic factors, medical treatment, and diagnostic indicators. *Archives of Dermatology, 138*, 370–379.

Chang, Y., Huang, F. C., & Tseng, S. H. (2007). Erythema multiforme, Stevens–Johnson syndrome, and toxic epidermal necrolysis: Acute ocular manifestations, causes, and management. *Cornea*, *26*, 123–129.

Charteris, D. G., Bonshek, R. E., & Tullo, A. B. (1995). Ophthalmic molluscum contagiosum: Clinical and immunopathological features. *The British Journal of Ophthalmology*, *79*(5), 476–481.

Chen, X., Anstey, A. V., & Bugert, J. J. (2013). Molluscum contagiosum virus infection. *The Lancet. Infectious Diseases*, *13*(10), 877–888.

Chin, G. N., & Hyndiuk, R. A. (1993). Parinaud's oculoglandular syndrome. In Clinical ophthalmology (vol. 4). Lippincott.

Compton, C. J., Melson, A. T., Clark, J. D., Shipchandler, T. Z., Nunery, W. R., & Lee, H. B. (2016). Combined medial canthopexy and lateral tarsal strip for floppy eyelid syndrome. *American Journal of Otolaryngology*, *37*(3), 240–244.

Culbertson, W. W., & Ostler, H. B. (1981). The floppy eyelid syndrome. *American Journal of Ophthalmology*, *92*, 568.

Culbertson, W. W., & Tseng, S. C. (1994). Corneal disorders in floppy eyelid syndrome. *Cornea*, *13*(1), 33–42.

Dev, S., McCallum, R. M., & Jaffe, G. J. (1999). Methotrexate treatment for sarcoid-associated panuveitis. *Ophthalmology*, *106*, 111–118.

Duke-Elder, W. S., & MacFaul, P. A. (1974). *Canaliculitis. Actinomycosis. WS Duke-Elder System of ophthalmology* (Vol. 13). Mosby.

Erdinest, N., & Solomon, A. (2014). Topical immunomodulators in the management of allergic eye diseases. *Current Opinion in Allergy and Clinical Immunology*, *14*(5), 457–463.

Glasser, D. B., & Hyndiuk, R. A. (1986). *Herpes simplex keratitis. KF Tabbara RA Hundiuk Infections of the eye*. Little Brown Boston.

Gonnering, R. S., & Kronish, J. W. (1988). Treatment of periorbital molluscum contagiosum by incision and curettage. *Ophthalmic Surgery*, *19*, 325–327.

Gregory, D. G. (2016). New grading system and treatment guidelines for the acute ocular manifestations of Stevens-Johnson syndrome. *Ophthalmology*, *123*(8), 1653–1658.

Hammerschlag. (1989). Chlamydia infections. *J Pediatr.*, *114*(727).

Hovakimyan, A., Kambulyan, L., Davtyan, A., Kirakosyan, A., & Tsarukyan, E. (2020). Vernal Keratoconjunctivitis with Atypical Localization of Shield Ulcer. *Journal of Advances in Medicine and Medical Research*, *32*(23), 245–248. https://doi.org/10.9734/jammr/2020/v32i2330742

Jabs, D. A., & Johns, C. J. (1986). Ocular involvement in chronic sarcoidosis. *American Journal of Ophthalmology*, *102*, 297–301.

Jain, R., Sharma, N., & Basu, S. (2016). Stevens-Johnson syndrome: The role of an ophthalmologist. *Survey of Ophthalmology*, *61*(4), 3.

Jones, L. T. (1966). The lacrimal secretory system and its treatment. *American Journal of Ophthalmology, 62*, 47.

Kaufman, H. E., & Haw, W. H. (2012). Ganciclovir ophthalmic gel 0.15%: Safety and efficacy of a new treatment for herpes simplex keratitis. *Current Eye Research, 37*(7), 654–660.

Kiliç, A., & Gürler, B. (2006). Topical 2% cyclosporine A in preservative-free artificial tears for the treatment of vernal keratoconjunctivitis. *Canadian Journal of Ophthalmology, 41*(6), 693–698.

Lemp, M. A., & Nichols, K. K. (2009). Blepharitis in the United States 2009: A survey-based perspective on prevalence and treatment. *The Ocular Surface, 7*(2, Suppl), S1–S14.

Li, J. Y. (2018). Herpes zoster ophthalmicus: Acute keratitis. *Current Opinion in Ophthalmology, 29*(4), 328–333.

MacCallan, A. (1931). The epidemiology of trachoma. *The British Journal of Ophthalmology, 15*, 369.

McCulley, J. P., Moore, M. B., & Matoba, A. Y. (1985). Mucus fishing syndrome. *Ophthalmology, 92*, 1262.

Mingers, A. M., Heimburger, N., & Zeitler, P. (1997). Homozygous type I plasminogen deficiency. *Seminars in Thrombosis and Hemostasis, 23*(3), 259–269.

Mingers, A. M., Philapitsch, A., & Zeitler, P. (1999). Human homozygous type I plasminogen deficiency and ligneous conjunctivitis. *APMIS, 107*(1), 62–72.

Naderan, M., Rajabi, M. T., Zarrinbakhsh, P., & Bakhshi, A. (2017). Effect of allergic diseases on keratoconus severity. *Ocular Immunology and Inflammation, 25*(3), 418–423.

Nottage, J. M., Hammersmith, K. M., Murchison, A. P., Felipe, A. F., Penne, R., & Raber, I. (2013). Treatment of mucous membrane pemphigoid with mycophenolate mofetil. *Cornea, 32*(6), 810–815.

O'Brien, T. P. (2013). Allergic conjunctivitis: An update on diagnosis and management. *Current Opinion in Allergy and Clinical Immunology, 13*, 543–549.

Oray, M., & Toker, E. (2013). Tear cytokine levels in vernal keratoconjunctivitis: The effect of topical 0.05% cyclosporine a therapy. *Cornea, 32*(8), 1149–1154.

Owen, C. G., Shah, A., Henshaw, K., Smeeth, L., & Sheikh, A. (2004). Topical treatments for seasonal allergic conjunctivitis: Systematic review and meta-analysis of efficacy and effectiveness. *The British Journal of General Practice, 54*(503), 451–456.

Periman, L. M., & Sires, B. S. (2002). Floppy eyelid syndrome: A modified surgical technique. *Ophthalmic Plastic and Reconstructive Surgery, 18*(5), 370–372.

Perkins, R. E., Kundsin, R. B., Pratt, M. V., Abrahamsen, I., & Leibowitz, H. M. (1975). Bacteriology of normal and infected conjunctiva. *Journal of Clinical Microbiology, 1*(2), 147–149. doi:10.1128/jcm.1.2.147-149.1975 PMID:1176598

Perry, H. D., Doshi-Carnevale, S., Donnenfeld, E. D., & Kornstein, H. S. (2003). Topical cyclosporine A 0.5% as a possible new treatment for superior limbic keratoconjunctivitis. *Ophthalmology, 110*(8), 1578–1581.

Perry, H. D., Doshi-Carnevale, S., Donnenfeld, E. D., & Kornstein, H. S. (2003). Topical cyclosporine A 0.5% as a possible new treatment for superior limbic keratoconjunctivitis. *Ophthalmology, 110*(8), 1578–1581.

Prutsky, G., Domecq, J. P., & Mori, L. (2013). Treatment outcomes of human bartonellosis: A systematic review and meta-analysis. *International Journal of Infectious Diseases, 17*, e811–e819.

Pucci, N., Caputo, R., & di Grande, L. (2015). Tacrolimus vs. cyclosporine eyedrops in severe cyclosporineresistant vernal keratoconjunctivitis: A randomized, comparative, double-blind, crossover study. *Pediatric Allergy and Immunology, 26*(3), 256–261.

Rapoza, P. A., Quinn, T. C., Kiessling, L. A., Green, W. R., & Taylor, H. R. (1986). Assessment of neonatal conjunctivitiswith a direct immunofluorescent monoclonal antibody stain for Chlamydia. *Journal of the American Medical Association, 255*(24), 3369–3373. doi:10.1001/jama.1986.03370240039033 PMID:2423718

Saw, V. P., Dart, J. K., & Rauz, S. (2008). Immunosuppressive therapy for ocular mucous membrane pemphigoid strategies and outcomes. *Ophthalmology, 115*(2), 253–261.

Schachter, J. (1990). Chlamydia infections. *The Western Journal ofMedicine, 153*, 523. PMID:2260289

Solomon, A. W., Holland, M. J., & Alexander, N. D. (2004). Mass treatment with single-dose azithromycin for trachoma. *The New England Journal of Medicine, 351*(19), 1962–1971.

Steinemann, T. L., Sheikholeslami, M. R., & Brown, H. H. (1999). Oculoglandular tularemia. *Archives of Ophthalmology, 117*, 132–133.

Sun, Y. C., Hsiao, C. H., Chen, W. L., Wang, I. J., Hou, Y. C., & Hu, F. R. (2008). Conjunctival resection combined with tenon layer excision and the involvement of mast cells in superior limbic keratoconjunctivitis. *American Journal of Ophthalmology, 145*(3), 445–452.

Szeto, S. K., Chan, T. C., Wong, R. L., Ng, A. L., Li, E. Y., & Jhanji, V. (2017). Prevalence of ocular manifestations and visual outcomes in patients with herpes zoster ophthalmicus. *Cornea, 36*(3), 338–342.

Tabbara, K. F., & Jarade, E. F. (2001). Ganciclovir effects in adenoviral keratoconjunctivitis. *ARVO, 42*, S579.

Tarnvik, A., & Berglund, L. (2003). Tularaemia. *The European Respiratory Journal, 21*, 361–373.

Vastine, D. W. (1987). *Viral diseases: adenovirus and miscellaneous viral infections. In The cornea.* Little Brown Boston.

Watts, P., Suresh, P., & Mezer, E. (2002). Effective treatment of ligneous conjunctivitis with topical plasminogen. *American Journal of Ophthalmology, 133*(4), 451–455.

West, E. S., Munoz, B., & Mkocha, H. (2005). Mass treatment and the effect on the load of Chlamydia trachomatis infection in a trachoma-hyperendemic community. *Investigative Ophthalmology & Visual Science, 46*(1), 83–87.

Wilhelmus, K. R. (2015). Antiviral treatment and other therapeutic interventions for herpes simplex virus epithelial keratitis. *Cochrane Database of Systematic Reviews, 1.*

Wilkins, M. R., & Dart, J. K. (2008). Mycophenolate mofetil for the treatment of severe inflammatory external eye diseases. *The British Journal of Ophthalmology*, *92*(4), 578–579.

Workowski, K. A. (2010). S Berman Centers for Disease Control and Prevention: Sexually transmitted diseases treatment guidelines. *MMWR. Recommendations and Reports*, *59*(RR–12), 1–110. PMID:21160459

Chapter 4
Non-Inflammatory Pathologies of Conjunctiva

ABSTRACT

Non-inflammatory pathologies of conjunctiva refer to conjunctival diseases or conditions that do not have infectious or immune inflammatory origin. This chapter includes disorders such as conjunctivochalasis, conjunctival cysts, conjunctival lymphangiectasias, conjunctival lymphoma, dermoids, papilloma, intraepithelial neoplasia, nevi and other rarely seen tumors, conjunctival degenerations and changes related to aging, xerosis, as well as interesting cases of fastidious conjunctivitis. Some cases of neoplasia have before and after treatment illustration to highlight the possibility of medical treatment against surgical interventions. At the end of this chapter, some observations are added to show the anatomical changes of conjunctiva without any underlying disease or inflammation.

INTRODUCTION

Non-Inflammatory Pathologies of Conjunctiva

Conjunctivochalasis represents redundant, loose conjunctiva, usually located above the lower lid margin as a prolapsed bulbar conjunctiva (Fig 1). Conjunctivochalasis is a bilateral condition, often asymptomatic, but can cause irritation, lacrimation, dryness, redness, etc (Hughes, 1942). Asymptomatic patients do not require treatment. The treatment of symptomatic patients includes lubrication and/or topical corticosteroids. Surgical management involves excision of the redundant conjunctiva (Otaka et al, 2000).

Conjunctival cysts can be acquired or congenital. Histologically, cysts consist of the nonkeratinizing conjunctival epithelium with goblet cells (Boynton et al, 1992). Usually, cysts are asymptomatic, stable, and they may rarely enlarge (Fig 2, 3). The treatment of symptomatic conjunctival cysts is excision. Visualization of the cyst may be more obvious by preoperative injection of a dye such as trypan blue or indocyanine green (Kobayashi et al, 2004).

DOI: 10.4018/978-1-7998-6937-5.ch004

Figure 1. Conjunctivochalasis. You can see the loose conjunctiva above inferior lid margin associated with poliosis

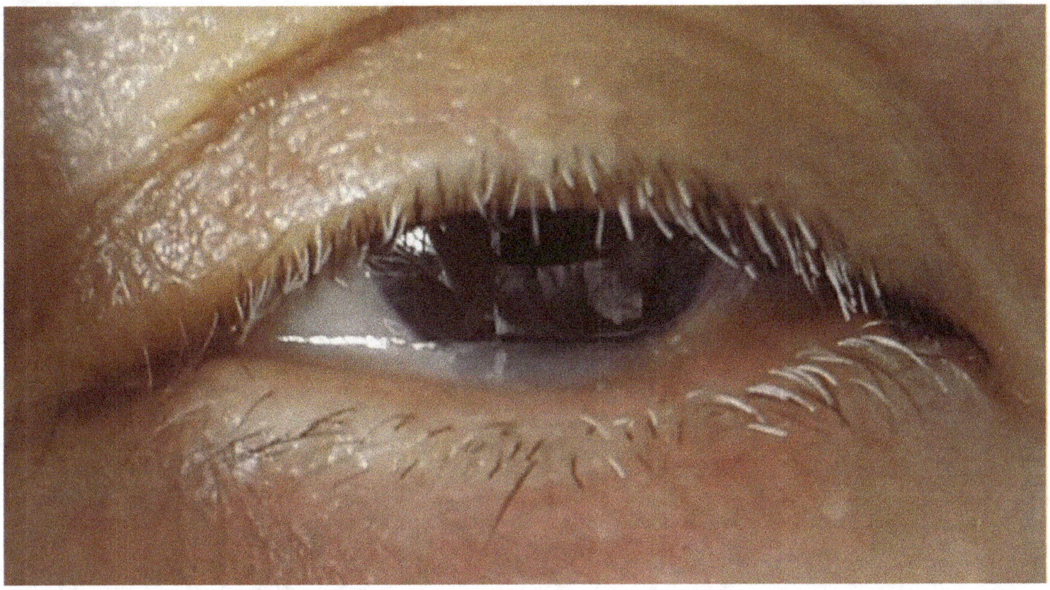

Figure 2. Conjunctival cyst. You can see a small round elevated cyst on bulbar conjunctiva

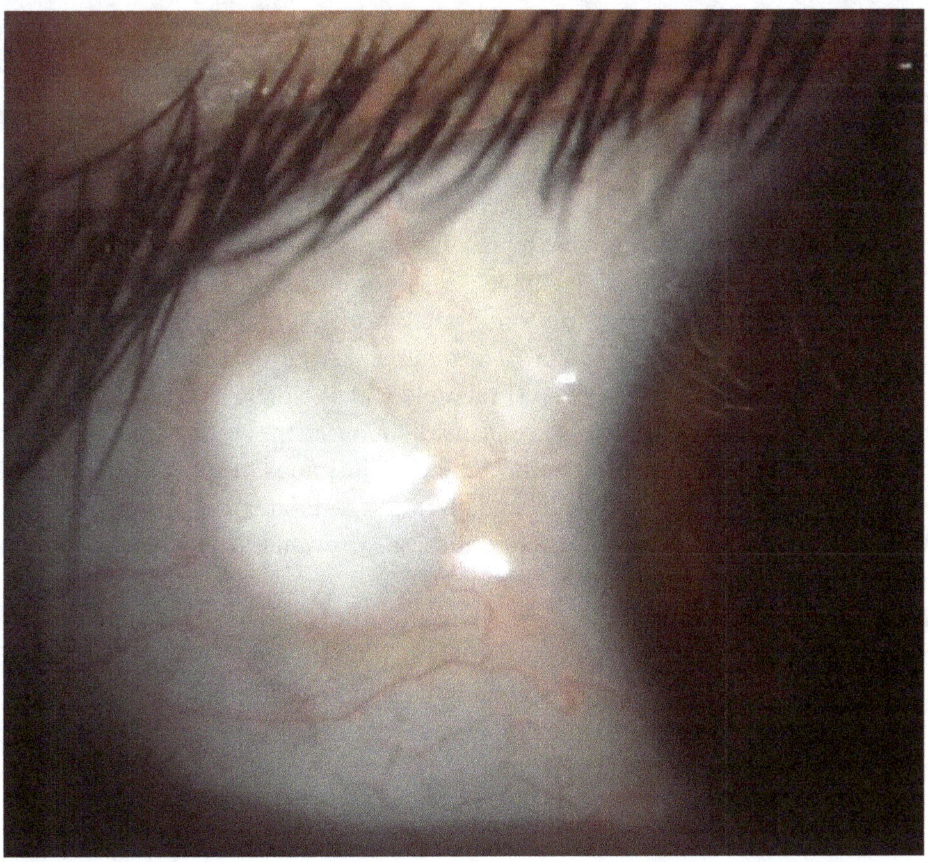

Figure 3. Conjunctival cyst on the lower tarsal conjunctiva

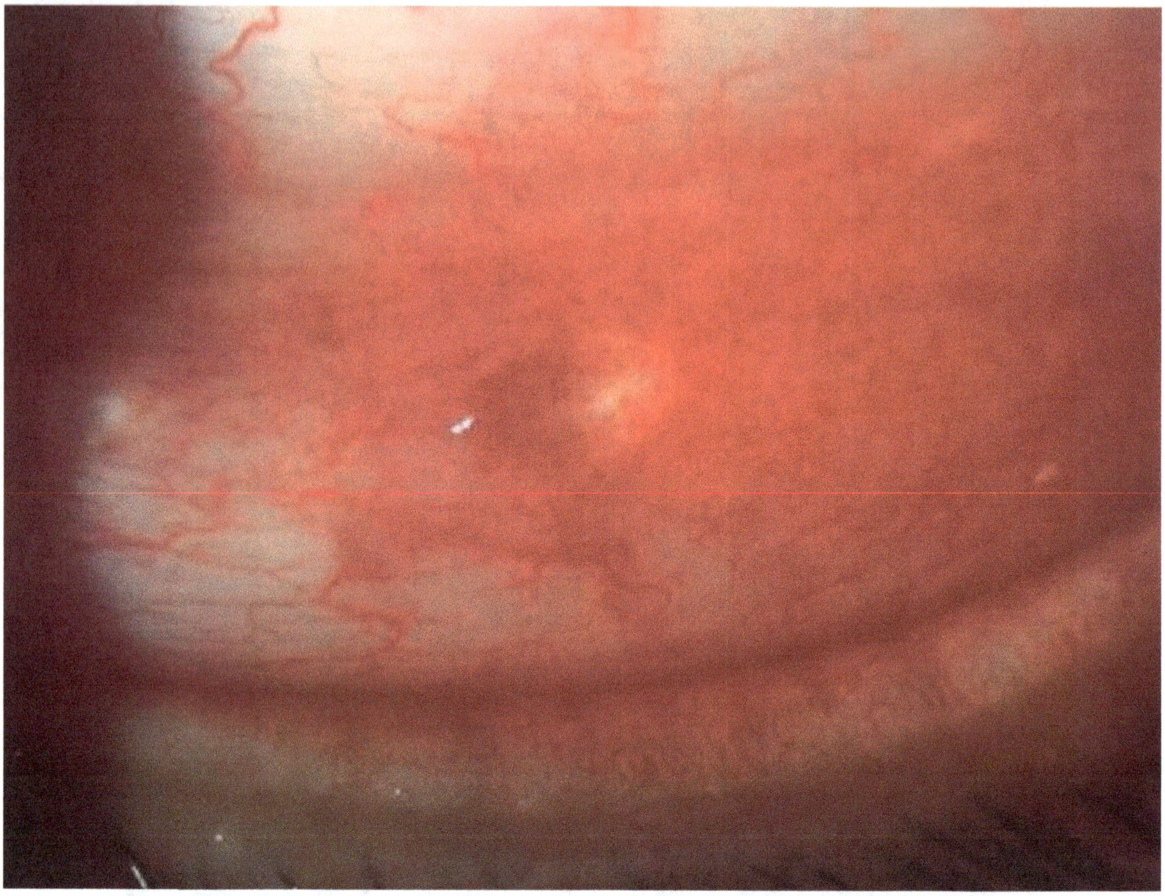

Lymphangiectasia is a rare condition that represents swelling of the conjunctiva caused by enlarged lymphatics. The exact cause is unknown; it can be a result of obstruction of the lymphatic ducts. Lymphangiectasia can cause tearing and ocular discomfort. Clinically, lymphangiectasia looks like irregular, dilated, and sausage-shaped channels (Fig 4, 5). The treatment is surgical excision (Meisler et al, 2003), but cryotherapy of the lesion is also described (Fraunfelder et al, 2009).

Conjunctival lymphoid tumors usually have an insidious onset; they represent asymptomatic, sharply demarcated masses that have salmon-pink coloring and an insidious onset (Shields et al, 2001). They are non-tender, nonulcerated, freely moveable, and often can be bilateral at presentation (6, 7). Patients should be evaluated for the presence of systemic disease. If evaluation reveals systemic lymphoma, systemic chemotherapy is indicated (Salepci et al, 2009).

Dermoids are bilateral and congenital lesions; they are mainly located on the inferotemporal limbal-corneal and epibulbar region (Elsas et al, 1975). Histologically, dermoids are solid, placoid tumors arising from the outer third of the cornea. They may contain hair, sebaceous glands, sweat glands, and/or fat lobules (Fig 8). The treatment includes surgically removal of the lesion. Dermoids that are incompletely excised can recur in the future.

Figure 4. Conjunctival lymphangiectasia

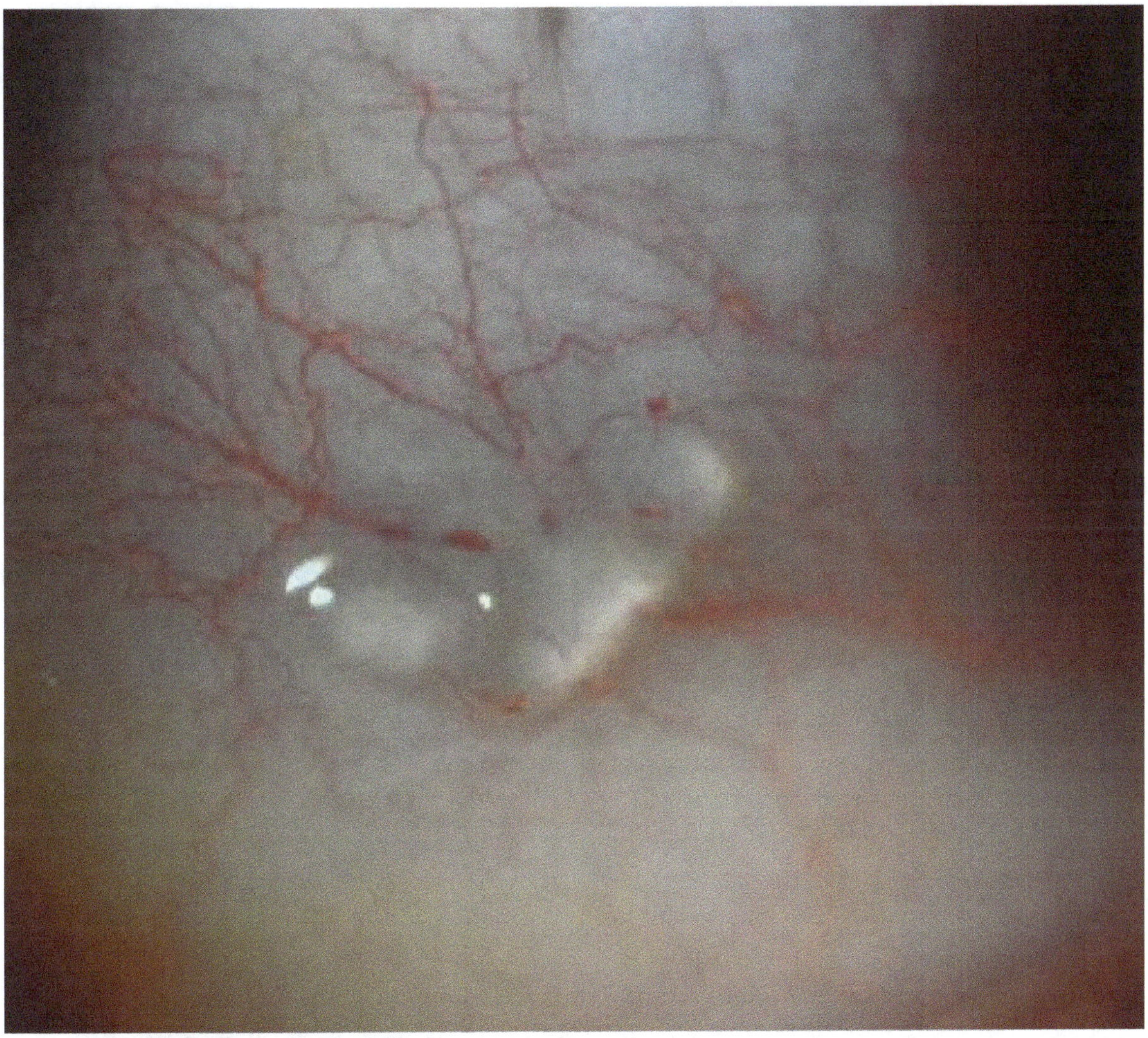

Figure 5. Multiple lymphangiectasias

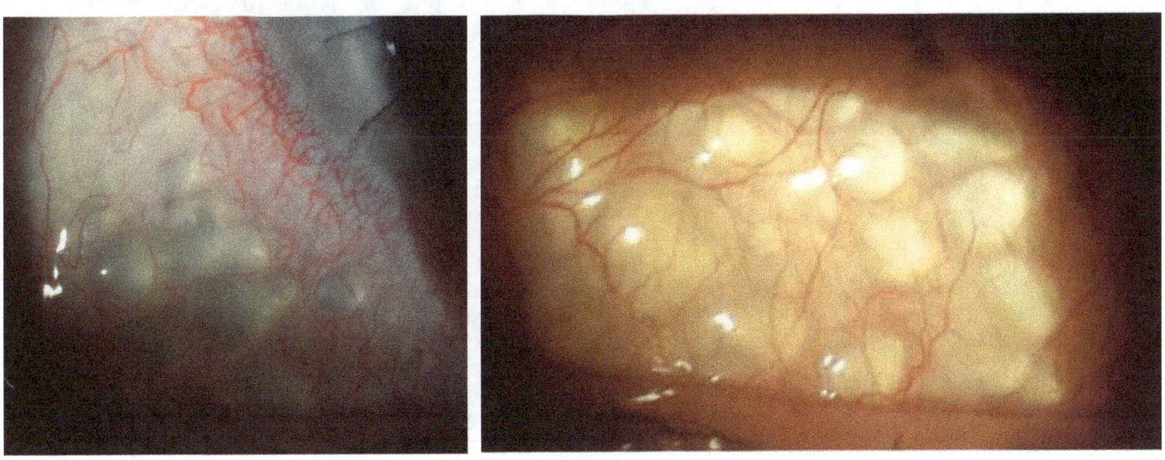

Figure 6. Patient with Non-Hodgkin lymphoma (NHL)

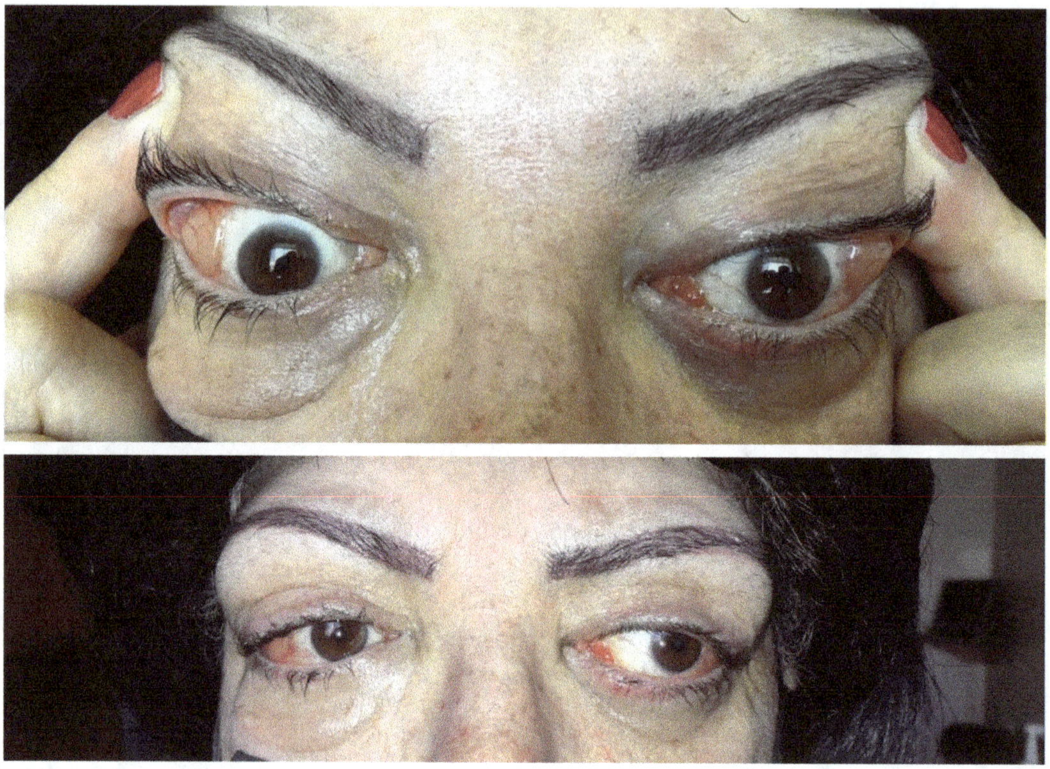

Figure 7. The same patient, close-up photo

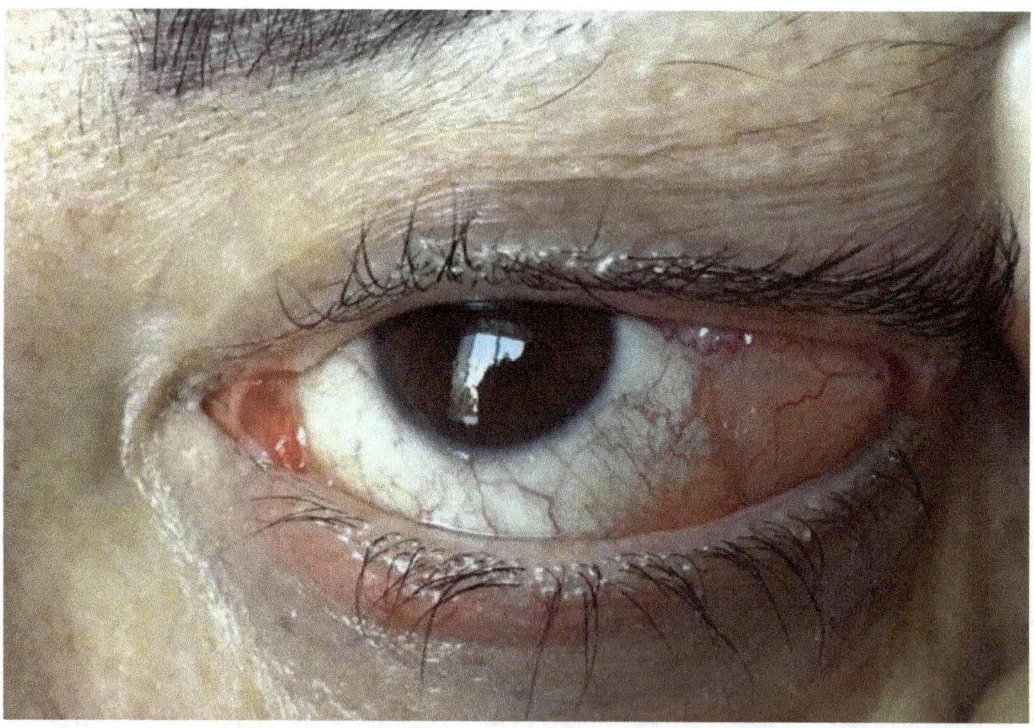

Figure 8. Dermoid. Growing hairs are on the surface

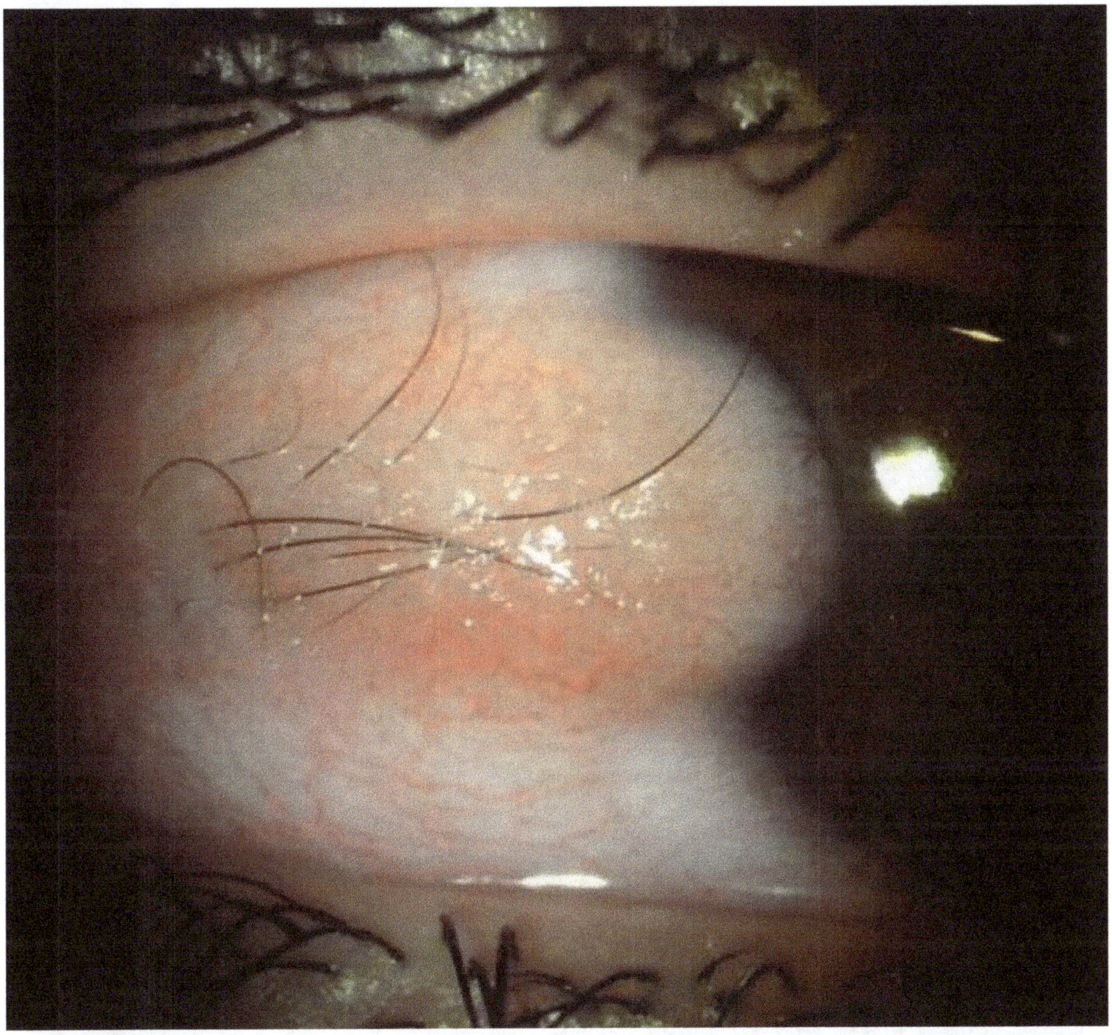

Goldenhar syndrome presents a version of the oculo-auriculo-vertebral sequence that includes malformation of the external ear, preauricular skin tags and pits, vertebral hypoplasia, micrognathia, and epibulbar dermoids (Fig 9,10). The presence of epibulbar dermoids is necessary for the confirmation of the diagnosis. It is usually unilateral, but it can occur bilaterally as well. Epibulbar dermoids are primarily located at the limbus inferotemporally (Baum et al, 1973) If desired, treatment is surgical excision. Main indications for the removal of epibulbar dermoids are continued growth and persistent irritation. Also, dermoids can be removed for cosmetic reasons in order to restore the normal ocular appearance (Kaufman et al, 1999).

Juvenile xanthogranuloma is a histiocytic proliferation that usually occurs among infants less than three years old. These non-neoplastic lesions almost always occur in the head and neck region and may also affect the eye, including the conjunctiva, the iris, and the ciliary body (Fig 11) (Roper et al, 1985). Treatment of ocular lesions includes steroids (Treacy et al, 1990), Bevacizumab injection (Ashkenazy et al, 2014) irradiation and surgery.

Figure 9. Goldenhar syndrome. You can see the epibulbar dermoid inferotemporall

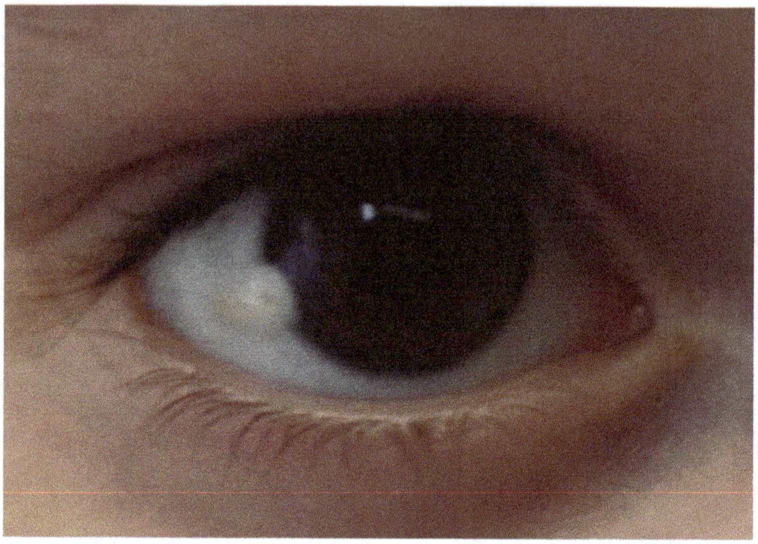

Figure 10. The same patient. Periauricular tag is seen (right photo)

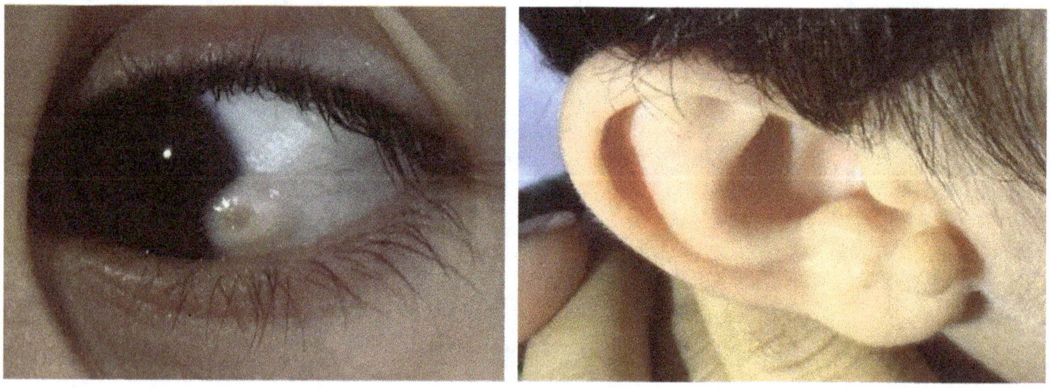

Figure 11. Presumed xanthogranuloma of the conjunctiva

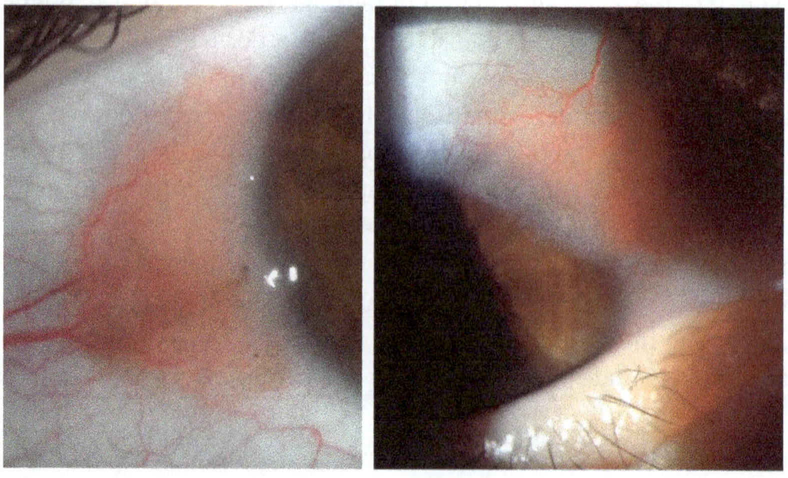

Figure 12. Presumed Rosai-Dorfman syndrome. The enlarged, fleshy conjunctival lesion is seen

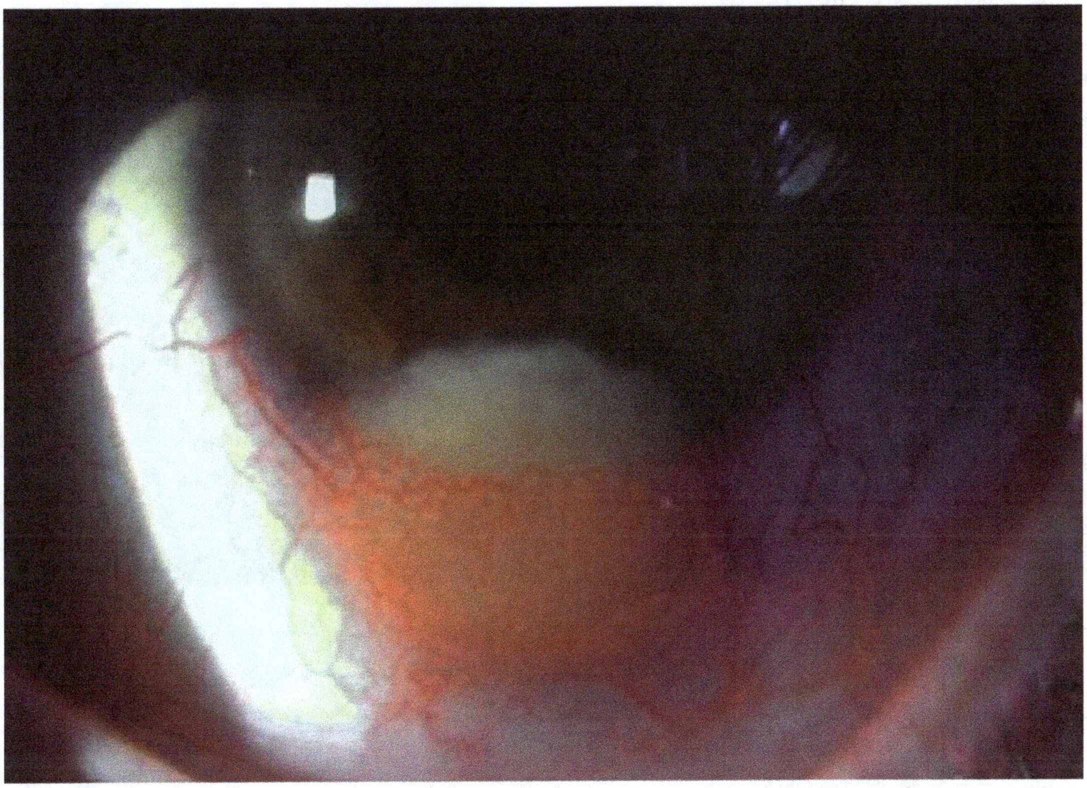

Rosai-Dorfman disease (RDD) is a rare, benign, histioproliferative disorder of unknown etiology. It is most frequently characterized by massive painless cervical lymphadenopathy (Ottaviano et al, 2006). Eye involvement is infrequent; mostly, the orbit or the eyelids are affected. Rarely, epibulbar masses are seen (Fig 12).

Conjunctival squamous papillomas may originate anywhere on the conjunctiva. Clinically, the lesions may be pedunculated and sessile. Lesions can appear solely, or they may multiply. In the case of multiple lesions, the infection is most likely indicative of human papillomavirus (Fig 13, 14, 15, 16) (McDonnell et al, 1987; Sjo et al, 2007; Buggage et al, 2002). Multiple regimens including α-interferon and mitomycin C have been tried with variable success. The most effective treatment is simple excision the base and surround of the lesion with cryotherapy (Muralidhar et al, 2009).

Conjunctival nevi are usually benign lesions that have variations in clinical and histopathological characteristics. The degree of pigmentation is variable in conjunctival nevi. Some nevi are entirely amelanotic. They may become more noticeable during puberty. Inclusions of conjunctival epithelium in the form of solid islands or cysts are usually observed (Hawkins et al, 1999). Management of conjunctival nevi includes observation and surgical resection (Shields et al, 2013).

Melanosis is a disorder that arises when excessive melanin production occurs together with the retention of pigment by epithelial melanocytes. This process does not elevate the conjunctival surface. Melanosis is classified as congenital (epithelial or subepithelial) or acquired (epithelial, primary, and secondary). Subepithelial congenital melanosis predisposes to the development of malignant melanoma not only in the conjunctiva, but also in other parts of the ocular system (Fig 21).

Figure 13. Conjunctival squamous papillomas. The same patient with 2 lesions; pedunculated (left photo) and sessile (right photo)

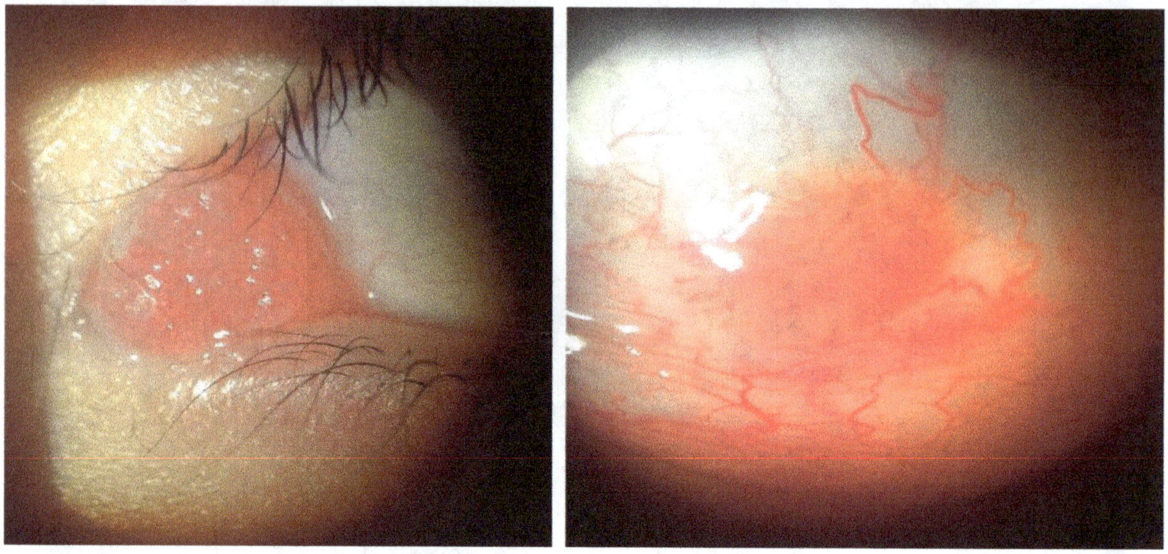

Figure 14. The same patient without slit lamp magnification

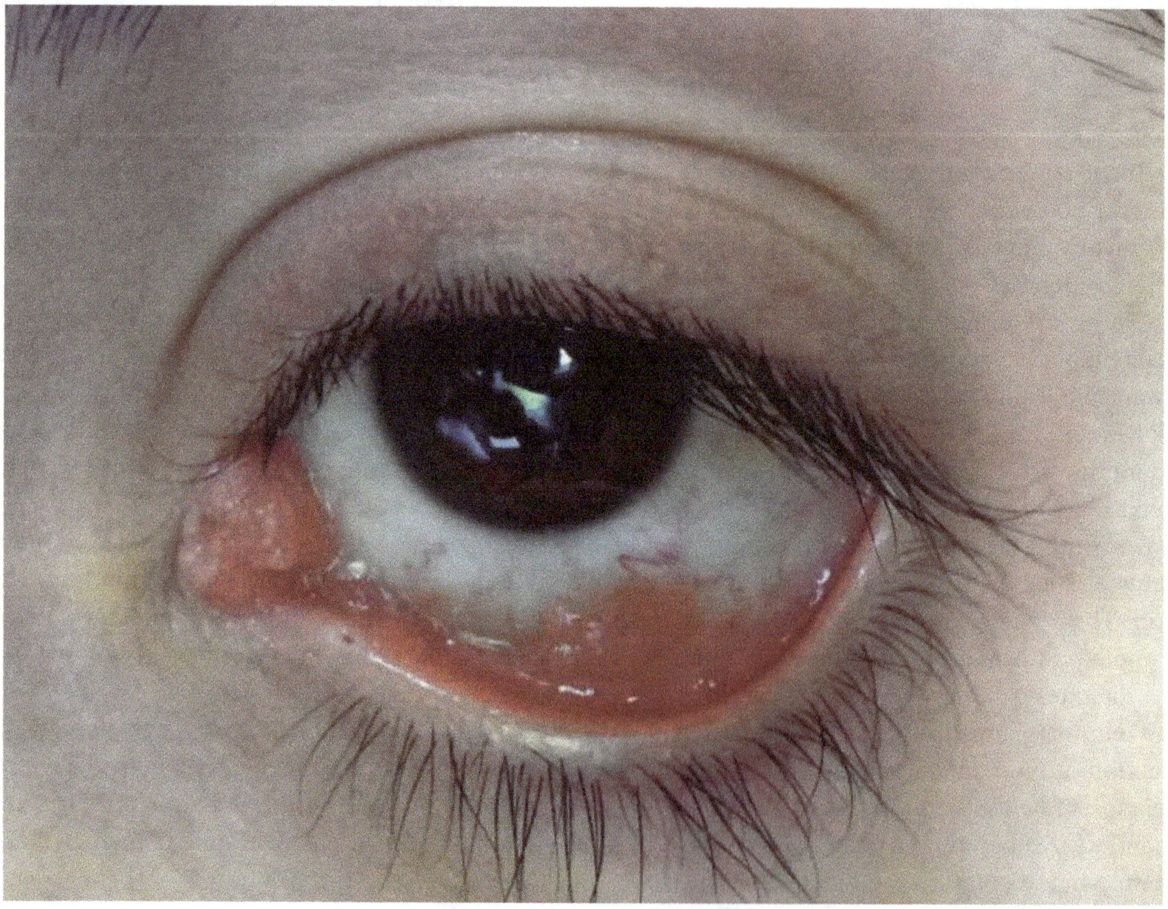

Figure 15. The same patient after 3 months of medical treatment with only Interferon alpha2B (1 MU/ml) dosage. No recurrences during 6 years of follow-up

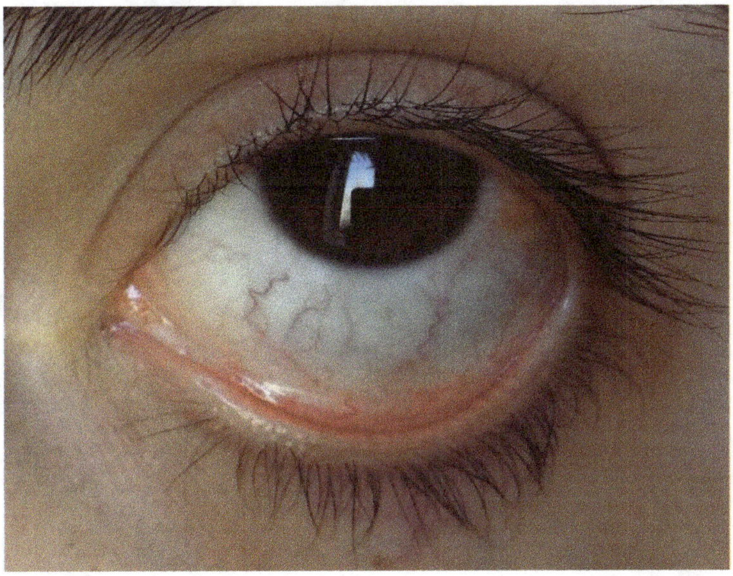

Figure 16. Angular papilloma mainly involving caruncle

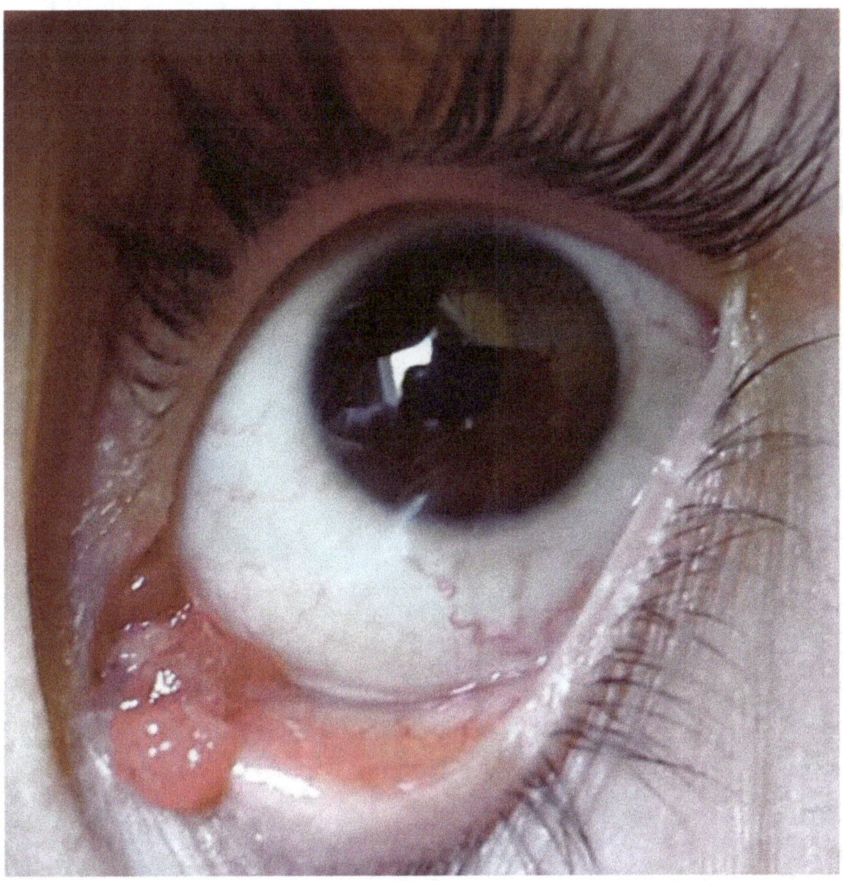

Figure 17. Conjunctival nevus. Small cysts within nevi are seen

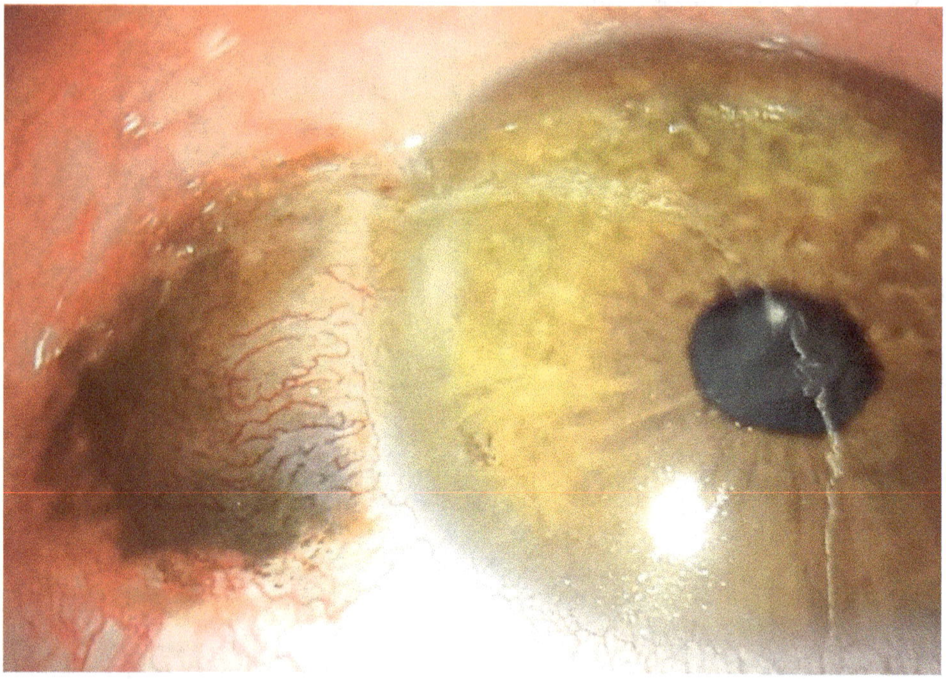

Figure 18. Conjunctival nevus with a variable degree of pigmentation

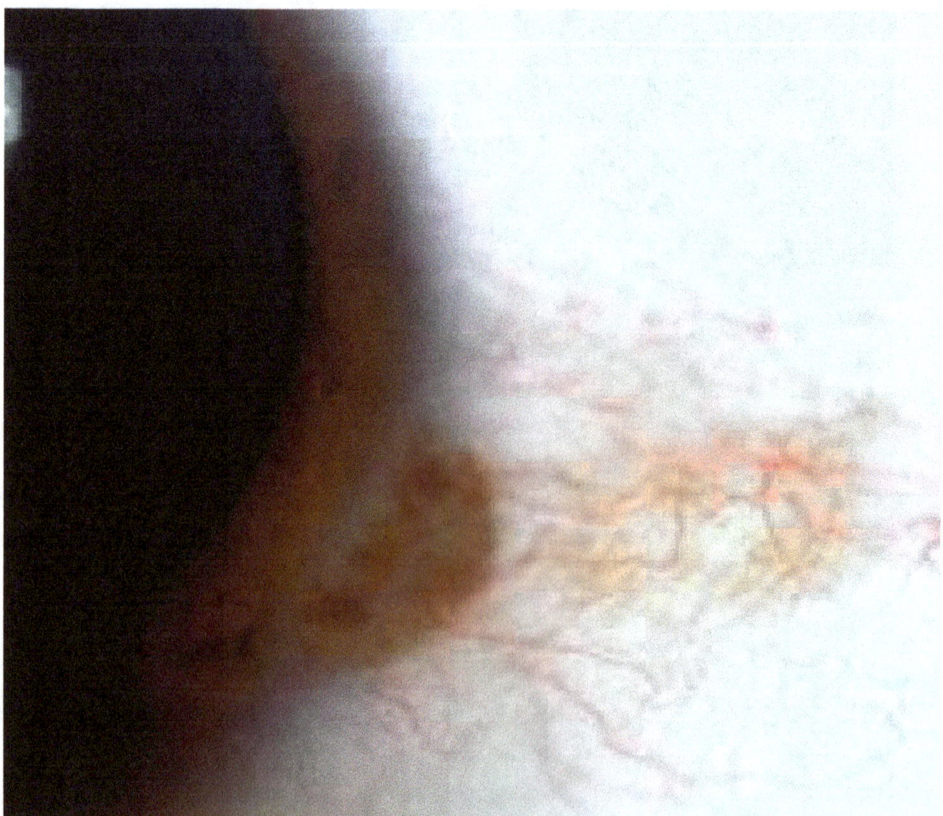

Figure 19. Caruncle nevus

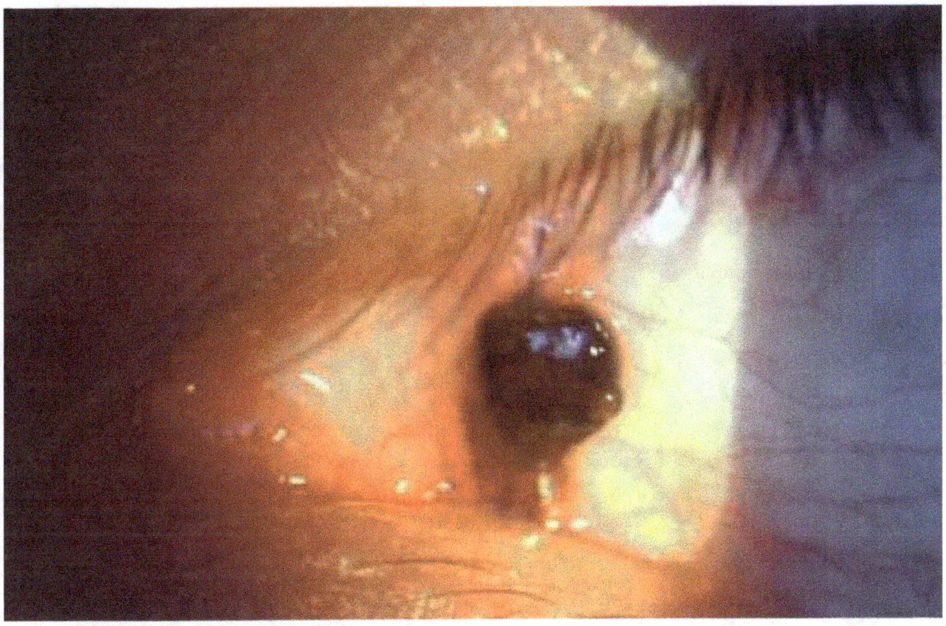

Figure 20. Presumed amelanotic nevus of conjunctiva

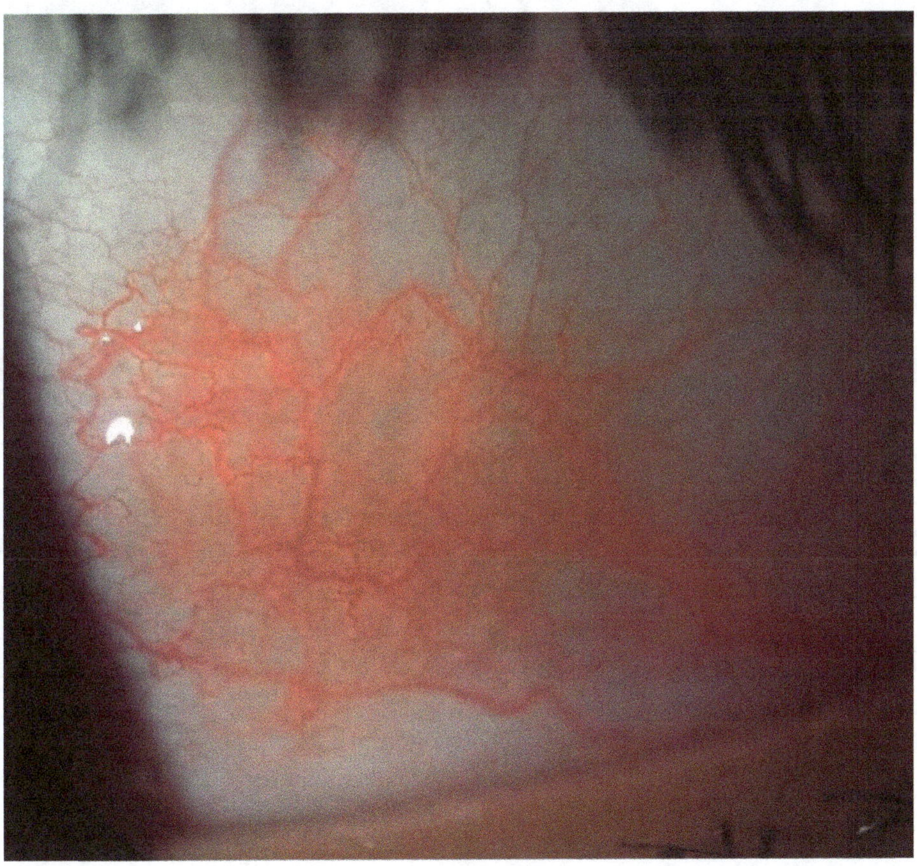

Figure 21. Congenital melanosis

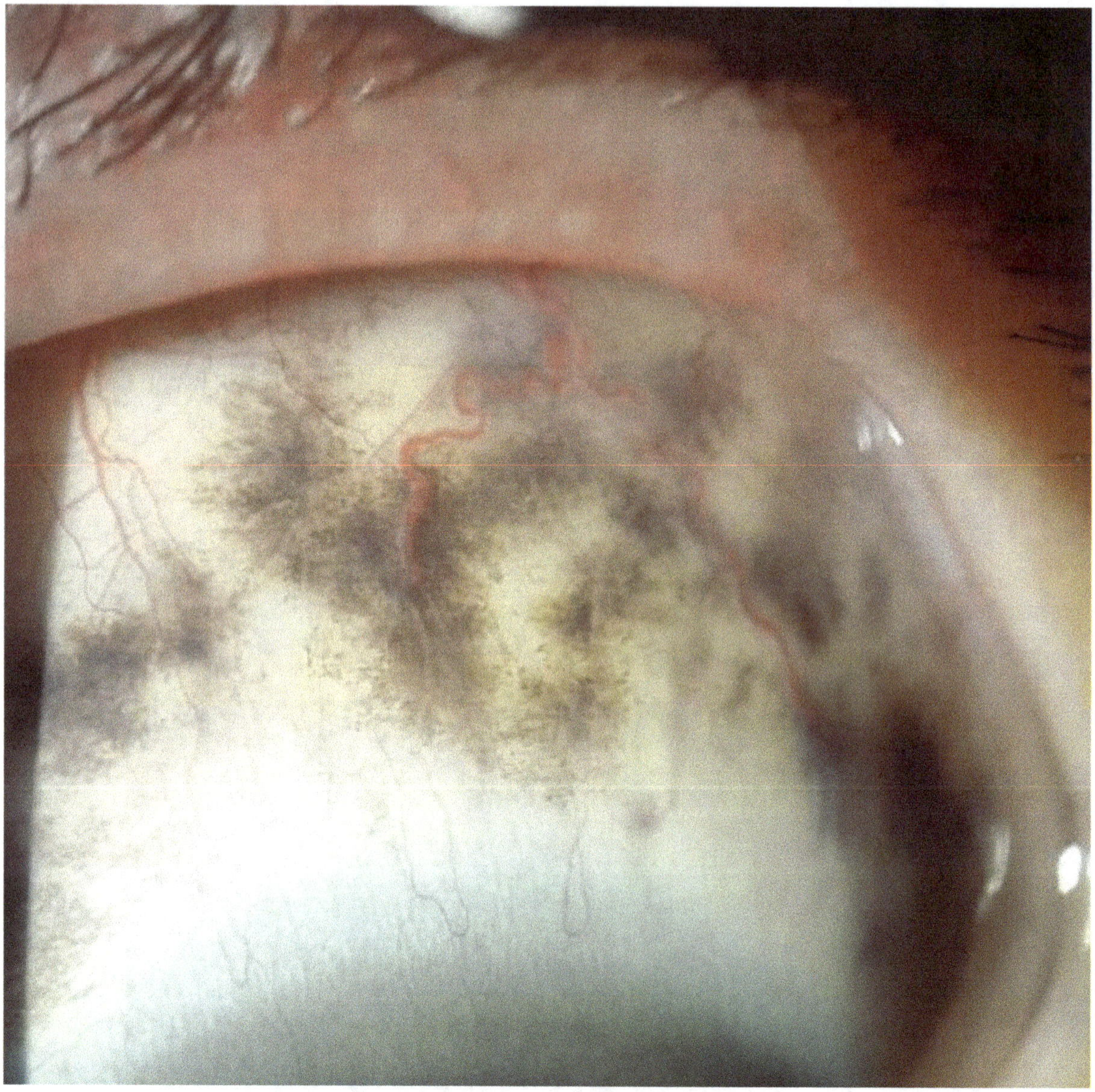

Primary acquired melanosis (PAM) is a neoplastic proliferation with the potential for malignancy within the conjunctival epithelium (Fig 22). It can progress to melanoma (Fig 23). This condition most often occurs as a unilateral lesion in middle-aged Caucasians (Folberg et al, 1986). All lesions, especially with high-risk histological features, should be completely resected, if applicable, without damaging the eye. Cryotherapy (Brownstein et al, 1981), mitomycin C (Chalasani et al, 2006) and interferon α-2b as extra therapy have also been used.

Conjunctival intraepithelial neoplasia (CIN) is a noninvasive neoplasia; it was previously named by terms like Bowen's disease, conjunctival squamous dysplasia, intraepithelial epithelioma, carcinoma in situ, and dyskeratosis. Usually, lesions occur at the limbal region, especially within the sun-exposed

Figure 22. Primary acquired melanosis. Granular, golden, brown pigmentation of the bulbar conjunctiva is seen

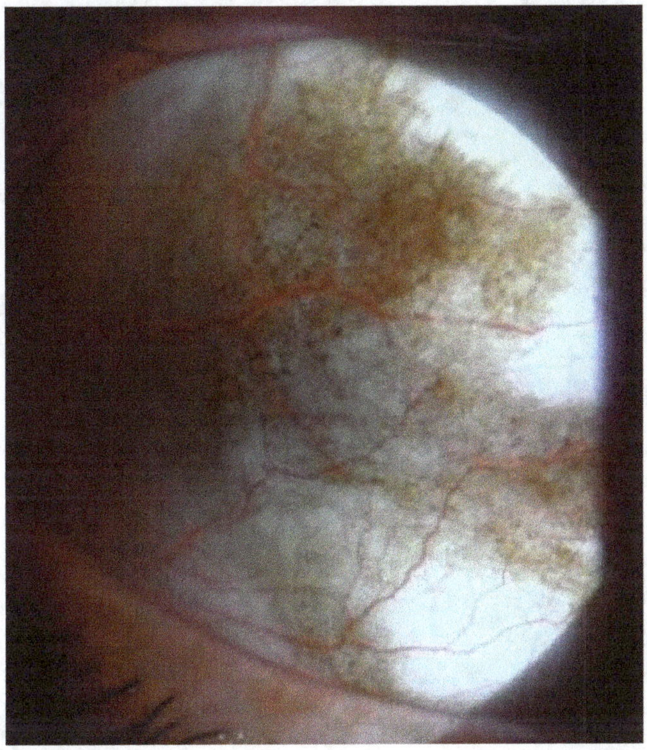

Figure 23. Corneolimbal melanoma

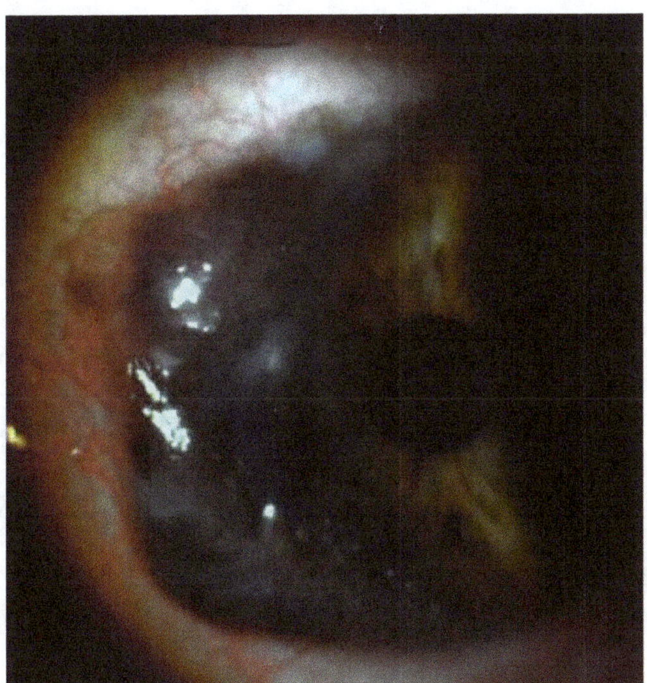

Figure 24. CIN

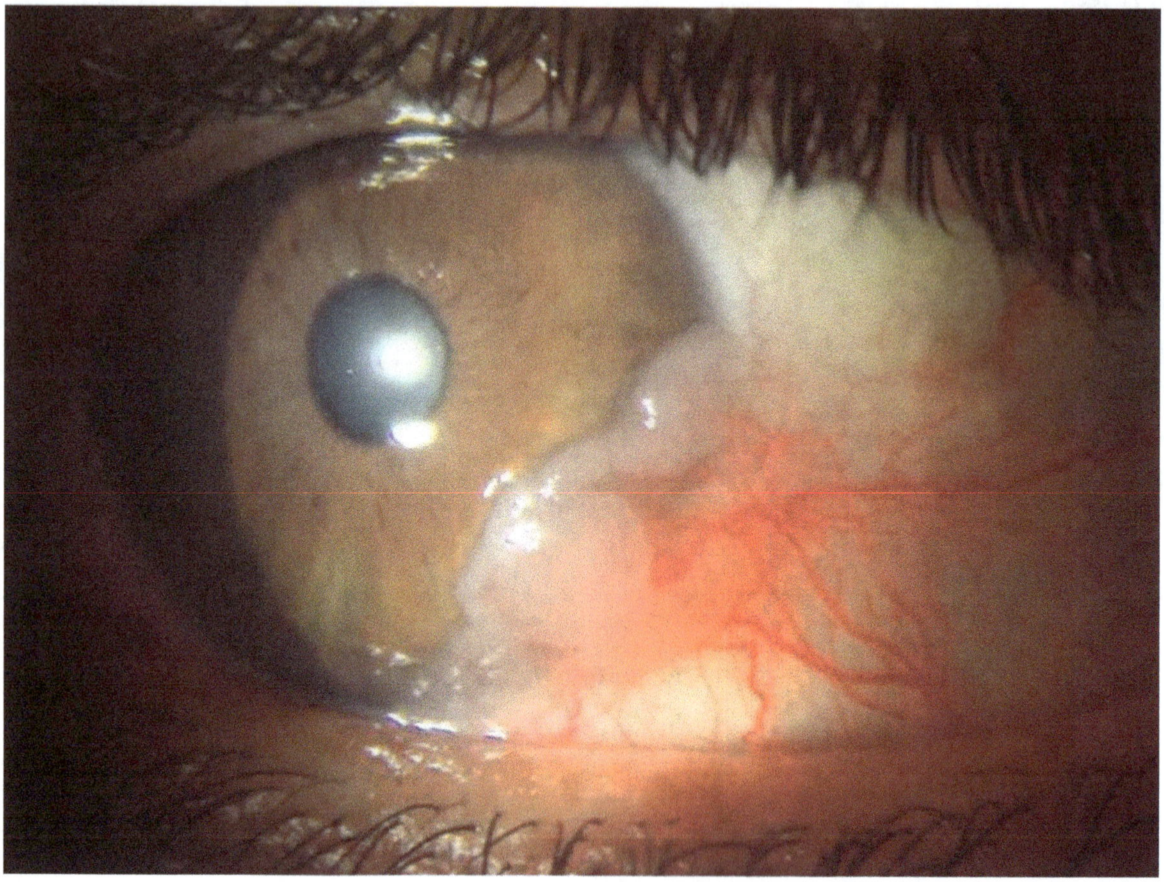

Figure 25. CIN (left eye) and the same eye 1-year post treatment (right eye). The treatment included surgical removal of the lesion with 4 months of topical chemotherapy with Interferon alfa2B (1 MU/ml) dosage (left photo)

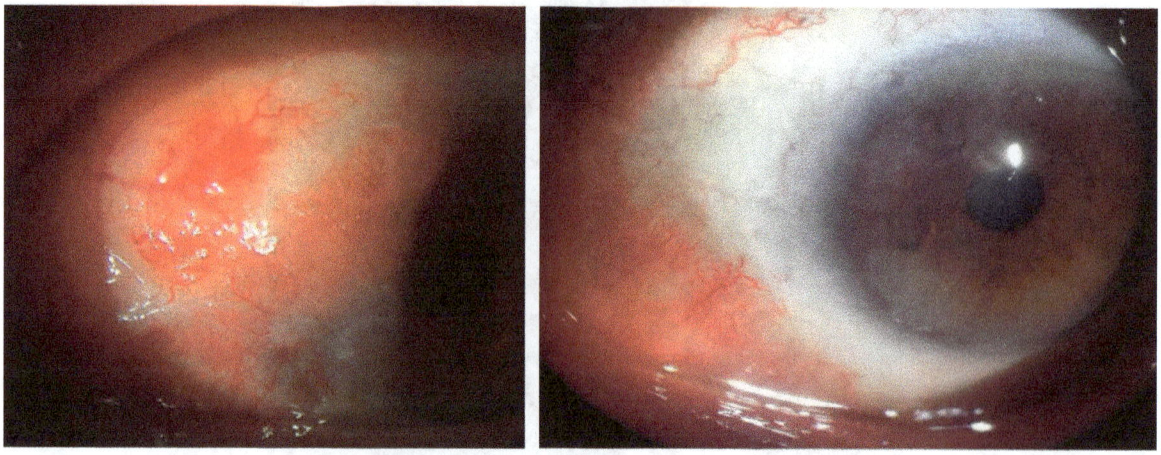

Figure 26. CIN of cornea, coast of Japan is seen (left photo) and the same eye after 2 months of medical treatment with topical Interferon alfa2B (1 MU/ml) dosage (right photo)

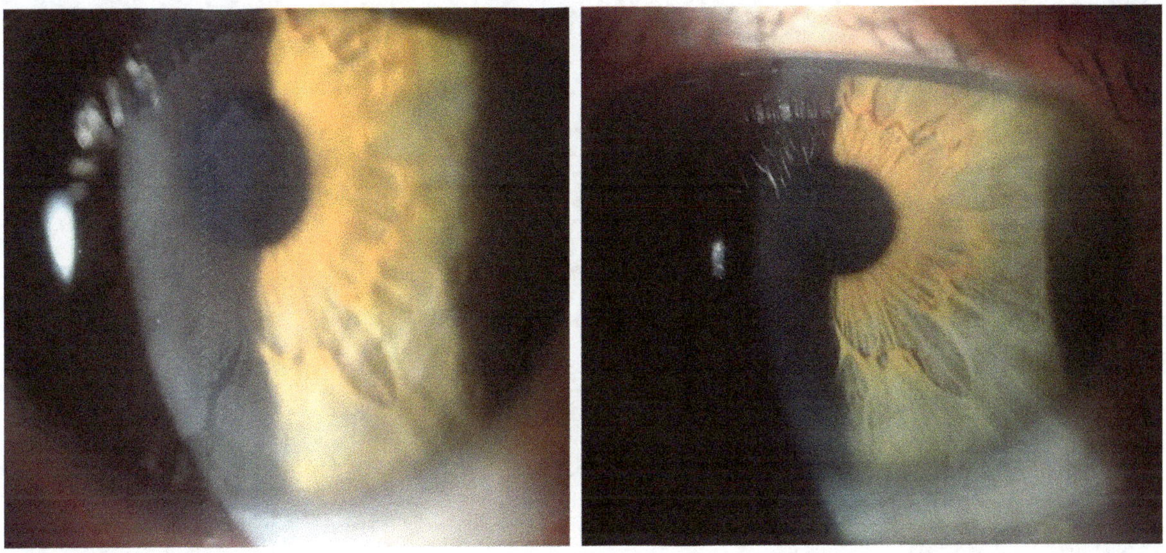

interpalpebral fissure. Clinically, the lesions are slow-growing tumefactions (Fig 24, 25). CIN lesions often spread from the adjacent limbus and involve the adjacent corneal surface, anterior to Bowman's layer. The abnormal epithelium has a frosted appearance with a fimbriated ("coast of Japan") margin (Fig 26). (Erie et al, 1986; Waring et al, 1984). Treatment includes surgical excision and topical chemotherapeutic agents. Topical mitomycin C, 5-flourouracil, or interferon alpha2B is helpful for the treatment of incompletely excised, recurrent or large lesions (Khong et al, 2006; Schechter et al, 2008; Nanji et al, 2014).

Adrenochrome deposits are usually found within the conjunctiva. These brown-black deposits occur in patients treated with epinephrine eye drops for a long period of time (Fig 27). Mascara can frequently accumulate in the conjunctival sac and mimic adrenochrome deposits (Fig 28). No treatment is required.

Concretions represent white to yellow spots and are found on the palpebral conjunctiva. They can develop because of chronic inflammation and are usually observed in elderly patients. This degeneration may be commonly seen in later stages of trachoma (Chumbley et al, 1988). Concretions are composed of mucopolysaccharide and mucin and may also contain calcium and cell debris (Fig 42, 43). If they are exposed and causing stinging and foreign body sensation, they can be easily removed for patient's comfort.

Xerosis represents metaplasia of the conjunctival epithelium from its normal columnar to a stratified squamous type. Vitamin A deficiency is one of the major causes of xeropthalmia. It leads to keratinizing metaplasia in mucosal surfaces throughout the body (29). Bitot spots are considered initial stages of vitamin A deficiency and represents tangles of keratin admixed with saprophytic bacteria and, sometimes, fungi (Rodger et al, 1963). Corynebacterium xerosis is often responsible for the typical "foamy" spots observed (Fig 30). Treatment includes massive systemic supplementation of vitamin A35. Surgical intervention is indicated when ulceration/perforation of cornea is observed. Amniotic membrane transplantation for corneal perforation in xerophthalmia has been shown to be effective with oral vitamin A supplementation as an alternative of corneal grafting (WY, 2003).

Figure 27. Adrenochrome deposits are seen

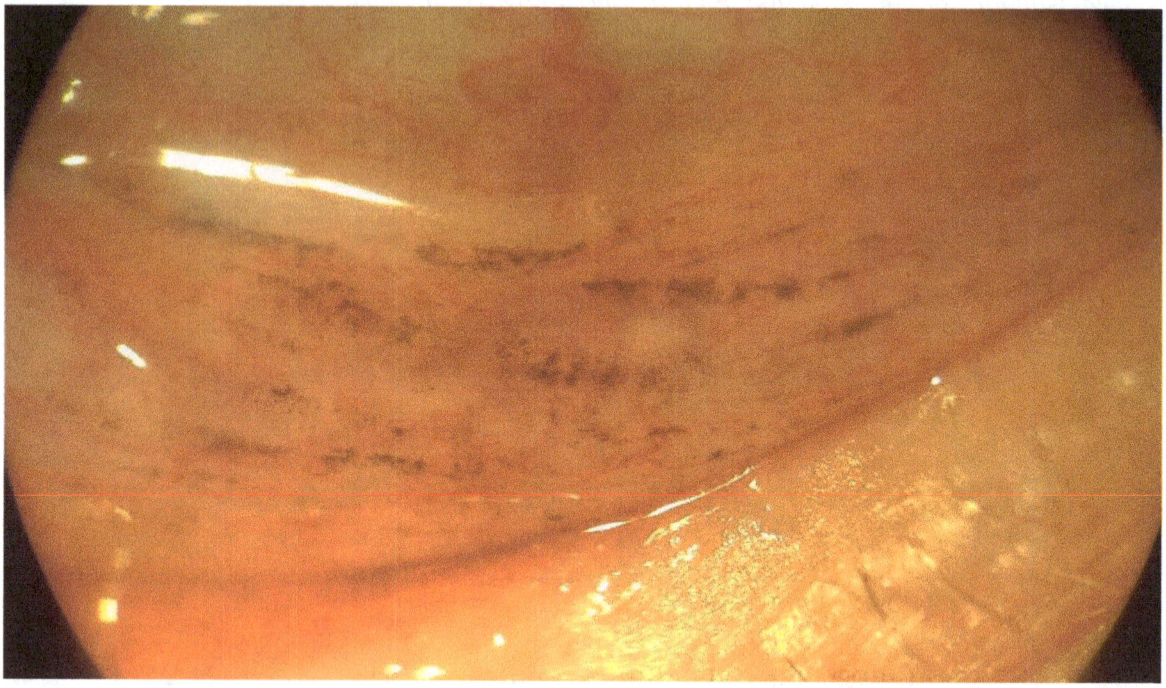

Figure 28. Deposits from mascara

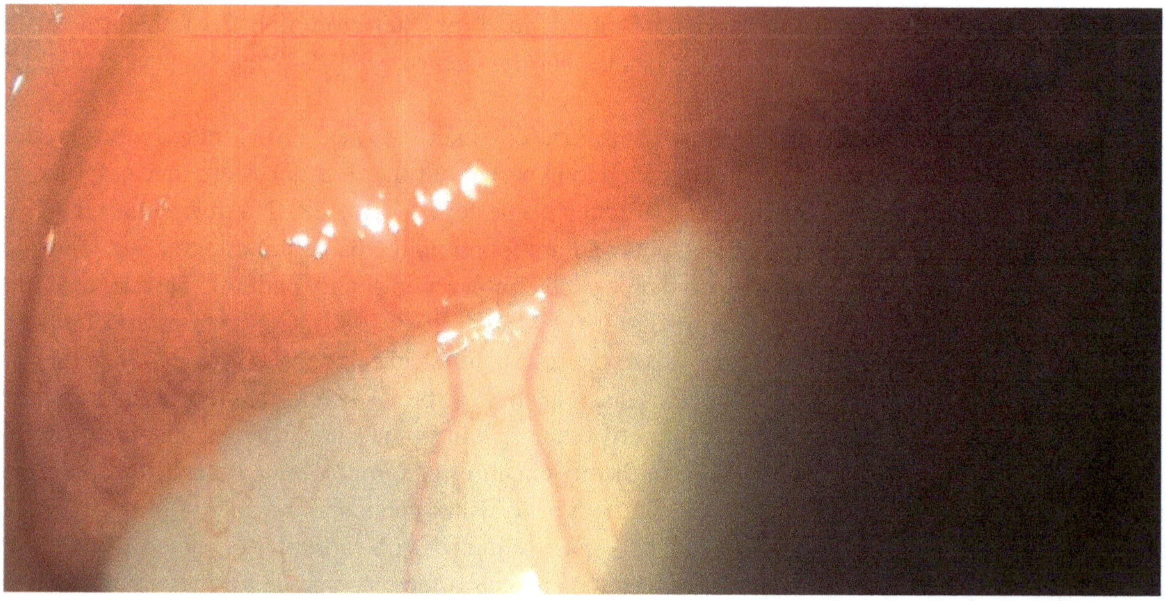

Figure 29. Xerosis of conjunctiva. Keratinized epithelium of lesion is seen

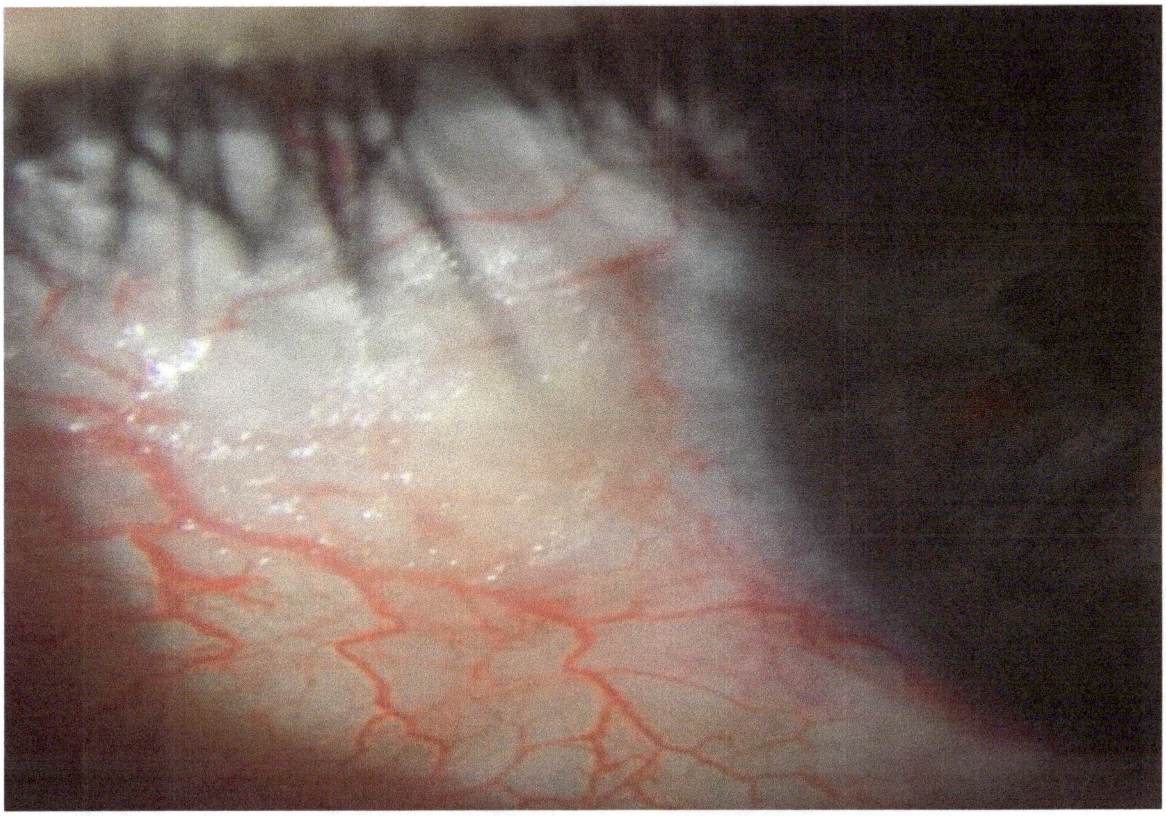

Figure 30. Bitot spots. The foamy appearance over the lesion is seen

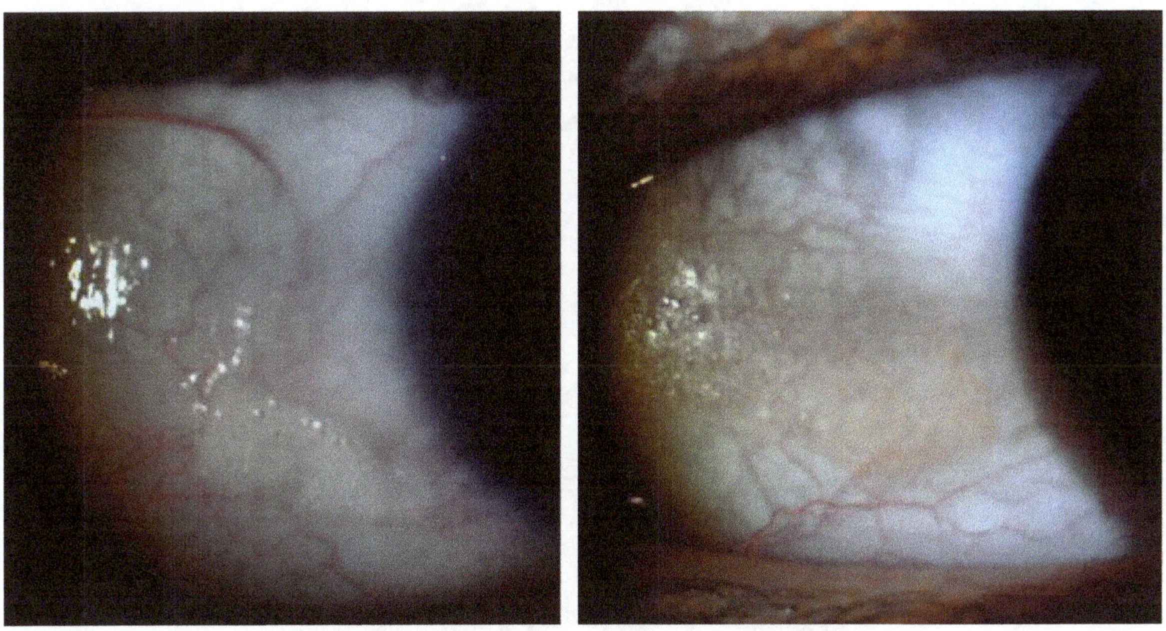

Figure 31. Xerophthalmia due to chemical injury

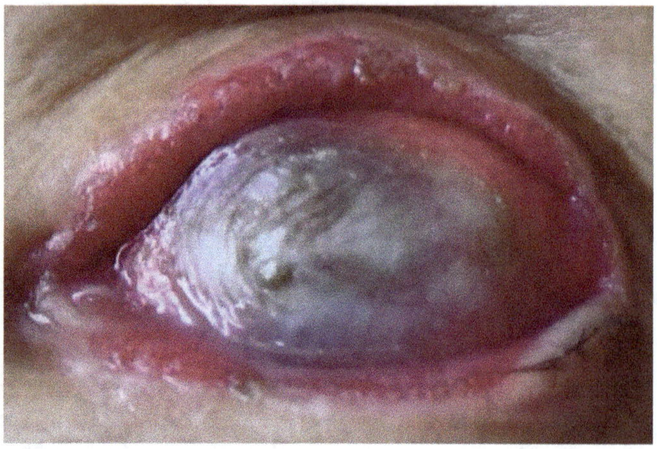

Figure 32. Patient with factitious conjunctivitis. Conjunctival hemorrhage or bleeding has never been revealed on examination. All systemic workup which can lead to this condition were negative. Photo was provided by patient when she was alone. It turned out that she was faking the condition by putting her finger blood in the eye

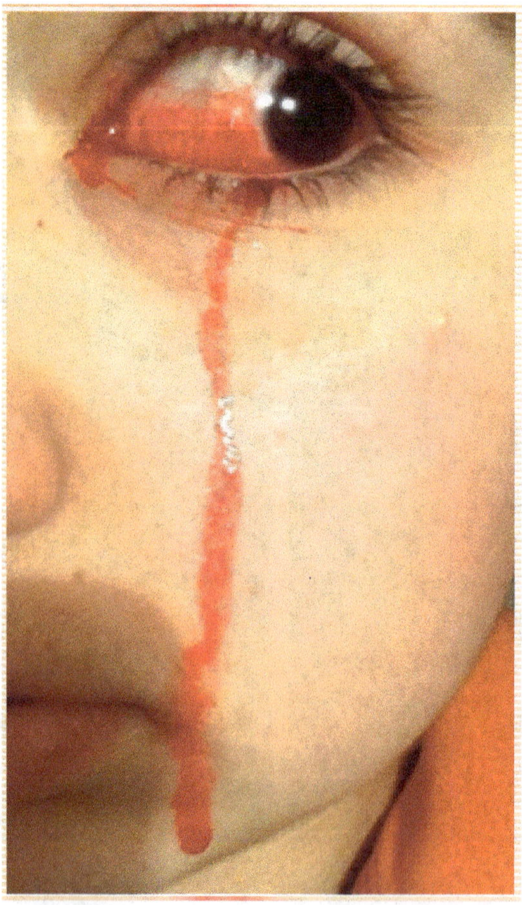

Figure 33. Patient imitates having crystal production when crying. It turned out later she was filling her conjunctival sack with shattered glass

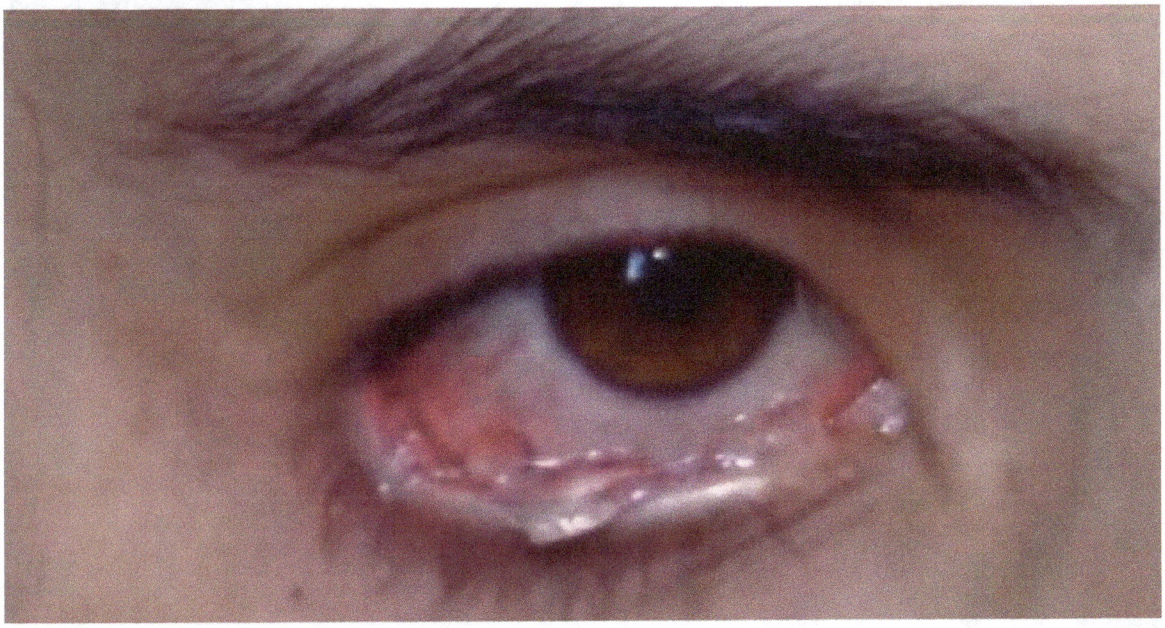

Self-inflicted (Factitious) Conjunctivitis is a factitious disorder in which a person repeatedly and deliberately represents signs and symptoms of diseases when he/she is not actually sick. It is associated with Munchhausen syndrome, which is considered a mental illness due to its association with serious emotional hardships. Patients may lie about or fake symptoms, hurt themselves to bring on symptoms, or even alter tests (Fig 32, 33) (Noel et al, 1987). Psychiatric referral should be considered in all cases, since various psychosocial stresses and internal conflicts are often present.

Atypical Observations for Reference

Figure 34. Prominent conjunctival vessels without any h/o underlying systemic or ocular disease

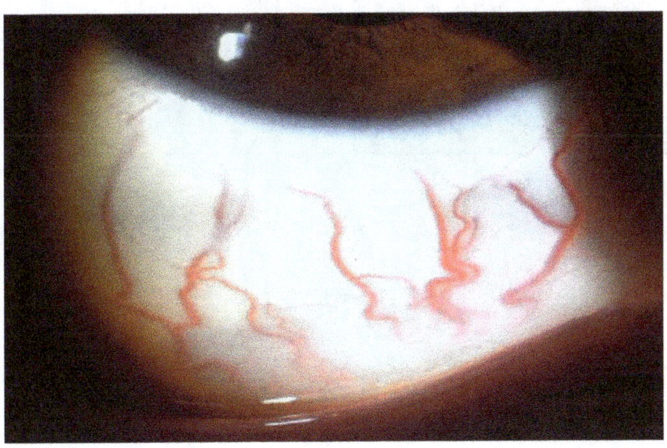

Figure 35. Additional layer of conjunctiva without any h/o ocular pathology

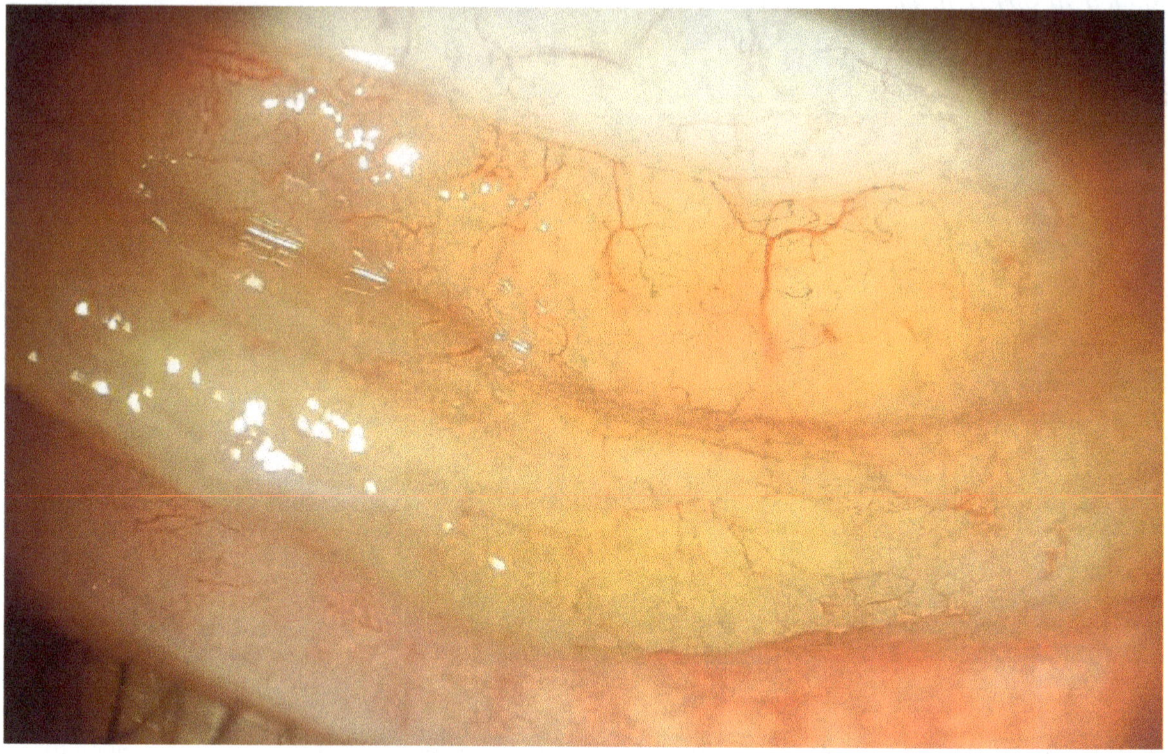

Figure 36. Additional caruncle with slit lamp (left photo) and without magnification (right photo)

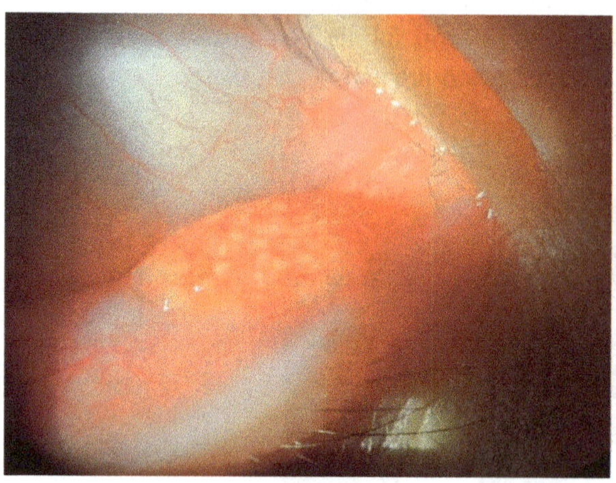

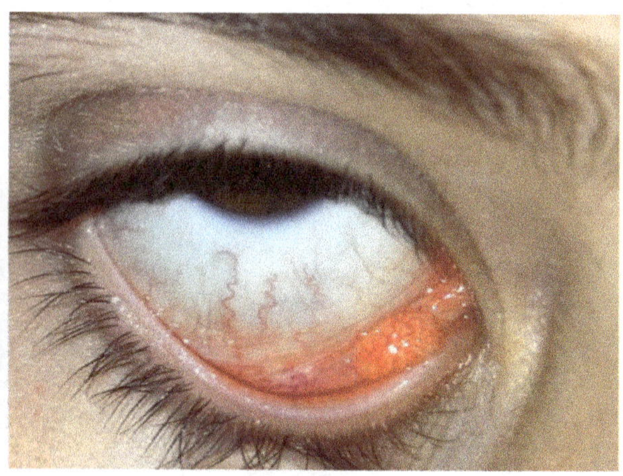

Conjunctival Degeneration

Pinguecula represents an elevated lesion on the conjunctiva, gray-white to yellow in color. It is usually located in the intrapalpebral zone, parallel to the limbus, in 3 and 9 o'clock positions. Pinguecula is usually bilateral and is more commonly found nasally than temporally (Fig 37) (Taylor et al, 1989). A Pinguecula is considered an elastotic degeneration and the cause is believed to be actinic, originating from UV radiation exposure. Asymptomatic patients do not require any treatment. Surgical excision can be performed if cosmetic appearance bothers the patient, although recurrence may occur.

Figure 37. Pingueculae. Elevated yellow masses are seen in the perilimbal nasal region

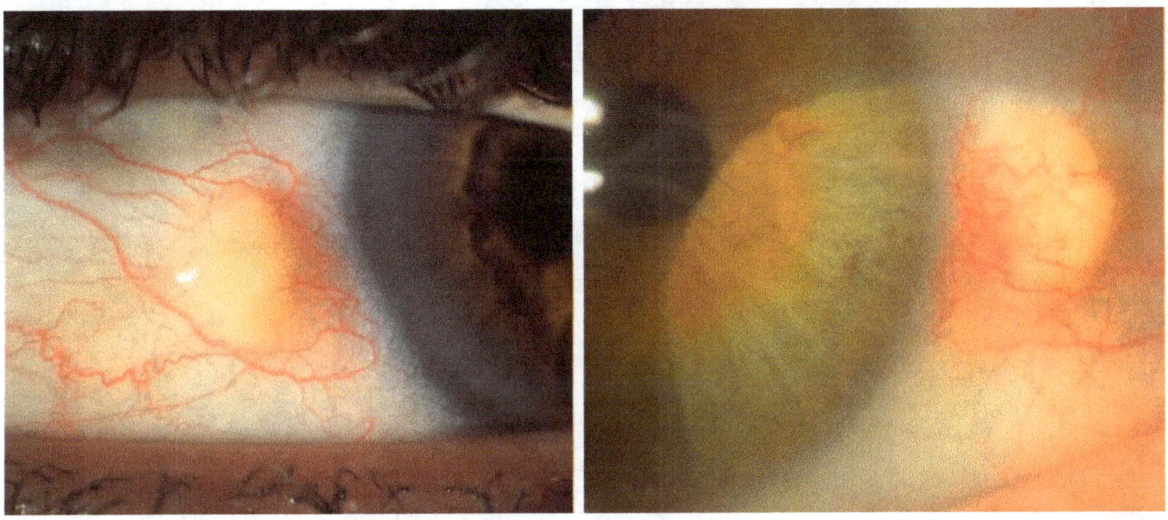

Pterygium is a winglike mass of fibrovascular tissue that extends from conjunctiva to the cornea. This lesion is highly vascular compared to pingueculae. Pterygia may arise from pingueculae, thus they are histologically similar (Coster et al, 1995). Pterygium is usually located in the interpalpebral fissure, in the horizontal meridian, often nasally than temporally (Fig 38, 39). A true pterygium should be differentiated from pseudopterygium, which may occur after trauma or inflammatory cornea disease (Fig 40, 41). The management of pterygium is surgical excision. Techniques vary from the simplest procedure of bare sclera excision to the more complex and extensive conjunctiva and sub-Tenon's excisions coupled with large conjunctiva autografts. Recurrence is the most common cause of pterygium surgery failure, and recurrence rates vary widely from 0% to 89% depending on the techniques used (Prabhasawat et al, 1997).

Figure 38. Pterygium. The fibrovascular winglike tissue is seen

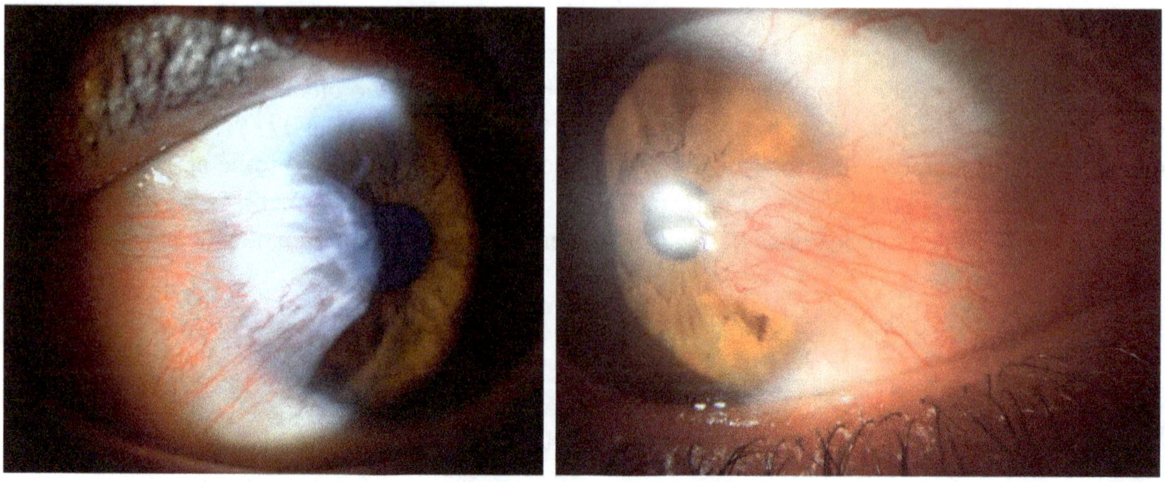

Figure 39. Advanced pterygium reaching to pupillary region

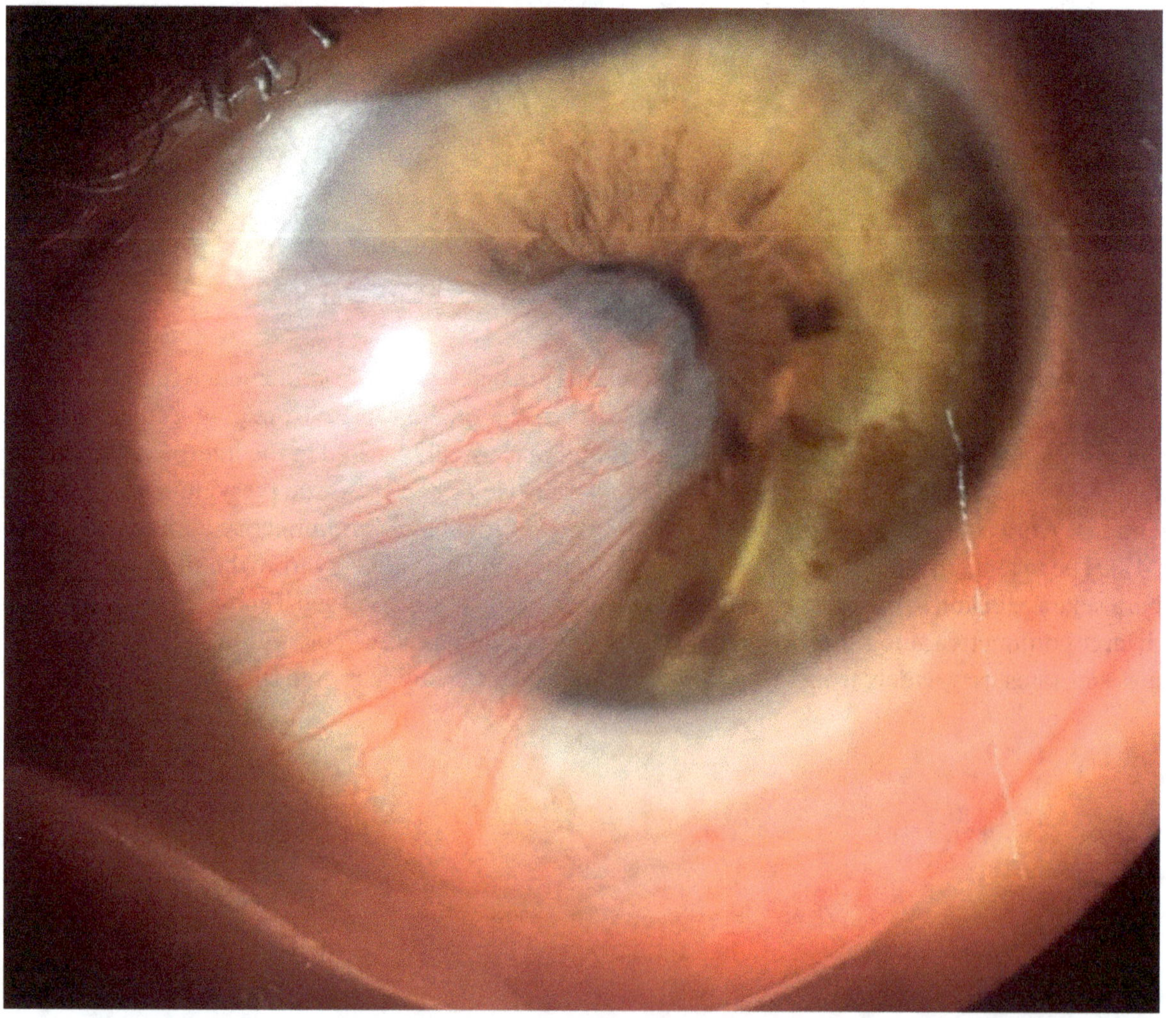

Figure 40. Pseudopterygium, developed after chemical injury, located temporally

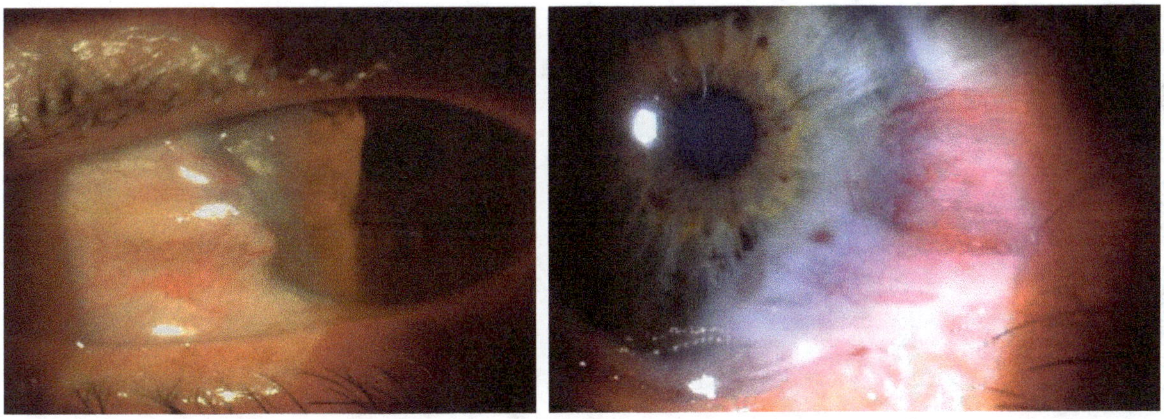

Figure 41. Temporal Pseudopterygium under slit lamp (right photo) and without magnification (left photo)

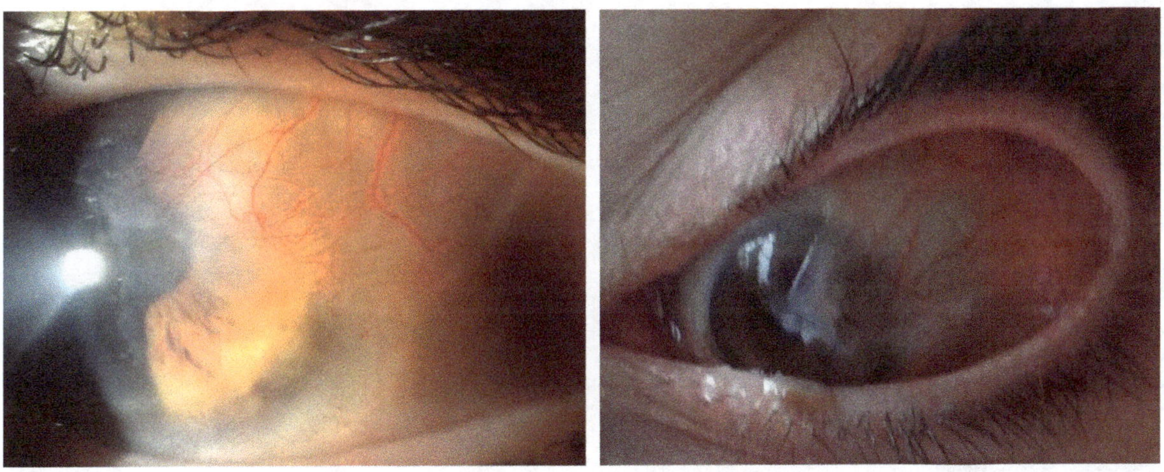

Figure 42. Multiple concretions on the upper tarsal conjunctiva

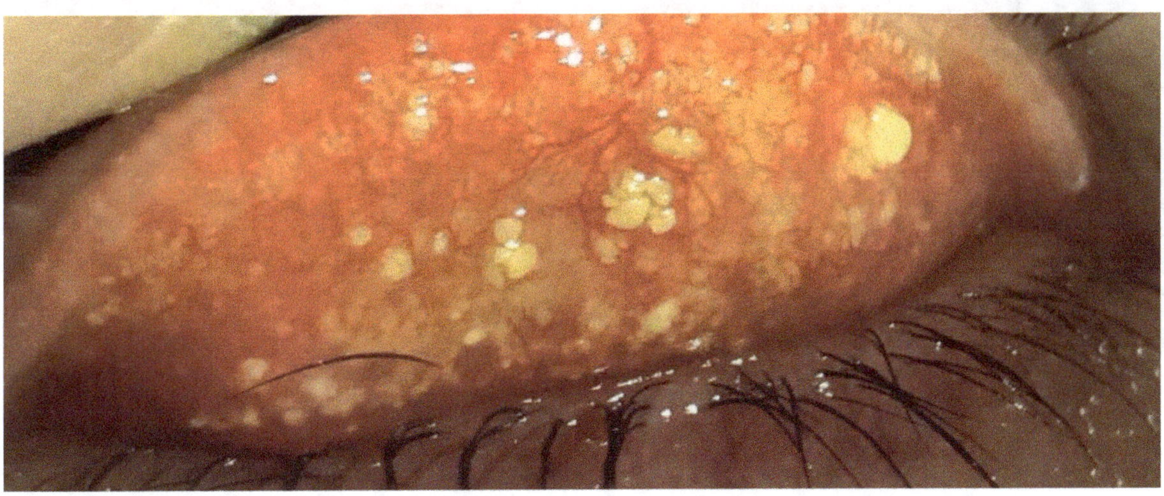

Figure 43. Concretions. The right and left eyes of the same patient

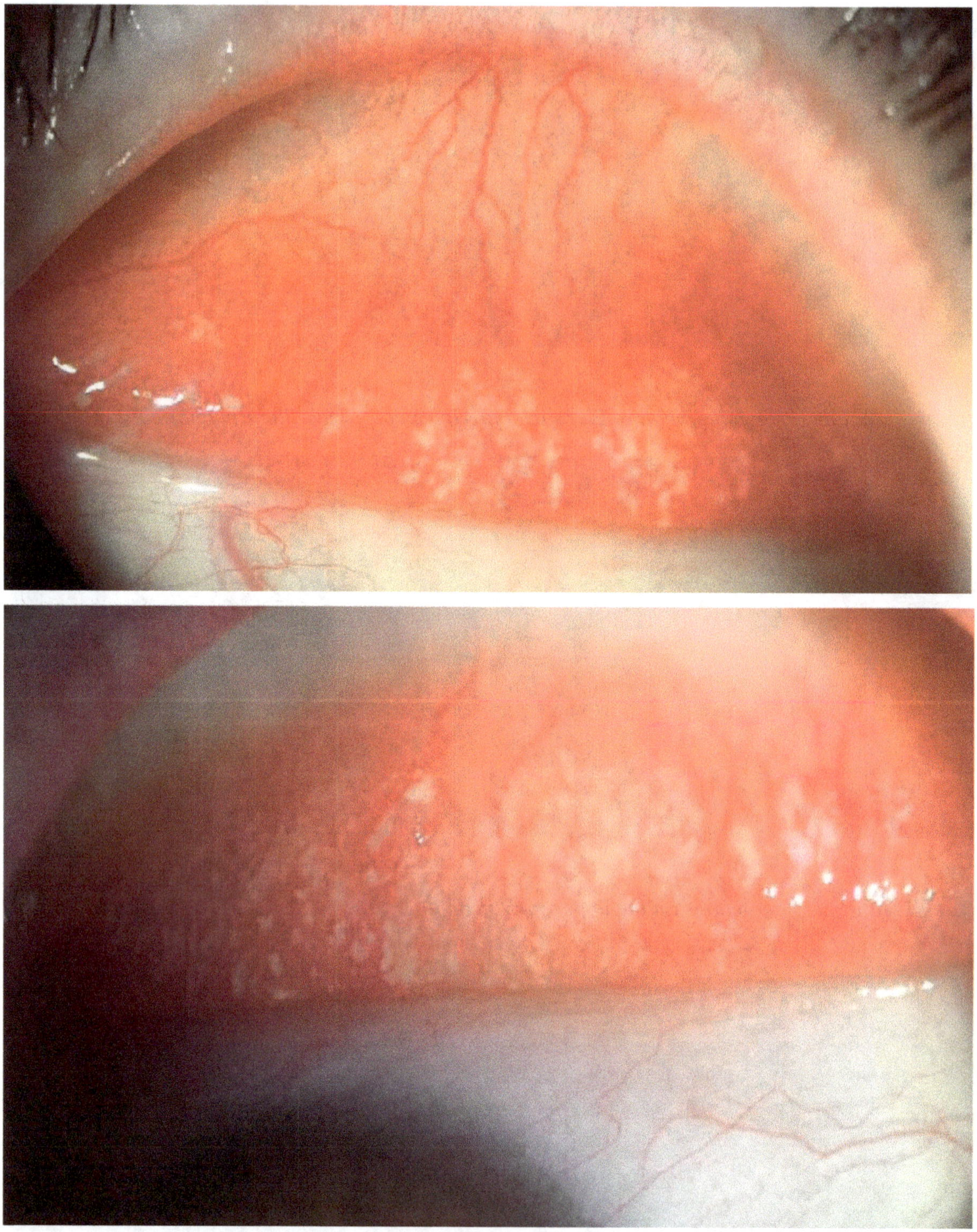

REFERENCES

Ashkenazy, N., Henry, C. R., & Abbey, A. M. (2014). Successful treatmenet of juvenile xanthogranuloma using bevacizumab. *Journal of AAPOS*, *18*, 295–297.

Baum, J. L., & Feingold, M. (1973). Ocular aspects of Goldenhar's syndrome. *American Journal of Ophthalmology*, *25*(2), 250–257.

Boynton, J. R., Searl, S. S., & Ferry, A. P. (1992). Primary nonkeratinized epithelial ('conjunctival') orbital cysts. *Archives of Ophthalmology*, *110*(9), 1238–1242. doi:10.1001/archopht.1992.01080210056024 PMID:1381579

Brownstein, S., Jakobiec, F. A., & Wilkinson, R. D. (1981). Cryotherapy for precancerous melanosis (atypical melanocytic hyperplasia) of the conjunctiva. *Archives of Ophthalmology*, *99*(7), 1224–1231.

Buggage, R. R., Smith, J. A., & Shen, D. (2002). Conjunctival papillomas caused by human papillomavirus type 33. *Archives of Ophthalmology*, *120*(2), 202–204.

Chalasani, R., Giblin, M., & Conway, R. M. (2006). Role of topical chemotherapy for primary acquired melanosis and malignant melanoma of the conjunctiva and cornea: Review of the evidence and recommendations for treatment. *Clinical & Experimental Ophthalmology*, *34*(7), 708–714.

Chumbley, L. C. (1988). Herbert's pits and lid secretions: An important association. *Eye (London, England)*, *2*, 476–477.

Coster, D. (1995). Pterygium–an ophthalmic enigma. *The British Journal of Ophthalmology*, *79*(4), 304–305.

Elsas, F. J., & Green, W. R. (1975). Epibulbar tumors in childhood. *American Journal of Ophthalmology*, *79*, 1001.

Erie, J. C., Campbell, R. J., & Liesegang, T. J. (1986). Conjunctival and corneal intraepithelial and invasive neoplasia. *Ophthalmology*, *93*(2), 176–183.

Folberg, R., Jakobiec, F. A., & Bernardino, V. B. (1989). Benign conjunctival melanocytic lesions. Clinicopathologic features. *Ophthalmology*, *96*(4), 436–461.

Folberg, R., & McLean, I. W. (1986). Primary acquired melanosis and melanoma of the conjunctiva: Terminology, classification, and biologic behavior. *Human Pathology*, *17*(7), 652–654.

Fraunfelder, F. W. (2009). Liquid nitrogen cryotherapy of conjunctival lymphangiectasia: A case series. *Archives of Ophthalmology*, *127*(12), 1686–1687. doi:10.1001/archophthalmol.2009.306 PMID:20008729

Hawkins, A. S., Yu, J., & Hamming, N. A. (1999). Treatment of recurrent conjunctival papillomatosis with mitomycin C. *American Journal of Ophthalmology*, *128*(5), 638–640.

Hirst, L. W. (2012). Recurrence and complications after 1000 surgeries using pterygium extended removal followed by extended conjunctival transplant. *Ophthalmology*, *119*(11), 2205–2210.

Hughes, W. L. (1942). Conjunctivochalasis. *American Journal of Ophthalmology*, *25*(1), 48–51. doi:10.1016/S0002-9394(42)93297-5

Jan, J. E., Good, W. V., & Freeman, R. D. (1994). Eye-poking. *Developmental Medicine and Child Neurology*, *36*(4), 321–325.

Kaufman, A., Medow, N., & Phillips, R. (1999). Treatment of epibulbar limbal dermoids. *Journal of Pediatric Ophthalmology and Strabismus*, *36*, 136–140.

Khong, J. J., & Muecke, J. (2006). Complications of mitomycin C therapy in 100 eyes with ocular surface neoplasia. *The British Journal of Ophthalmology*, *90*(7), 819–822.

Kobayashi, A., & Sugiyama, K. (2005). Visualization of conjunctival cyst using Healon V and trypan blue. *Cornea*, *24*(6), 759–760. doi:10.1097/01.ico.0000154238.87230.05 PMID:16015101

McDonnell, P. J., McDonnell, J. M., & Kessis, T. (1987). Detection of human papillomavirus type 6/11 DNA in conjunctival papillomas by in situ hybridization with radioactive probes. *Human Pathology*, *18*(11), 1115.

Meisler, D. M., Eiferman, R. A., Ratliff, N. B., & Burns, C. D. (2003). Surgical management of conjunctival lymphangiectasis by conjunctival resection. *American Journal of Ophthalmology*, *136*(4), 735–736. doi:10.1016/S0002-9394(03)00398-2 PMID:14516817

Muralidhar, R., Sudan, R., & Bajaj, M. S. (2009). Topical interferon alpha-2b as an adjunctive therapy in recurrent conjunctival papilloma. *International Ophthalmology*, *29*(1), 61–62.

Nanji, A. A., Moon, C. S., & Galor, A. (2014). Surgical versus medical treatment of ocular surface squamous neoplasia: A comparison of recurrences and complications. *Ophthalmology*, *121*(5), 994–1000.

Noel, L. P., & Clarke, W. N. (1982). Self-inflicted ocular injuries in children. *American Journal of Ophthalmology*, *94*, 630–633.

Otaka, I., & Kyu, N. (2000). A new surgical technique for management of conjunctivochalasis. *American Journal of Ophthalmology*, *129*(3), 385–387. doi:10.1016/S0002-9394(99)00384-0 PMID:10704560

Ottaviano, G., Doro, D., & Marioni, G. (2006). Extranodal Rosai-Dorfman disease: Involvement of eye, nose and trachea. *Acta Oto-Laryngologica*, *126*(6), 657–660.

Paton, D., & McLaren, D. S. (1960). Bitot's spots. *American Journal of Ophthalmology*, *50*, 568–574.

Prabhasawat, P., Barton, K., & Burkett, G. (1997). Comparison of conjunctival autografts, amniotic membrane grafts, and primary closure for pterygium excision. *Ophthalmology*, *104*(6), 974–985.

Rodger, F. C., Saiduzzafar, H., & Grover, A. D. (1963). A reappraisal of the ocular lesion known as Bitot's spots. *British Journal of Nutrition*, *17*, 475–485.

Roper, S. S., & Spraker, M. K. (1985). Cutaneous histiocytosis syndromes. *Pediatric Dermatology*, *3*, 19.

Salepci, Seker, & E Kurnaz. (2009). Conjunctival malt lymphoma successfully treated with single agent rituximab therapy. *Leukemia Research*, *33*, e10–e13.

Schechter, B. A., Koreishi, A. F., & Karp, C. L. (2008). Long-term follow-up of conjunctival and corneal intraepithelial neoplasia treated with topical interferon alfa-2b. *Ophthalmology*, *115*(8), 1291–1296.

Shields, C. L., Regillo, A. C., & Mellen, P. L. (2013). Giant conjunctival nevus: Clinical features and natural course in 32 cases. *JAMA Ophthalmology*, *131*(7), 857–863.

Shields, C. L., Shields, J. A., Carvalho, C., Rundle, P., & Smith, A. F. (2001). Conjunctival lymphoid tumors: Clinical analysis of 117 cases and relationship to systemic lymphoma. *Ophthalmology*, *108*(5), 979–984. doi:10.1016/S0161-6420(01)00547-4 PMID:11320031

Shields, J. A., Shields, C. L., & Luminais, S. (2003). Differentiation of pigmented conjunctival squamous cell carcinoma from melanoma. *Ophthalmic Surgery, Lasers & Imaging*, *34*(5), 406–408.

Sjo, N. C., von Buchwald, C., & Cassonnet, P. (2007). Human papillomavirus in normal conjunctival tissue and in conjunctival papilloma: Types and frequencies in a large series. *The British Journal of Ophthalmology*, *91*(8), 1014–1015.

Sommer, A., Muhilal, H., & Tarwatjo, I. (1982). Treatment of xerophthalmia. *Archives of Ophthalmology*, *100*, 785–787.

Su, W. Y., Chang, S. W., & Huang, S. F. (2003). Amniotic membrane transplantation for corneal perforation related to vitamin A deficiency. *Ophthalm Surg Las Imag.*, *34*, 140–144.

Taylor, H. R., West, S. K., & Rosenthal, F. S. (1989). Corneal changes associated with chronic UV irradiation. *Archives of Ophthalmology*, *107*, 1481–1484.

Treacy, K. W., Letson, R. D., & Summers, C. G. (1990). Subconjunctival steroid in the management of uveal juvenile xanthogranuloma: A case report. *Journal of Pediatric Ophthalmology and Strabismus*, *27*, 126.

Waring, G. O. III, Roth, A. M., & Ekins, M. B. (1984). Clinical and pathologic description of 17 cases of corneal intraepithelial neoplasia. *American Journal of Ophthalmology*, *97*(5), 547–559.

Young, A. L., Ho, M., & Jhanji, V. (2013). Ten-year results of a randomized controlled trial comparing 0.02% mitomycin C and limbal conjunctival autograft in pterygium surgery. *Ophthalmology*, *120*(12), 2390–2395.

Chapter 5
Corneal Ulcers (Infectious Keratitis)

ABSTRACT

Microbial keratitis is an infectious process that occurs due to the proliferation of microorganisms (bacteria, fungi, viruses, and parasites) and associated inflammation and tissue destruction. Smears and cultures are indicated for the isolation of microorganisms and for making the correct diagnosis and immediate initiation of antimicrobial therapy, especially in cases where corneal infiltrate is chronic, large, deep, or atypical. Microbial keratitis is considered a vision-threatening ocular emergency. Therefore, this chapter, which consists of almost all cases studied before and after treatment, highlights the importance of early recognition, isolation of specific microorganisms, and sensitivity-based therapy. Also, the evaluation of these cases helps to show the appearance of the eye after the therapeutic treatment and demonstrates the emergency of immediate surgery to save the eyeball in cases where medical treatment is ineffective. The authors have summarized the treatment options they have used for bacterial, fungal, acanthamoeba, and herpetic keratitis cases.

INTRODUCTION

Bacterial Keratitis

A wide variety of pathogens can cause bacterial keratitis. Predisposing factors include trauma, contact lens wear, surgery, ocular surface disease, systemic disease, and immunosuppression (Wilhelmus et al, 1987). These may alter the defense mechanisms of the ocular surface, thus making it possible for the infection to invade the cornea. According to AAO, the most common Gram-positive organisms are Staphylococcus aureus, Streptococcus pneumoniae and viridians group, Propionibacterium species, Mycobacterium species and Gram-negative isolates are Pseudomonas aeruginosa, Serratia marcescens, Proteus mirabilis, Enteric gram-negative bacilli, Moraxella species and Haemophilus influenzae and other Haemophilus species.

DOI: 10.4018/978-1-7998-6937-5.ch005

In all our cases, cultures and smears were studied at SIRMED Diagnostic Medical Center with a VITEK 2 Compact, Automated ID/AST instrument. We have always started the initial treatment with broad spectrum antibiotic drops before the results of the cultures were received. In cases with huge epithelial defect, Chloramphenicol 0.5% eye drops were used as it's a very friendly medication for the epithelium. We have always prescribed cycloplegic/mydriatic drops and oral Doxycycline for 3-4 weeks (100mg bid for 2 weeks, followed by 100mg qd) depending on the size of the epithelial defect and the corneal melt/stromal lysis. Antibiotic ointment has always been prescribed at bedtime. In most cases we have injected Betamethasone sub-Tenon (0.2-0.3 ml) initially after 7 days of sensitivity-based antibiotic treatment and have repeated after 5-7 days with increased dose (0.5-0.7ml) upon response. We have never prescribed oral steroids to avoid possible systemic complications. After total epithelization of the ulcer, mild steroid drops were added 3-4 times a day. Later, after scar formation, stronger steroids (Dexamethasone 0.1%, Prednisolone acetate 1% with tapering in 6-8 weeks) and Vit C orally (500mg bid for 2 months) were prescribed so the patient is left with as mild fibrosis as possible. In cases with severe thinning (70-90%) with pending perforation or already microperforation, amniotic membrane transplantation was performed to enhance the healing process and obtain time until donor cornea (we used to receive from US from Corneagen Eye bank) arrives in case transplant surgery becomes absolutely necessary to save the eyeball.

Staphylococcus is the most common Gram-positive organism and is present in normal ocular flora. Staphylococcus aureus produces progressive corneal infiltration, usually associated with endothelial plaque and moderate or severe (hypopyon) anterior chamber reaction (Fig 1,2,3) (Lichtinger et al, 2012).

Figure 1. Corneal infiltrate and hypopyon are seen

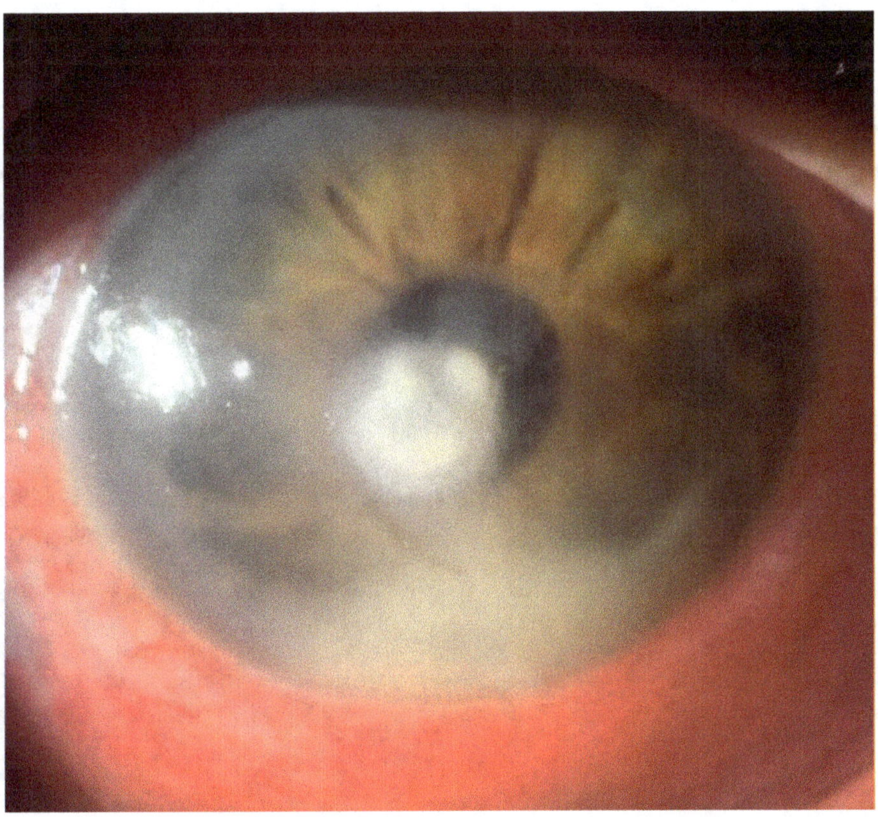

Figure 2. Dense stromal infiltrate with treatment

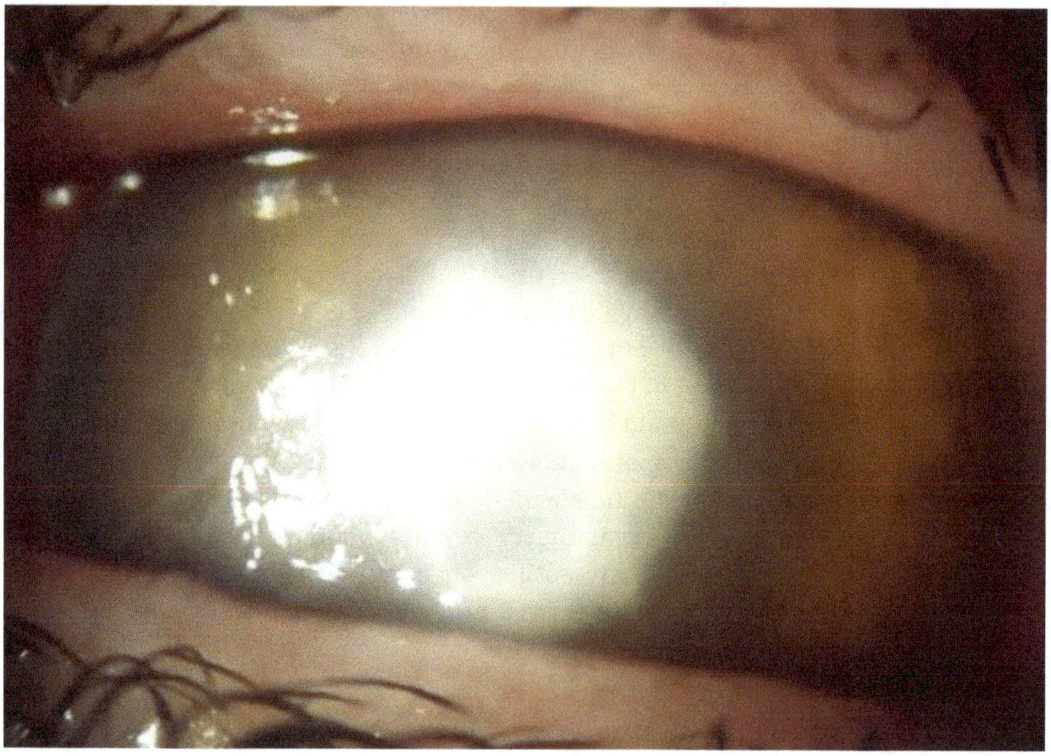

Figure 3. Mild stromal scar after 3 months of corneal edema

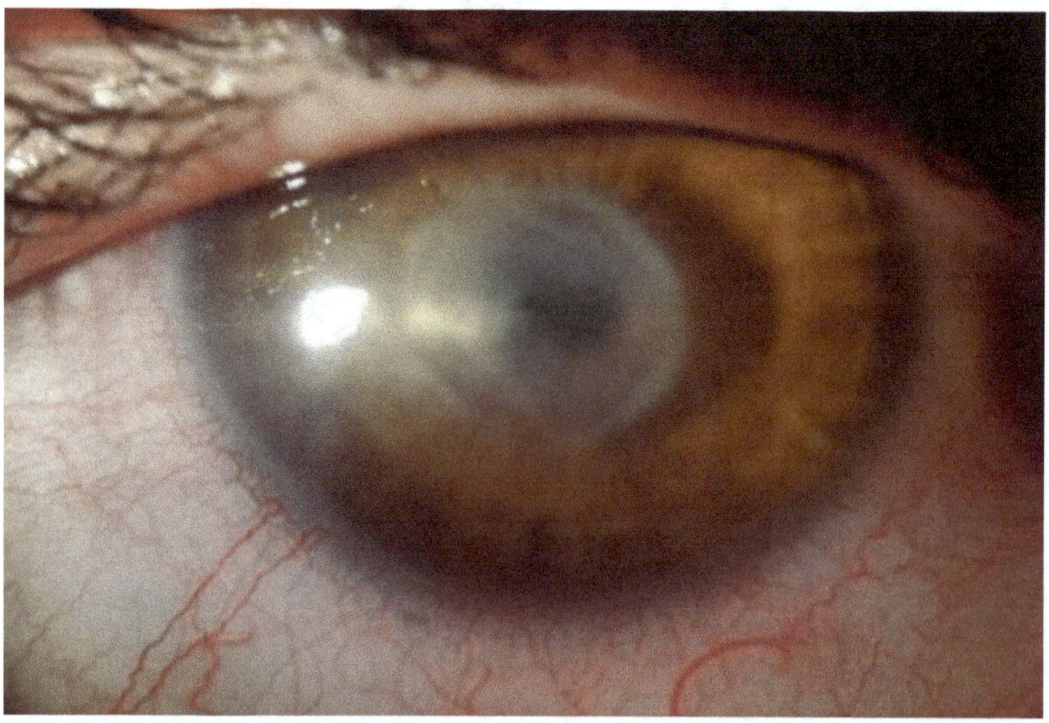

Staphylococcus xylosus is a Gram-positive coagulase-negative microorganism. It exists as a commensal on the skin of humans and animals and in the environment (Fig 4,5,6) (Schleifer et al, 1975).

Figure 4. Large vertical peripheral corneal epithelial defect, atypial oblique hypopyon are seen

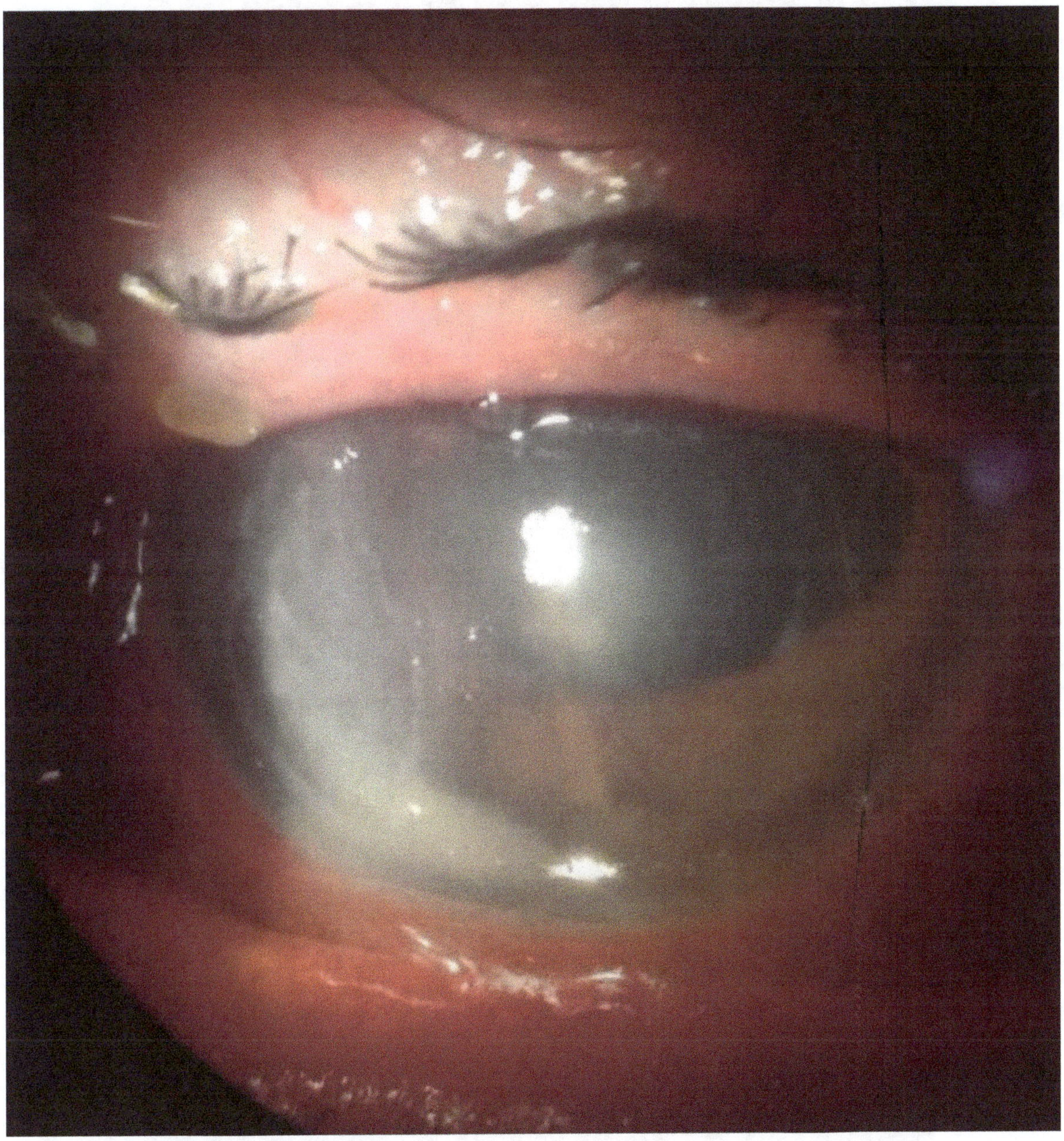

Figure 5. The same eye with amniotic membrane in OR

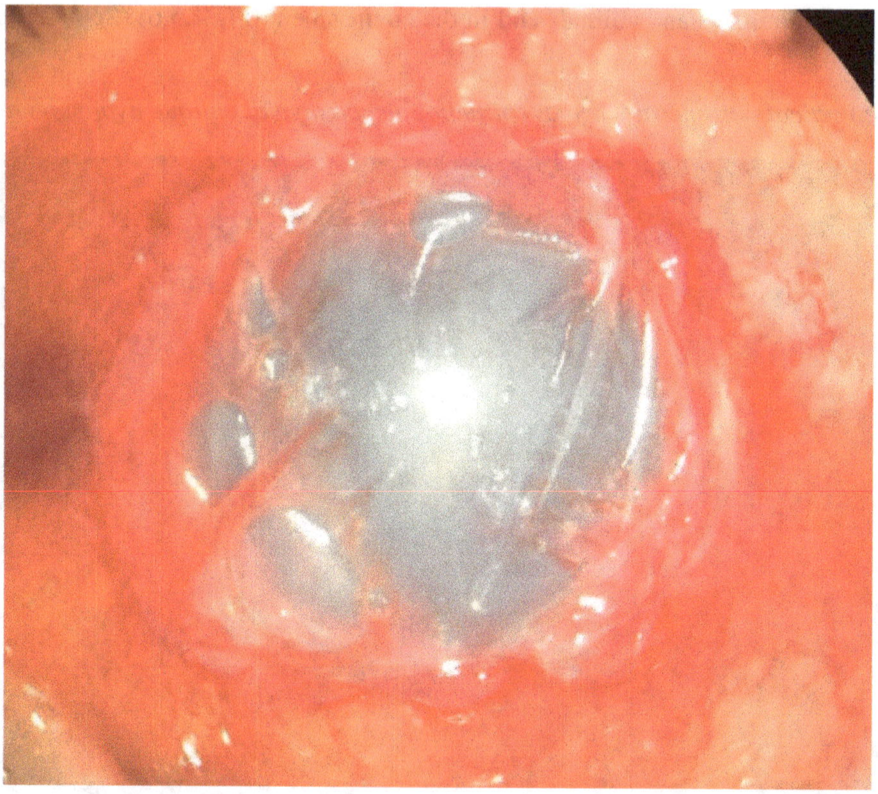

Figure 6. Mild stromal scar 2 months after surgery and medical treatment

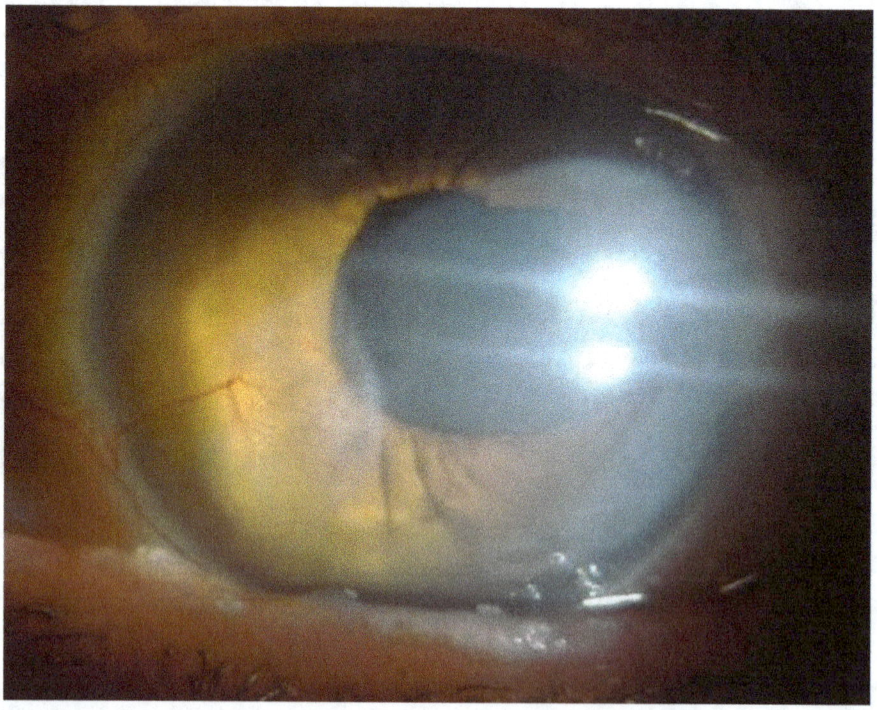

Staphylococcus haemolyticus is a member of the coagulase-negative staphylococci (CoNS) and part of the human skin flora. It is a well-known opportunistic pathogen, and is the second most frequently isolated CoNS after S. epidermidis_(Fig 7,8) The patient's past ocular history was remarkable for bacterial keratitis caused by kocuria kristinae two years ago (Fig 40, 41, 42).

Figure 7. Corneal perforation, total corneal stromal melt/ necrosis, hyphema. Please note sutures from previous PK perfomred for keratitis caused by kocuria kristinae unresponsive to medical treatment

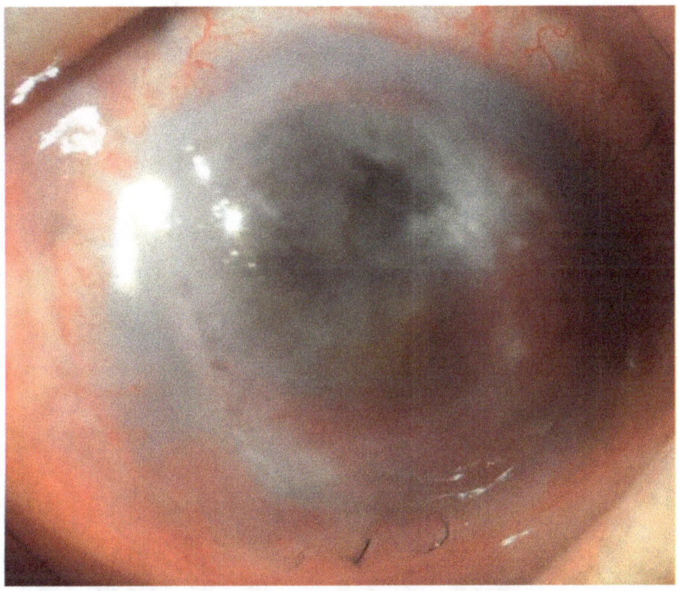

Figure 8. The same eye after PK the next day, residual hyphema

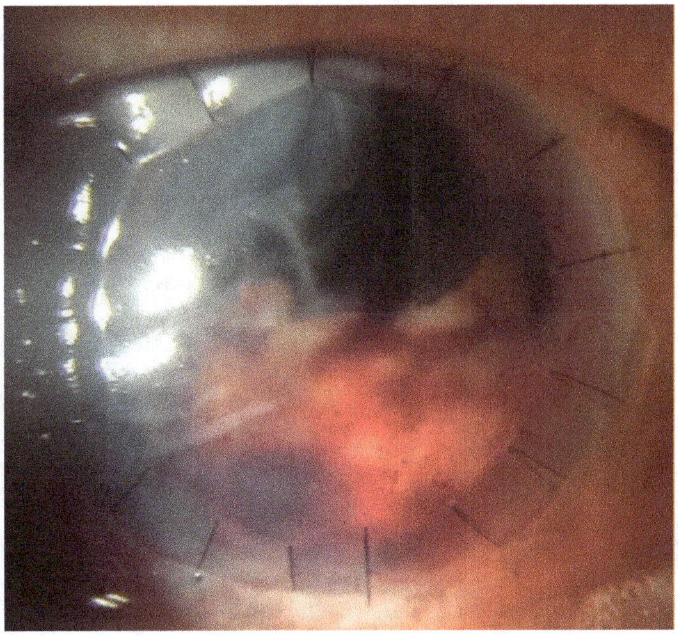

Streptococcus pneumoniae, or pneumococcus, is a Gram-positive facultative anaerobic bacterium. They are usually found in pairs (diplococci) and do not form spores and are nonmotile (Ryan KJ, 2004). pneumoniae resides asymptomatically in healthy carriers, typically colonizing the respiratory tract, sinuses, and nasal cavity. Streptococcus pneumoniae keratitis usually occurs after corneal trauma, dacryocystitis, or filtering bleb surgery. The ulcer tends to be acute, purulent, and rapidly progressive with deep stromal abscess. The anterior chamber reaction can be severe with marked hypopyon (Fig 9, 10).

Figure 9. Note large epithelial defect, stromal infiltrate, marked hypopyon

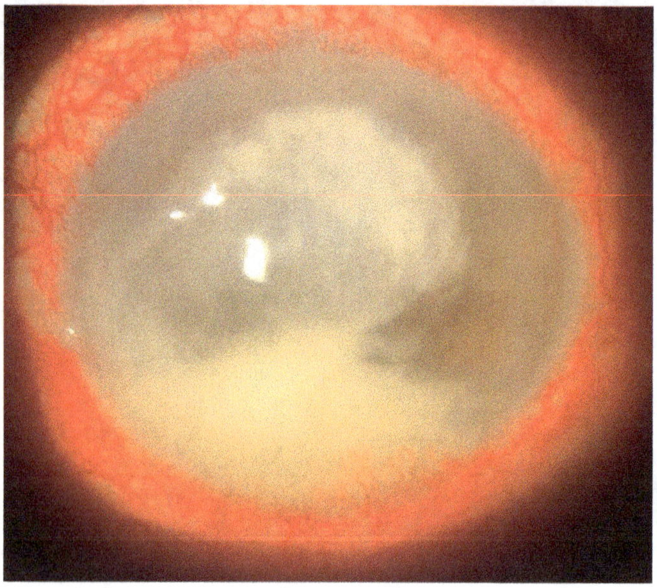

Figure 10. Mild anterior stromal scar after 9 weeks of treatment

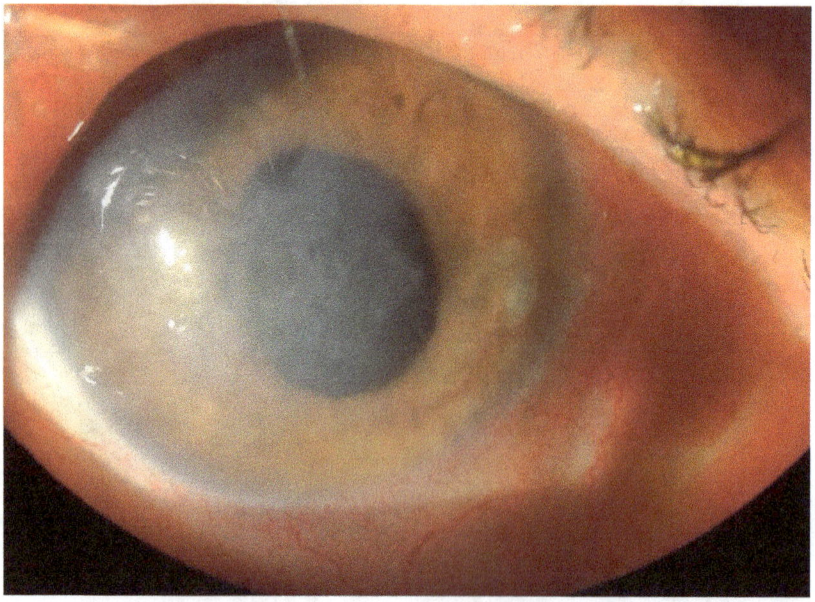

Streptococcus sanguinis is a Gram-positive facultative anaerobic bacterium and a member of the Viridans Streptococcus group (Paik et al, 2005). S. sanguinis is a normal inhabitant of the healthy human mouth. It may gain entrance to the bloodstream when opportunity presents, such as during dental cleanings or surgeries.

Figure 11. Clinical presentation at first visit resembles a herpetic georgraphic ulcer

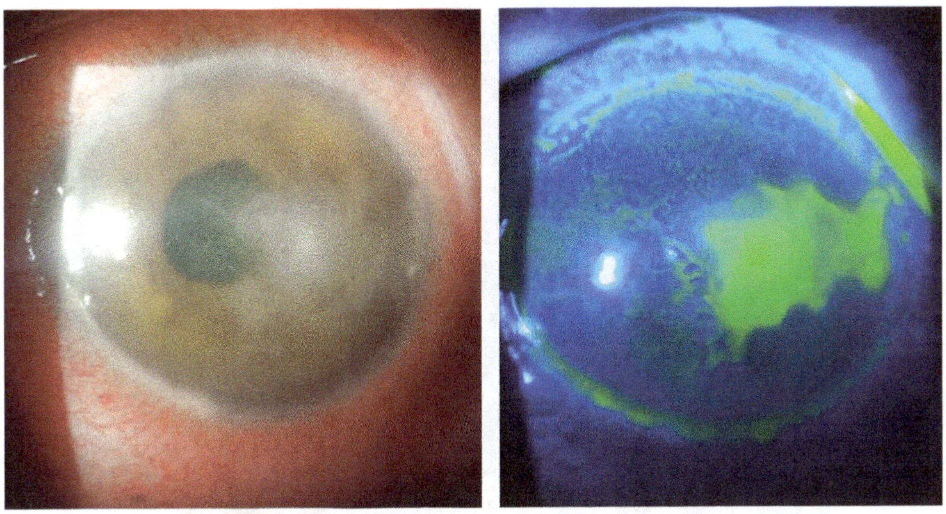

Figure 12. The same eye 10 days later. Ovoid-shaped corneal ulcer with epithelial defect, stromal infiltrate surrounding edema and hypopyon, non-responding to medical treatment. The patient was advised to get PK, but she was visiting from Russia and she decided to leave, so was lost for follow-up

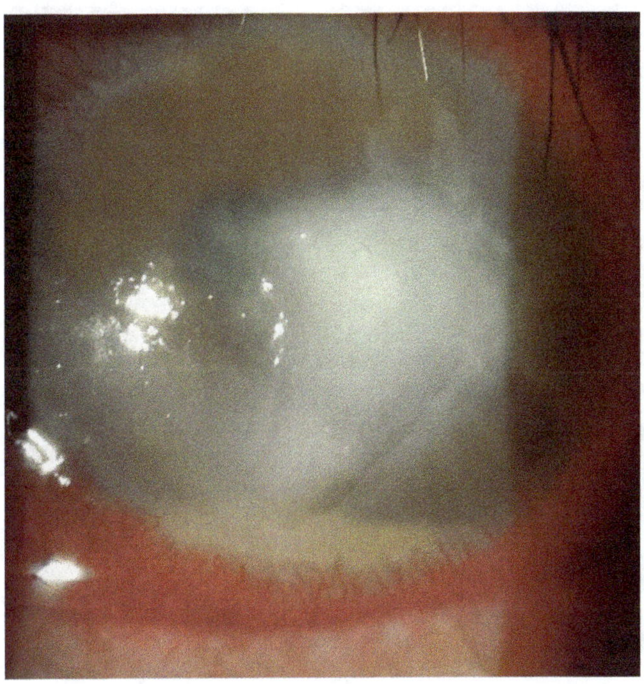

Streptococcus mitis are commensal bacteria that colonize hard surfaces in the oral cavity such as dental hard tissues as well as mucous membranes and are part of the oral flora (Streptococcus et al, 2011). They are not usually pathogenic but commonly cause bacterial endocarditis (Figure 13, 14). It is extremely rare for this microorganism to cause ulcerative keratitis.

Figure 13. Large epithelial defect, hypopyon, stromal edema

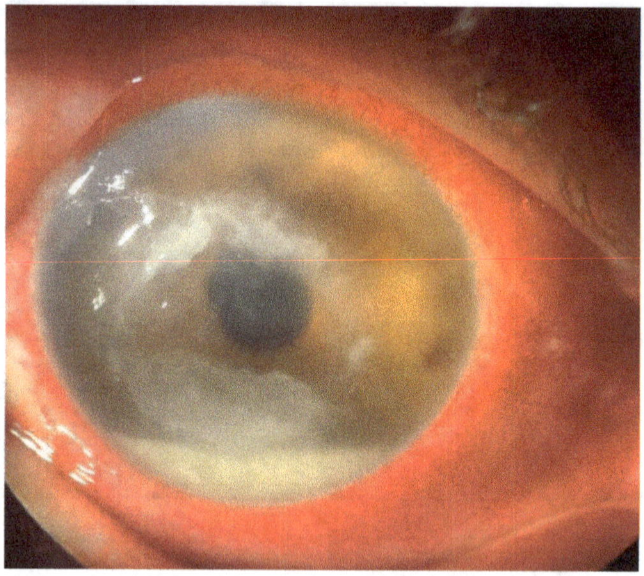

Figure 14. The same eye 2 weeks after treatment (in healing process)

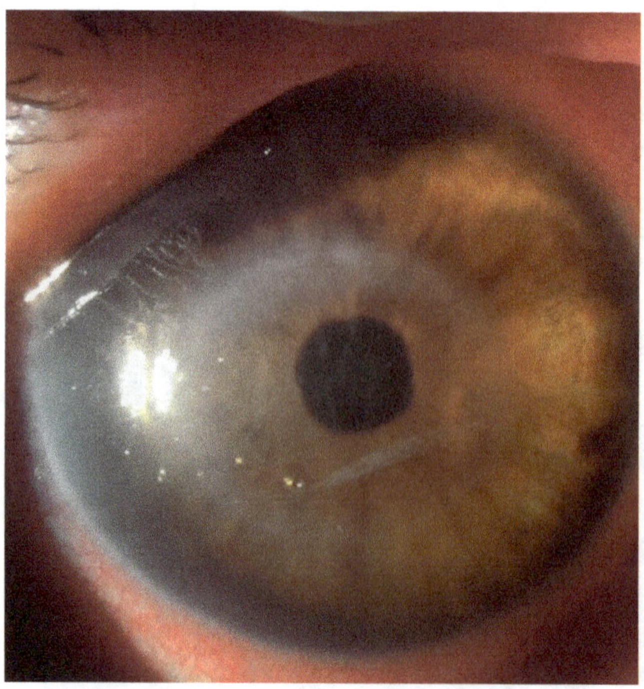

Streptococcus anginosus group (also known as the S. milleri group) is a subgroup of viridans streptococci (Morita et al, 2005). The organisms were subsequently recognized as normal human flora (cultures of the oral cavity, throat, stool, and vagina have all yielded S. milleri strains) with the ability to cause abscesses and systemic infections (Fig 15, 16).

Figure 15. Corneal perforation due to corneal abscess caused by Stp. Anginousus. Note the IOL extrusion

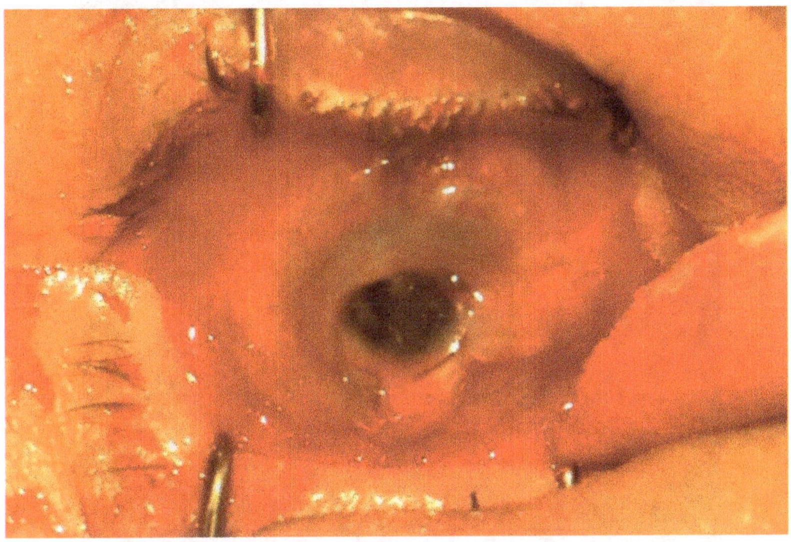

Figure 16. The same eye one month after PK, residual hyphema, aphakia

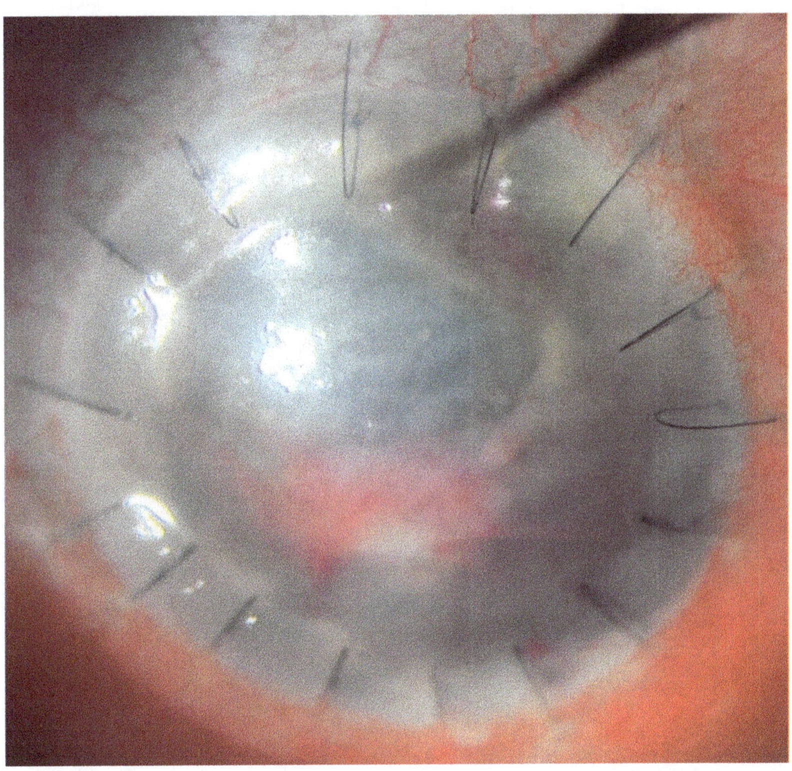

Granulicatella adiacens, a recently nomenclatured bacterium, was considered one of the nutritionally variant streptococci (NVS) and is a mouth commensal (Fig 17, 18) (Collins et al, n.d.).

Figure 17. Total corneal melt/abscess, mucopurulent discharge

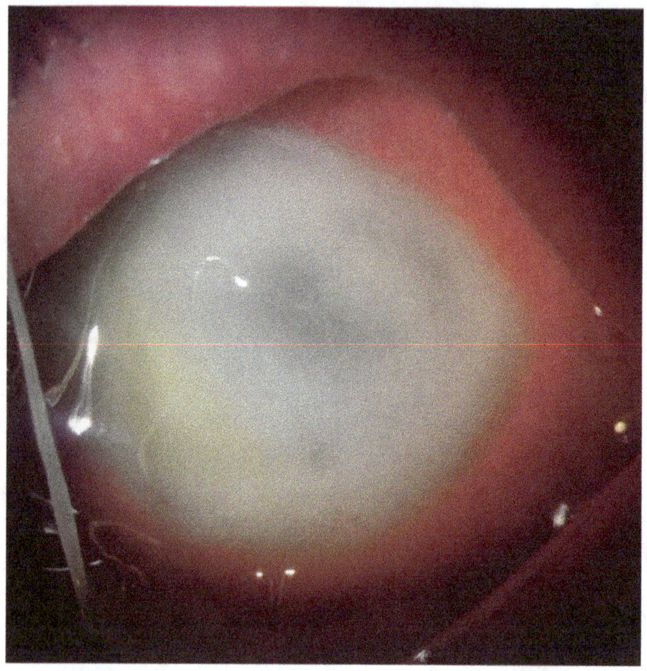

Figure 18. The same eye 4 months post PK

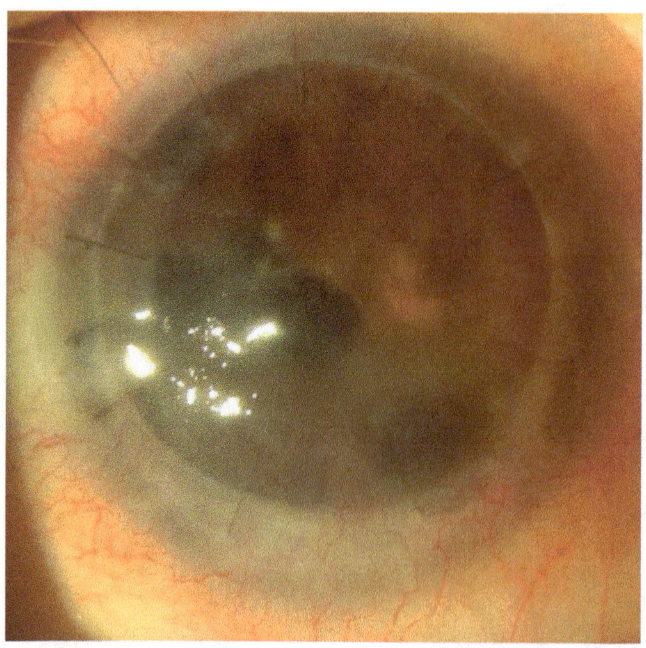

Pseudomonas aeruginosa is the most common Gram-negative isolated microorganism in severe corneal ulcers. The prevalence of pseudomonas keratitis associated with the use of contact lenses has increased recently (McLeod et al, 1998). Rapid progression, dense stromal infiltrate, and necrosis are considered very characteristic of Pseudomonas keratitis, often leading to stromal keratolysis and corneal perforation. The corneal ring infiltrate is usually observed (Fig 19, 20).

Figure 19. Total epithelial defect is seen with underying stromal infiltrate and central thinning, pending perforation

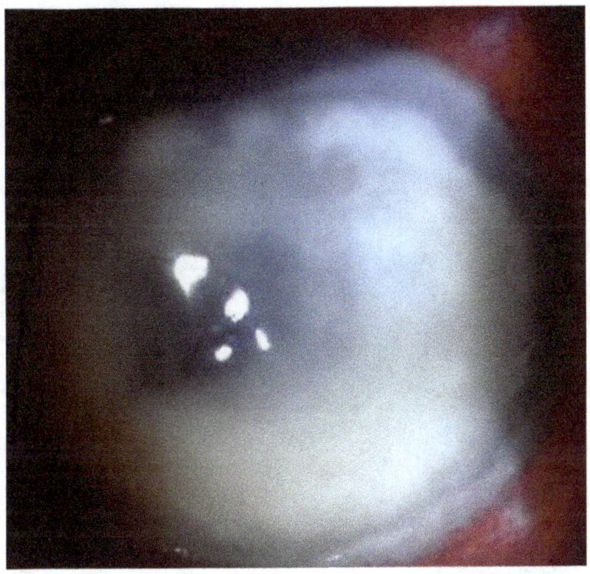

Figure 20. The same eye. Photo is taken 6 months post PK and medical treatment

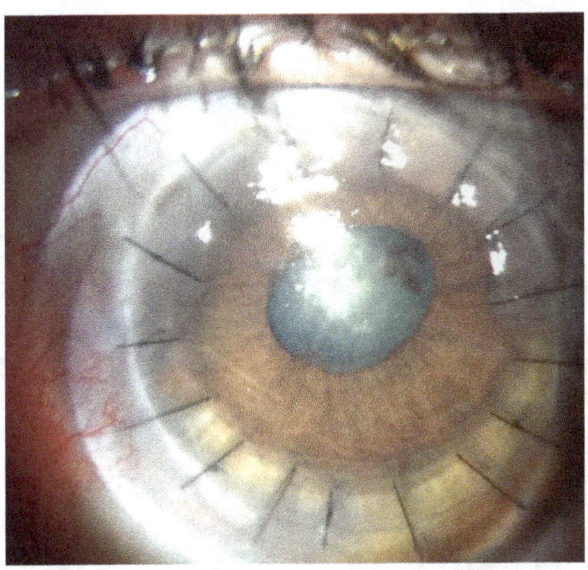

Serratia marcescens is a rod-shaped, facultative, anaerobic Gram-negative bacterium, and belongs to family Klebsielleae. Because of its abundant presence in the environment, especially in damp conditions, S. marcescens is commonly found growing in bathrooms where it appears like a pink-to-orange discoloration (Fig 21, 22) (Hejazi et al, 1997). Keratitis caused by Serratia marcescens is usually associated with corneal surface diseases and contact lens wear.

Figure 21. Infectious keratitis caused by Serratia marcescens. Severe injection, ring infiltrate with hypopyon are seen

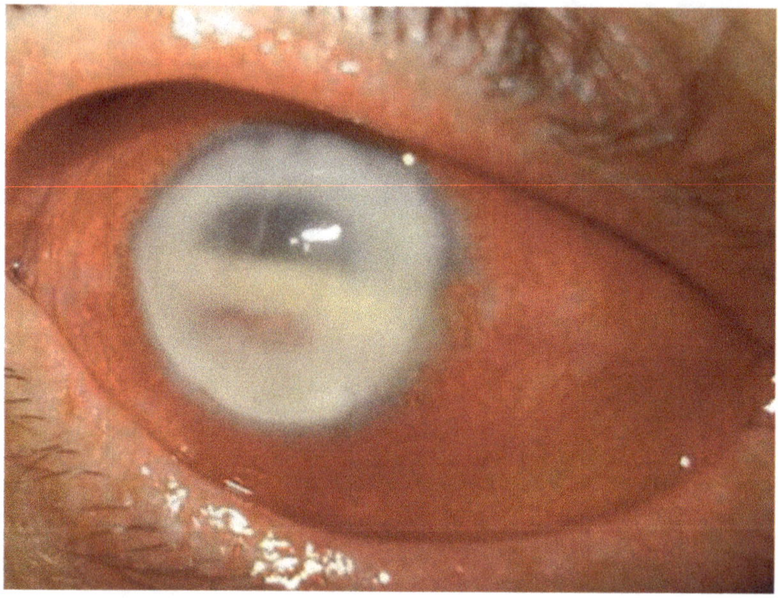

Figure 22. The same eye 1-month post PK

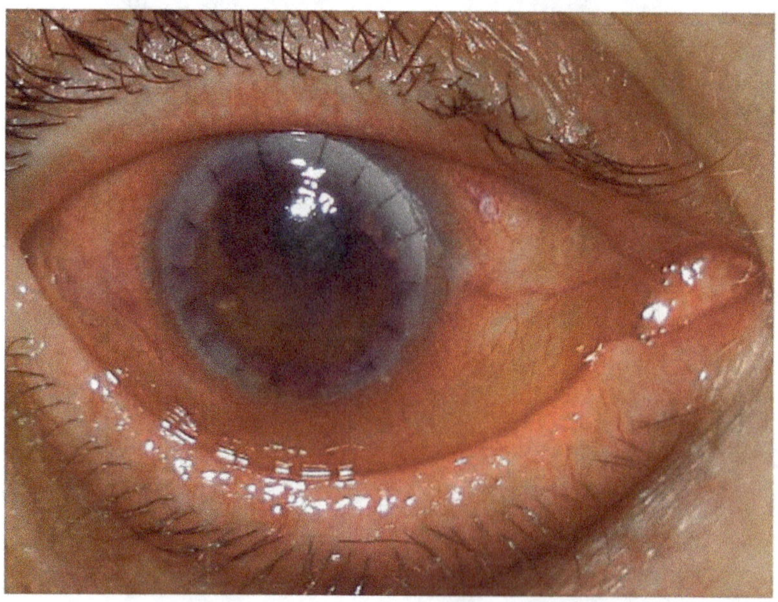

Acinetobacter baumannii is a Gram-negative coccobacillus. Many species of the genus Acinobater are often found in soil samples, but A. baumanii is almost always isolated from hospital environments (Fig 23, 24) (Antunes et al, 2014).

Figure 23. Comma-shaped corneal infiltrate with overlying epithelial defect and surrounded stromal edema is seen

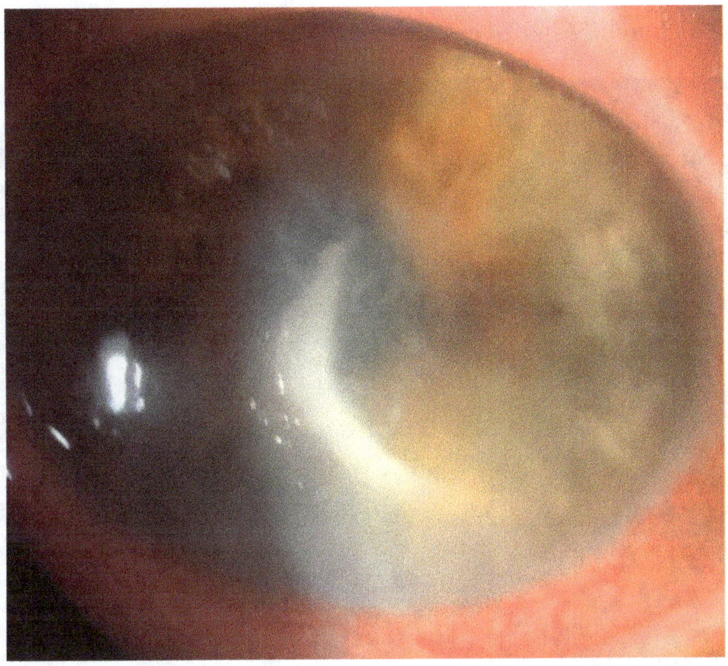

Figure 24. The same eye after 6 weeks of treatment. Mild stromal scar is noted

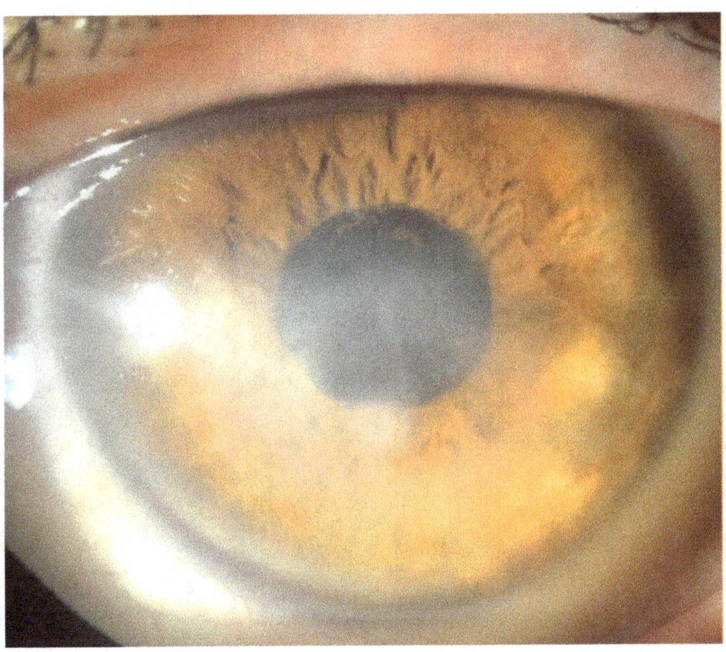

Nontuberculous mycobacteria: the most common pathogens are Mycobacterium fortuitum and Mycobacterium chelonae, which are usually found in soil and water. They cause a slowly progressive keratitis, mainly occurring after corneal surgery (particularly after LASIK) and corneal trauma (Velotta et al, 2005; Tenailon et al, 2017; Ryan KJ et al, 2004). This keratitis is usually associated with delayed onset of symptoms, corticosteroids use, and severe ocular pain, which can develop 2 to 8 weeks after exposure. The organisms' isolation is difficult, which explains the reason for delayed diagnosis (Fig 25-29).

Figure 25. Crystalline looking like peripheral corneal lesion caused by Mycobacterium chelonae

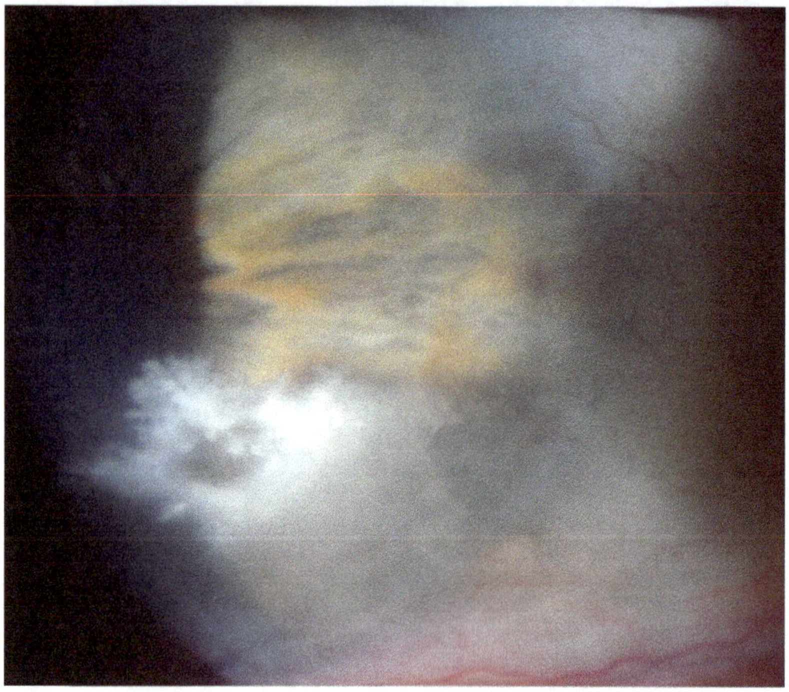

Figure 26. The same eye after 3 months (left photo) and after 5 months (right photo), nonresponsive to medical treatment, hypopyon developed

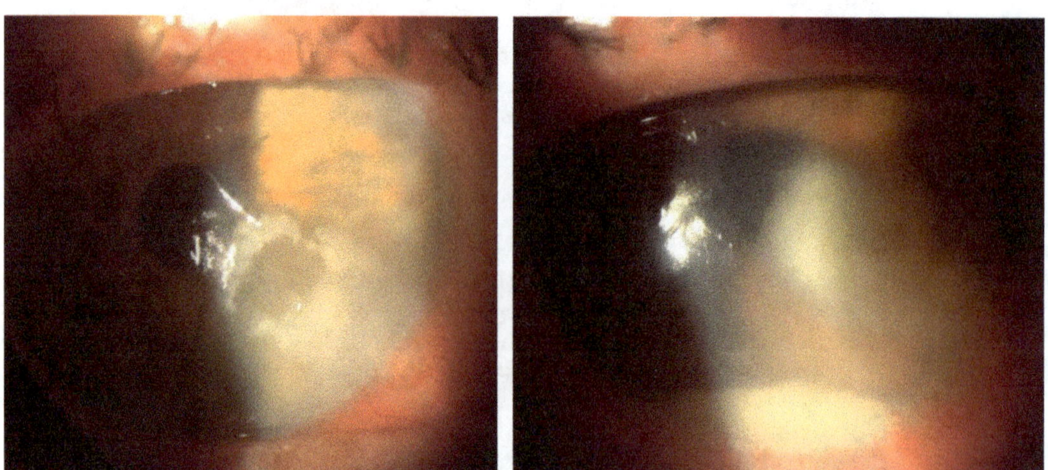

Figure 27. Two weeks post PK, recurrence of infection on the graft

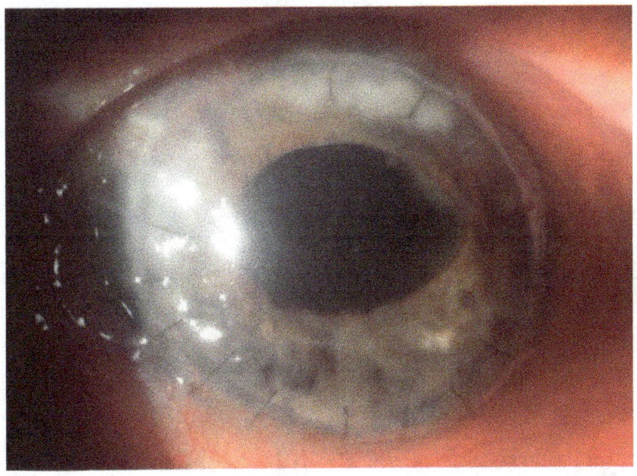

Figure 28. The same eye after 1-month, scleral involvement is seen, although on Amikacin treatment

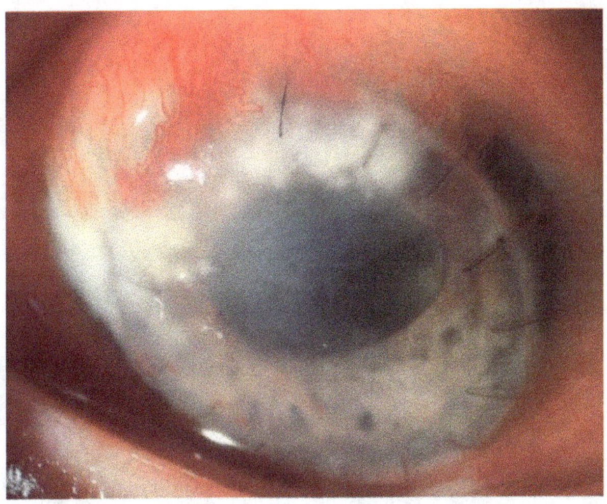

Figure 29. The same eye 5 months post Amikacin treatment (left photo) and 1 year later (right photo)

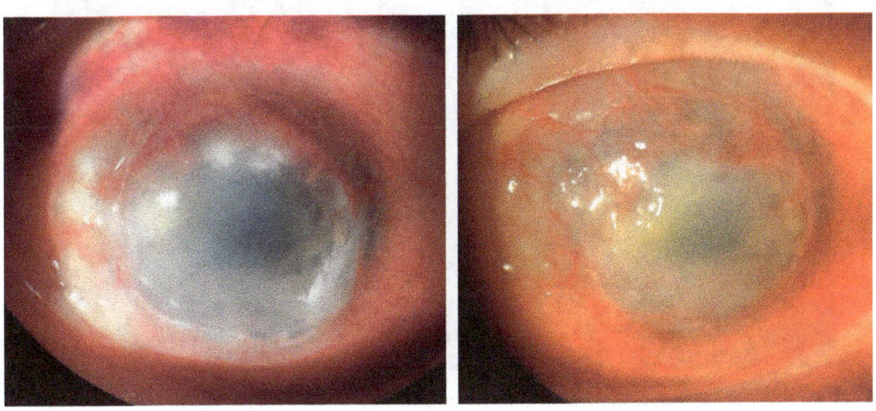

Escherichia coli is a Gram-negative, facultative anaerobic, rod-shaped bacterium, found in the normal flora of the gastrointestinal track (Fig 30, 31) (Tenanilon et al, 2017). It can also cause corneal ulcer and endophthalmitis.

Figure 30. Central and corneolimbal infiltrates, paracentral severe thinning, neovascularization

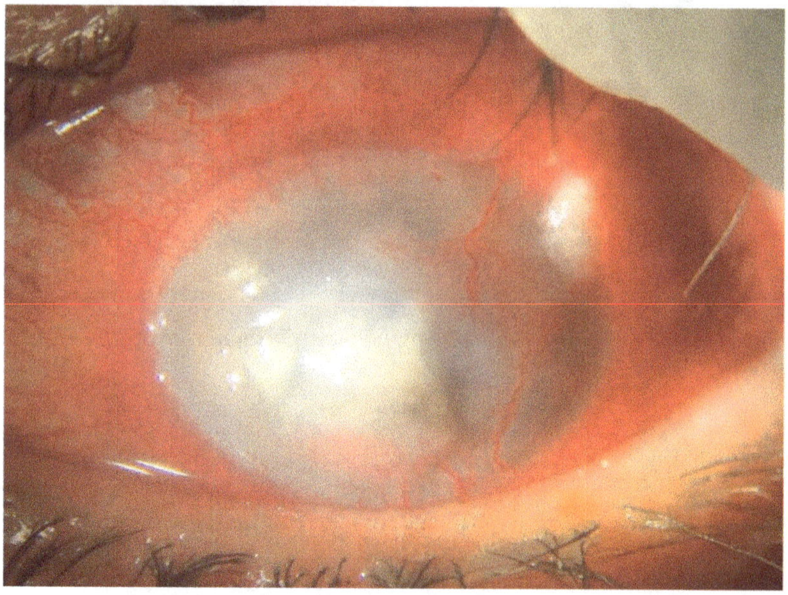

Figure 31. Stromal scar formation after 6 weeks of treatment

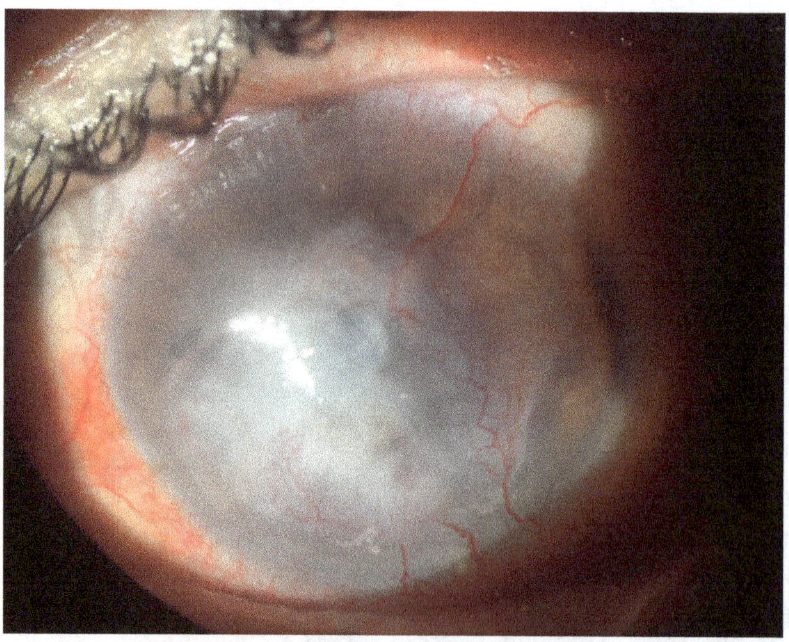

Enterococcus faecalis is a Gram-positive, commensal bacterium inhabiting in the gastrointestinal tracts of humans. Like other species in the genus Enterococcus, E. faecalis is found in healthy humans, but can cause life-threatening infections, especially in hospitals (Fig 32,33 34) (Ryan KJ et al, 2004).

Figure 32. Corneal perforation associated with E.faecalis infection (photo taken in OR). Amniotic membrane transplantation being performed till the availability of donor cornea

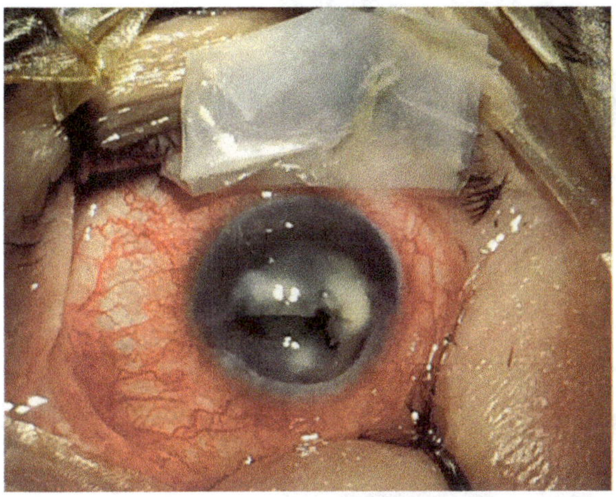

Figure 33. The same eye 10 days later during PK surgery. Opaque lenc extrusion from perforated cornea is seen

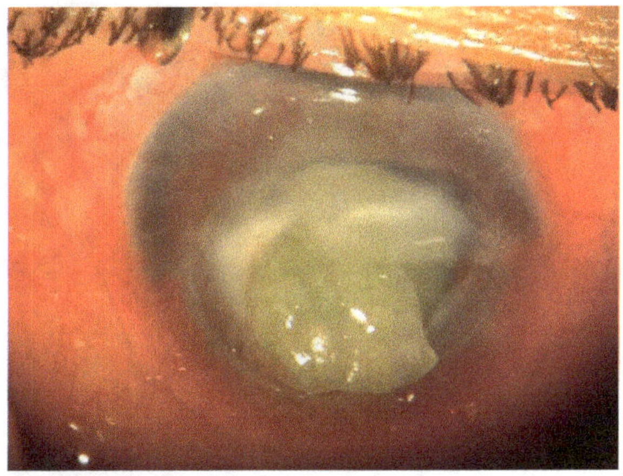

Figure 34. The same eye at the end of PK surgery. Patient was left aphakic for placement of IOL later

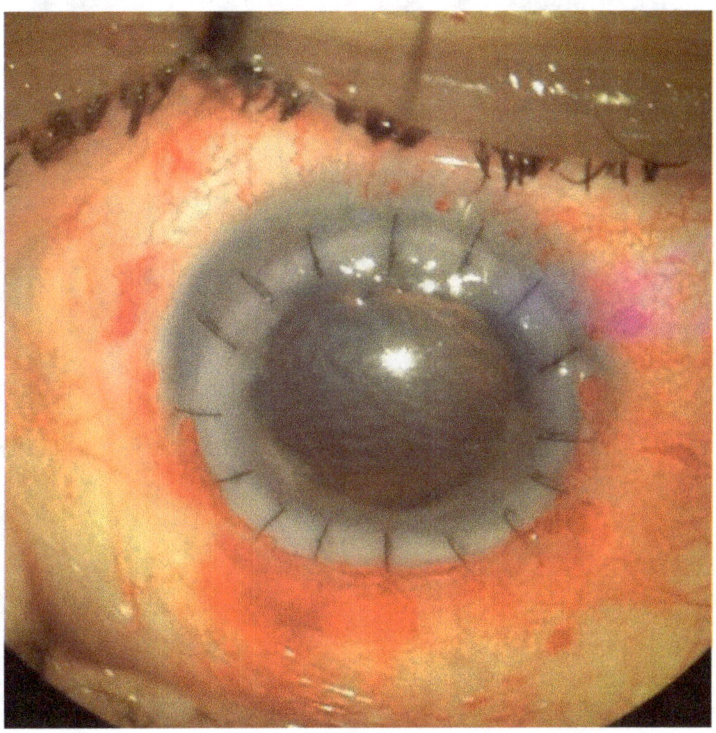

Clostridium bifermentans is an anaerobic, spore-forming, Gram-positive bacillus (Ryan K et al, 2004). This organism is infrequently reported as a cause of infection in humans and can be a cause of septic arthritis, osteomyelitis, soft tissue infection, abdominal infections, brain abscess, bacteremia and endocarditis (Fig 35, 36).

Figure 35. Large stromal infiltrate with overlying epithelial defect and 5mm of hypopyon with severe conjunctival injection are seen

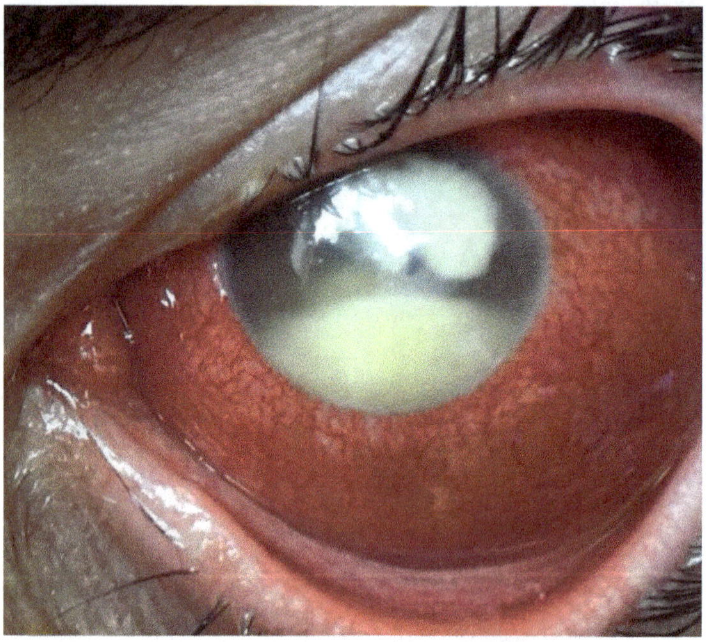

Figure 36. The same eye after 10 days of treatment (left photo, under slit lamp) and 1 month later, healing stage, stromal scar formation (right photo)

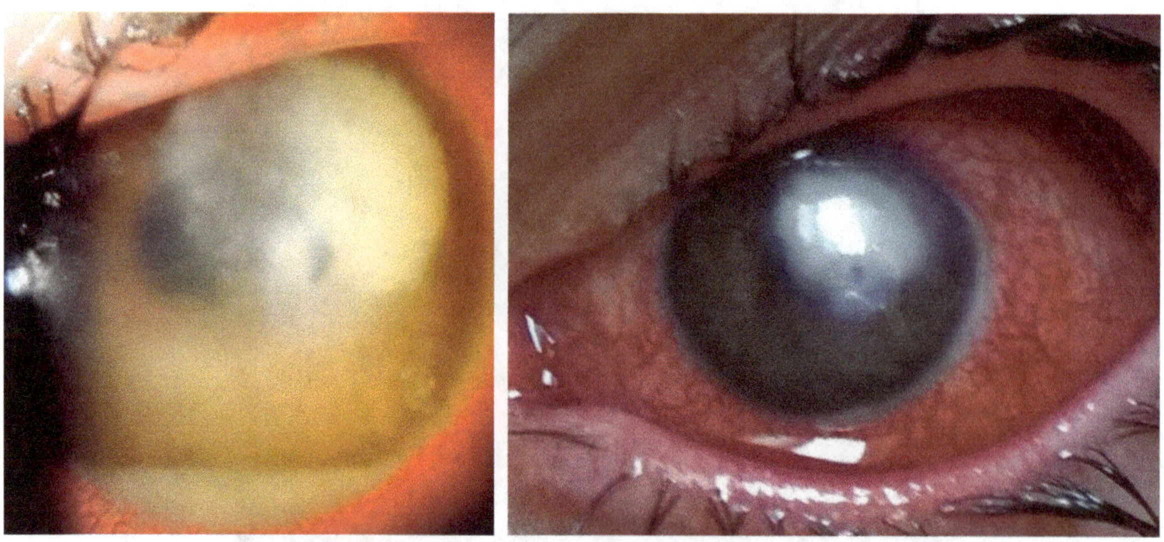

Sphingomonas paucimobilis (*S. paucimobilis*) is a non-fermentative, aerobic, Gram-negative, non-spore-forming bacillus, first described in 1990. It has been reported to proliferate in distilled water, hemodialysis fluids, and sterile drug solutions (Ryan MP et al, 2010) it can infect persons with chronic diseases or immunosuppression, particularly (Fig 37, 38).

Figure 37. Total epithelial defect, stromal infiltrate, severe peripheral thinning and neovascularization are seen on the photo

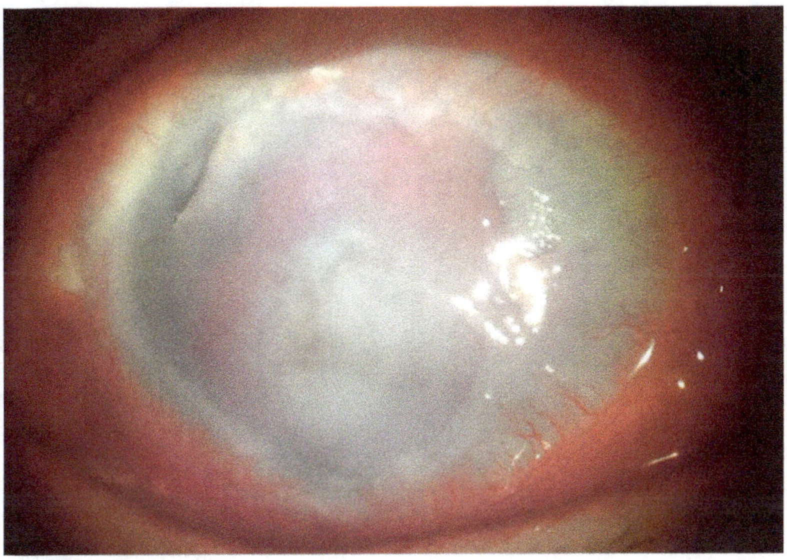

Figure 38. Four weeks later; post medical treatment. Total epithelization ocurred, stromal scar formation is noted

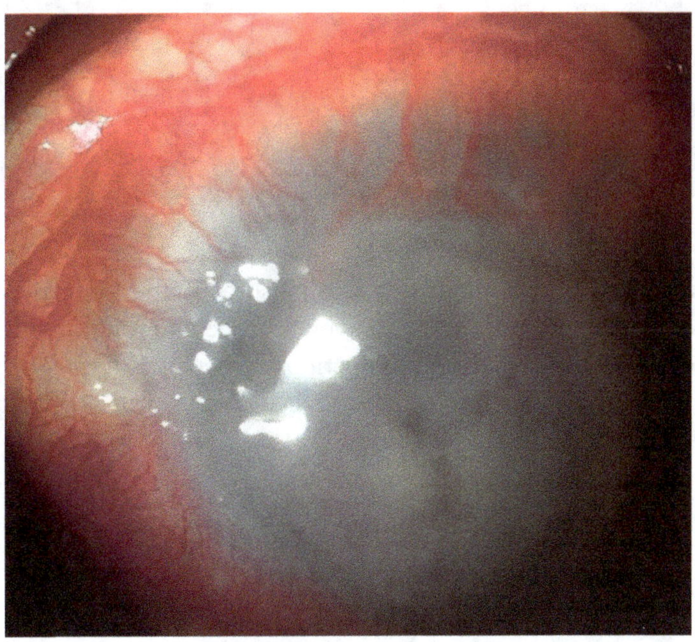

Veillonella species are anaerobic, Gram-negative cocci that are part of the normal mouth, gastrointestinal, and urogenital flora in humans. Veillonella species have been isolated from skin, dental, and respiratory tract infections, where they are often part of a mixed flora (Arif et al, 2008). Rarely, Veillonella can cause severe infections like meningitis, endocarditis, and osteomyelitis (Figure 39).

Figure 39. Stromal infiltrate with paracentral stromal lysis, neovascularization and hypopyon are seen. Patient had terminal glaucoma and asked for evisceration due to severe pain

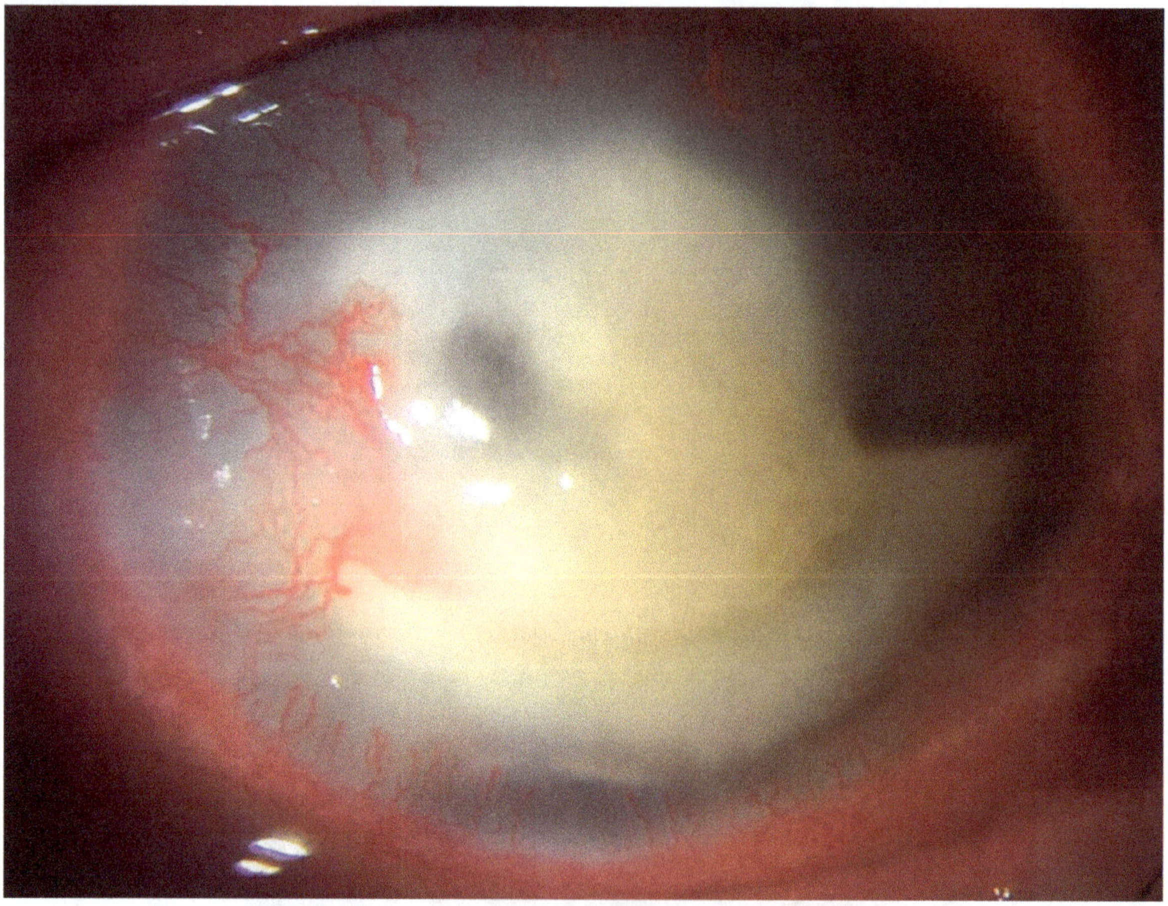

Kocuria spp. are ubiquitous in nature, and they can also be found as normal skin flora in humans and other mammals. Kocuria kristinae is a facultative anaerobe and a non-motile, coagulase-negative and Gram-positive coccus. Documented cases of infections caused by Kocuria spp. are rare. K. Kristinae was not considered to be a primary pathogen, but in recent years, well documented cases of catheter related bacteremia were reported (Fig 40-44) (Basaglia et al, 2002).

Figure 40. Stromal infiltrate, epithelial defect, hypopyon

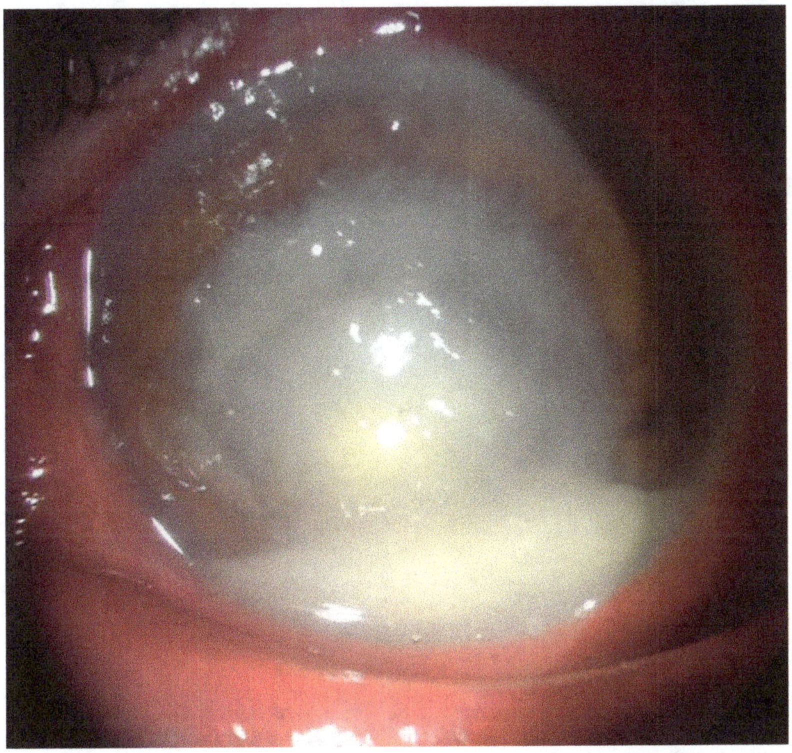

Figure 41. The same eye unresponsive to medical treatment, photo is taken in OR before PK

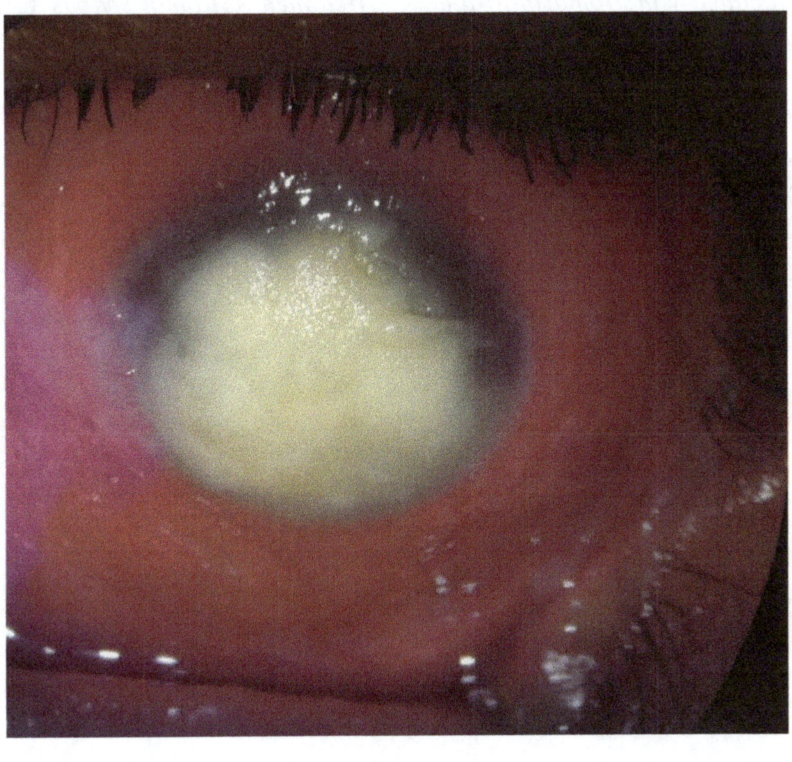

Figure 42. The same eye after PK, photo is taken in OR

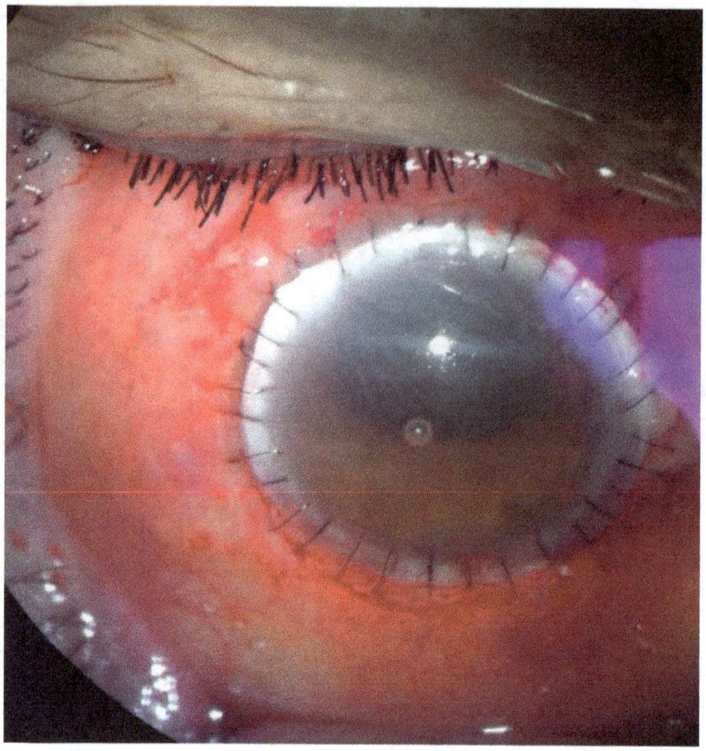

Figure 43. Different patient with large round epithelial defect associated with stromal infiltrate superiorly, stromal edema and marked hypopyon on corneal transplant (the patient had undergone PK for acanthamoeba keratitis 5 years ago)

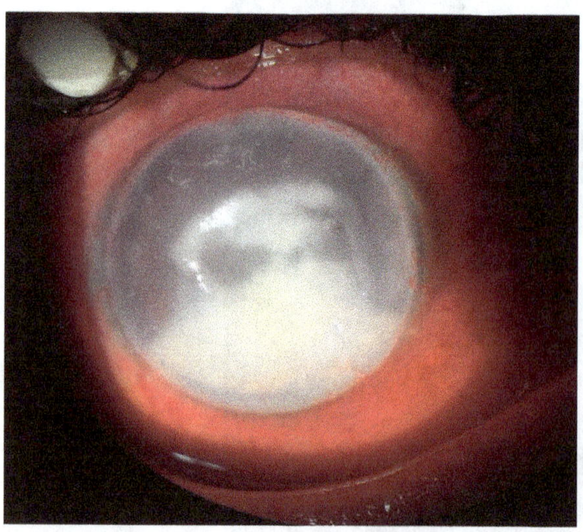

Figure 44. The same eye after 8 weeks of medical treatment. Stromal scar is seen with neovascularization

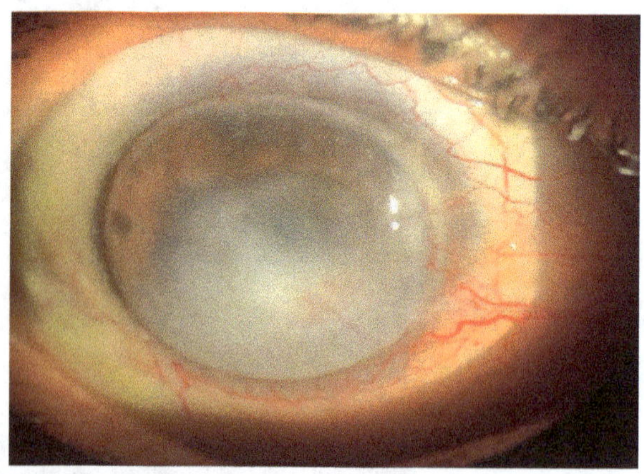

Micrococcus luteus is a Gram-positive, nonmotile, saprotrophic bacterium[23]. An obligate aerobe, M. luteus, is found in soil, dust, water and air. The bacterium also colonizes the human mouth, mucosae, oropharynx and upper respiratory tract. It was discovered by Sir Alexander Fleming before he discovered penicillin in 1928 (Fig 45, 46).

Figure 46. Mild anterior stromal scar after 2 months of medical treatment is seen

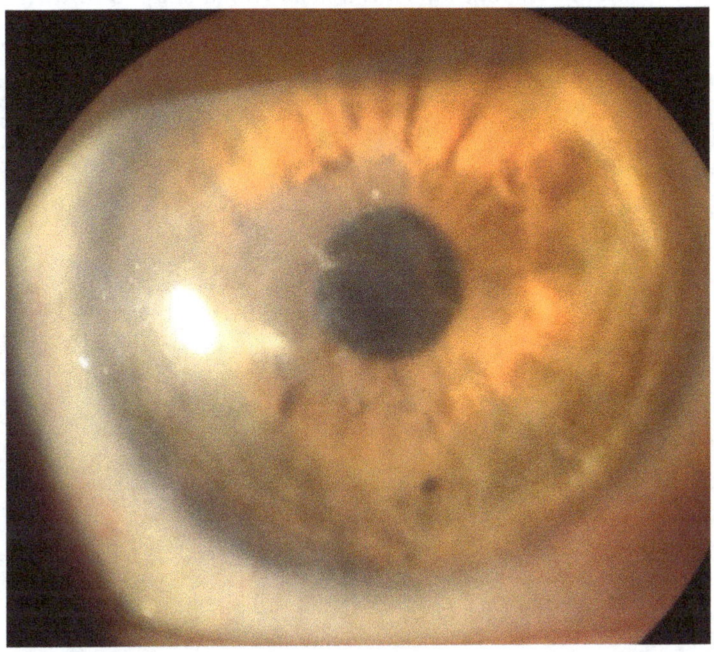

Figure 45. Dens arcus-shaped stromal infiltrate, edema, epithelial defect, hypopyo are seen

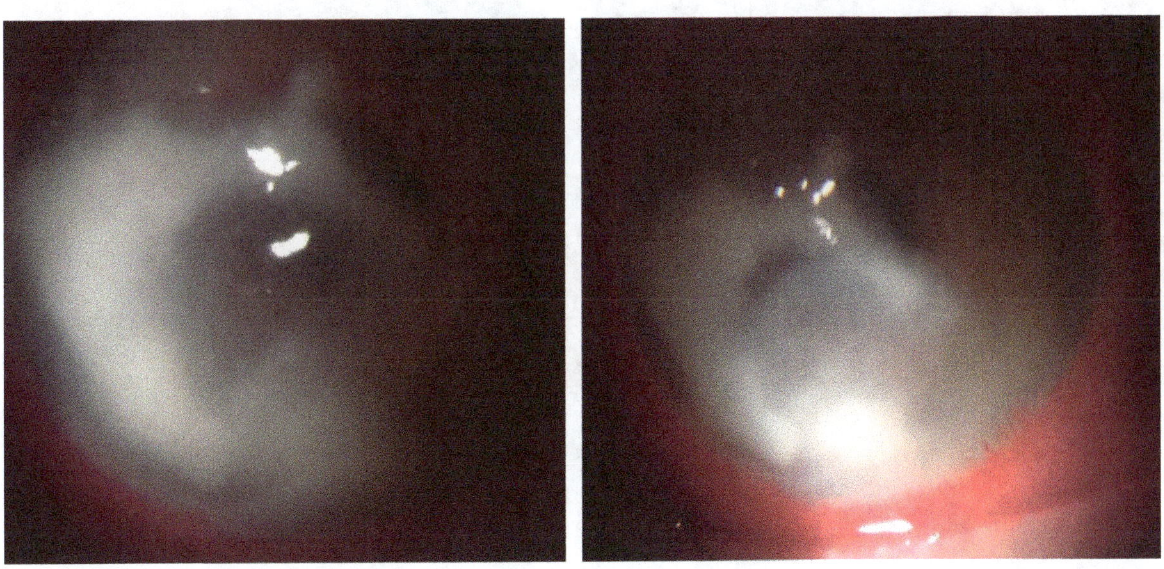

Actinomyces are all gram-positive, facultatively anaerobic bacteria, and they grow best under anaerobic conditions. Actinomyces colonies form fungus-like branched networks of hyphae24. The aspect of these colonies initially led to the incorrect assumption that the organism was a fungus. Certain species are commensal in the skin flora, oral flora, gut flora, and vaginal flora of humans and livestock (Figure 47, 48, 49).

Figure 47. Total stromal, epithelial edema, inferior, dense, round shaped infiltrate with moderate thinning is seen

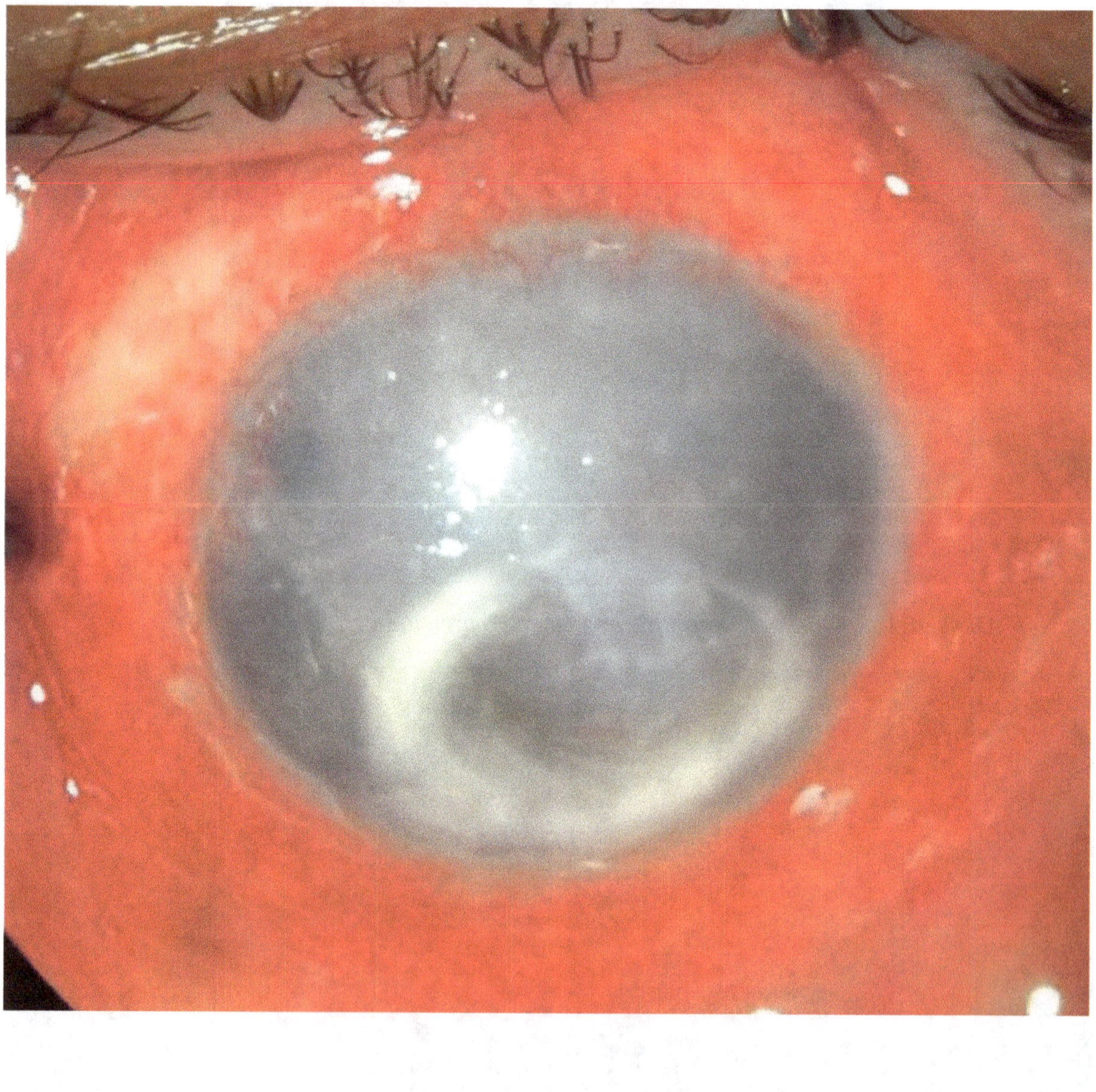

Figure 48. The same eye covered with amniotic membrane

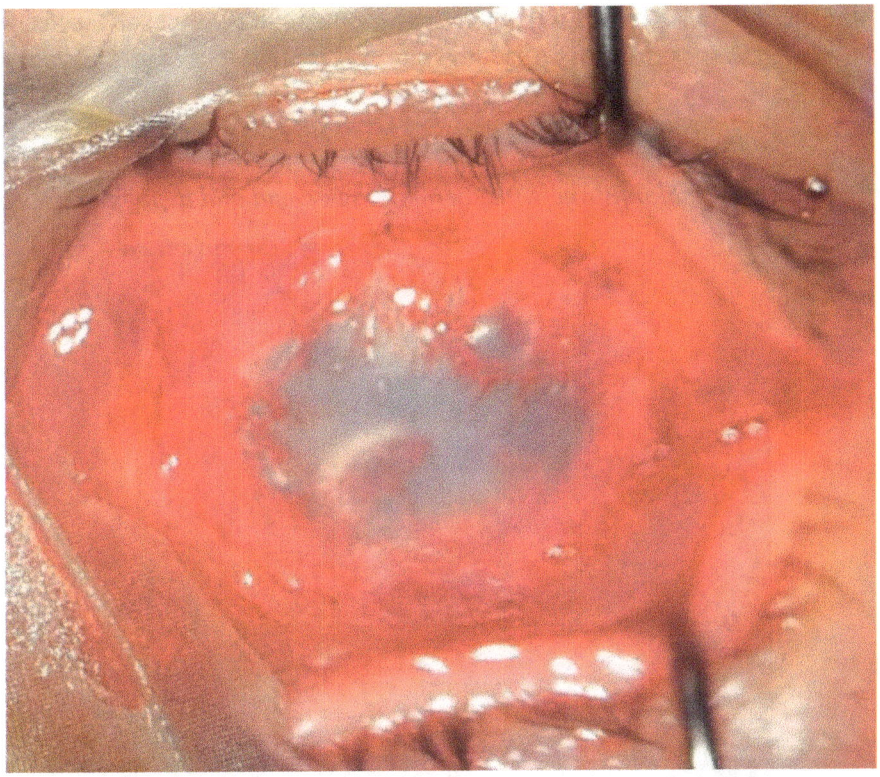

Figure 49. The same eye 10 weeks post treatment. Mild anterior stromal scar left inferiorly

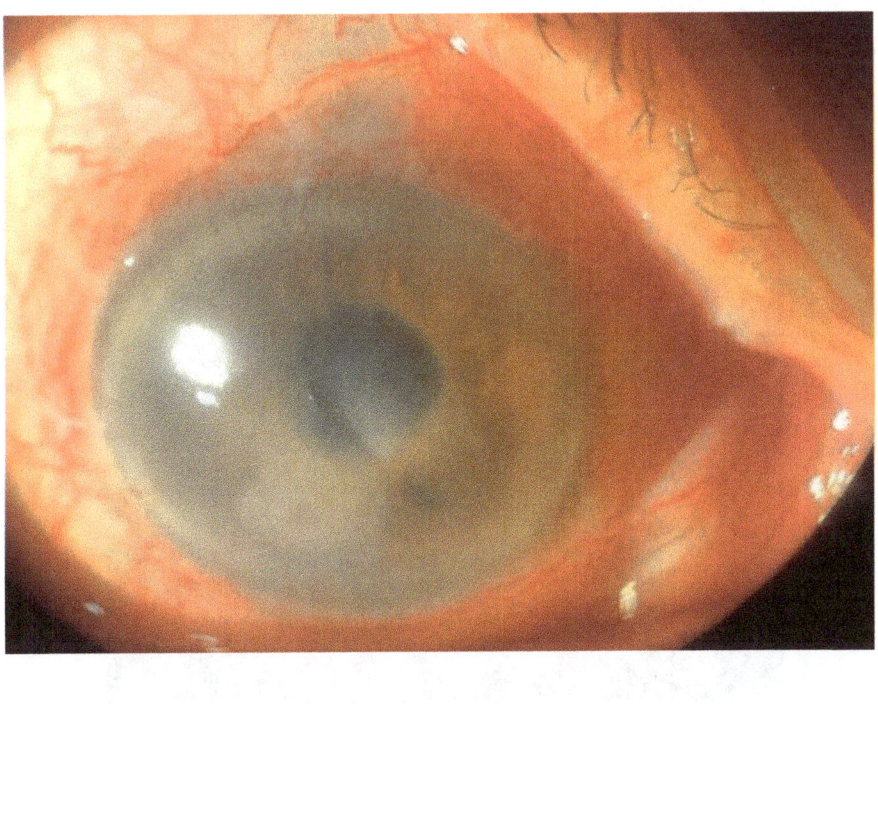

Corynebacterium striatum is a Gram-positive facultative anaerobe. It is generally found as a ubiquitous microorganism, and, as a commensal of humans, colonizing the nasopharynx Recent interest has been sparked in the microorganism as it is known to be resistant to and gaining resistance to many antibiotics (Fig 50, 51, 52, 53).

Figure 50. Dense central stromal infiltrate with surrounding edema and hypopyon are seen

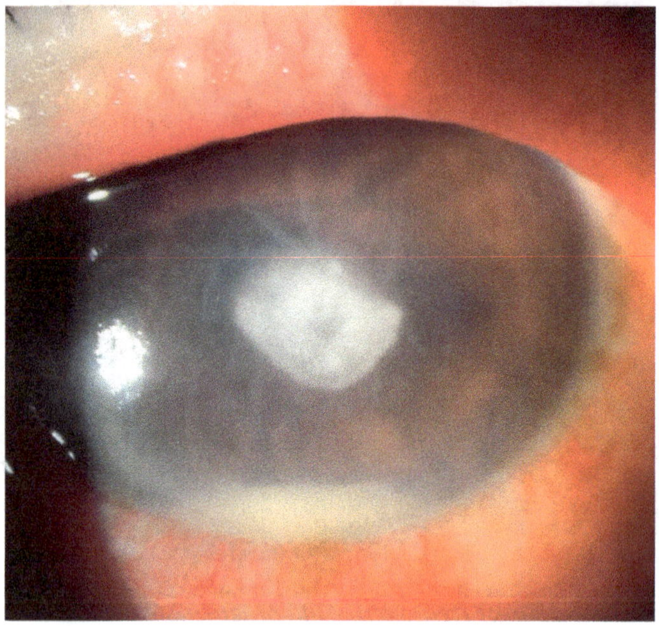

Figure 51. The same eye 1-month post treatment. Anterior stromal scar is seen

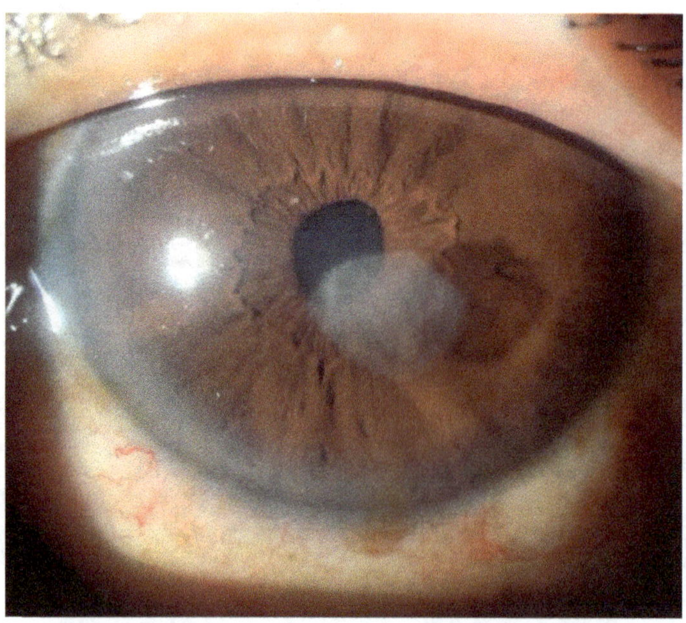

Figure 52. Fine crystal-looking like lesions with overlying epithelial defect caused by Corynebacterium spp

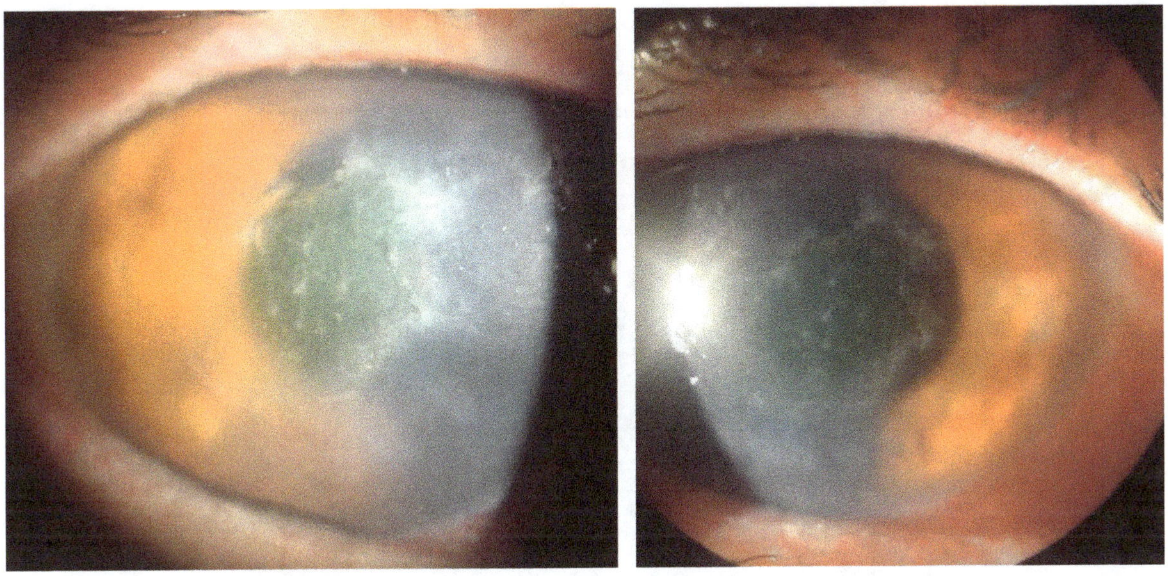

Figure 53. The same eye after 3 months of medical treatment, left with subepithelial fibrosis

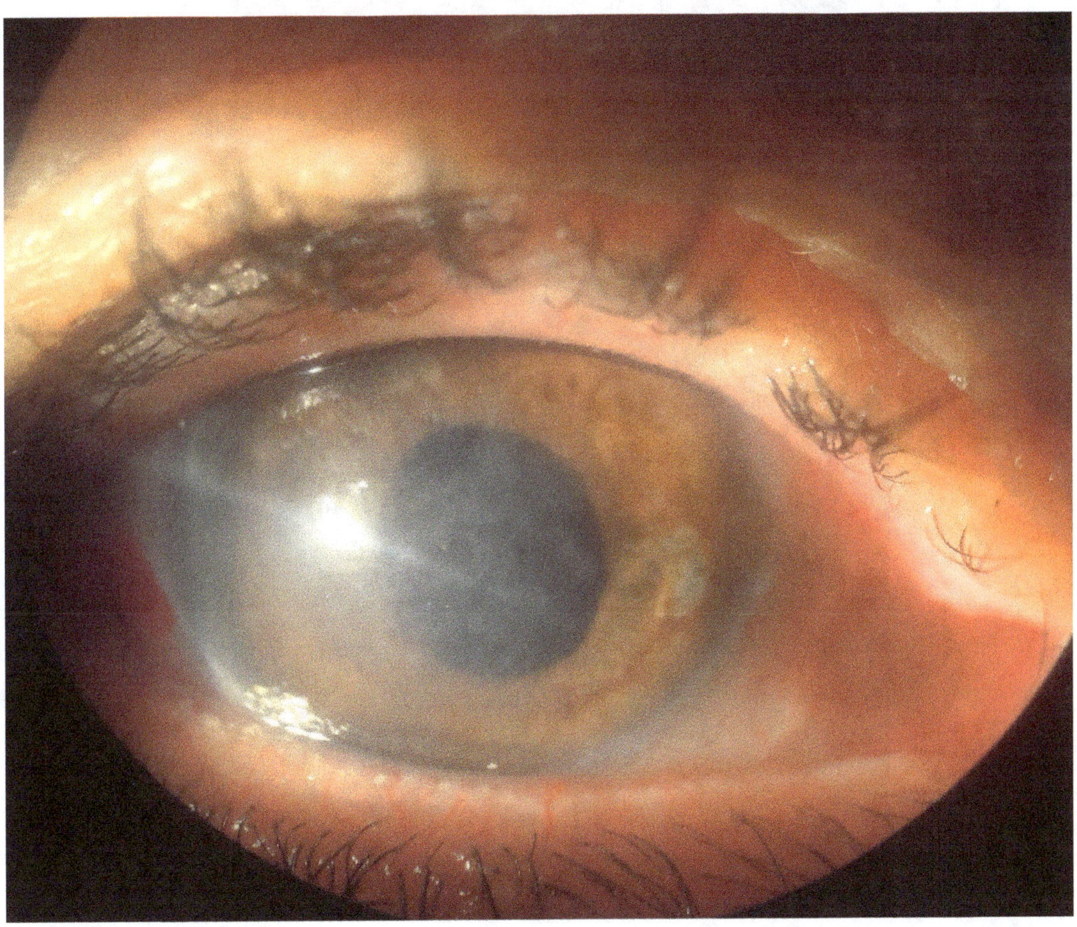

Alloiococcus otitis is a newly recognized species of Gram-positive bacterium, which was recently discovered as a pathogen associated with some types of acute otitis (Fig 54, 55) (Harimaya e tal, 2006).

Figure 54. Dense central stromal infiltrate with oblique hypopyon

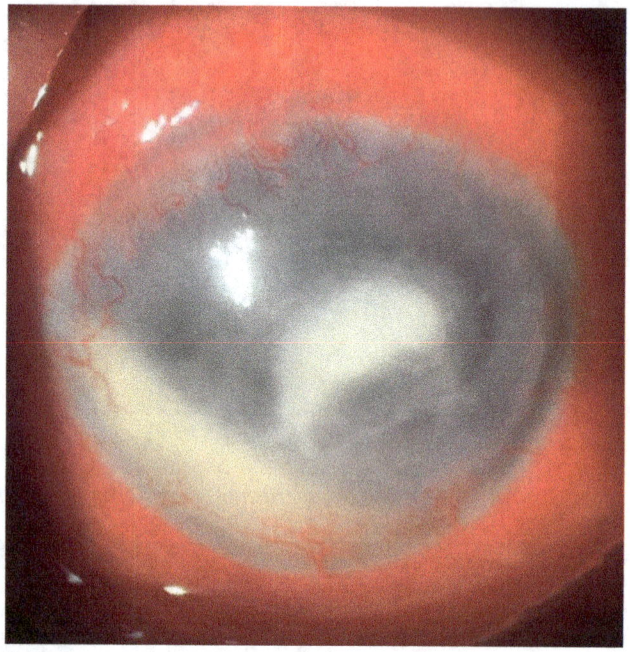

Figure 55. The same eye after 8 weeks of treatment, mild anterior stromal scar is formed

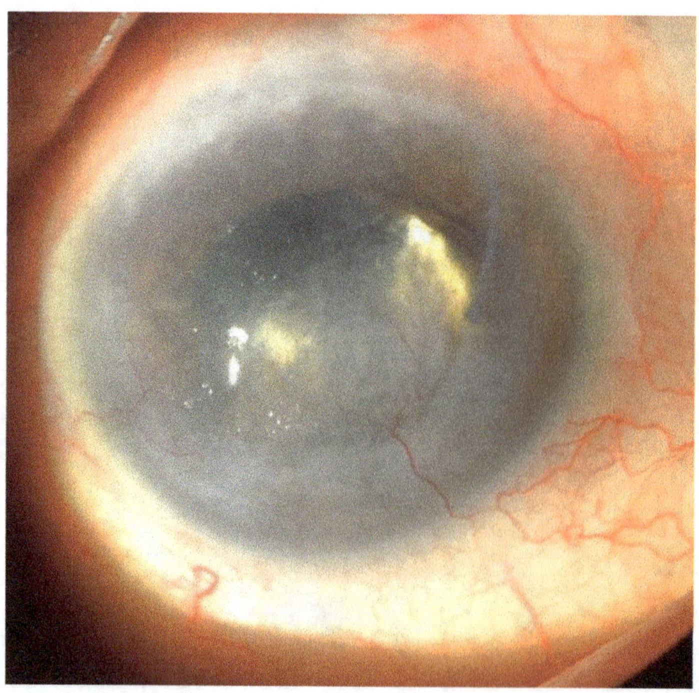

Stenotrophomonas maltophilia is an aerobic, non-fermentative, Gram-negative bacterium. It is an uncommon bacterium, and human infection is difficult to treat (Gilligan et al, 2003) It is a multidrug-resistant Gram-negative bacillus that is an opportunistic pathogen, particularly among hospitalized patients. *S. maltophilia* infections have been associated with high morbidity and mortality in severely immunocompromised and debilitated individuals (Fig 56, 57).

Figure 56. Round epithelial defect with stromal infiltrate inside and hypopyon are seen

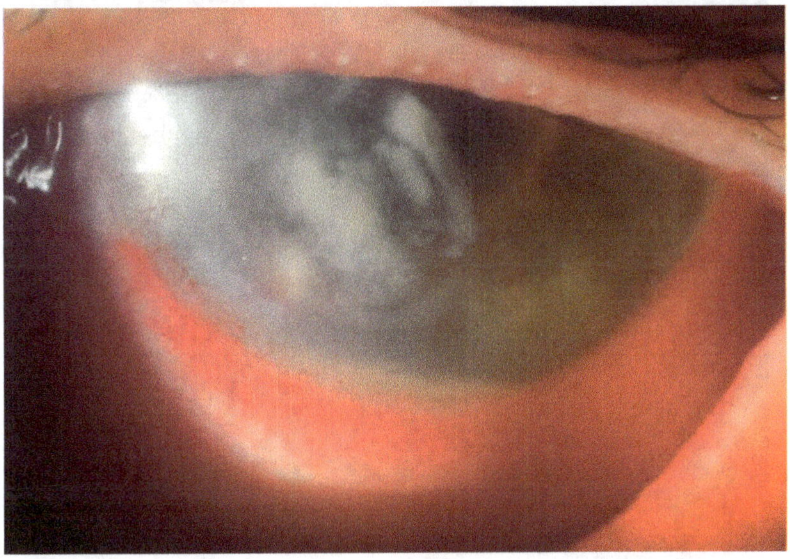

Figure 57. The same eye 3 months post PK

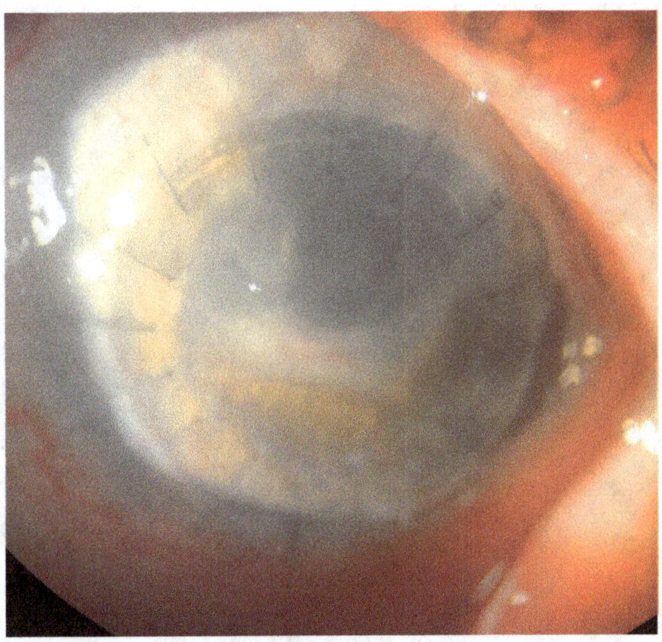

The most common causative agents of **bleb-associated endophthalmitis** are streptococci faecalis, viridans, pneumoniae, H. Influenza (Fig 58, 59, 60).

Figure 58. Total corneal edema, bleb purulent infiltrate, hypopyon. Pathology was caused by H. Influenza

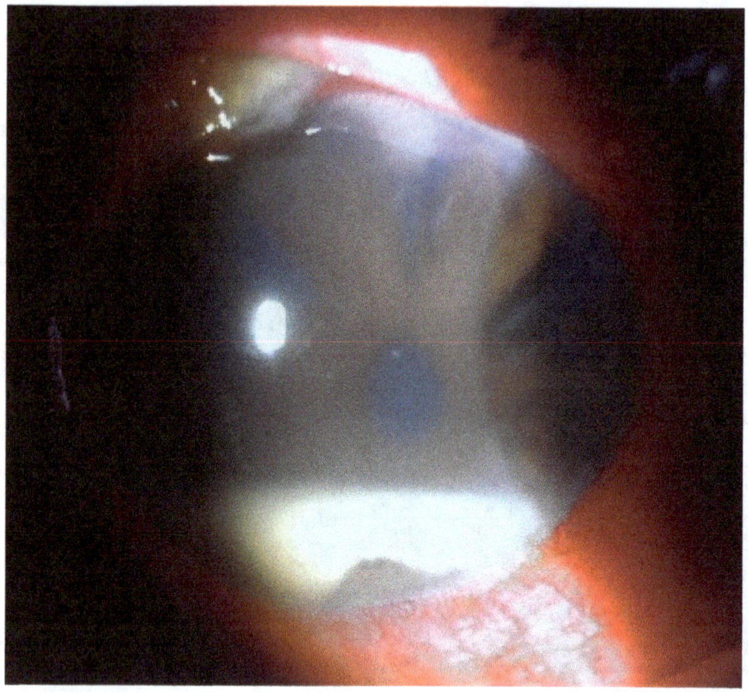

Figure 59. Same eye. Bleb purulent infiltrate

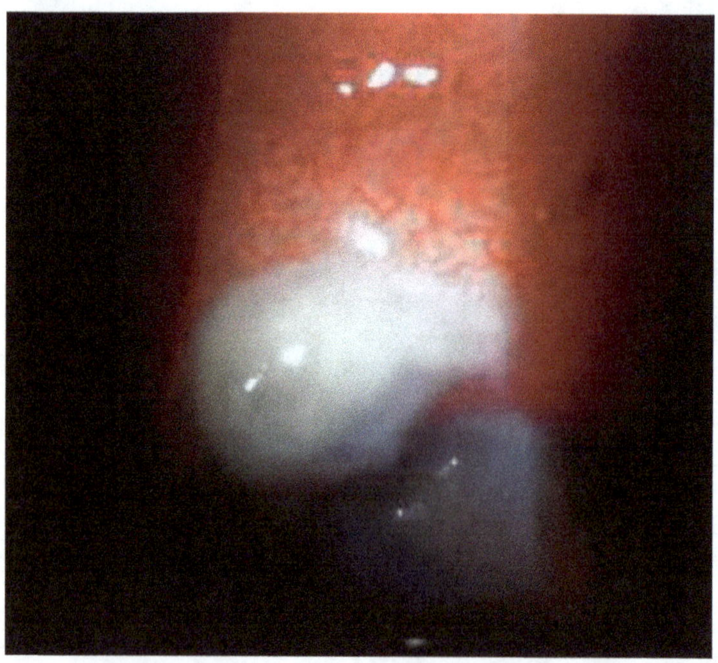

Figure 60. The same patient after 6 weeks of treatment. Hypopyon resolved, conjunctival scar formation in the bleb region is seen

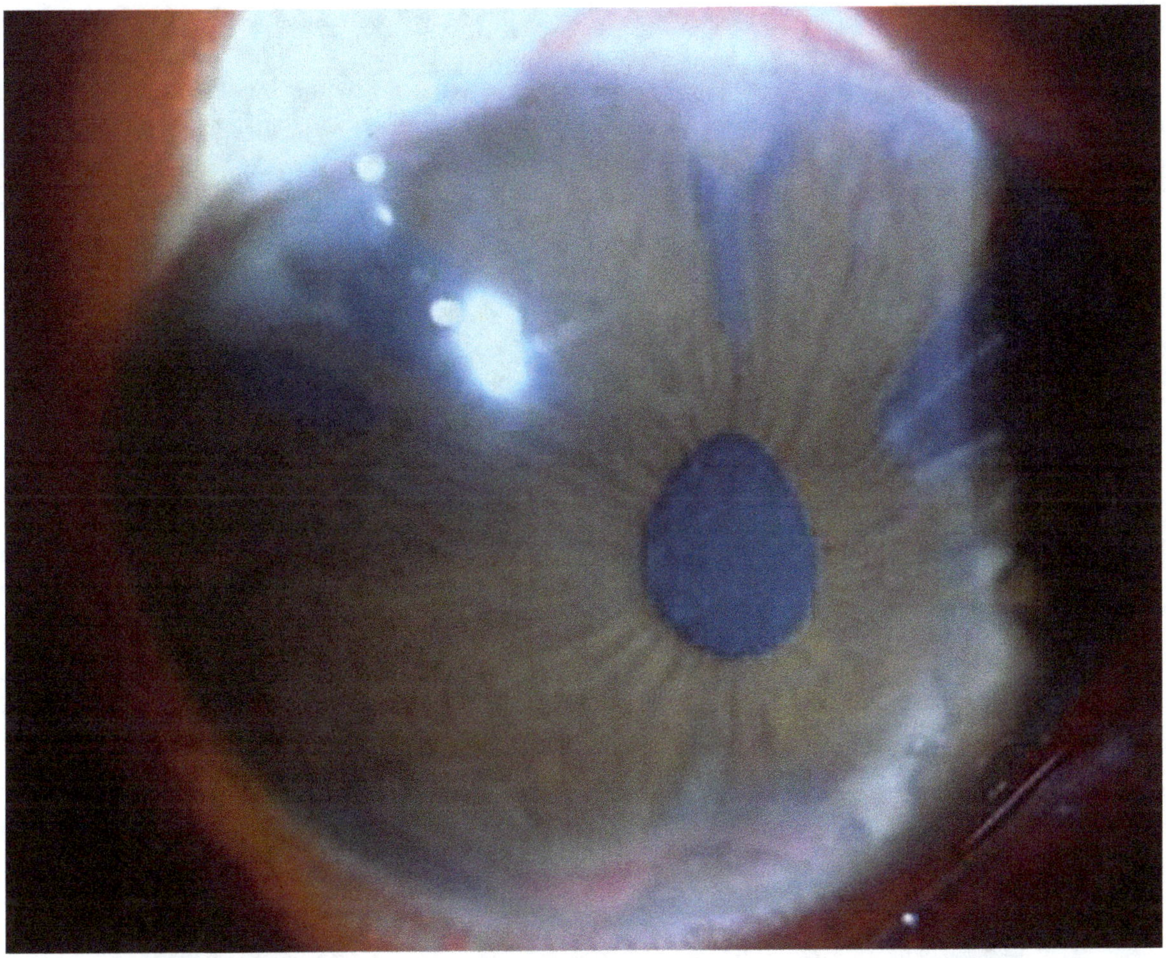

Acanthamoeba Keratitis

Acanthamoeba keratitis is caused by free-living protozoa found in water and soil. It is a usual contact lens-related infection, which is the primary risk factor in otherwise healthy individuals of any age (Gilligan et al, 2003). Acanthamoeba keratitis usually presents as pseudodendrites, often resembling herpetic epithelial keratitis. The most common signs and symptoms include severe pain, presence of ring infiltrate, and radial keratoneuritis. The visible ring infiltrate represents an immune reaction. Before the formation of a ring, herpetic stromal keratitis, interstitial keratitis, and anesthetic abuse may also mimic this clinical appearance (Fig 61-66).

Our country lacks medications, except Chlorhexidine 0.02% eye drops compounded here, used to treat acanthamoeba keratitis. Therefore, when this diagnosis is given, we always warn the patient that transplant surgery may be required as an emergency to save the eyeball. The case shown below was the only case that responded to Chlorhexidine 0.02% eye drops and Brolene 0.15% eye ointment, which the patient was able to obtain from abroad. Topical cycloplegics and lubricants were prescribed as well.

Figure 61. Ring infiltrate, epithelial demarcation line, hypopyon and 360-degree of neovascularization are seen on the photo

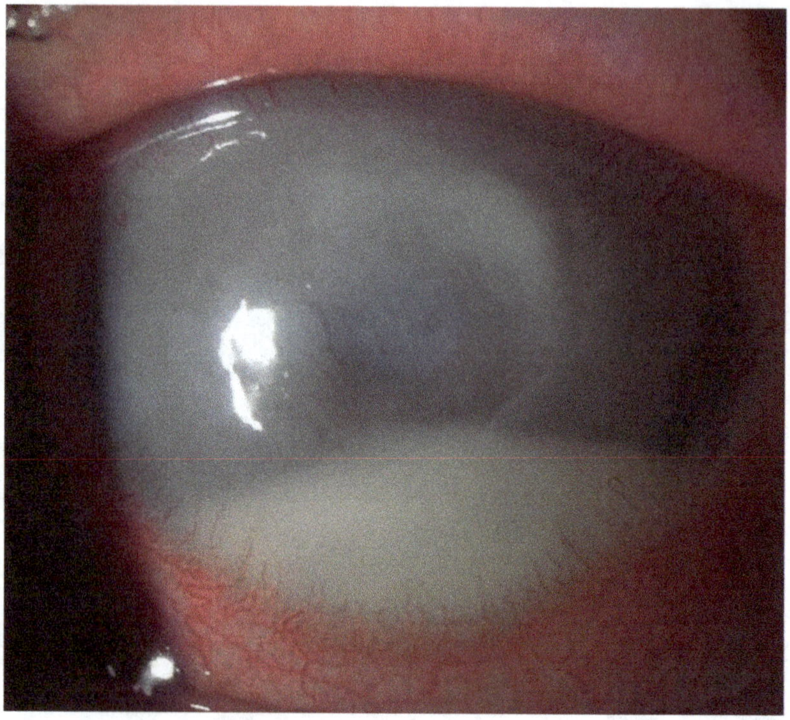

Figure 62. The same eye after 3 months of medical treatment

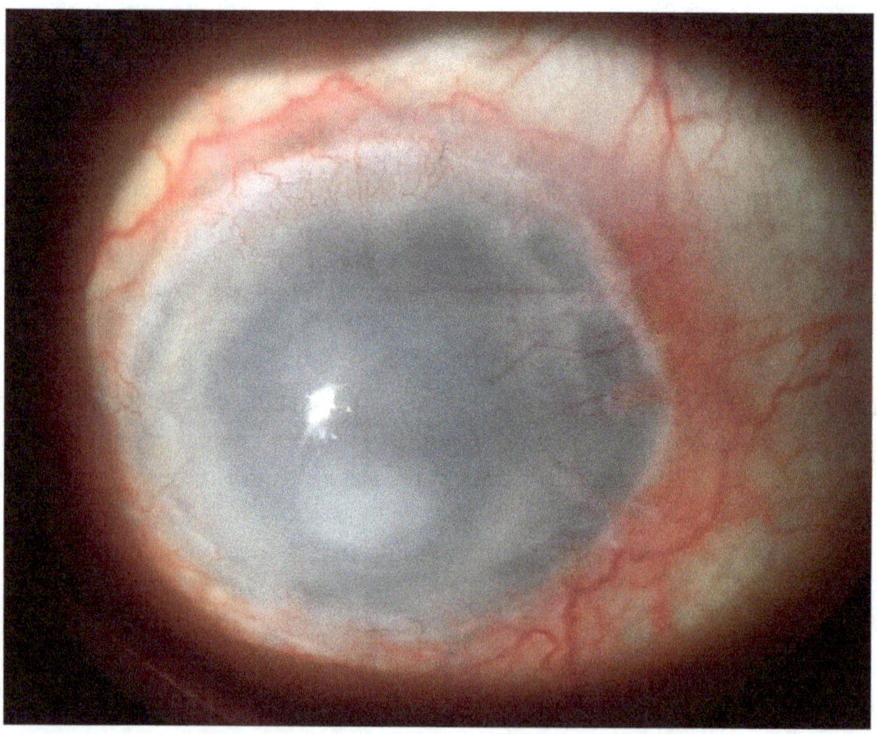

Figure 63. Acanthamoeba keratitis with ring infiltrate, non-responding to medical treatment

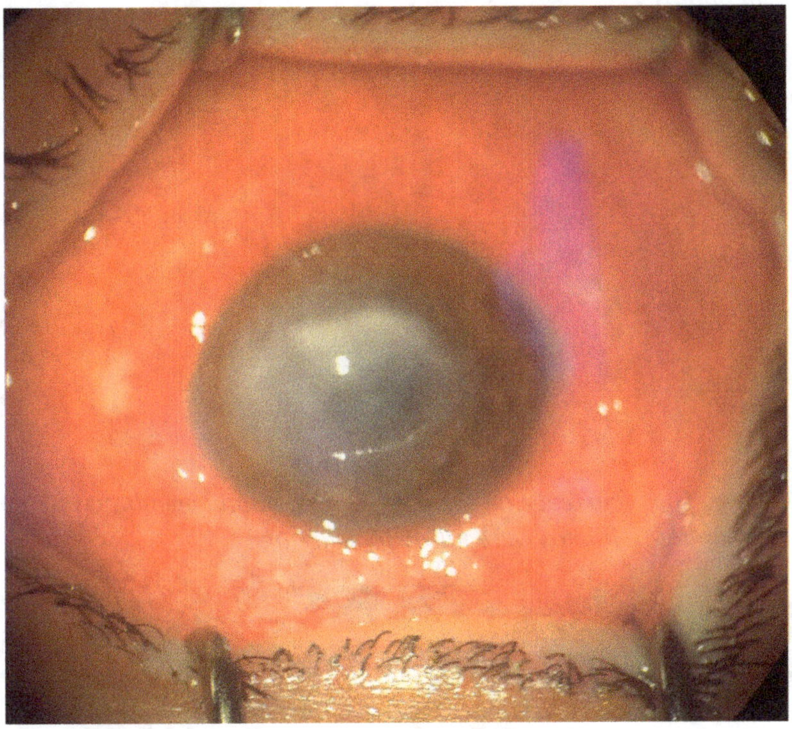

Figure 64. The same patient after PK

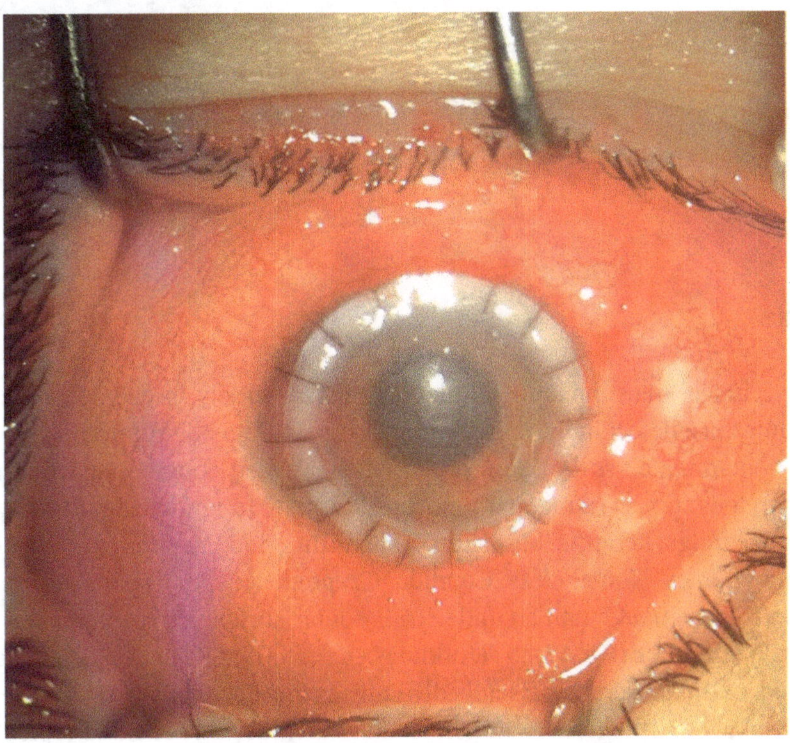

Figure 65. Acanthamoeba keratitis. Ring infiltrate is seen (left eye), the same eye progressed to total corneal abscess (right photo)

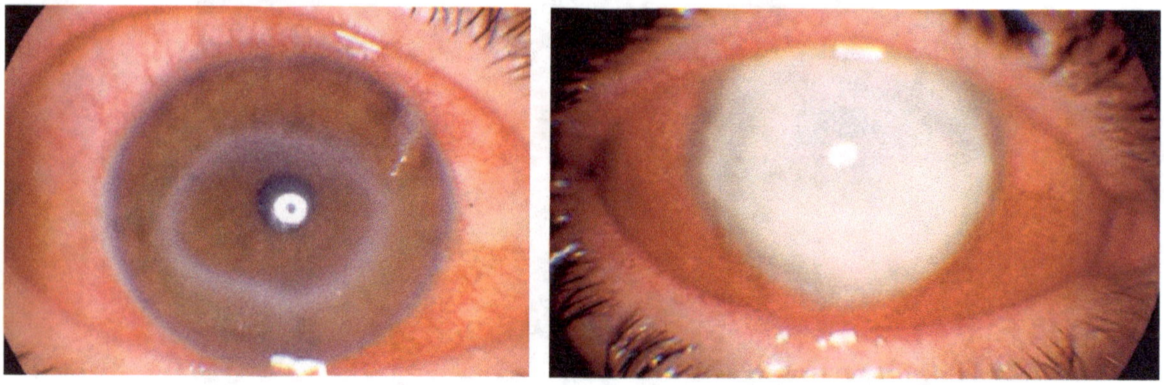

Figure 66. The Same eye. The recurrence on the graft with amniotic membrane (left eye) and 6 months after repeated PK (right photo). Photos were taken 16 years ago

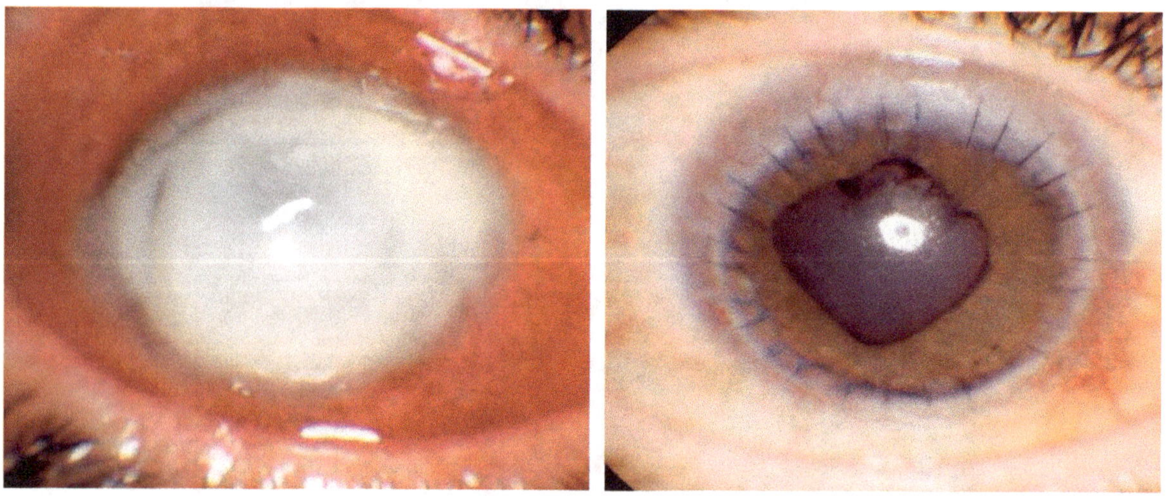

Fungal Keratitis

Fungi are eukaryotic, unicellular, and multicellular organisms, widely spread in nature. Fungi can access into the cornea stroma via a defect in the epithelial barrier. Epithelial disruption may be due to traumatic implantation with contaminated soil or plant materials, damaged contact lens wearing, compromised ocular surface, or previous surgery. Among the more than 250.00 fungal species that have been identified, less than 100 can cause fungal keratitis. Fusarium, Aspergillus, and Paecilomyces species are considered to be the most common ones. Nonetheless, Candida, Cryptococcus, or Trichosporum species are more likely to be isolated from patients with an underlying ocular surface disease and chronic use of ocular anesthetic drops and antibiotics (Fig 67-89) (Jurkunas et al, 2009; DG et al, 2011; Thomas et al, 2013). Medical management of fungal keratitis is really difficult, as there are no standard guidelines for selecting and administering current antifungals. Treatment usually includes one or more topical antifungals with systemic support of oral antifungal medications. The most common classes of antifungal medications used for medical therapy include polyenes, azoles, and echinocandins. Among topical antifungals, only Fluconazole 0.3% eye drops are available in our country. When needed, patients obtain Amphotericin B and Voriconazole from abroad, mainly from Russia. The pharmacies compound the needed dosage for topical use here in Armenia. We have treated our cases mainly with Amphotericin B 0.15% eye drops, and intracameral injections, Fluconazole eye drops with Fluconazole subconjunctival injections (sensitivity-based), Voriconazole eye drops, intrastromal injections and systemic Itraconazole. Topical cycloplegics were given in almost every case. In our cases around 80% of fungi were non sensitive to Fluconazole, thus, mostly Amphotericin B eye drops were used as topical medications, whereas Itraconazole was sensitive in about 70% of cases. PK was performed to save the eyeball and provide possible vision in cases when the arrival of required medications was delayed, and the disease progressed.

Figure 67. Fungal keratitis caused by Fusarium. Hypopyon and epithelial ulcer with underlying stromal infiltrate and edema are seen

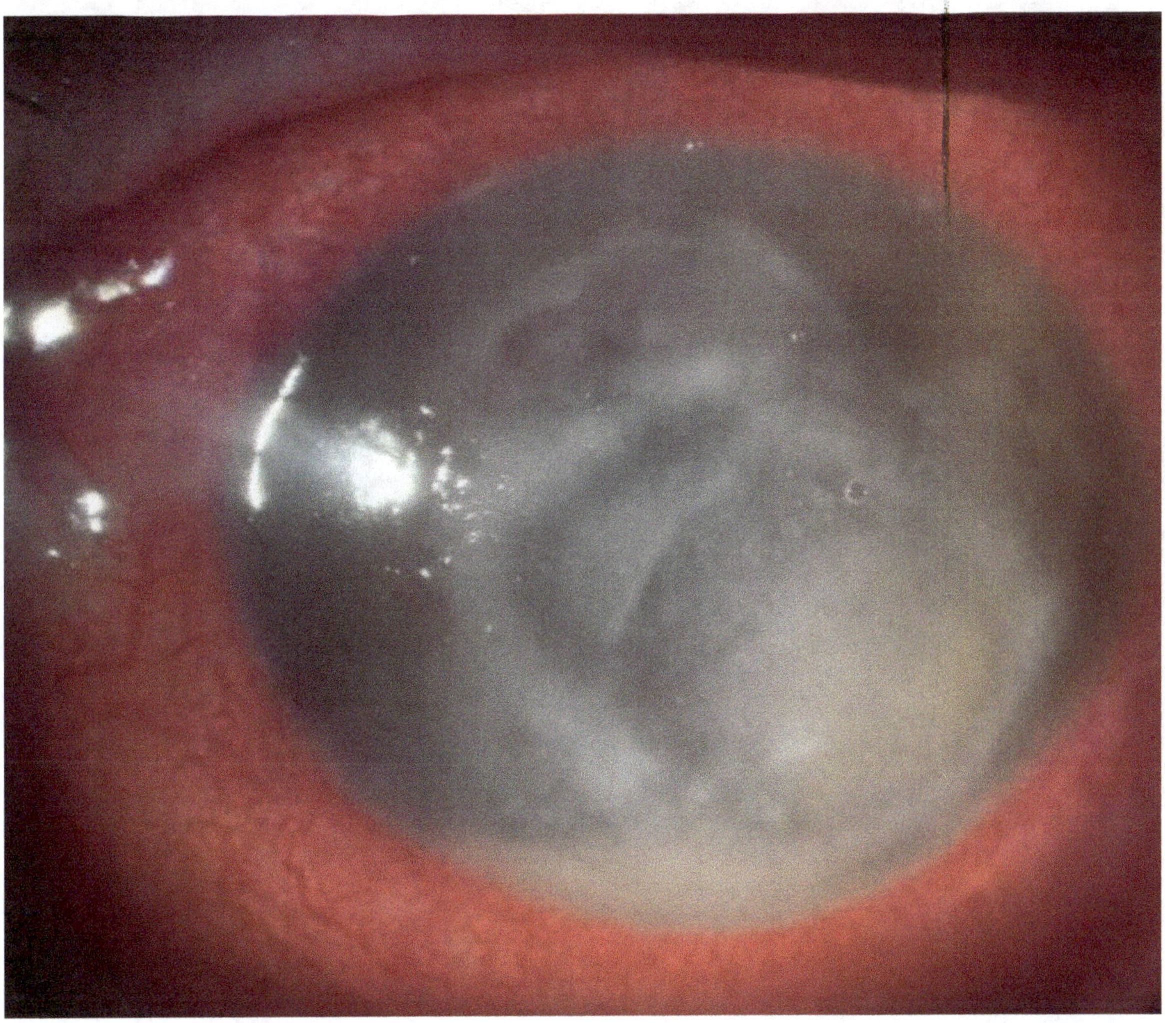

Figure 68. The same eye unresponsive to medical treatment with total corneal abscess (in OR)

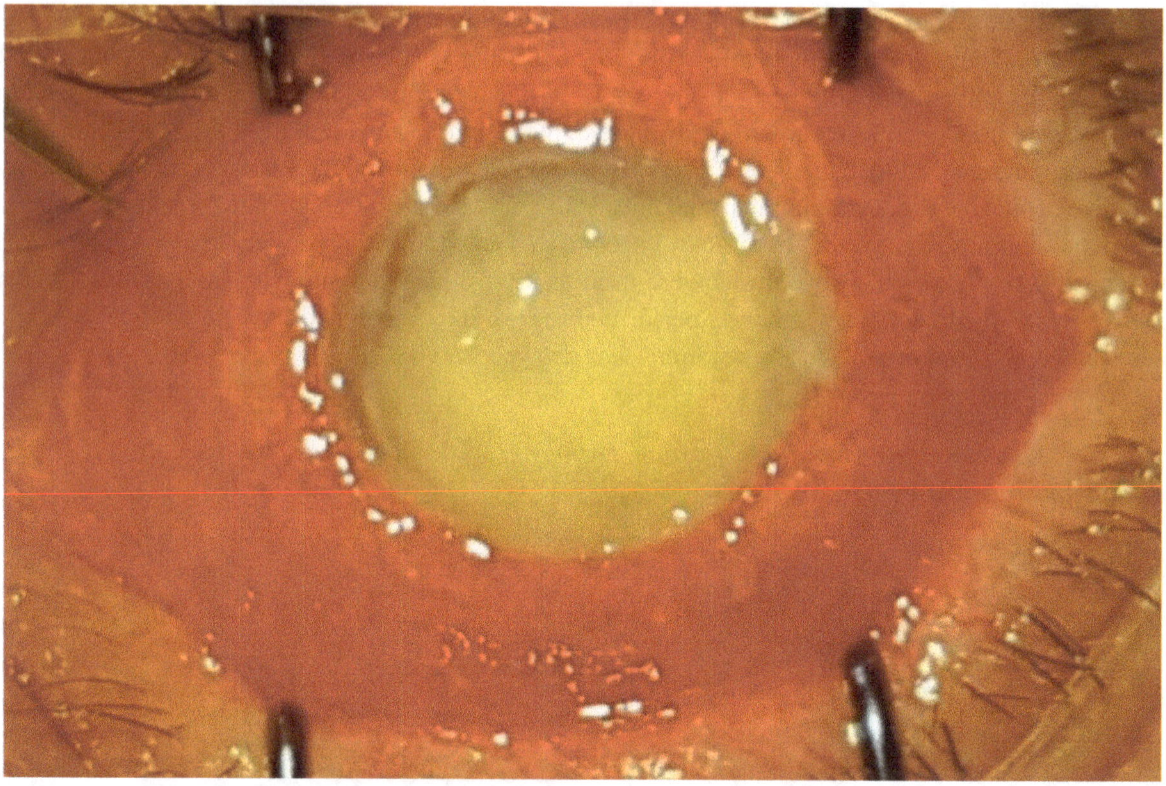

Figure 69. The same patient the next day after PK

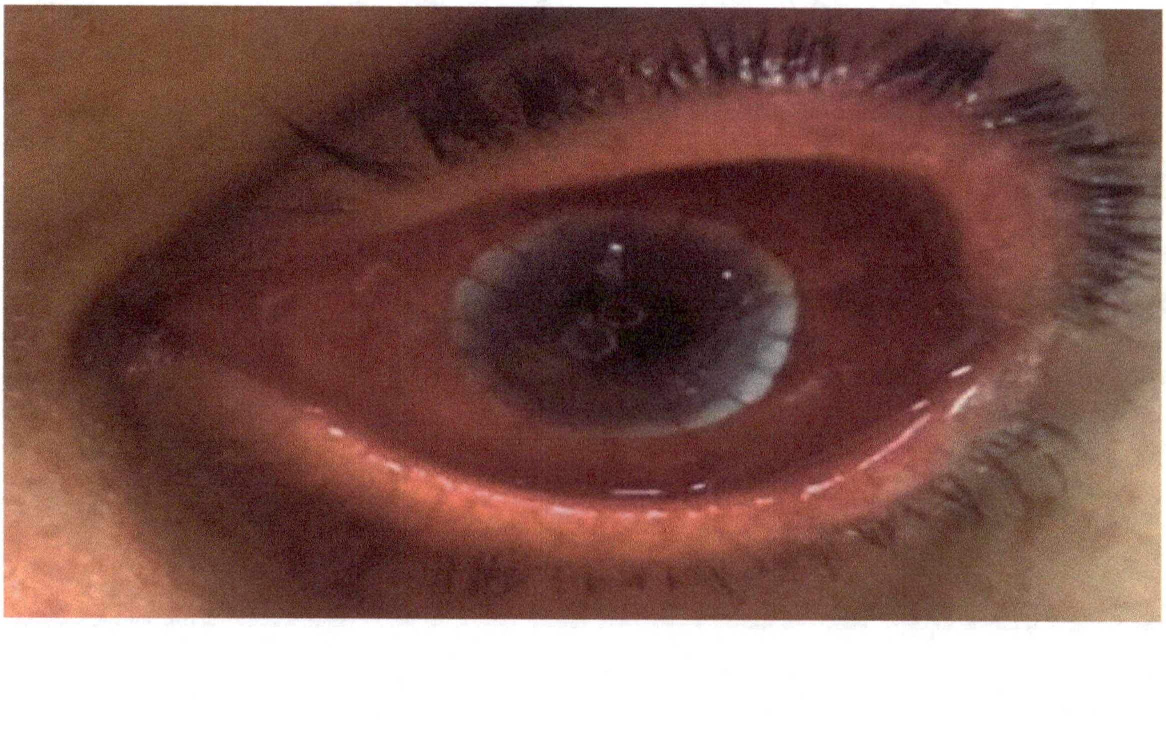

Figure 70. Keratitis caused by Fusarium unresponsive to the treatment. Marked hypopyon and stromal infiltrate are seen (left photo) along with microscopic view of smears (right photo)

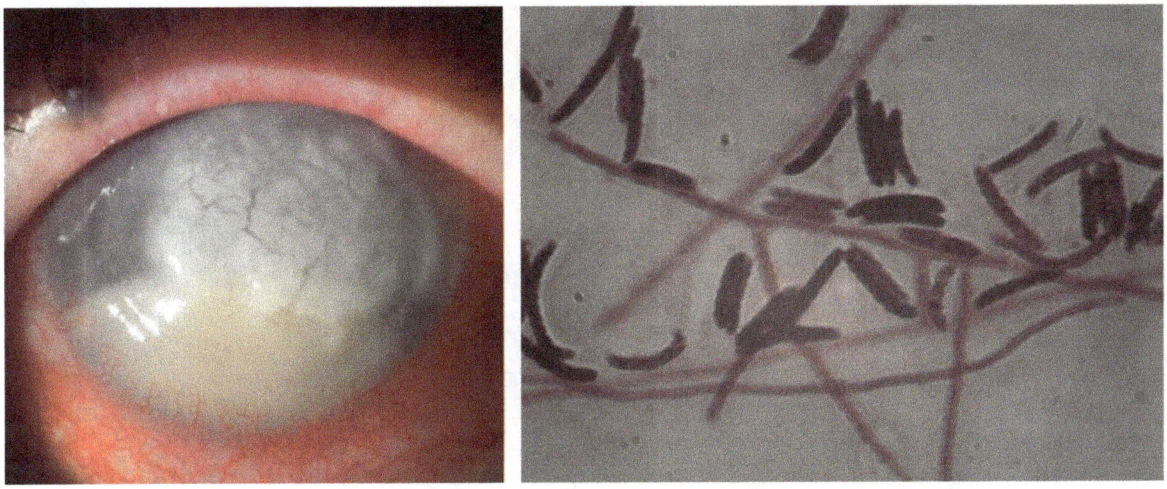

Figure 71. The same eye after PK (in OR)

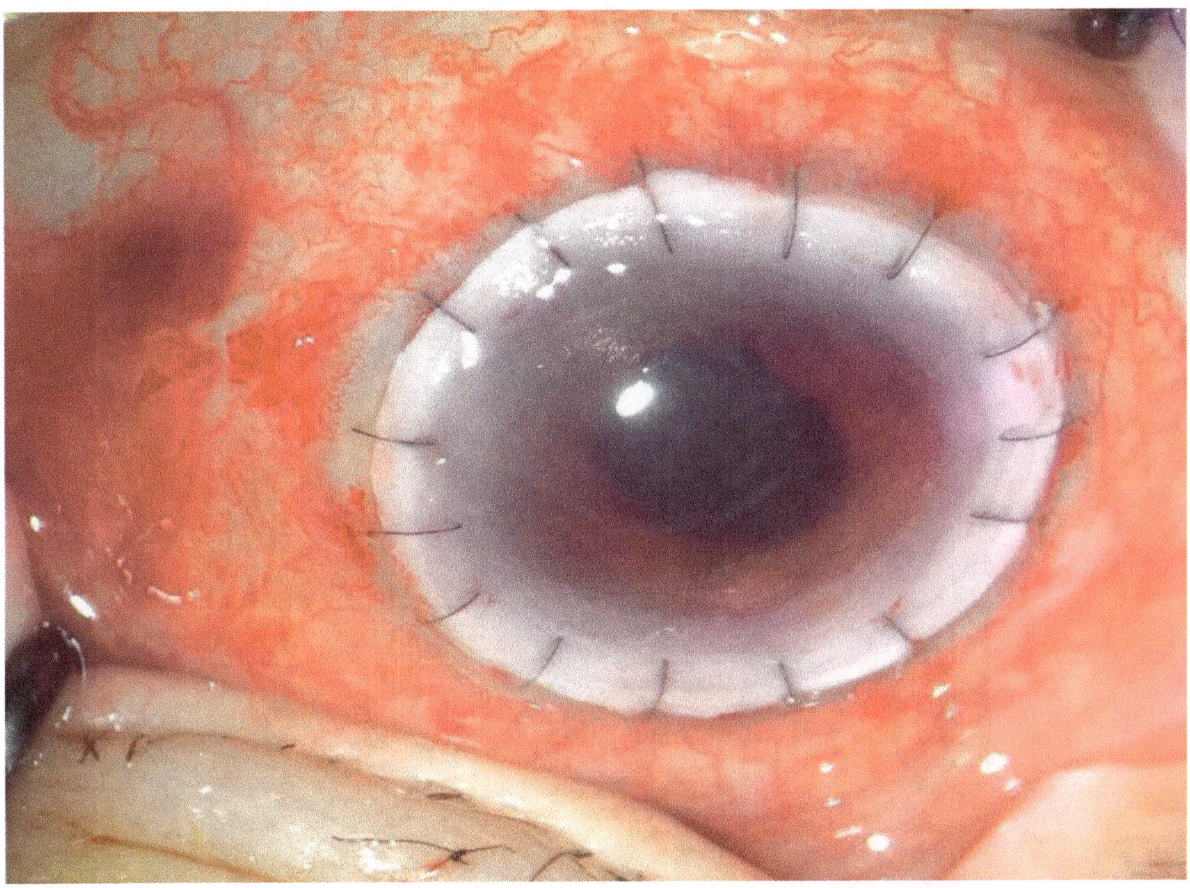

Figure 72. Fusarium fungal keratitis 1 week after extracapsular cataract extraction. Subtotal stromal infiltrate with hypopyon are seen

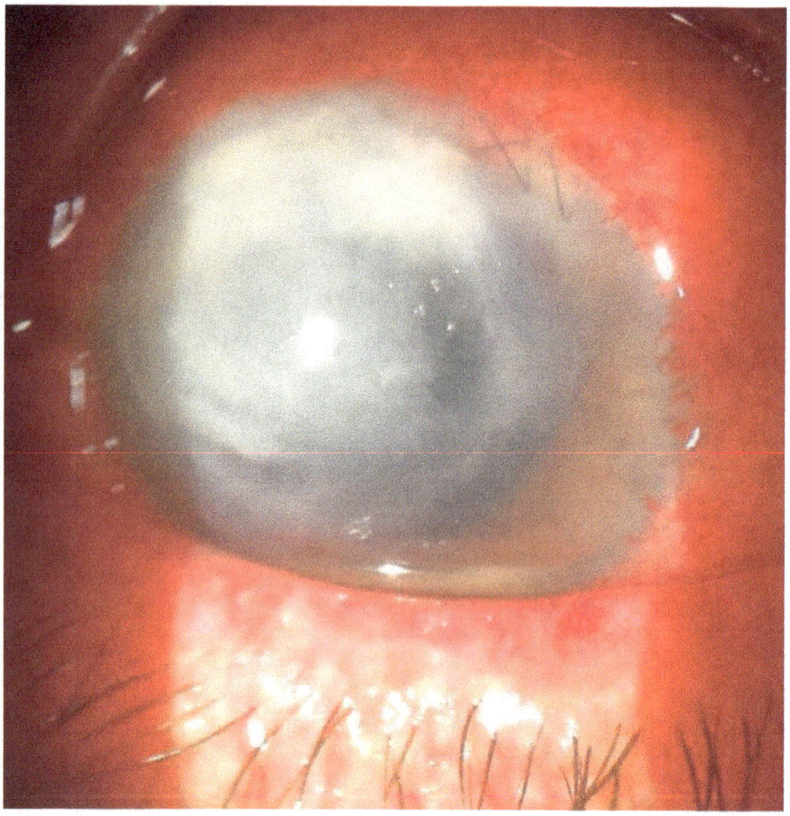

Figure 73. The same eye 1 month after PK

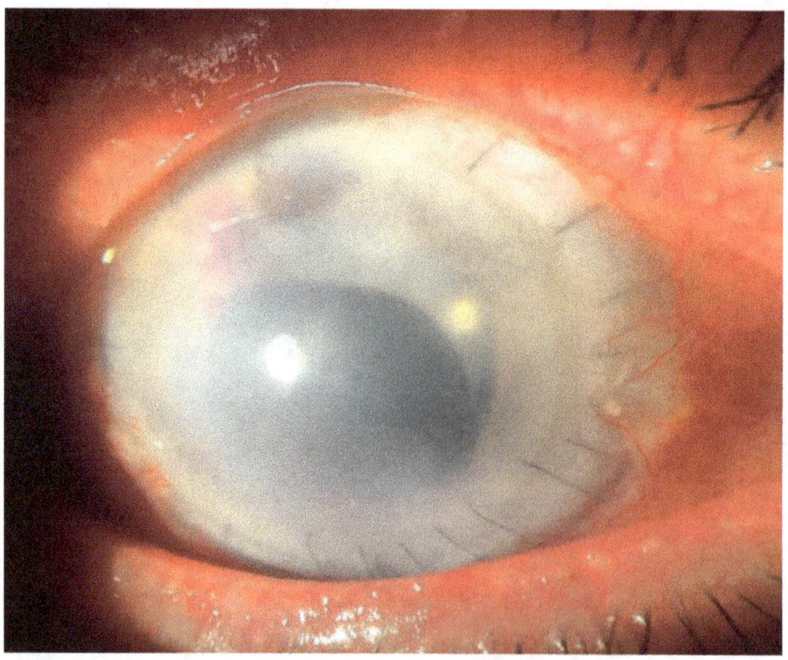

Figure 74. Fungal keratitis caused by Aspergillus. Oval-shaped epithelial defect with underlying stromal infiltrate and marked hypopyon are seen

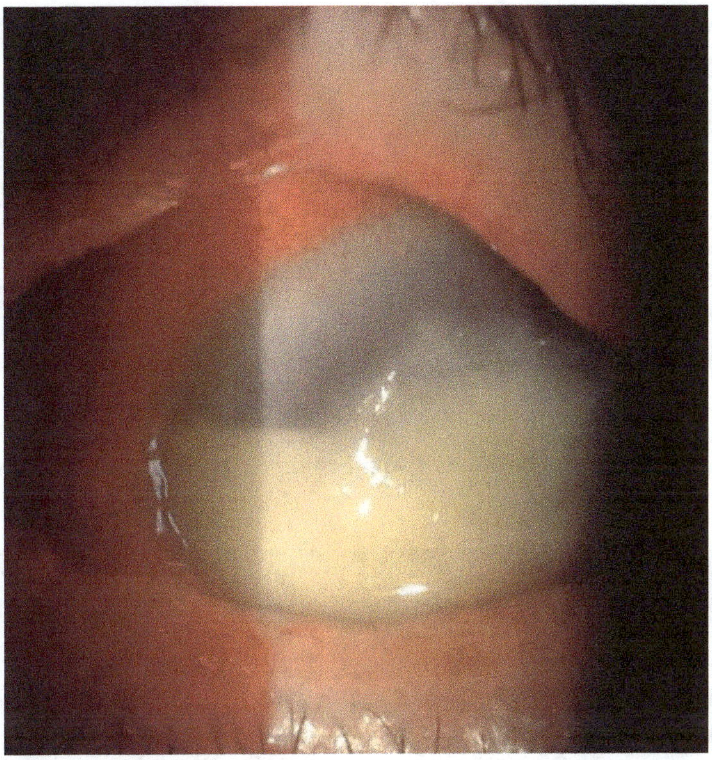

Figure 75. The same eye 10 days after PK

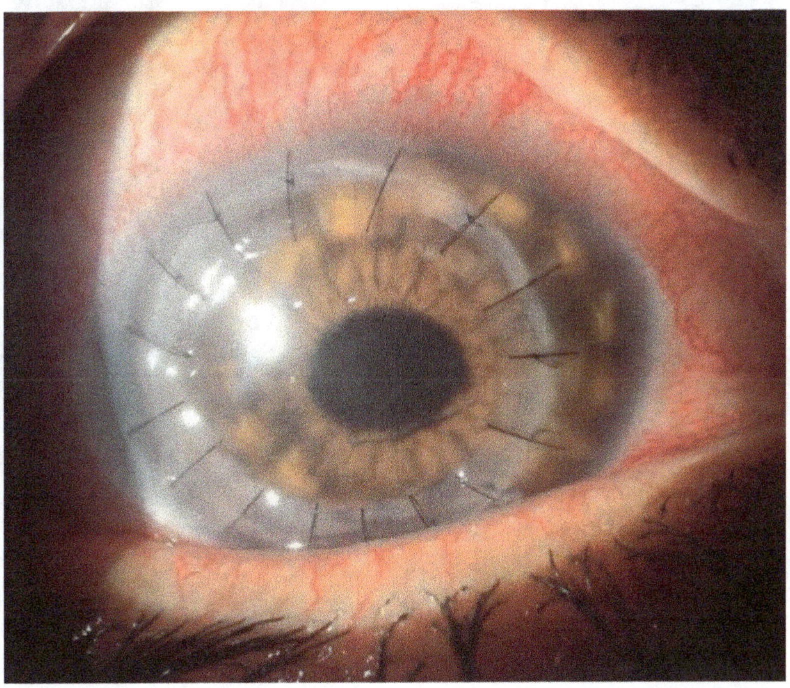

Figure 76 Fungal keratitis caused by Aspergillus (right photo – microscopic view). Small round temporal paracentral lesion with marked hypopyon and hyphema are seen (left photo)

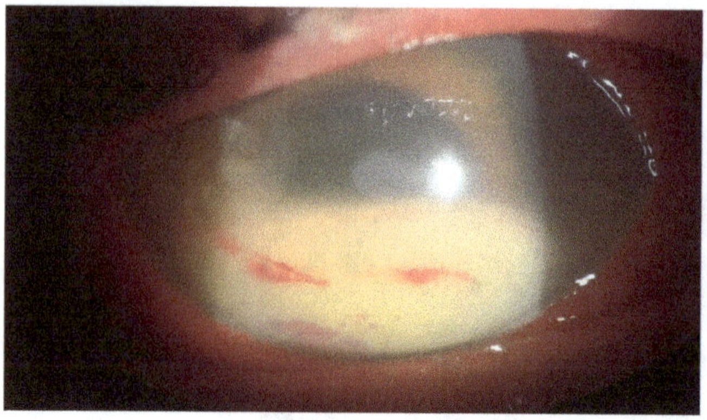

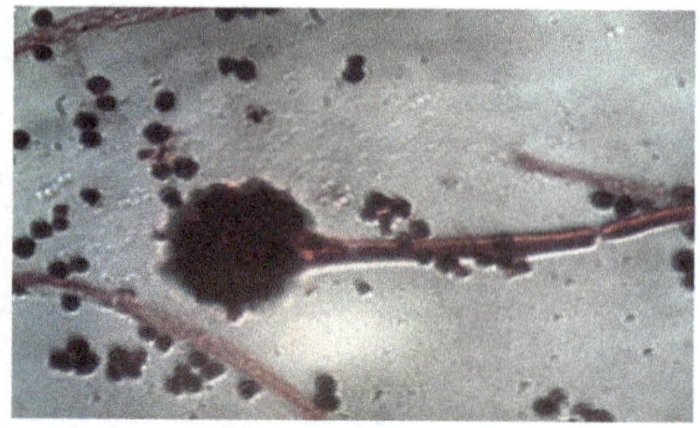

Figure 77. The same patient 3 months after medical treatment. The paracentral subepithelial fibrosis is seen

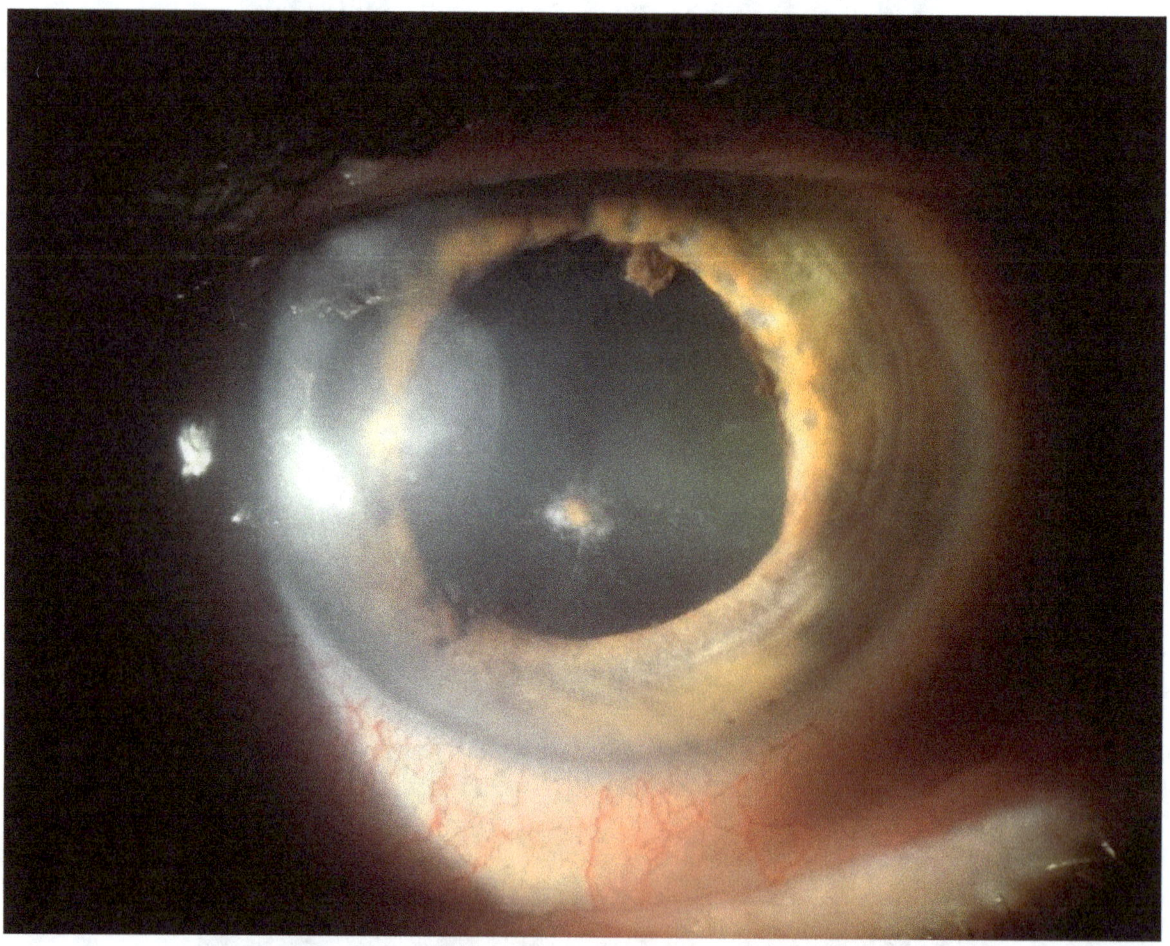

Figure 78. Fungal keratitis caused by Aspergillus. Dens central infiltrate, stromal edema and hypopyon are seen on the photo

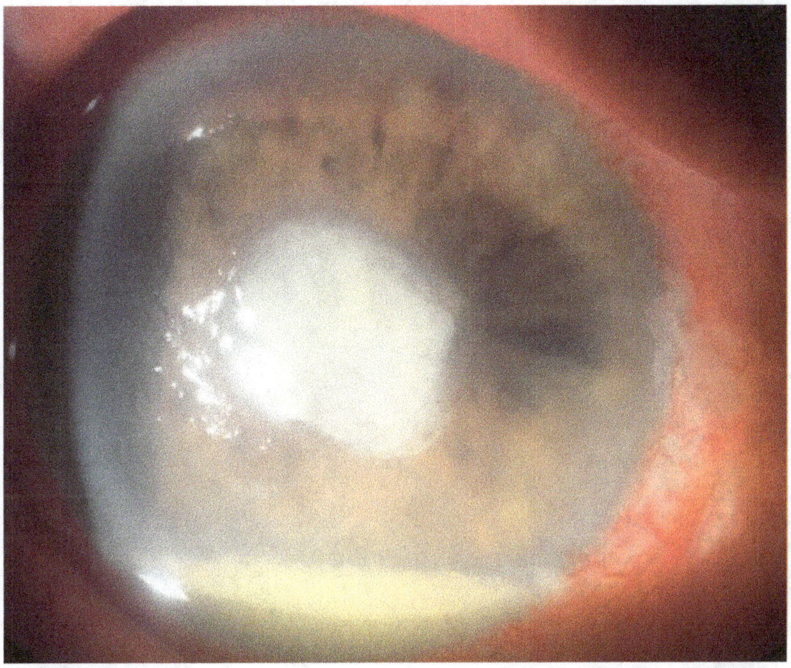

Figure 79. The same eye after 1 week of treatment with worsening condition

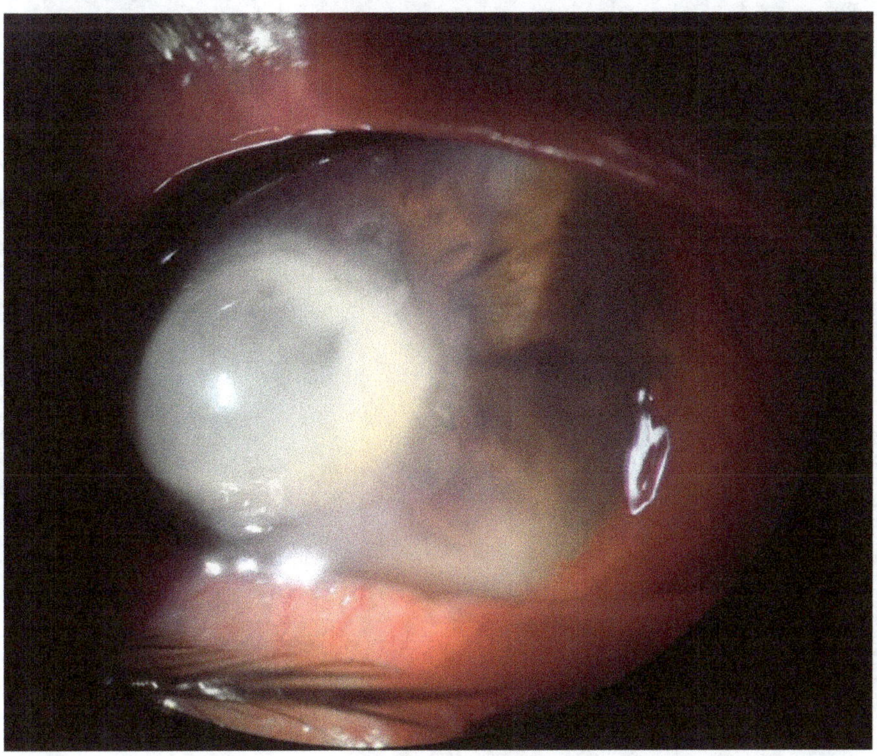

Figure 80. The same eye 1 month after PK

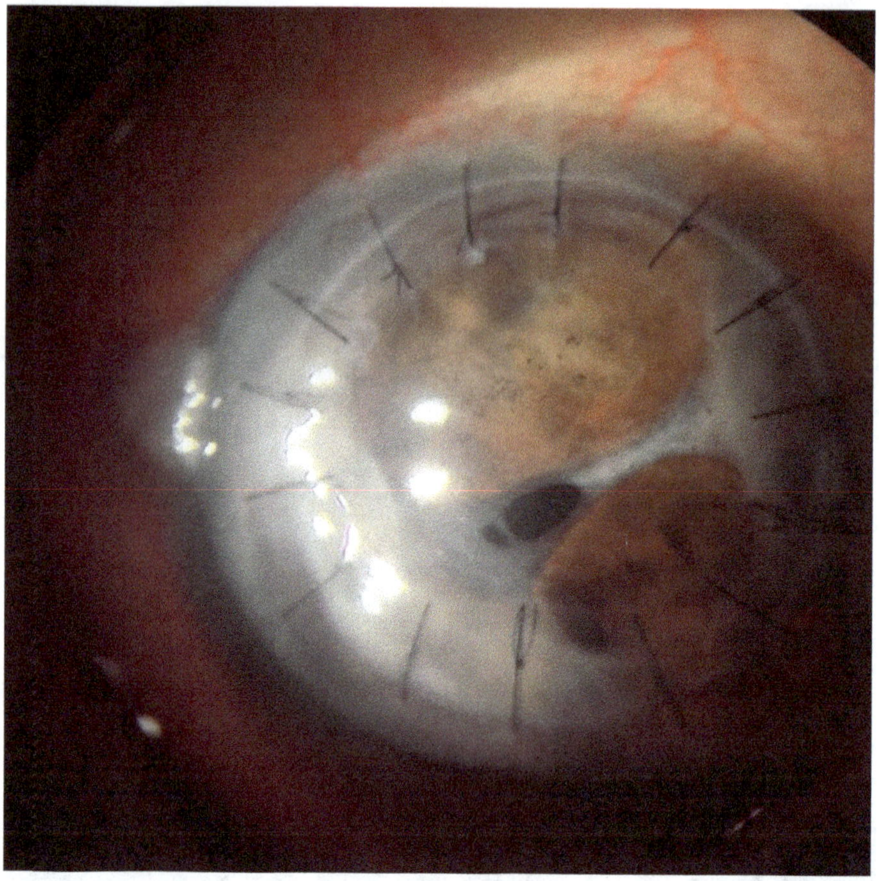

Figure 81. Fungal keratitis caused by Aspergillus. Note the feathery borders and 1mm hypopyon

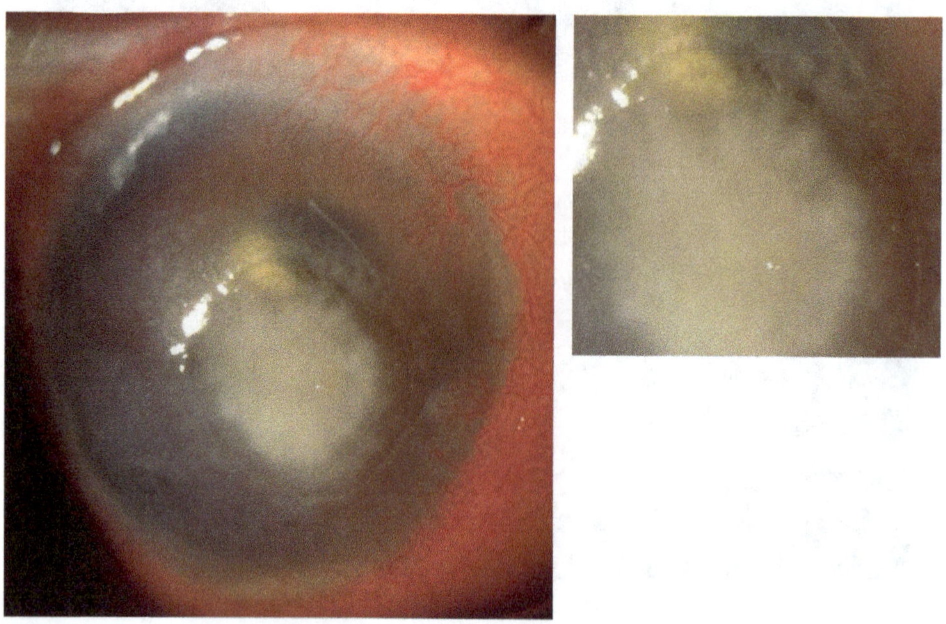

Figure 82. The same eye after 3 weeks of medical treatment; hypopyon got resolved, persistent epithelial defect (left photo). The same eye covered with amniotic membrane (right photo in OR)

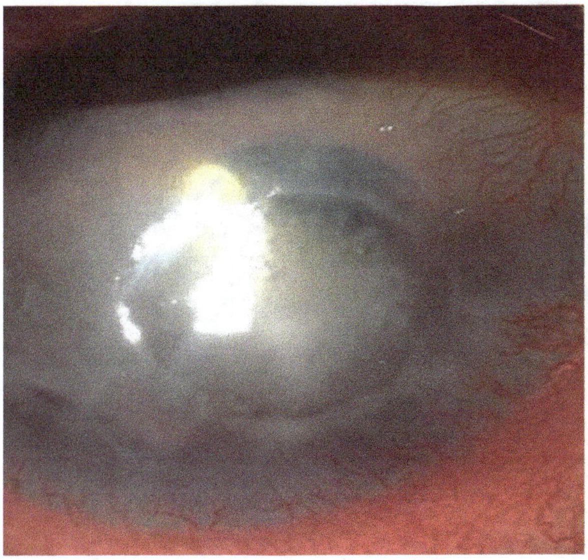

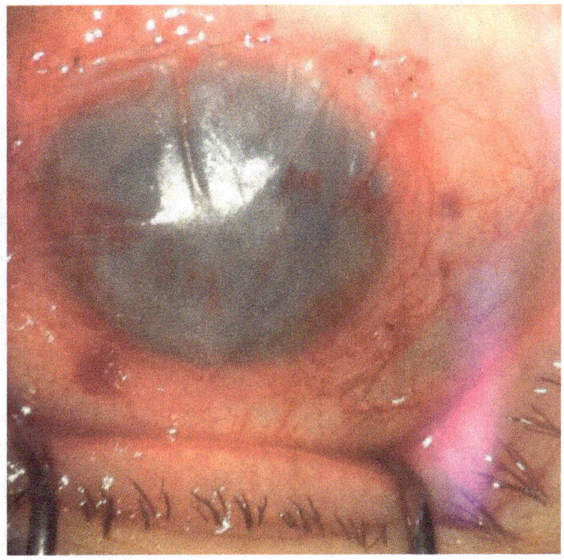

Figure 83. The same eye after 2 months. Patient left with mild subepithelial scarring

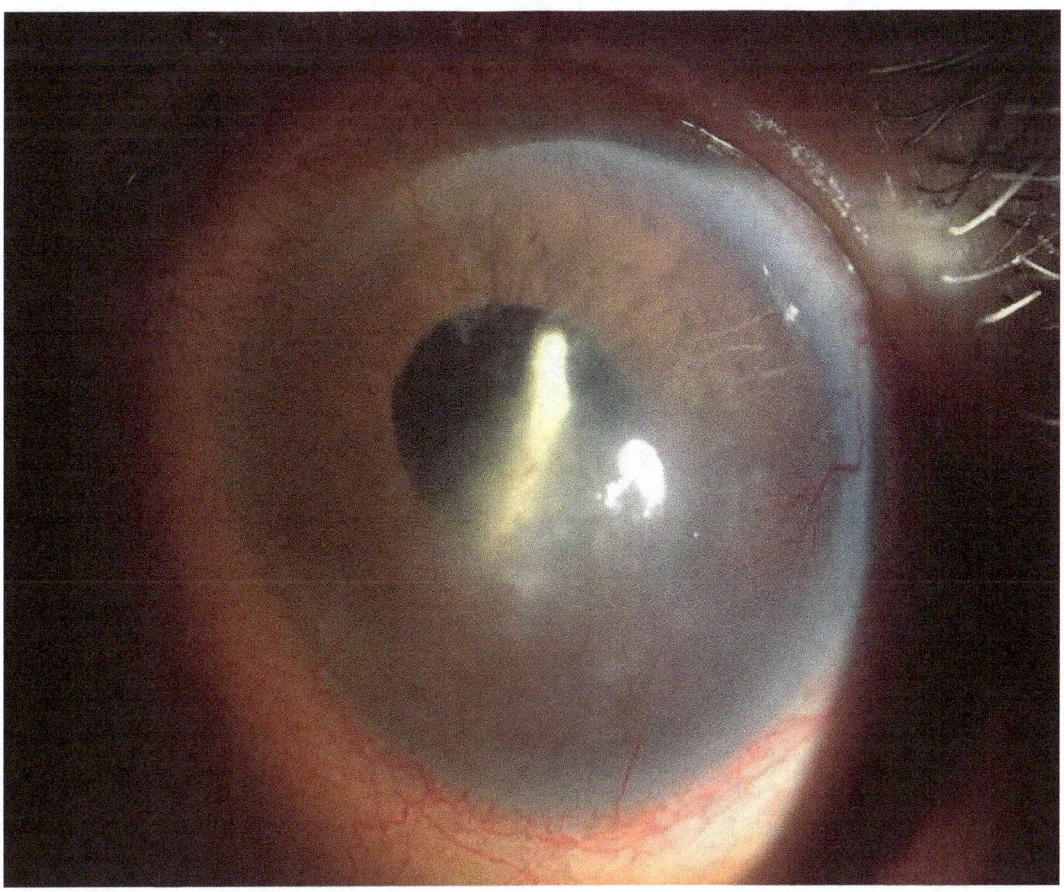

Figure 84. Fungal keratitis caused by Candida albicans. A stromal lesion with feathery borders and hypopyon is seen. This patient was visiting from Persia and was lost for follow-up

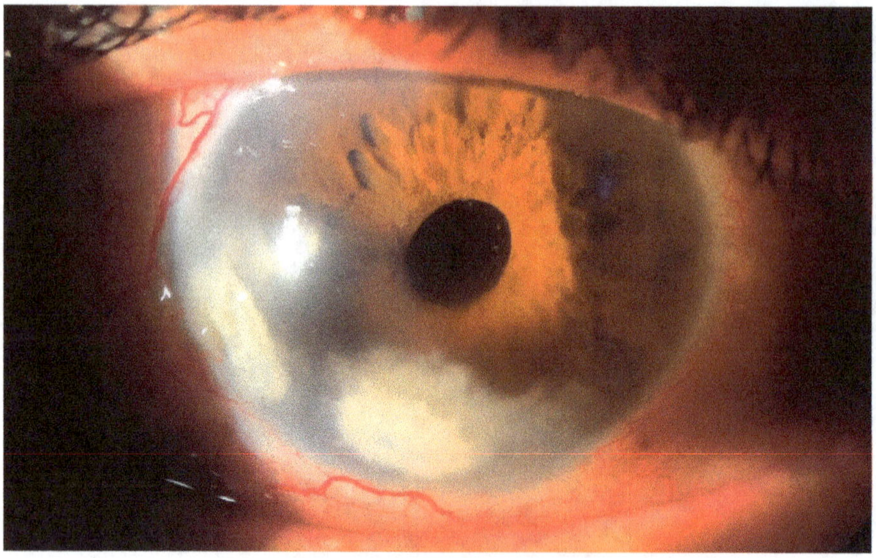

Figure 85. Fungal keratitis caused by Candida albicans with satellite lesions

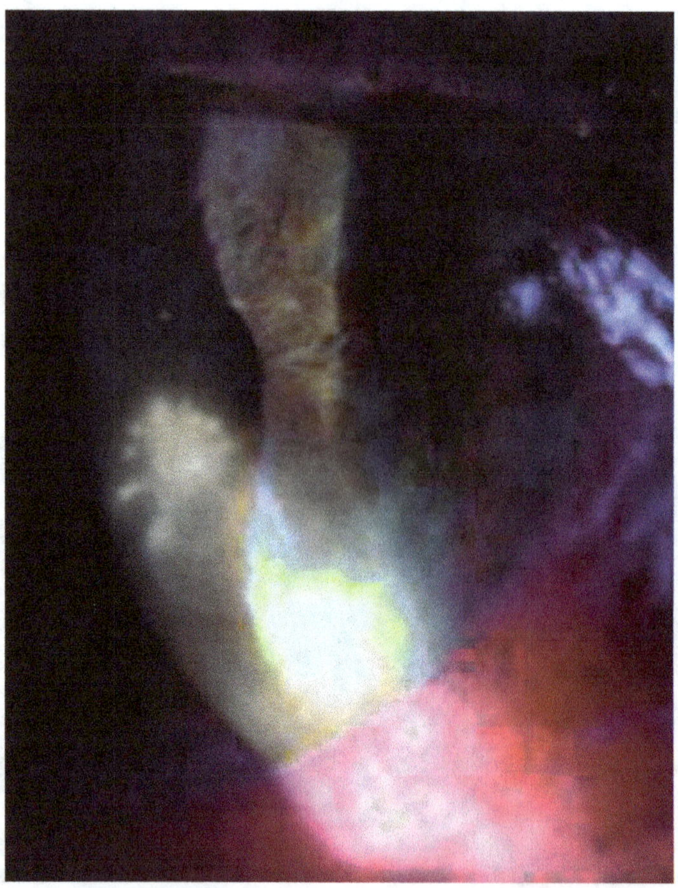

Figure 86. The same eye after treatment. A mild anterior stromal scar is formed

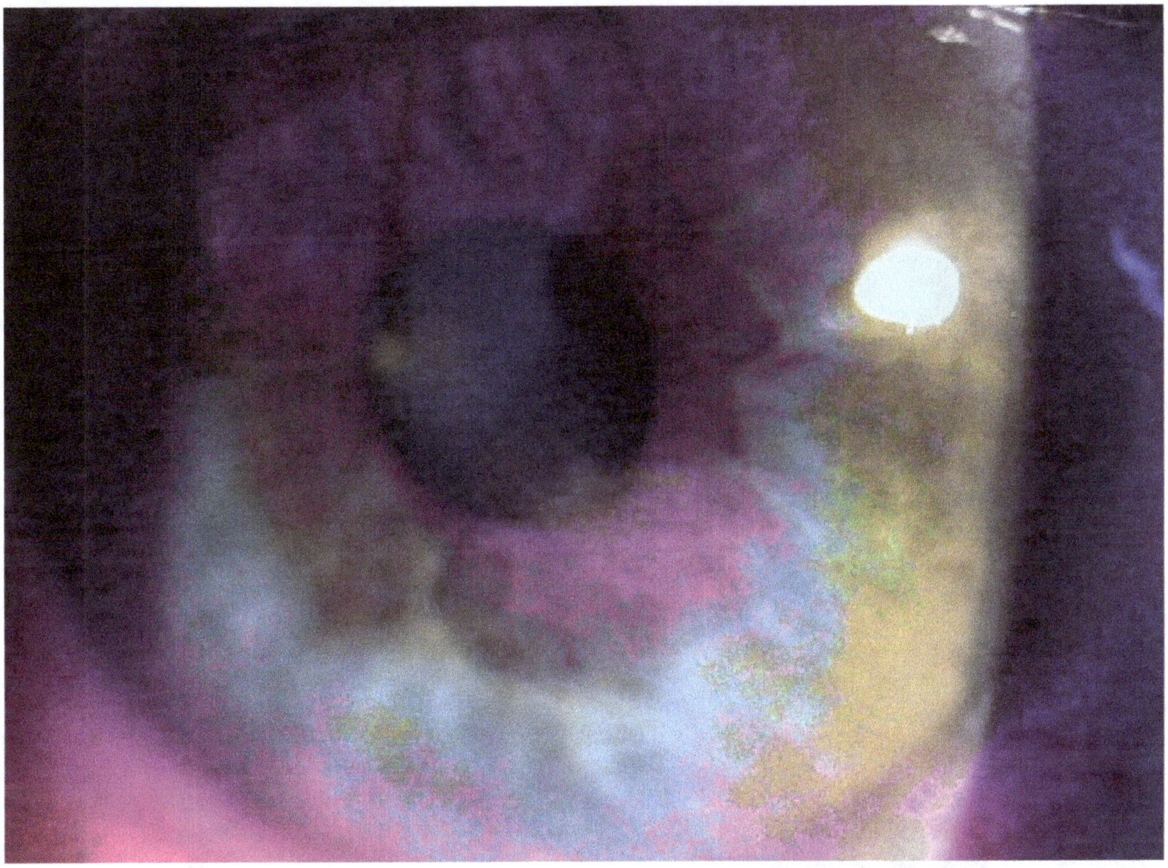

Figure 87. Candida fungal keratitis with satellite lesions and hypopyon

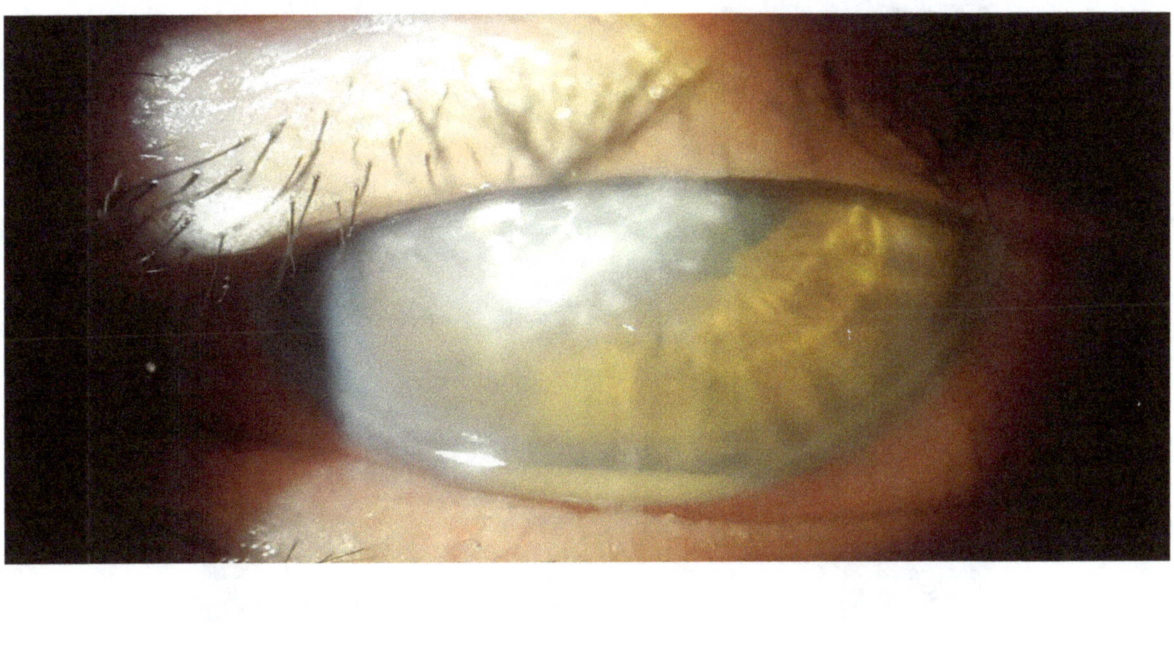

Figure 88. 6 weeks after medical treatment. A stromal scar is noted

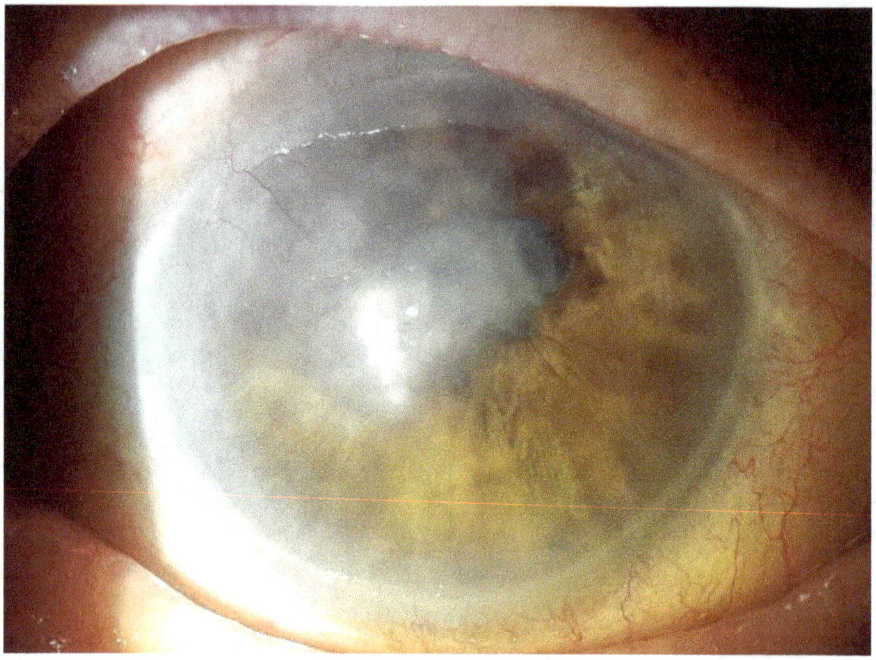

Figure 89. Multiple Candida-caused lesions with crystalline-like and feathery borders are seen on the corneal graft

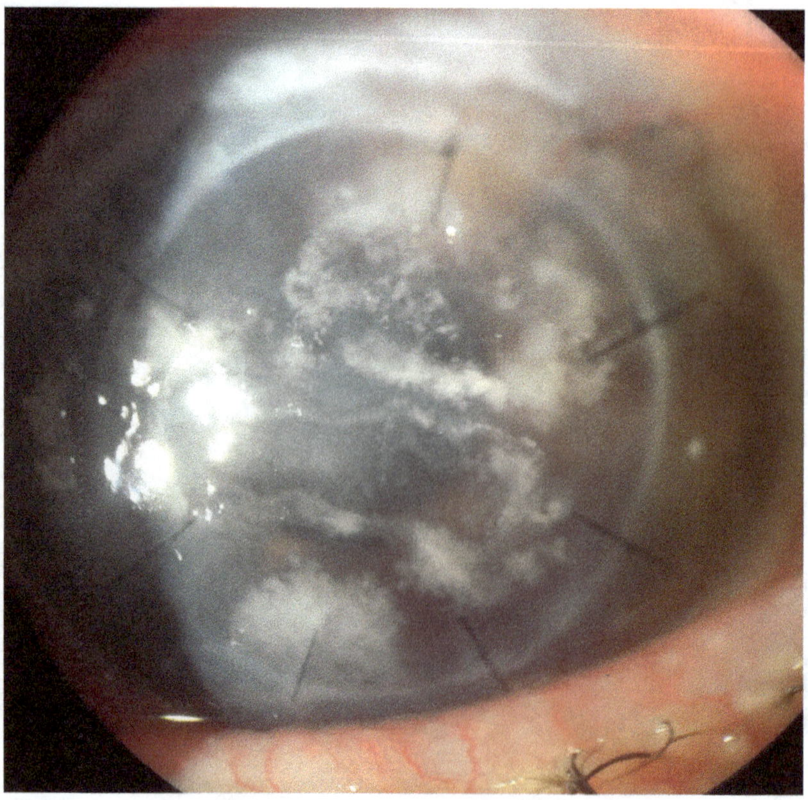

Figure 90. The same eye after 8 weeks of treatment

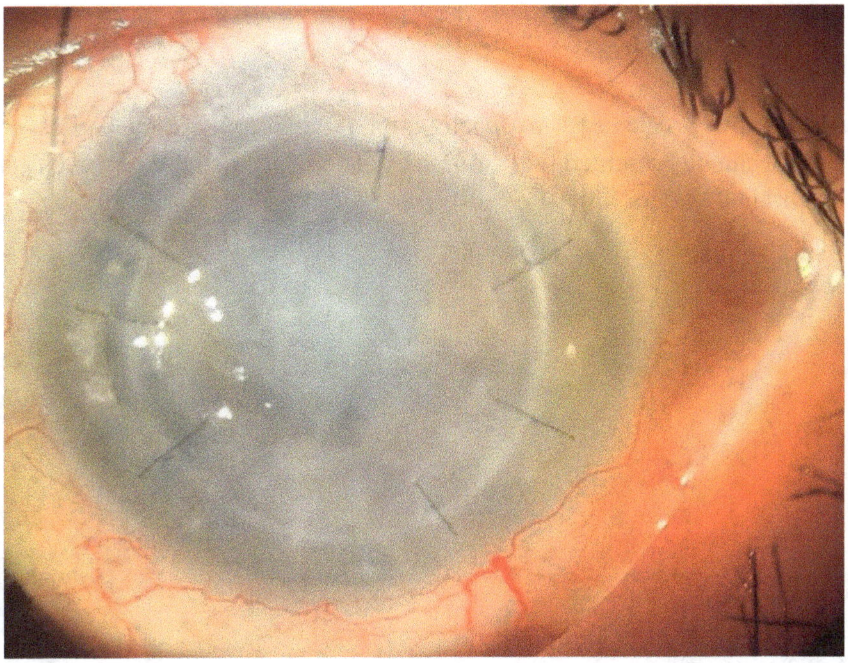

Herpes Simplex Keratitis

Humans are considered the only natural reservoir of HSV. HSV usually spreads via close personal contact because of the physical instability of the virus and the fact that the significant sites of the entrance are the mucous membranes and the skin. The eye can get involved when the trigeminal ganglion is affected. About 60% of the population is already infected with HSV by the age of 5 years, but only 6% develop clinical manifestation.

Classification of HSV Keratitis

1. Infectious epithelial keratitis
    a. Corneal vesicles
    b. Dendritic ulcer
    c. Geographic ulcer
    d. Marginal ulcer
2. Neurotrophic keratopathy
3. Stromal keratitis
    a. Necrotizing stromal keratitis
    b. Immune stromal (interstitial) keratitis
4. Endotheliitis
    a. Disciform
    b. Diffuse
    c. Linear

The treatment approach to each subtype is discussed below.

Infectious Epithelial Keratitis

Infectious epithelial keratitis is caused by the reactivation of the live virus. The earliest epithelial lesions of the reactivated HSV can be presented with small vesicles, which usually become typical geographic or dendritic ulcers within 24 hours (Fig 91).

Figure 91. Fine herpetic vesicles are seen

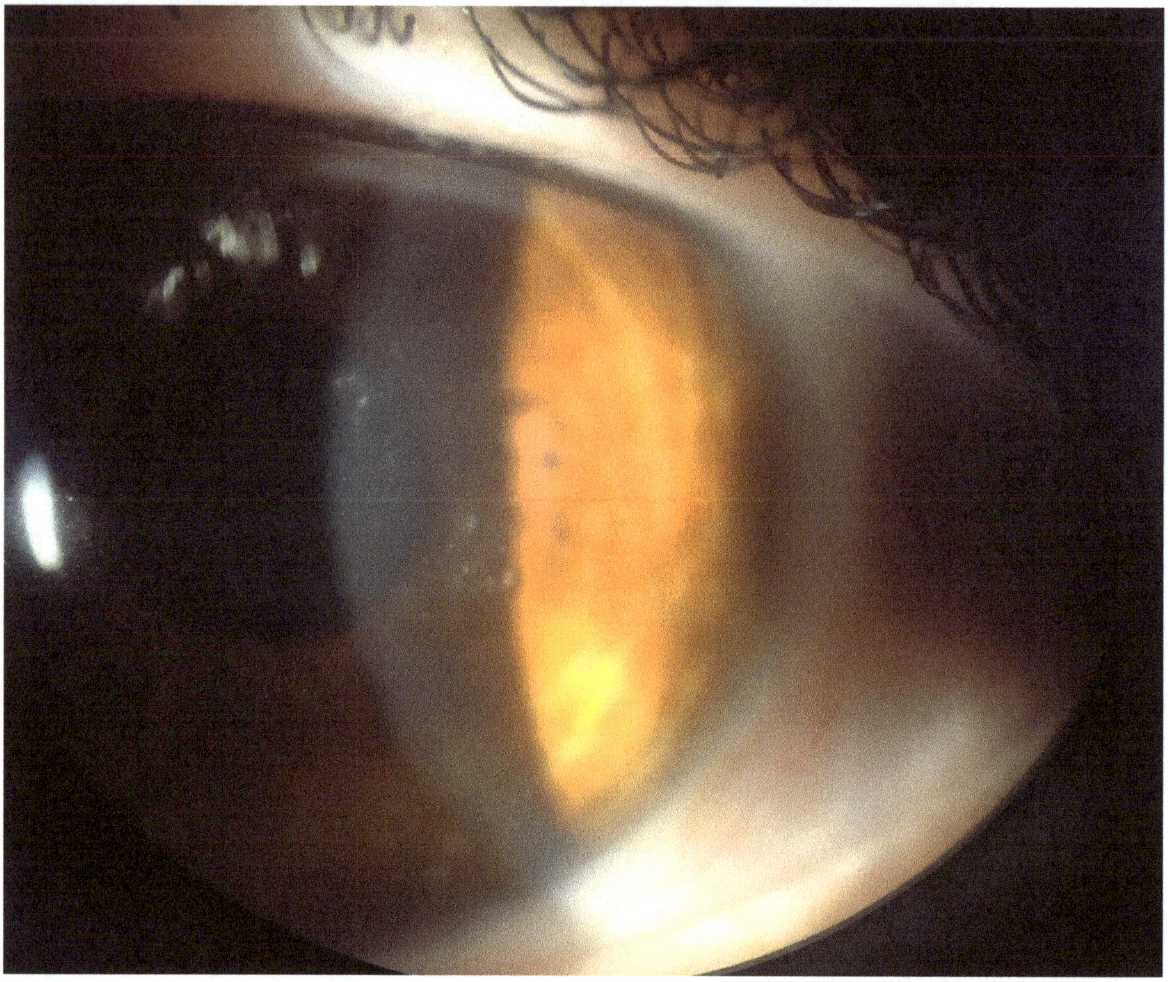

The most common presentation of HSV keratitis is the **dendritic ulcer**. The dendritic lesion is a branching, linear, true ulcer with terminal bulbs and swollen epithelial borders that contain the live virus (Fig 92, 93) (Pavan-Langston et al, 1994).

Figure 92. Herpes simplex dendrite with terminal bulbs

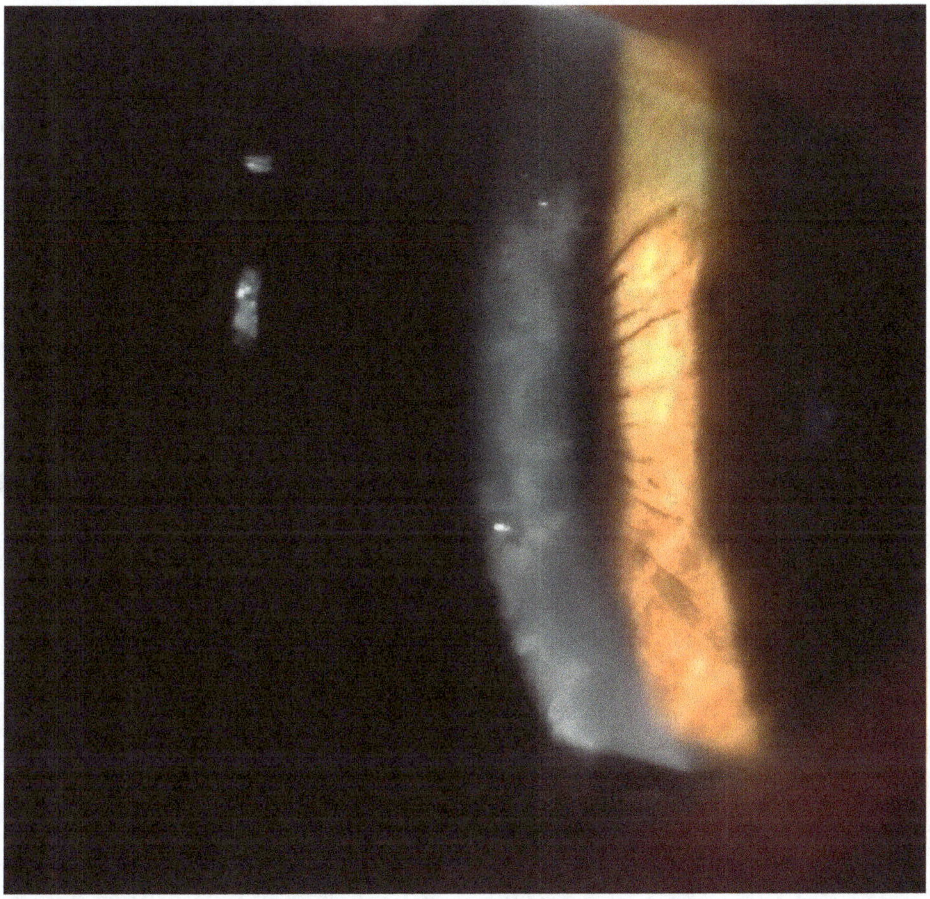

Figure 93. The same eye stained with fluorescein

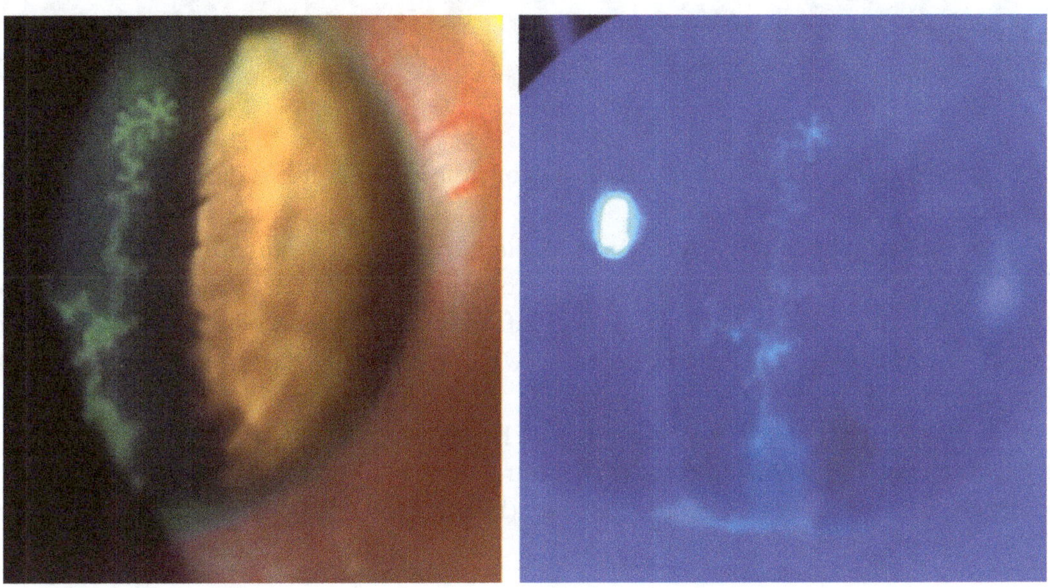

The infectious ulcers in our cases responded to Ganciclovir (Virgan) 0.15% eye gel, 5 times a day for a week, tapered to 3 times a day for the next week, and once a day for the week after. In few cases of a geographic ulcer, systemic Acyclovir was administered too, usually for 2-3 weeks. Topical lubricants were always prescribed as well.

HSV dendritic ulcer may result in an abnormal-appearing epithelium for several weeks after the ulcer heals and is called HSV dendritic epitheliopathy (Fig 94). The lesion is dendritic in shape, is not ulcerated and simply represents healing epithelium after the infection.

Figure 94. HSV dendritic epitheliopathy

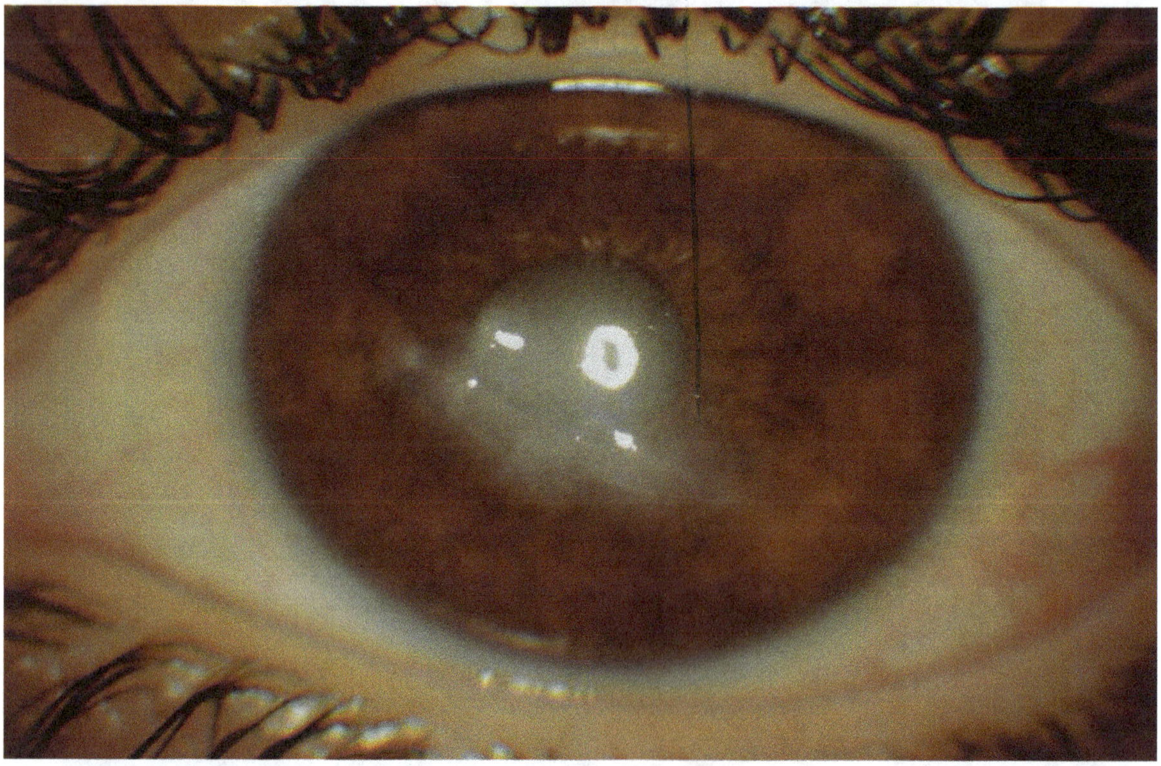

An enlarged dendritic ulcer is referred to as a **geographic ulcer**. It is a true ulcer and contains the live virus (Fig 95, 96, 97).

Another manifestation of HSV infectious epithelial keratitis is the **marginal ulcer**. The epithelial lesion is quickly infiltrated with white blood cells from limbal blood vessels nearby. The lesion, typically seen on presentation, has an anterior stromal infiltrate with an underlying ulcer and adjacent limbal injection. HSV marginal ulcer can be confused with the marginal (catarrhal) disease (Fig 98-101) (Thygeson et al, 1971).

Patients with a history of multiple recurrences of herpetic keratitis are at risk of developing **neurotrophic keratopathy**. The epithelial defect in neurotrophic keratopathy has a round or oval shape, and smooth borders, usually with a paracentral location. (Fig 102-104).

Figure 95. HSV dendrite is seen, widened superiorly, representing geographic ulcer

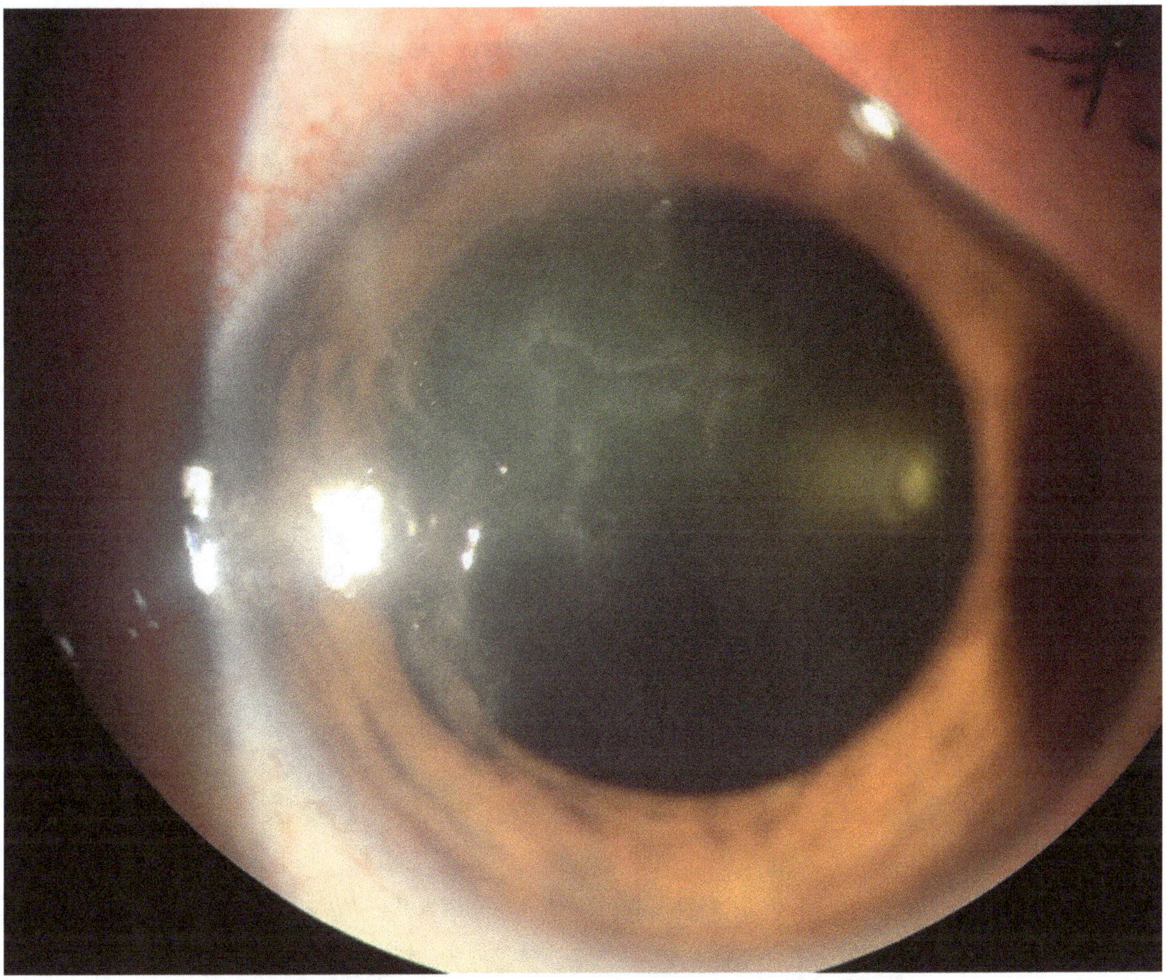

The treatment was initiated with oral Doxycycline, topical mild steroids 2-3 times a day, non-preserved tears, cycloplegics 2-3 times a day, topical antibiotic for prophylaxis (usually Chloramphenicol or Tobramycin 3 times a day), bandage contact lens, serum tears, NACL 0.5%. In severe cases amniotic membrane transplantation, conjunctival flap surgery or tarsorrhaphy were performed as well. Few cases, when already presented with complications of secondary infection and perforation, have undergone PK surgery.

Figure 96. HSV geographic ulcer with inferiorly extending dendrite with terminal bulbs, stained with Fluorescein

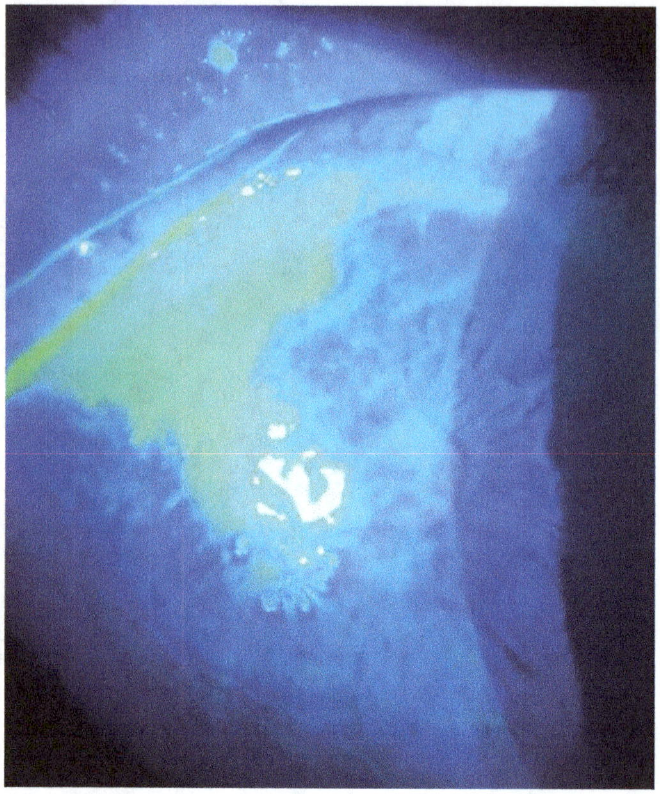

Figure 97. HSV geographic ulcer stained with Fluorescein, subtotal epithelial defect

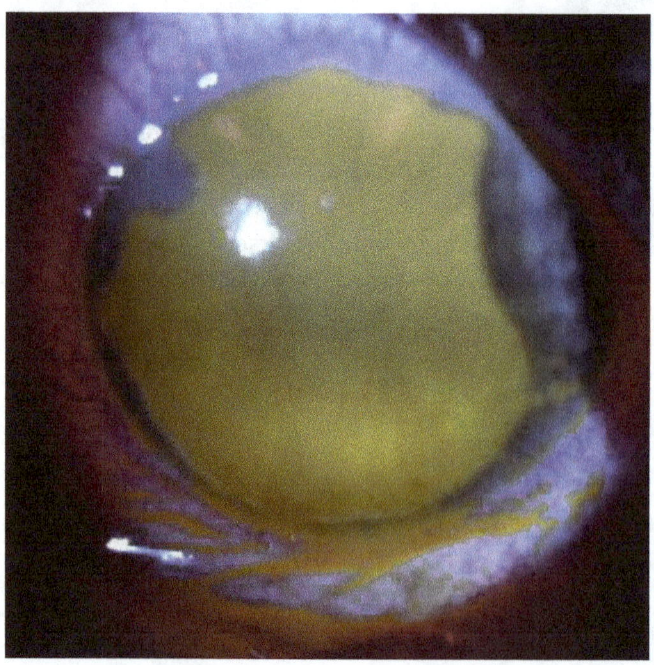

Figure 98. Marginal epithelial ulcer, limbal infiltrate, subepithelial fibrosis from previous episode is seen nasally (left photo), and after treatment (right photo)

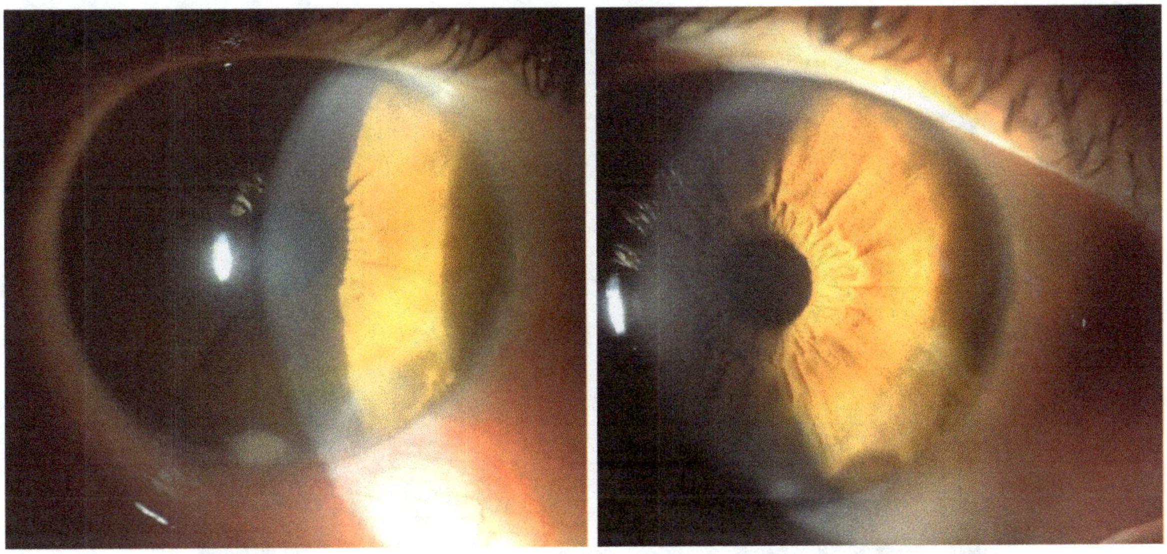

Figure 99. PCR proven HSV limbal epithelial keratitis stained with fluorescein

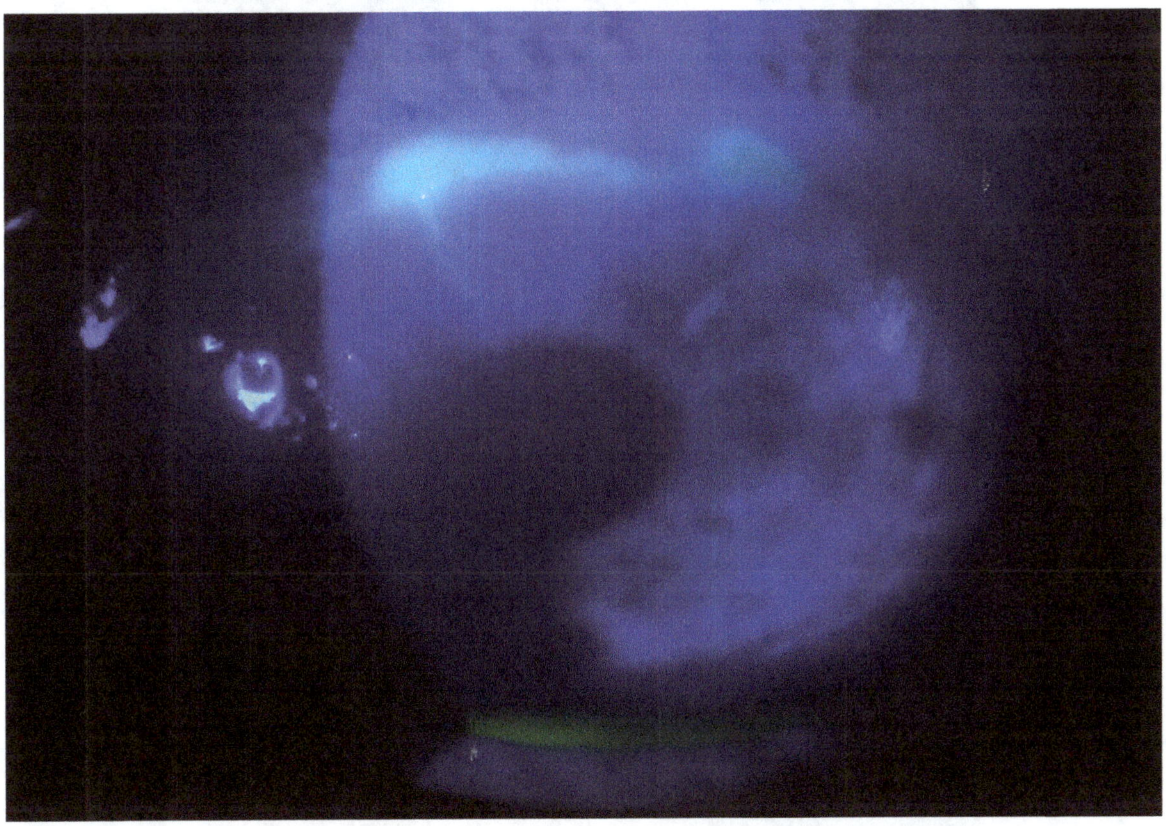

Figure 100. Peripheral PCR proven HSV keratitis resembling PUK. The crescent-shaped epithelial defect is seen surrounded by stromal edema, and severe, almost 90% thinning of the peripheral cornea

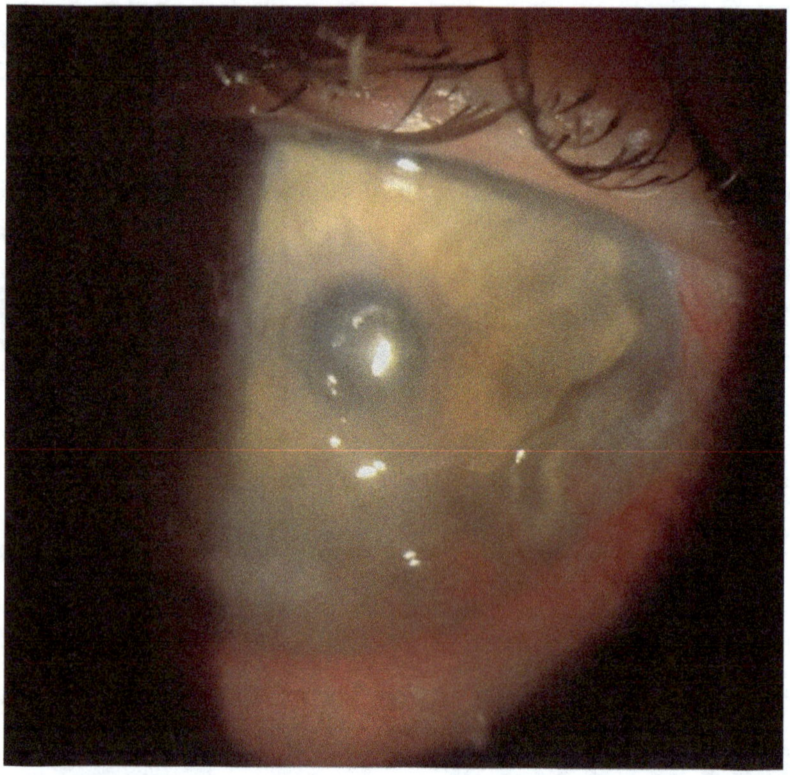

Figure 101. The same eye. Mild anterior stromal scar is seen after 3 months of medical treatment

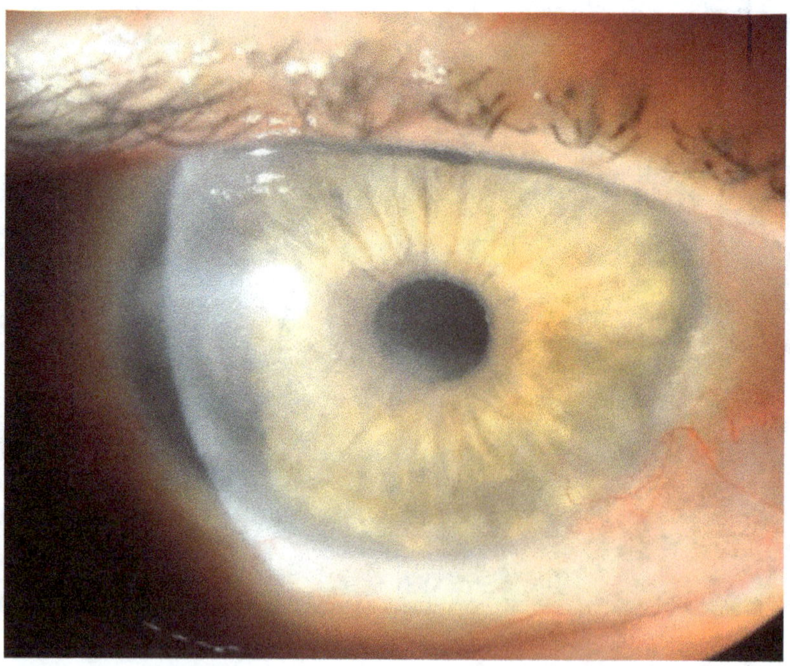

Figure 102. the round-shaped tropic ulcer with thickened, heaped-up epithelial borders and neovascularization

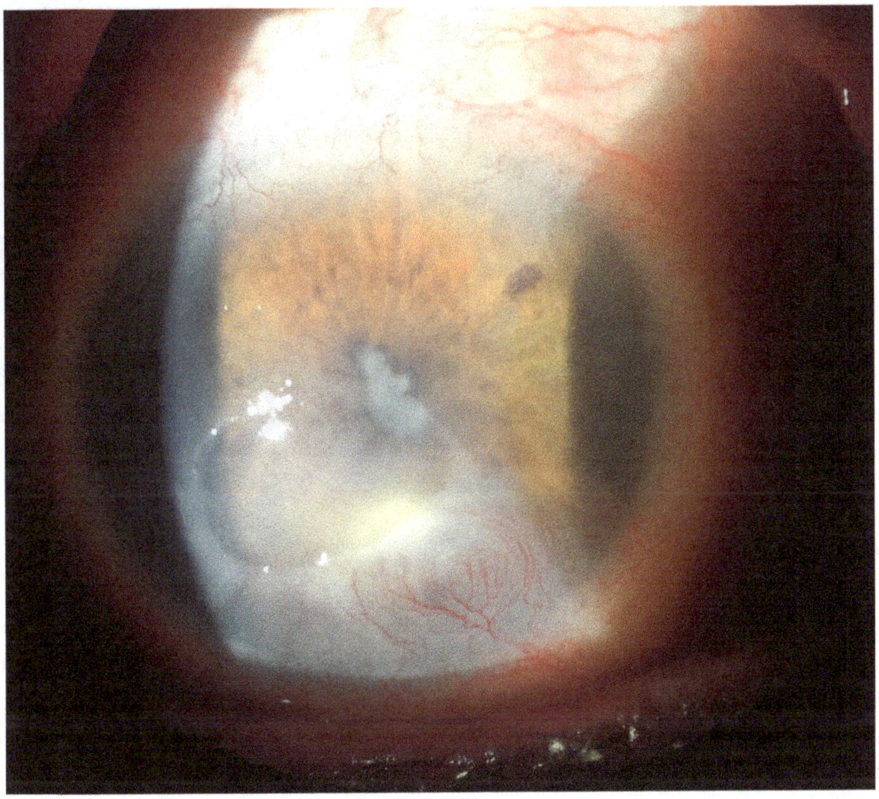

Figure 103. Postherpetic neurotrophic ulcer. A mild stromal scar is noted superiorly from previous HSV infection

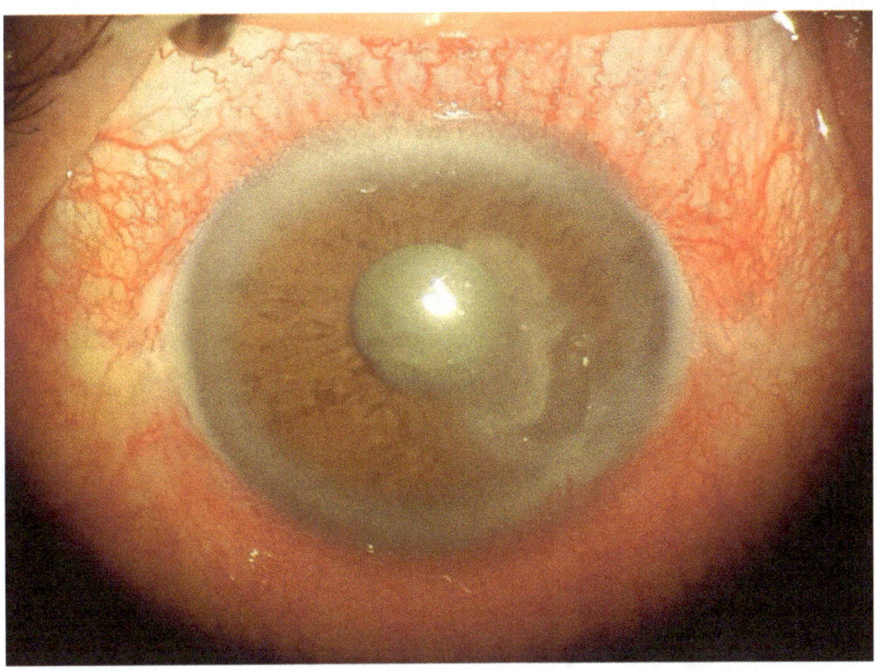

Figure 104. Central corneal graft perforation due to a neurotrophic ulcer (left photo), covered with a contact lens, and the same eye after repeated PK the next day, covered with a contact lens (right phot)

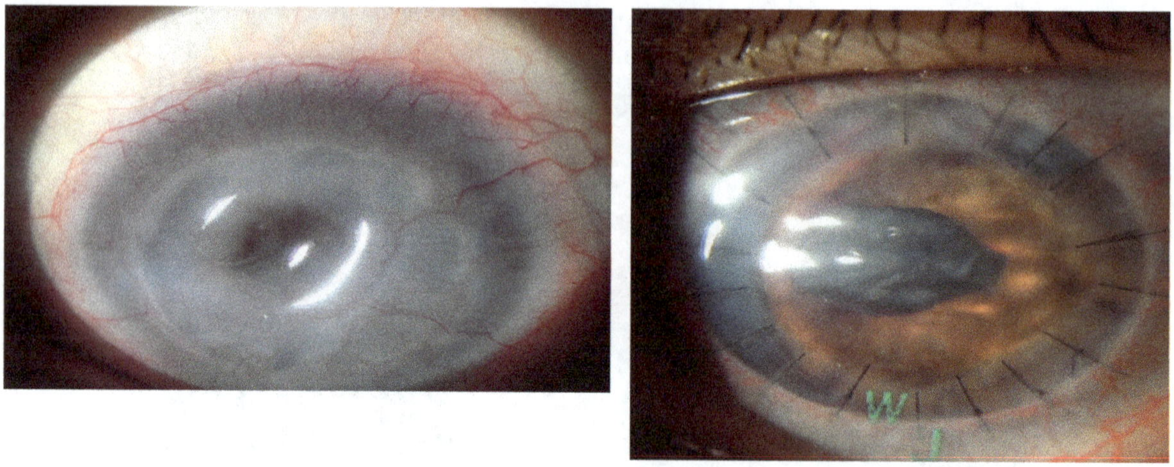

Stromal Disease

Necrotizing stromal keratitis is a rare manifestation of HSV that is thought to occur from direct viral invasion of the corneal stroma (Tuft, et al 2003). Clinical findings include necrosis, ulceration, and dense infiltration of the stroma with overlying epithelial defect, which can resemble those of infectious keratitis (Fig 105-111). The combination of replicating virus and severe host inflammatory response leads to destructive intrastromal inflammation. The severe inflammation may lead to thinning and perforation within a short period of time.

Figure 105. PCR proven Stromal necrotizing keratitis. Dens stromal infiltrate with overlying epithelial defect and neovascularization

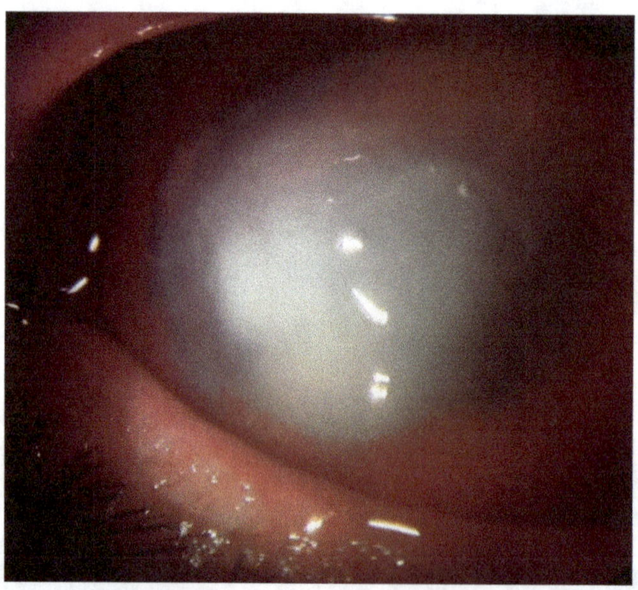

Figure 106. PCR proven Stromal necrotizing keratitis. Stromal infiltrate with overlying epithelial defect and hypopyon is seen

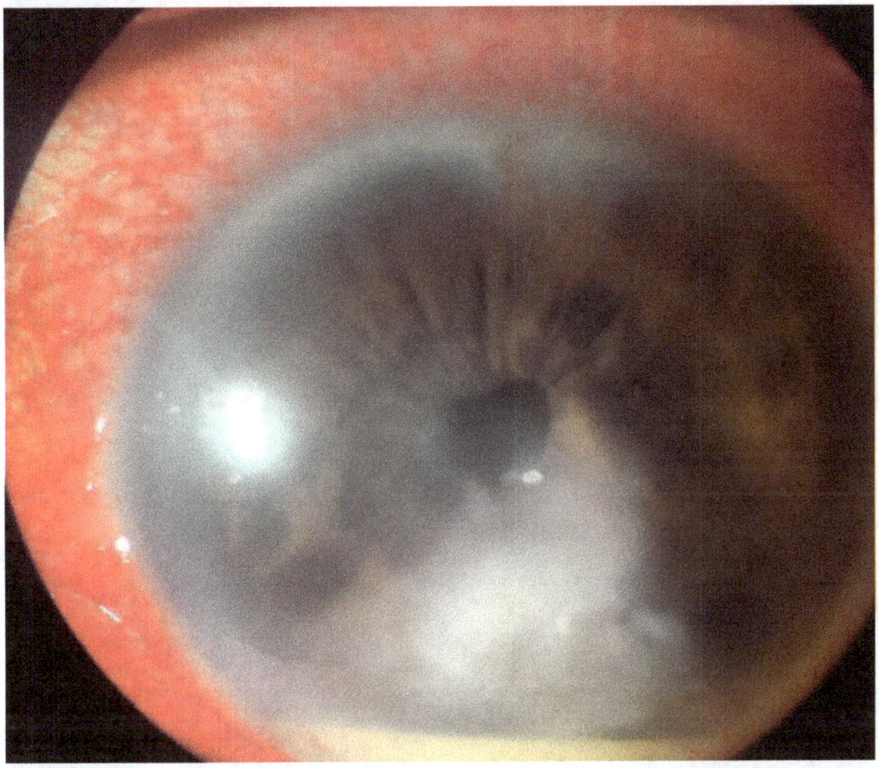

Figure 107. Recurrence of HSV stromal necrotizing keratitis on the graft. Stromal infiltrate and epithelial defect are seen in the photo

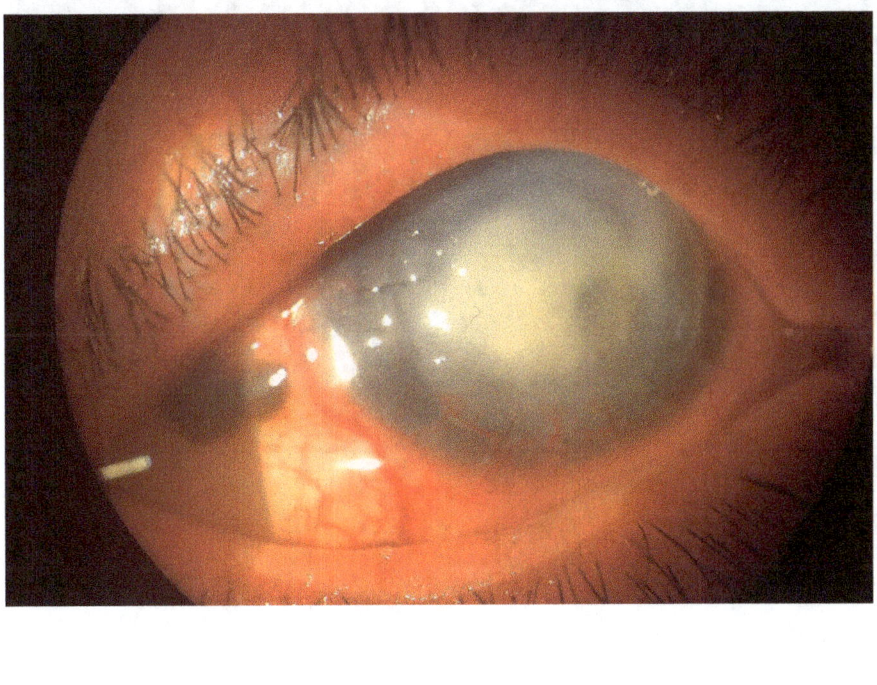

Figure 108. Same eye after 5 months of PK

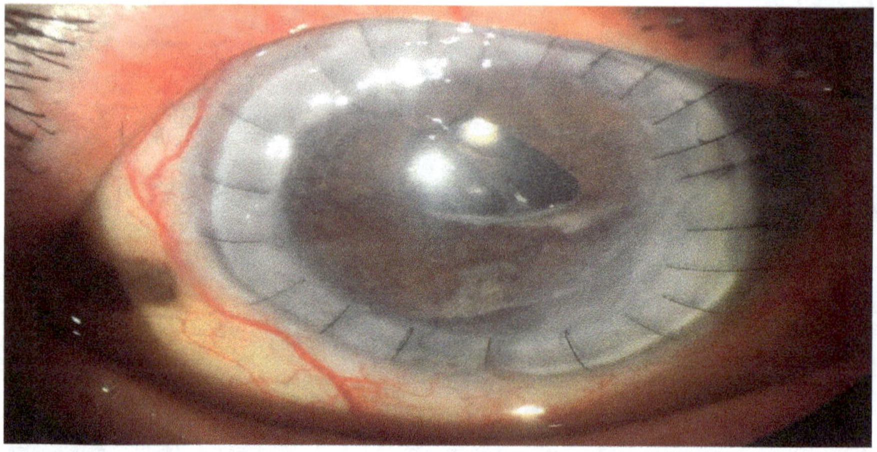

Figure 109. Necrotizing keratitis. PCR proven HSV, limbal epithelial defect is present with stromal lysis up to 90%, surrounded by stromal infiltrate and edema

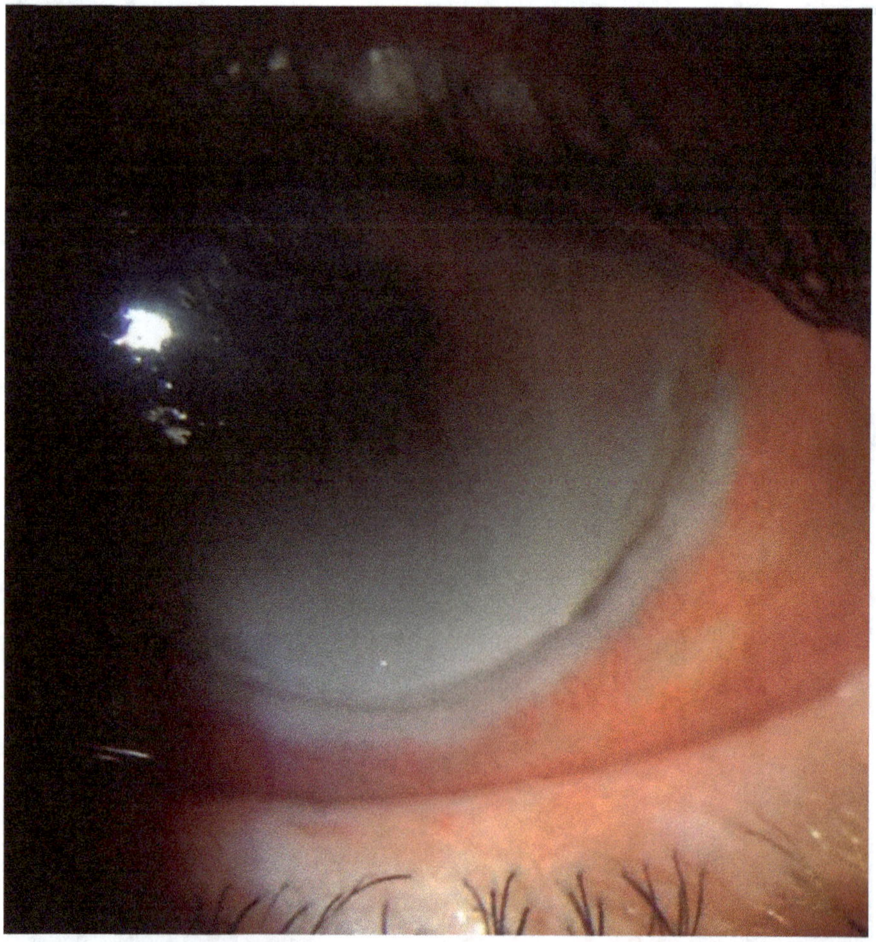

Figure 110. The same eye three weeks after treatment. Oval shaped epithelial defect got developed, amniotic membrane was transplanted

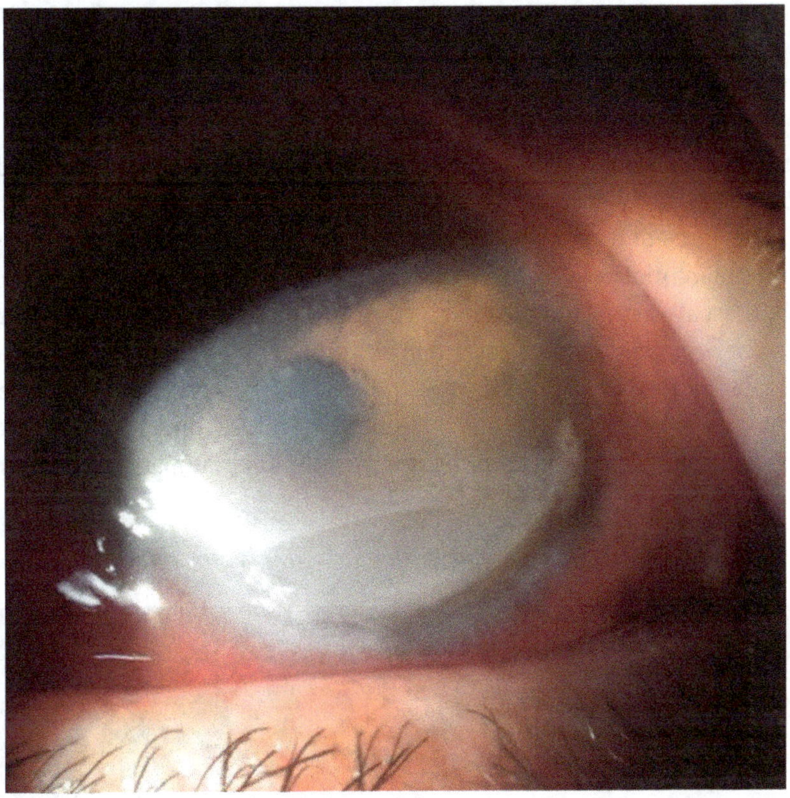

Figure 111. The same eye after 12 weeks of treatment. A stromal scar is formed

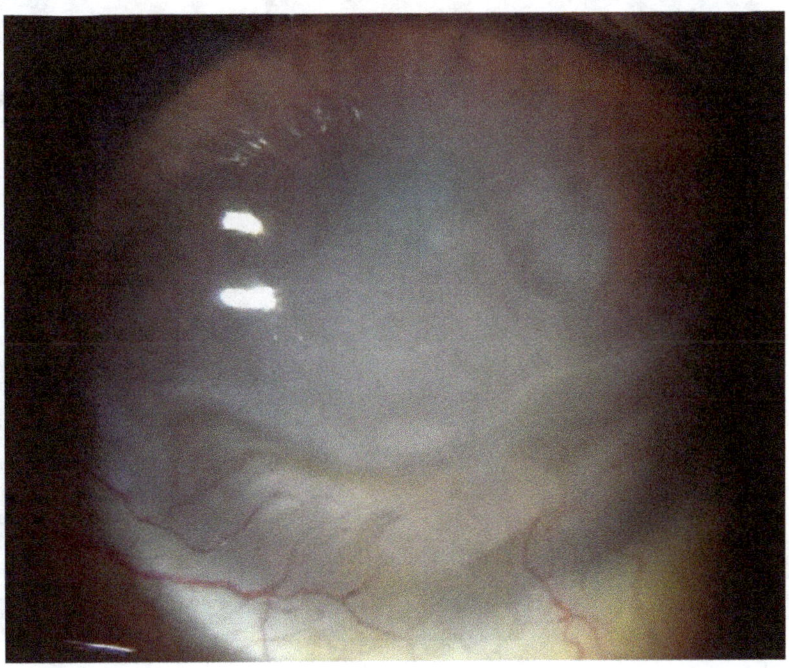

In our cases the treatment was initiated with topical Ganciclovir 0.15% 5 times a day, with tapering in 3 weeks, topical cycloplegics q2 hour, systemic Acyclovir 400mg 5 times a day for a week with tapering to 400mg 2-3 times a day for months, or Valacyclovir 500mg 3 times a day for 10 days, tapered to once a day for months, oral Doxycycline for 3-4 weeks in cases with stromal lysis more than 30-40%. Betamethasone sub-Tenon injection (0.2-0,3ml) was given after 7-10 days, repeated after a week with 0,5-0,7ml dosage. After the total epithelization, mild steroids were added 2-3 times a day along with oral antiviral coverage. Later, stronger topical steroids (Dexamethasone 0.1%) were added with oral Vit C 500mg bid for 2 months. In few cases with severe thinning, amniotic membrane transplantation was performed as well. The cases unresponsive to medical treatment have undergone PK surgery.

Immune stromal (interstitial keratitis) is a type of chronic recurrent manifestation of HSV. The overlying epithelium is almost always intact. Stromal infiltration can be focal, multifocal, or diffuse. Specific signs of immune stromal keratitis include stromal infiltration with complete or incomplete immune ring and stromal neovascularization (Fig 112). Ghost vessels, which represent empty vessel channels within the stroma, can occur if the inflammation and neovascularization are long-standing before subsiding (Fig 113). Stromal neovascularization can be complicated with lipid keratopathy (Wilhelmus et al, 1987).

Figure 112. Interstitial keratitis. Dense stromal infiltrate with neovascularization is visible

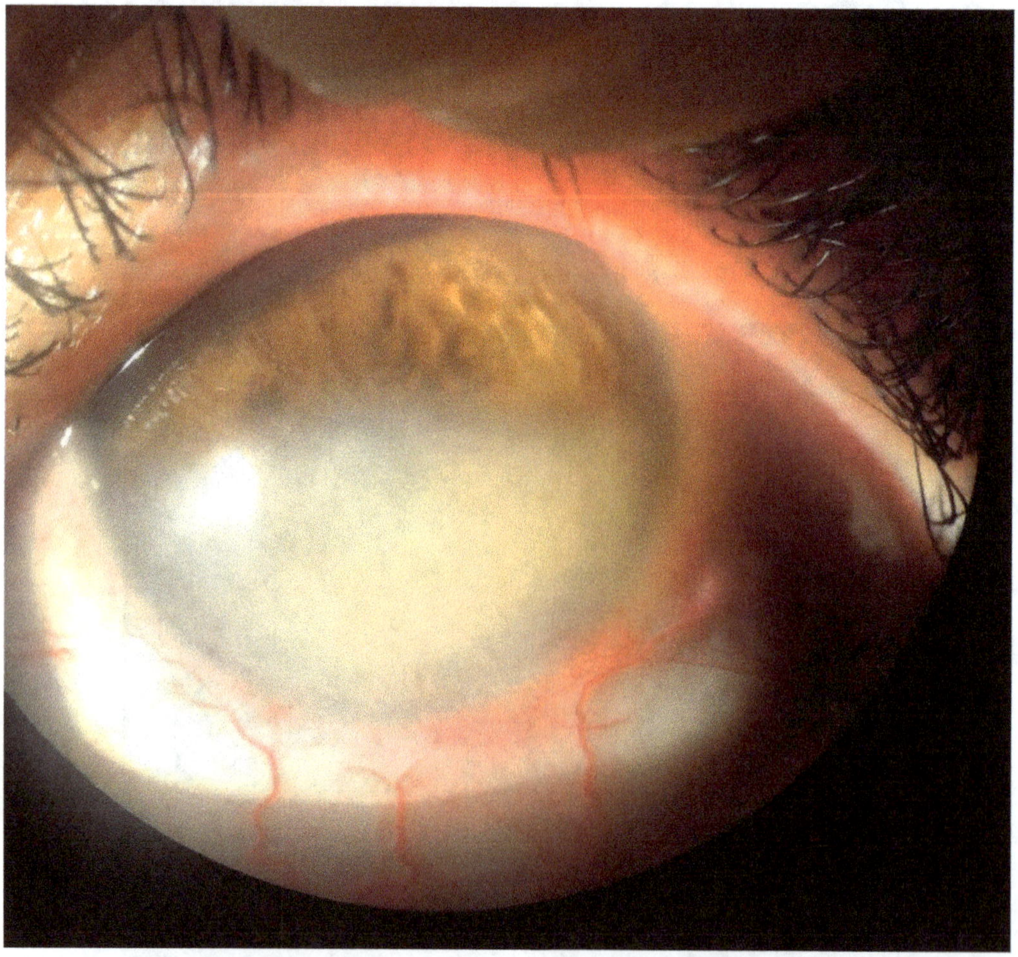

Figure 113. Ghost vessels after herpetic interstitial keratitis

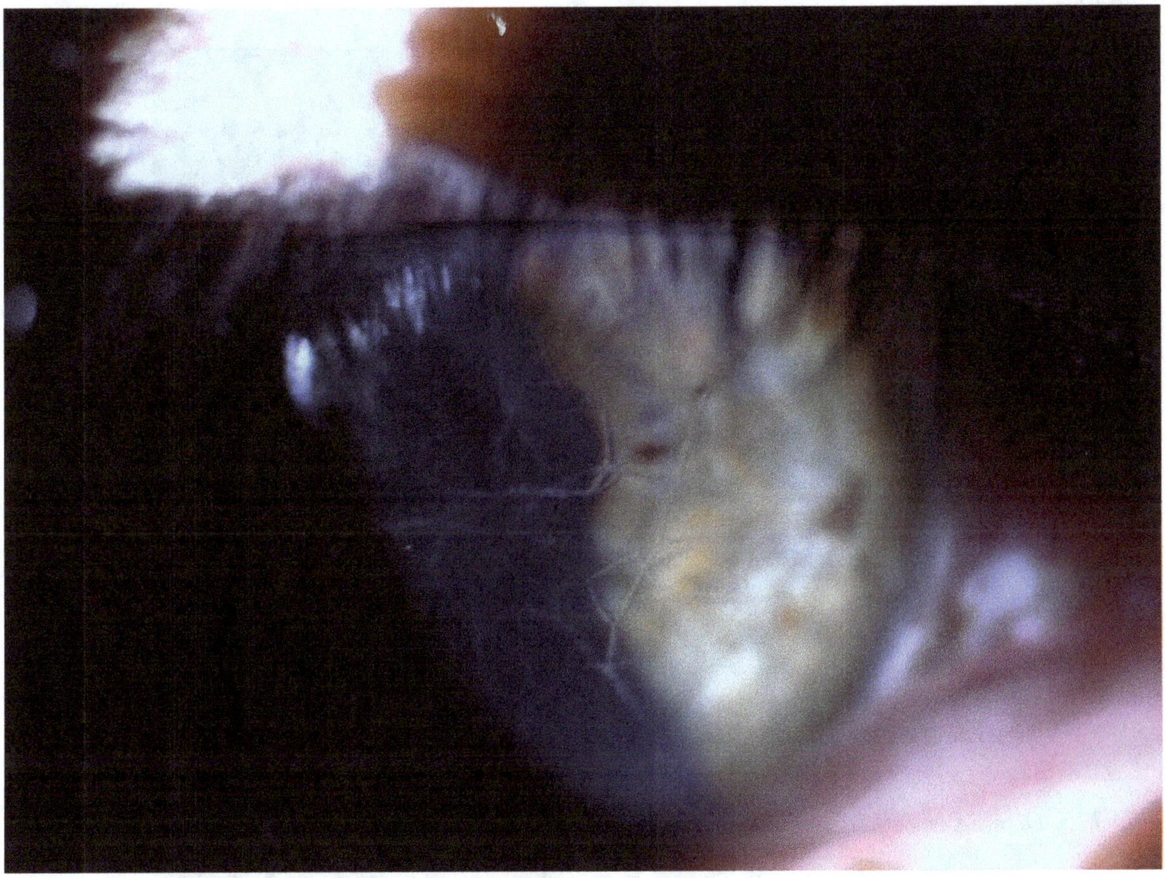

Our cases responded to topical steroids (mostly Dexamethasone 0.1% eye drops) q2h, tapered within 6-8 weeks depending on clinical response. Oral Acyclovir 400mg was administered 5 times a day for a week and tapered to 2-3 times a day for months. Topical cycloplegics and tears were prescribed as well. In cases of IOP elevation, topical antiglaucoma medication was added. Betamethasone sub-Tenon injection was given in rare cases when no clinical response was noted after 2 weeks of treatment.

Endotheliitis

The exact pathogenesis of endothelitis in HSV is unknown. It has an immune origin because of the clinical findings of KP and iritis, but the role of live virus has also been speculated (Robin et al, 1985).

Disciform endotheliitis: the most characteristic finding of disciform endotheliitis is a round-shaped or disk-shaped stromal edema, which can be central or paracentral, and always associated with KPs (Fig 114, 115).

Our cases responded to topical steroids (mostly Dexamethasone 0.1% eye drops) q2h, tapered in 6-8 weeks depending on clinical response. Oral Acyclovir 400mg was administered 5 times a day for a week and tapered to 2-3 times a day for months. Tears were prescribed as well. In cases of IOP elevation, topical antiglaucoma medication was added.

Figure 114. Disciform endotheliitis. Discoid edema with Descemet folds and underlying KP is seen on the photo

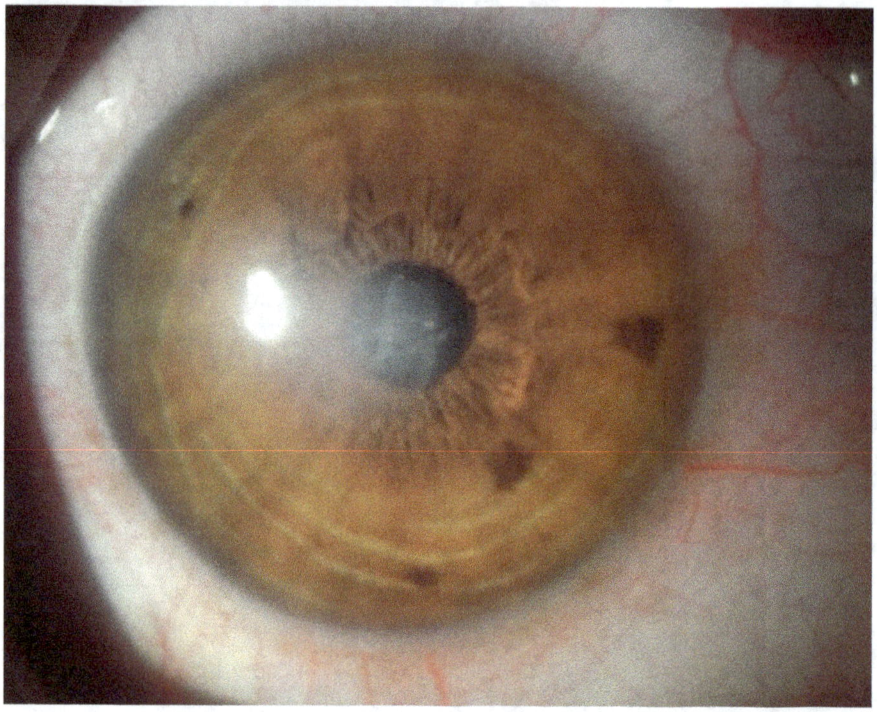

Figure 115. Discoid endotheliitis. Stromal discoid edema is seen with underlying fine KPs

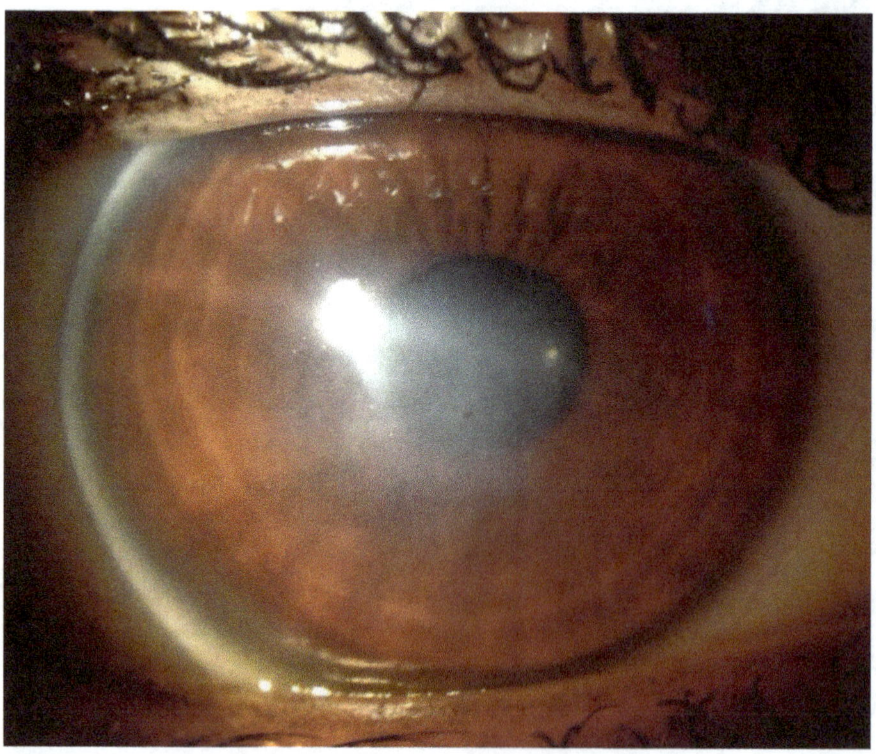

Patients with **diffuse endotheliitis** typically have scattered KPs over the entire cornea with overlying diffuse stromal edema. In severe cases, a dense retrocorneal plaque of inflammatory cells accompanied by hypopyon may be seen (Fig 116-120).

Our cases responded to topical Ganciclovir 0.15% eye gel, topical steroids (mostly Dexamethasone 0.1% eye drops) q2h, tapered in 6-8 weeks depending on clinical response. Oral Acyclovir 400mg was administered 5 times a day for a week and tapered to 2-3 times a day for months, or oral Valacyclovir 500mg 3 times a day for a week and tapered to once a day for months. Topical cycloplegics and tears were prescribed as well. In cases of IOP elevation, topical antiglaucoma medication was added. Betamethasone sub-Tenon injection was given in most cases where no clinical response was noted after 2 weeks of treatment.

Figure 116. Total edema with Descemet folds and fine KPs

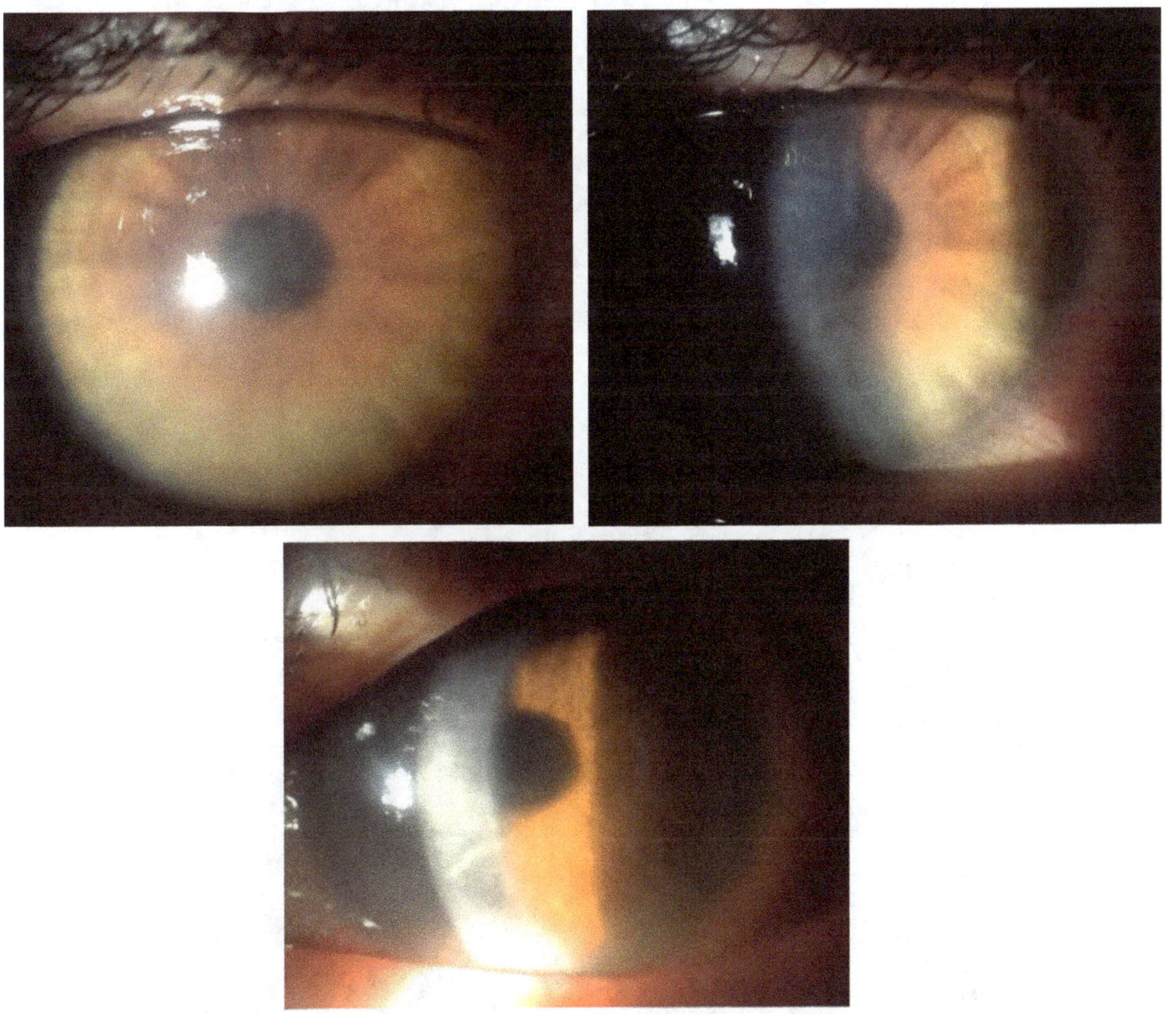

Figure 117. Diffuse total edema with fine KPs are seen

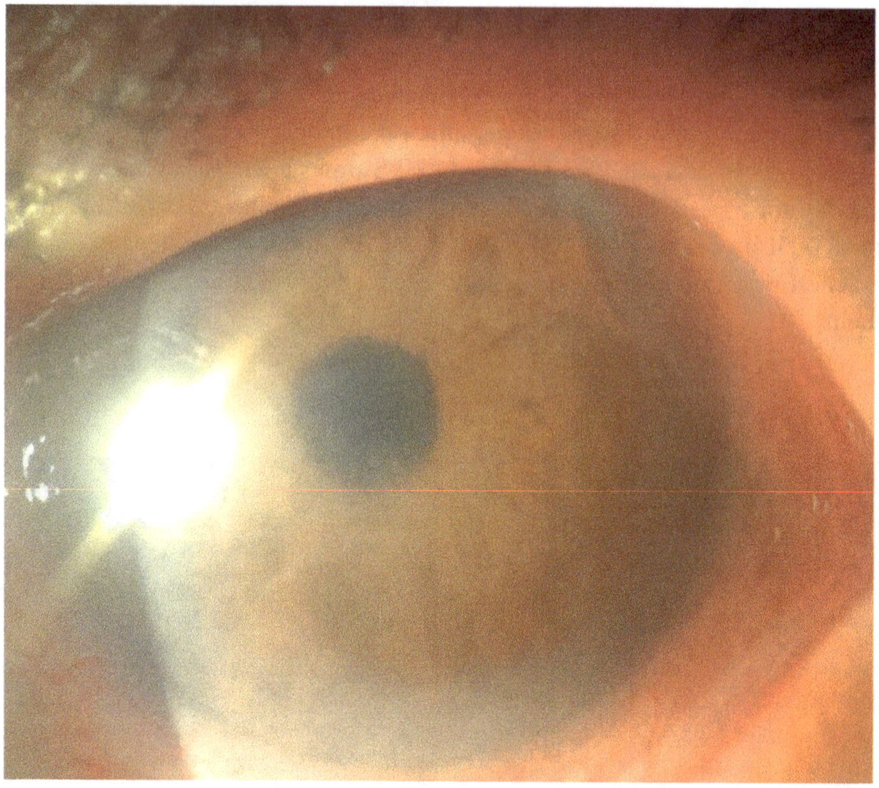

Figure 118. The same eye 3 weeks post treatment

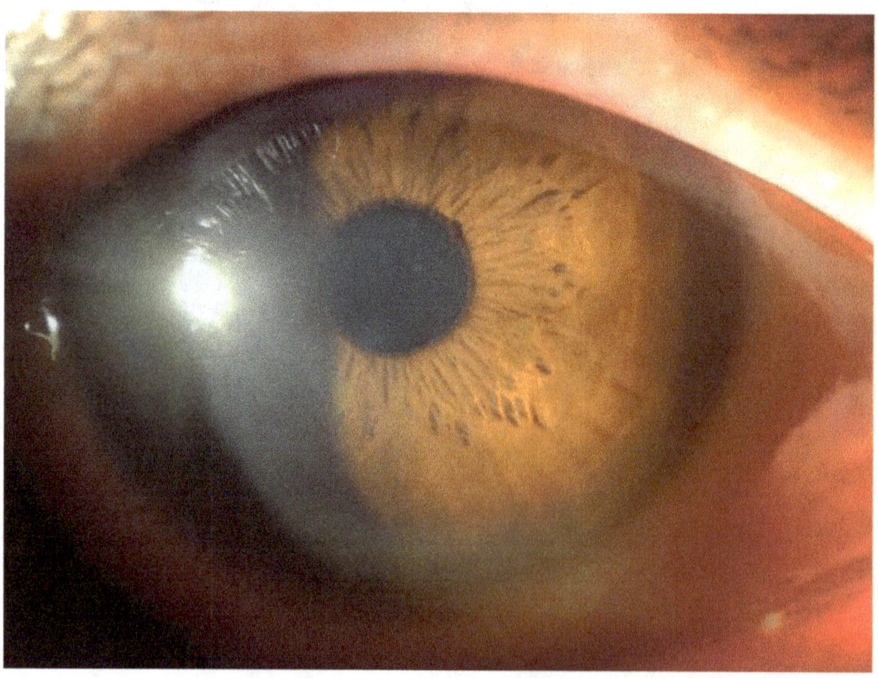

Figure 119. Diffuse endotheliitis in a patient with Sturge-Weber syndrome

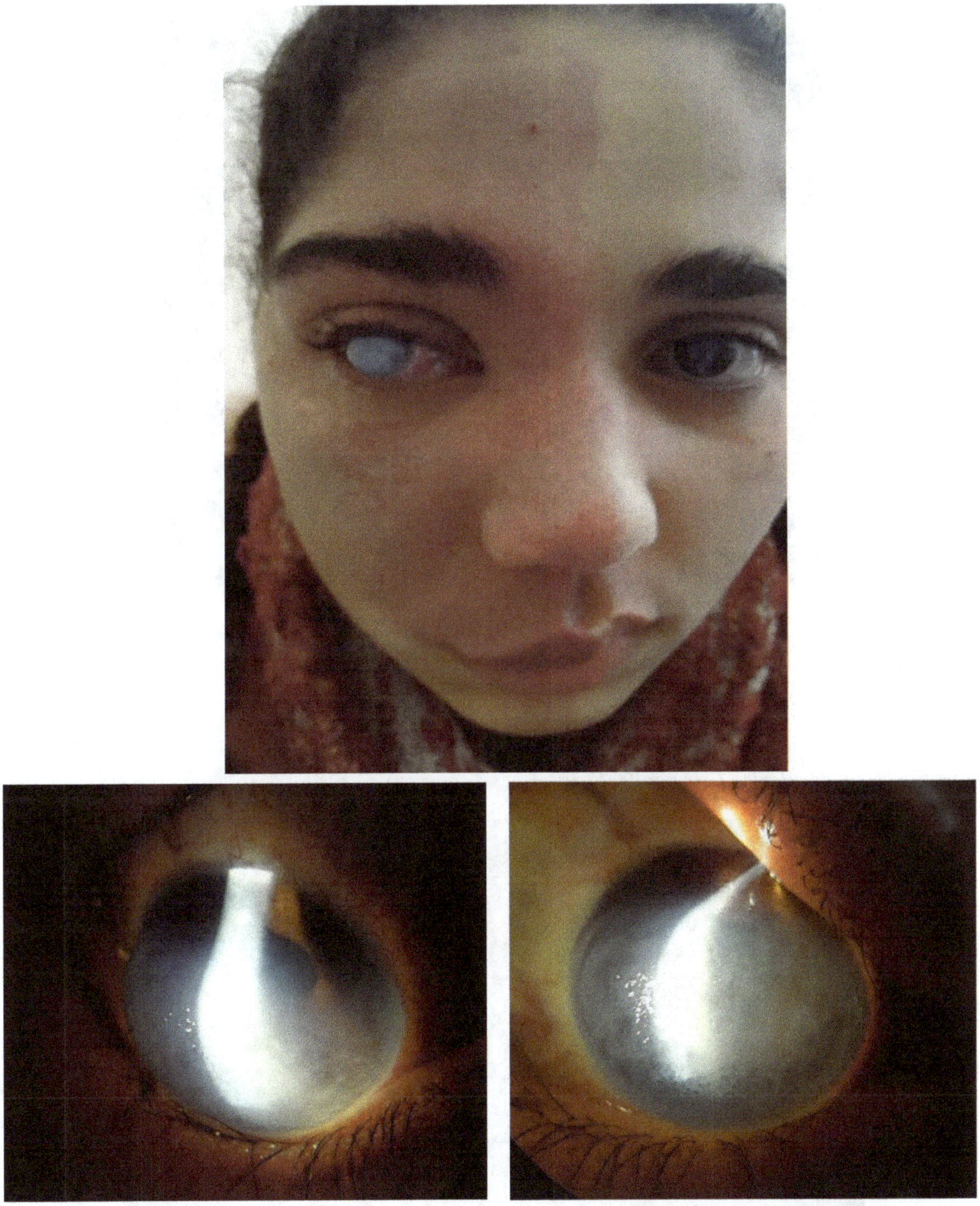

Figure 120. The same eye 3 months after treatment

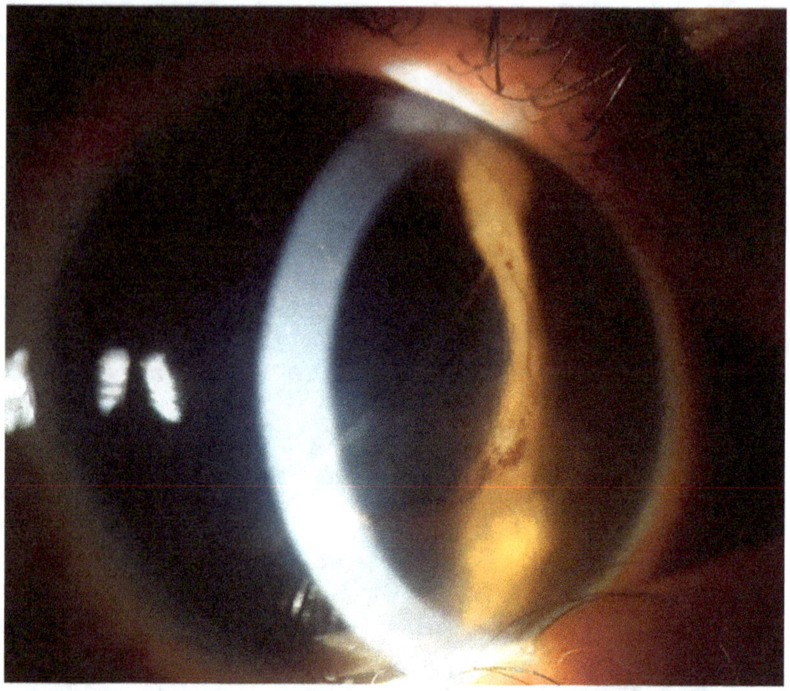

Postherpetic ectasia is a rare complication that can develop after multiple recurrences of herpetic disease (Fig 121-125).

Figure 121. Neovascularized corneal ectasia

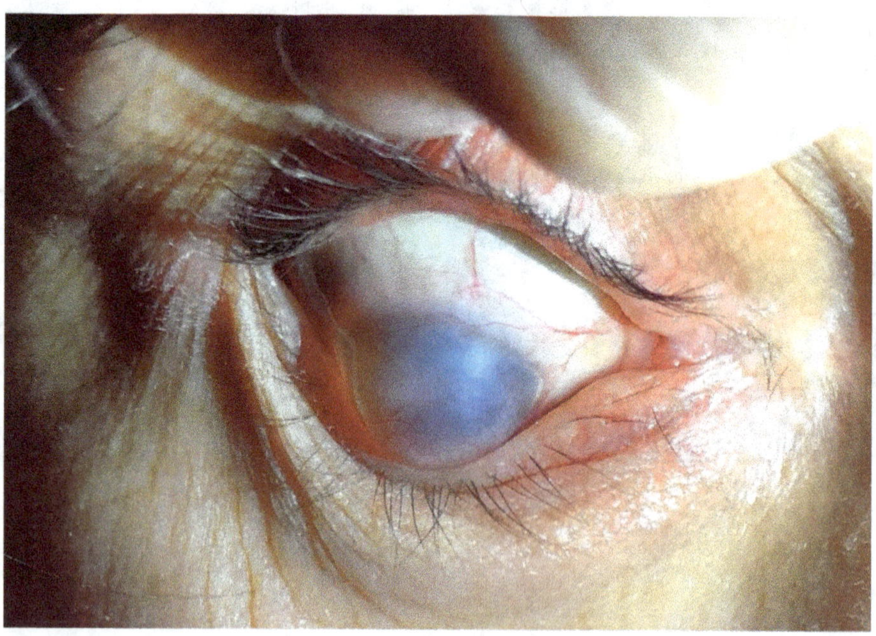

Figure 122. The same eye under slit lamp

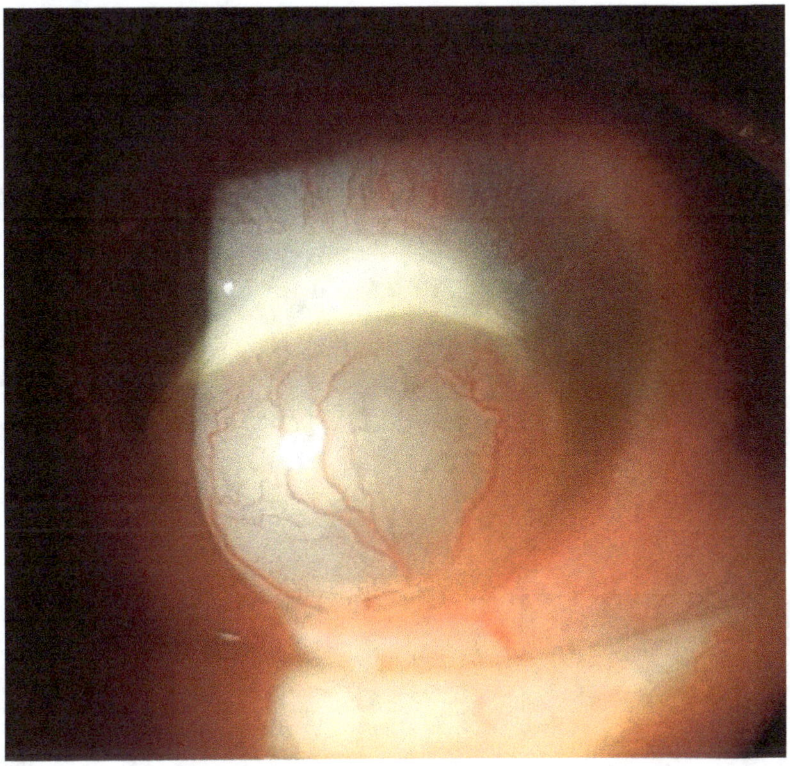

Figure 123. The same eye 2 weeks after PK

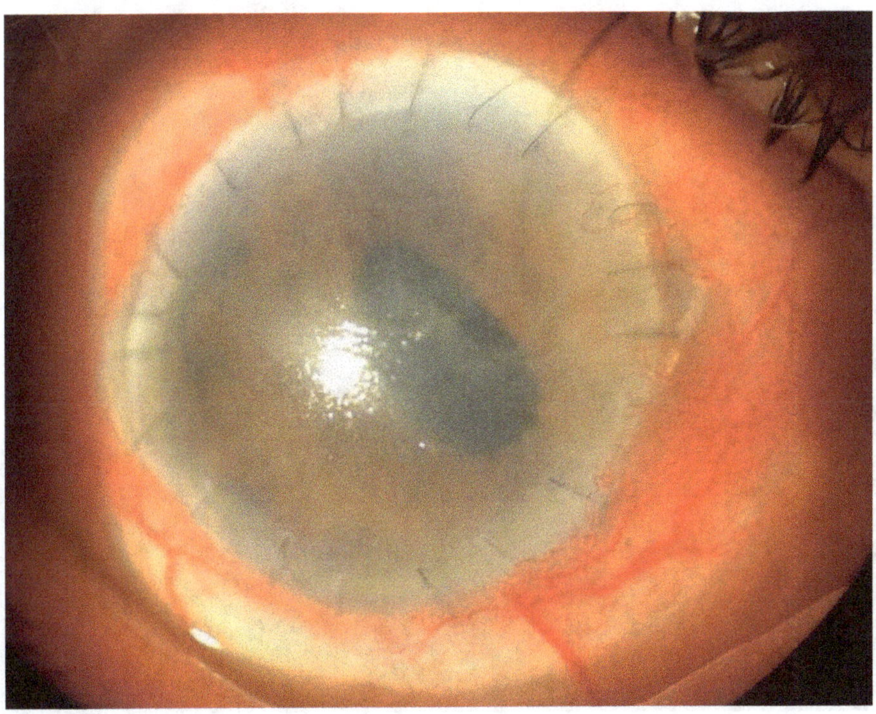

Figure 124. Severe ectasia due to multiple recurrences of herpetic disease. The same eye under a slit lamp (right photo)

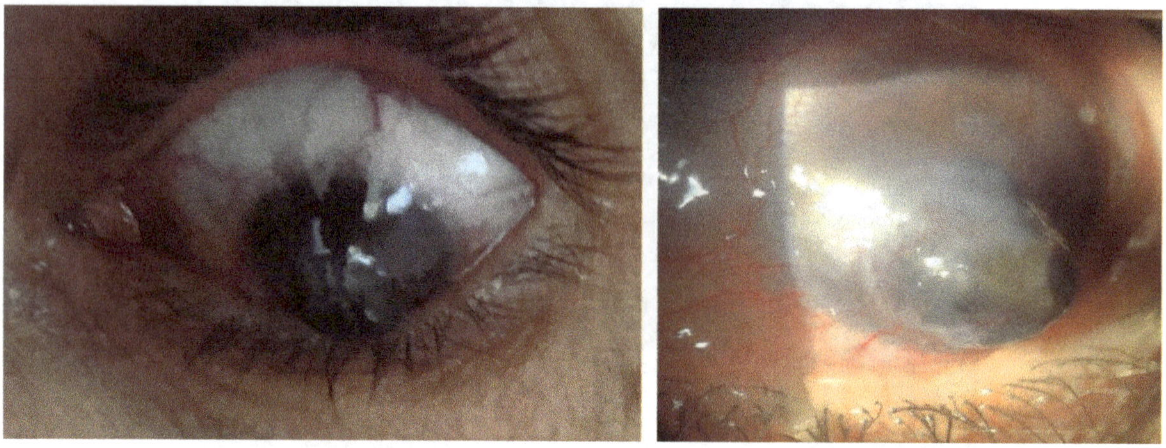

Figure 125. The same eye 3 weeks post PK

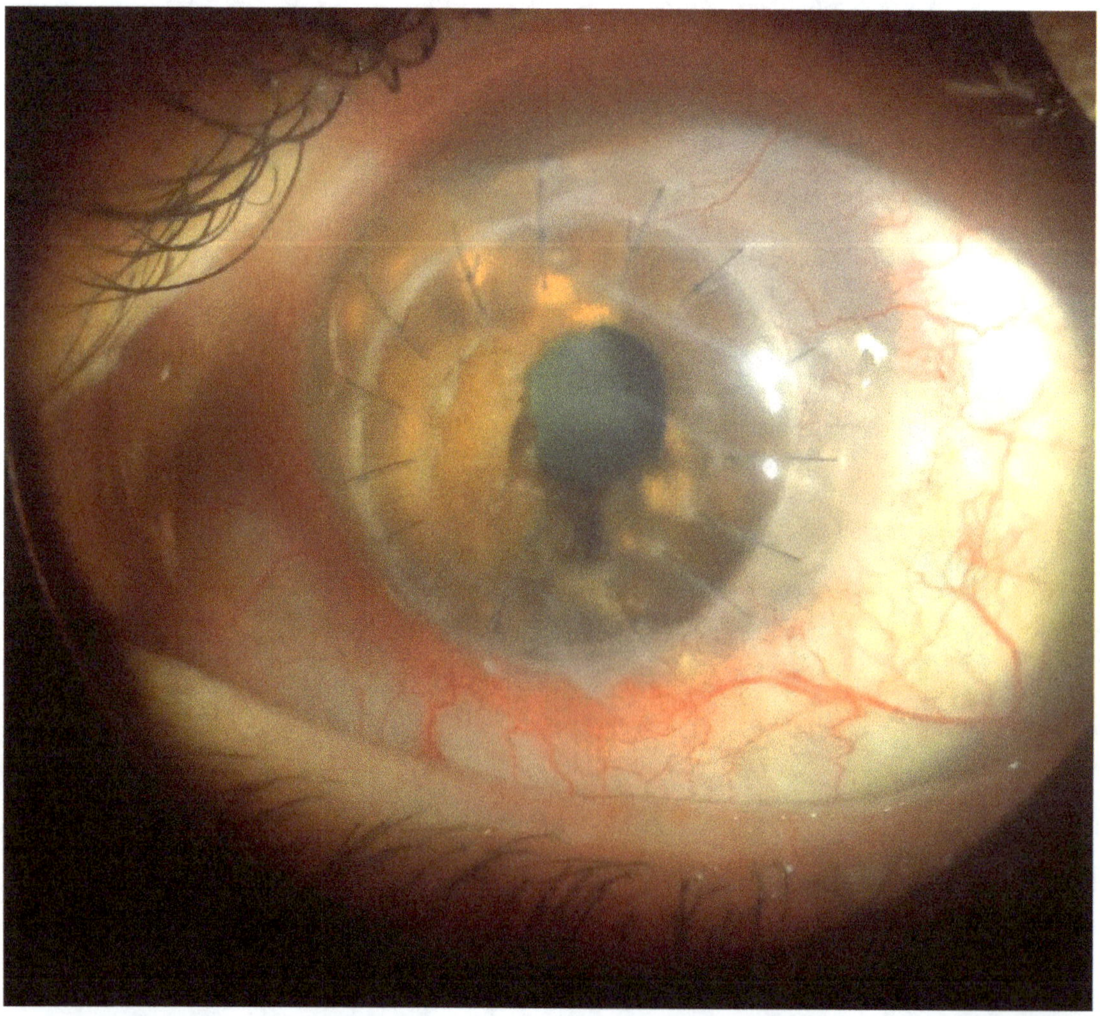

Herpes Zoster

Varicella zoster virus (VZV) infection is a highly contagious member of the herpes virus family that causes varicella (chickenpox) in children and herpes zoster in the elderly population (Mullooly et la, 2005). Vesicles at the side of the tip of the nose are known as Hutchinson sign, representing a nasociliary involvement, and are an indication of potential ocular involvement (Fig 126). Commonly, the frontal nerve is most involved. HZO manifestation includes punctate epithelial keratitis, early pseudodendrites, anterior stromal infiltrates, sclerokeratitis, keratouveitis/endotheliitis, neurotrophic keratopathy, etc (Liesegang et al, 2008). Recommended treatment of Herpes Zoster is acute oral antiviral treatment within 72 hours of the onset of the rash with medications such as; valacyclovir 1000 mg three times a day, famciclovir 500 mg three times a day, or acyclovir 800 mg 5 times a day for 1 week (Tyring et al, 2000). Management of anterior segment involvement of the eye in HZO (Herpes Zoster Ophthalmicus) is not standardized. Topical ganciclovir 5 times a day until healed, and then twice daily for 2 to 4 weeks is effective for dendriform keratitis, even in cases that have been unresponsive to oral antivirals (Aggarwal et al, 2014). Topical corticosteroids are used steadily in the management of stromal keratitis and uveitis. They often need to be continued at a low-dose chronically and require close monitoring for safety and efficacy (McLeod et al, 2012). In case of neurotrophic keratopathy development, the treatment is alike any type of neurotrophic keratopathy treatment.

Figure 126. Herpetic skin rash and Hutchinson sign associated with blepharoconjunctivitis

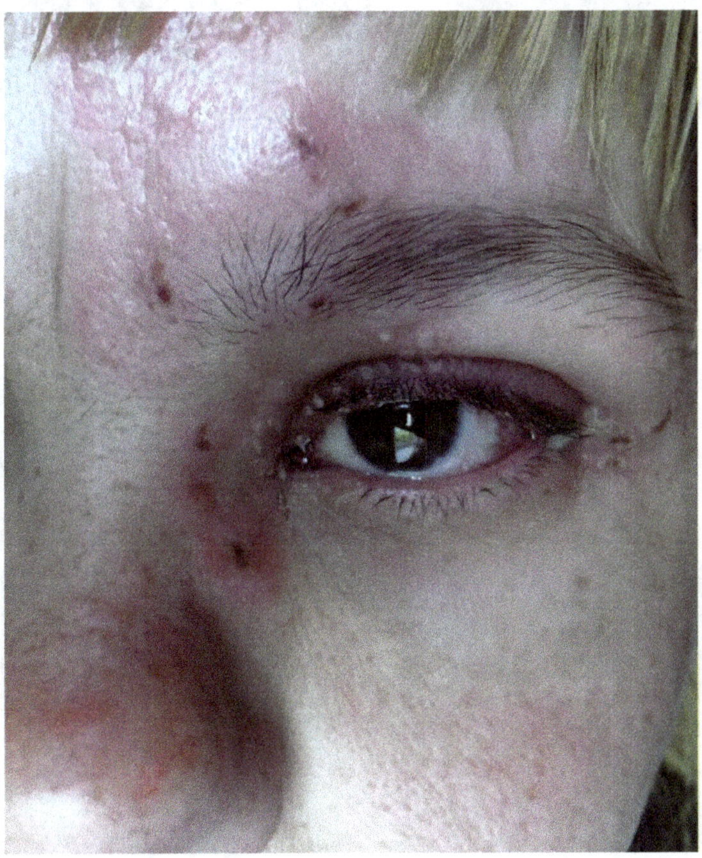

Pseudodendrites are usually found in the corneal periphery and most likely represent a coalescence of a previous punctate epithelial keratitis. Compared to herpes simplex viral dendrites, these lesions are more superficial, have blunt ends, lack central ulceration, and stain minimally with fluorescein and rose Bengal (Fig 127).

Figure 127. Pseudodendrite caused by Herpes zoster

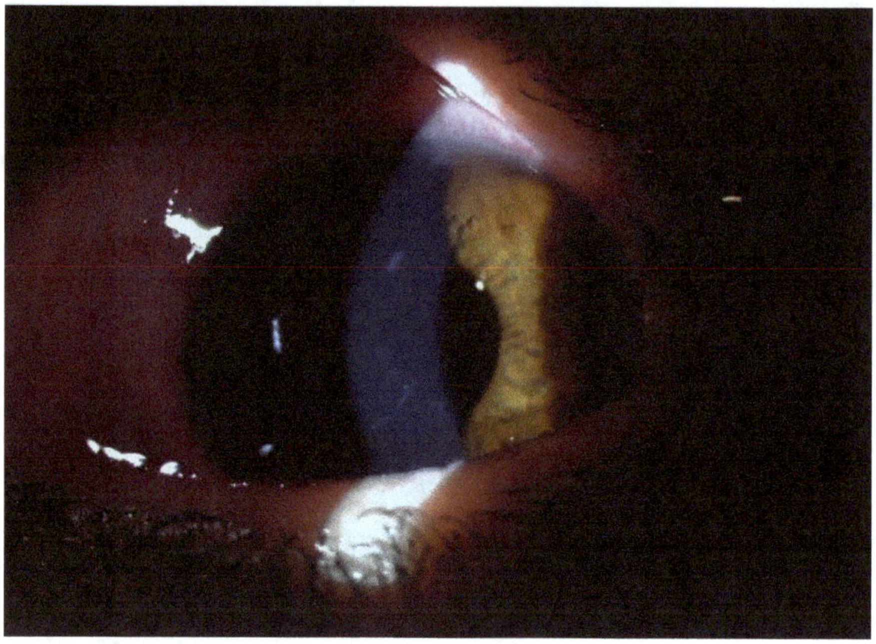

Figure 128. Anterior stromal keratitis with multiple, hazy, dry infiltrates (left photo) and the same eye 2 weeks after treatment with steroids drops (Dexamethasone 0.1% q2h) and Systemic Acyclovir 800mg tid (right photo)

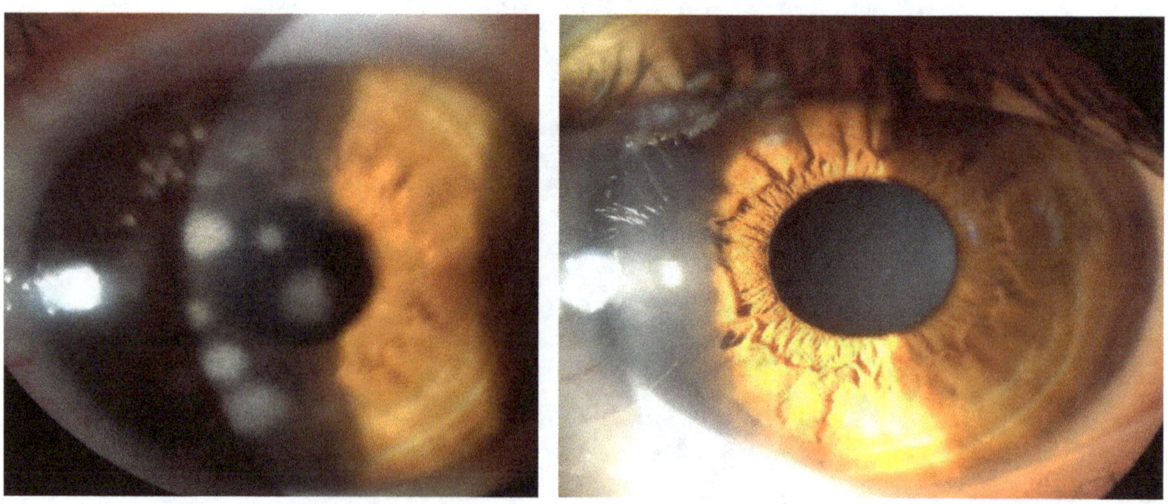

Anterior stromal keratitis represents either isolated or multiple patches of hazy, granular, dry infiltrate just under the Bowman's layer. The residual nummular scars are a marker of previous Herpes zoster corneal inflammation (Fig 128, 129). Neurotrophic ulcers can be observed in Herpes Zoster keratitis as well (Fig 128).

Figure 129. Stromal necrotizing keratitis due to HZV. Epithelial defect, stromal infiltrate, central thinning and hypopyon are seen

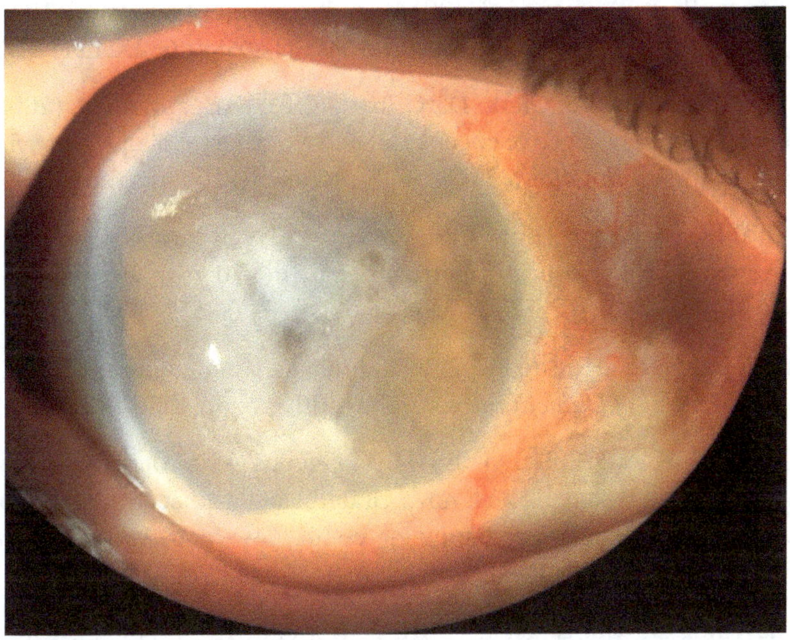

Figure 130. HZ skin rash (left photo) and the same patient with a neurotrophic ulcer and underlying stromal edema (right photo)

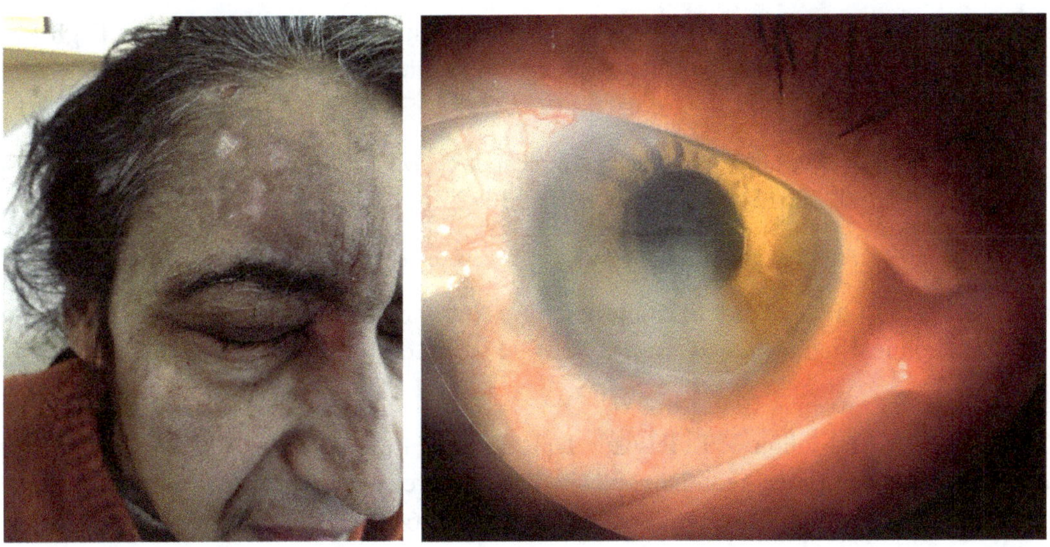

REFERENCES

(1986). Acanthamoeba keratitis associated with contact lenses–United States. *MMWR. Morbidity and Mortality Weekly Report*, *35*(25), 405–408. PMID:3088418

Aggarwal, S., Cavalcanti, B. M., & Pavan-Langston, D. (2014). Treatment of pseudodendrites in herpes zoster ophthalmicus with topical ganciclovir 0.15 gel. *Cornea*, *33*(2), 109–113. doi:10.1097/ICO.0000000000000020 PMID:24322809

Antunes, L. C. S., Visca, P., & Towner, K. J. (2014). Acinetobacter baumannii: Evolution of a global pathogen. *Pathogens and Disease*, *71*(3), 292–301. doi:10.1111/2049-632X.12125 PMID:24376225

Arif, A., Do, T., Byun, R., Sheehy, E., Clark, D., Gilbert, S. C., & Beighton, D. (2008). Veillonella rogosae sp. nov., an anaerobic Gram-negative coccus isolated from dental plaque. *International Journal of Systematic and Evolutionary Microbiology*, *58*(3), 581–584. doi:10.1099/ijs.0.65093-0 PMID:18319459

Basaglia, G., Carretto, E., Barbarini, D., Moras, L., Scalone, S., Marone, P., & De Paoli, P. (2002). Catheter-related bacteremia due to Kocuria kristinae in a patient with ovarian cancer. *Journal of Clinical Microbiology*, *40*(1), 311–313. doi:10.1128/JCM.40.1.311-313.2002 PMID:11773142

Burkholderia, Stenotrophomonas, Ralstonia, Brevundimonas, Comamonas, Delftia, Pandoraea, and Acidivorax. (2003). In *Manual of Clinical Microbiology* (8th ed., pp. 729–748). ASM Press.

Collins, M. D., & Lawson, P. A. (2000, January 1). The genus Abiotrophia (Kawamura et al.) is not monophyletic: Proposal of Granulicatella gen. nov., Granulicatella adiacens comb. nov., Granulicatella elegans comb. nov. and Granulicatella balaenopterae comb. nov. *International Journal of Systematic and Evolutionary Microbiology*, *50*(Pt 1), 365–369. doi:10.1099/00207713-50-1-365 PMID:10826824

Funke, G., von Graevenitz, A., Clarridge, J. E. III, & Bernard, K. A. (1997). Clinical microbiology of coryneform bacteria. *Clinical Microbiology Reviews*, *10*(1), 125–159. doi:10.1128/CMR.10.1.125 PMID:8993861

Hakin, Dart, & Sherrard. (n.d.). Sporadic diffuse corneal endotheliitis. *Am J Ophthalmol.*

Harimaya, A., Takada, R., Hendolin, P. H., Fujii, N., Ylikoski, J., & Himi, T. (2006). High Incidence of Alloiococcus otitidis in Children with Otitis Media, Despite Treatment with Antibiotics. *Journal of Clinical Microbiology*, *44*(3), 946–949. doi:10.1128/JCM.44.3.946-949.2006 PMID:16517881

Hejazi, A., & Falkiner, F. R. (1997). Serratia marcescens. *Journal of Medical Microbiology*, *46*(11), 903–912. doi:10.1099/00222615-46-11-903 PMID:9368530

Holt, J. G. (Ed.). (1994). *Bergey's Manual of Determinative Bacteriology* (9th ed.). Williams & Wilkins.

John, E., & Velotta, E. (2005). Velotta: Nontuberculous (atypical) mycobacterial keratitis after LASIK: current status and clinical implications. *Cornea*, *24*(3), 245–255. doi:10.1097/01.ico.0000151565.63107.64 PMID:15778593

Joslin, C. E., Tu, E. Y., McMahon, T. T., Passaro, D. J., Stayner, L. T., & Sugar, J. (2006). Epidemiological characteristics of a Chicago-area Acanthamoeba keratitis outbreak. *American Journal of Ophthalmology*, *142*(2), 212–217. doi:10.1016/j.ajo.2006.04.034 PMID:16876498

Jurkunas, U., Behlau, I., & Colby, K. (2009). Fungal keratitis: Changing pathogens and risk factors. *Cornea*, *28*(6), 638–643. doi:10.1097/ICO.0b013e318191695b PMID:19512908

Karl, H. (1975). Isolation and Characterization of Staphylococci from Human Skin I. Amended Descriptions of Staphylococcus epidermidis and Staphylococcus saprophyticus and Descriptions of Three New Species: Staphylococcus cohnii, Staphylococcus haemolyticus, and Staphylococcus xylosus. *International Journal of Systematic Bacteriology*, *25*(1), 50–61. doi:10.1099/00207713-25-1-50

Karp, C. L., Tuli, S. S., Yoo, S. H., Vroman, D. T., Alfonso, E. C., Huang, A. H., Pflugfelder, S. C., & Culbertson, W. W. (2003). Infectious keratitis after LASIK. *Ophthalmology*, *110*(3), 503–510. doi:10.1016/S0161-6420(02)01760-8 PMID:12623812

Lichtinger, A., Yeung, S. N., Kim, P., Amiran, M. D., Iovieno, A., Elbaz, U., Ku, J. Y. F., Wolff, R., Rootman, D. S., & Slomovic, A. R. (2012). Shifting trends in bacterial keratitis in Toronto: An 11-year review. *Ophthalmology*, *119*(9), 1785–1790. doi:10.1016/j.ophtha.2012.03.031 PMID:22627118

Liesegang, T. J. (2008). Herpes zoster ophthalmicus: Natural history, risk factors, clinical presentation, and morbidity. *Ophthalmology*, *115*(2), S3–S12. doi:10.1016/j.ophtha.2007.10.009 PMID:18243930

Madigan, M., & Martinko, J. (Eds.). (2005). *Brock Biology of Microorganisms* (11th ed.). Prentice Hall.

McLeod, S. D., Goei, S. L., Taglia, D. P., & McMahon, T. T. (1998). Nonulcerating bacterial keratitis associated with soft and rigid contact lens wear. *Ophthalmology*, *105*(3), 517–521. doi:10.1016/S0161-6420(98)93036-6 PMID:9499784

Mitchell, J. (2011). Streptococcus mitis: Walking the line between commensalism and pathogenesis. *Molecular Oral Microbiology*, *26*(2), 89–98. doi:10.1111/j.2041-1014.2010.00601.x PMID:21375700

Morita, E., Narikiyo, M., Yokoyama, A., Yano, A., Kamoi, K., Yoshikawa, E., Yamaguchi, T., Igaki, H., Tachimori, Y., Kato, H., Saito, D., Hanada, N., & Sasaki, H. (2005). Predominant presence of Streptococcus anginosus in the saliva of alcoholics. *Oral Microbiology and Immunology*, *20*(6), 362–365. doi:10.1111/j.1399-302X.2005.00242.x PMID:16238596

Mullooly, J. P., Riedlinger, K., Chun, C., Weinmann, S., & Houston, H. (2005). Incidence of herpes zoster, 1997–2002. *Epidemiology and Infection*, *133*(2), 245–253. doi:10.1017/S095026880400281X PMID:15816149

Paik, S., Senty, L., Das, S., Noe, J. C., Munro, C. L., & Kitten, T. (2005). Identification of Virulence Determinants for Endocarditis in Streptococcus sanguinis by Signature-Tagged Mutagenesis. *Infection and Immunity*, *73*(9), 6064–6074. doi:10.1128/IAI.73.9.6064-6074.2005 PMID:16113327

Pavan-Langston. (1994). Herpetic infections. In *The cornea*. Little, Brown.

Pepose, J. S., & Wilhelmus, K. R. (1992). Divergent approaches to the management of corneal ulcers. *American Journal of Ophthalmology*, *114*(5), 630–632. doi:10.1016/S0002-9394(14)74496-4 PMID:1443028

Robin, J. B., Steigner, J. B., & Kaufman, H. E. (1985). Progressive herpetic corneal endotheliitis. *American Journal of Ophthalmology*, *100*(2), 336–337. doi:10.1016/0002-9394(85)90811-6 PMID:2992281

Ryan, K., & Ray, C. (2004). *Sherris Medical Microbiology* (4th ed.). McGraw Hill.

Ryan, K. J., & Ray, C. G. (Eds.). (2004). *Sherris Medical Microbiology* (4th ed.). McGraw Hill.

Ryan, K. J., & Ray, C. G. (Eds.). (2004). Sherris Medical Microbiology. McGraw Hill.

Ryan, M. P., & Adley, C. C. (2010). Sphingomonas paucimobilis: A persistent Gram-negative nosocomial infectious organism. *The Journal of Hospital Infection*, *75*(3), 153–157. doi:10.1016/j.jhin.2010.03.007 PMID:20434794

Said, D. G., Otri, M., Miri, A., Kailasanathan, A., Khatib, T., & Dua, H. S. (2011). The challenge of fungal keratitis. *The British Journal of Ophthalmology*, *95*(12), 1623–1624. doi:10.1136/bjophthalmol-2011-301148 PMID:22096205

Shimeld, C., Tullo, A. B., Easty, D. L., & Thomsitt, J. (1982). Isolation of herpes simplex virus from the cornea in chronic stromal keratitis. *The British Journal of Ophthalmology*, *66*(10), 643–647. doi:10.1136/bjo.66.10.643 PMID:6288065

Solomon, A., Karp, C. L., & Miller, D. (2001). Mycobacterium interface keratitis after laser in situ keratomileusis. *Ophthalmology*, *108*(12), 2201–2208. doi:10.1016/S0161-6420(01)00851-X PMID:11733259

Sy, A., McLeod, S. D., Cohen, E. J., Margolis, T. P., Mannis, M. J., Lietman, T. M., & Acharya, N. R. (2012). Practice patterns and opinions in the management of recurrent or chronic herpes zoster ophthalmicus. *Cornea*, *31*(7), 786–790. doi:10.1097/ICO.0b013e31823cbe6a PMID:22269677

Tenaillon, O., Skurnik, D., Picard, B., & Denamur, E. (2017). The population genetics of commensal Escherichia coli. *Nature Reviews. Microbiology*, *8*(3), 207–217. doi:10.1038/nrmicro2298 PMID:20157339

Thomas, P. A., & Kaliamurthy, J. (2013). Mycotic keratitis: Epidemiology, diagnosis and management. *Clinical Microbiology and Infection*, *19*(3), 210–220. doi:10.1111/1469-0691.12126 PMID:23398543

Thygeson, P. (1971). Marginal herpes simplex keratitis simulating catarrhal ulcer. *Investigative Ophthalmology & Visual Science*, *10*, 1006.

Tuft, S. J. (2003). Suppurative keratitis. *The British Journal of Ophthalmology*, *87*(2), 127. doi:10.1136/bjo.87.2.127 PMID:12543733

Tyring, S. K., Beutner, K. R., & Tucker, B. A. (2000). Antiviral therapy for herpes zoster: Randomized, controlled clinical trial of valacyclovir and famciclovir therapy in immunocompetent patients 50 years and older. *Archives of Family Medicine*, *9*(9), 863–869. doi:10.1001/archfami.9.9.863 PMID:11031393

Wilhelmus, K. R. (1987). Review of clinical experience with microbial keratitis associated with contact lenses. *The CLAO Journal*, *13*(4), 211–214. PMID:3331130

Wilhelmus, K. R. (1987). Diagnosis and management of herpes simplex stromal keratitis. *Cornea*, *6*(4), 286–291. doi:10.1097/00003226-198706040-00011 PMID:3319411

Chapter 6
Noninfectious Corneal Disorders

ABSTRACT

This chapter discusses noninfectious corneal disorders, caused by an immune inflammation such as phlyctenular keratoconjunctivitis, marginal staphylococcal keratitis, peripheral ulcerative keratitis, Mooren's ulcer, interstitial keratitis, rosacea keratitis, etc. Mooren's ulcer, which is considered one of the most severe diseases, is presented with serial photos of follow-ups within 3 years with different complications, management of the condition, and results. A severe case of rosacea keratitis associated with anterior uveitis is included in this chapter too. Thygeson's superficial punctate keratitis case is shown as well, but the disease is very rare in Middle Eastern populations. The material in this chapter also includes filamentary, neurotrophic, and exposure keratitis. A rare disorder like anesthetic abuse keratopathy, caused by topical excess use of anesthetic drops, is presented with before and after treatment photos to illustrate that the condition, if treated appropriately, can leave minimal scarring.

NONINFECTIUOS CORNEAL DISORDERS

Filamentary keratitis (FK) is a disease, which clinically presents by the attachment of filaments (complexes of degenerated epithelial cells and mucus) to the corneal surface (Tanioka et al, 2009). FK is usually associated with many ocular and systemic diseases, most commonly dry eye disease with or without Sjogren syndrome, and herpetic keratitis. Filaments are visible as gelatinous strands of different sizes and distribution, attached to the corneal epithelium (Fig 1, 2, 3). Patients complain of foreign-body sensation, blurry vision, pain and photophobia. Control of the underlining disease is very important for treating this condition. Treatment includes administration of non-preserved lubricants, topical steroidal and nonsteroidal anti-inflammatory agents, punctal occlusion, hypertonic saline solutions, mucolytic agents, mechanical removal of filaments, and bandage contact lenses. Treatment with 5% sodium chloride topically 3-4 times daily resulted in improved symptoms and a decrease or elimination of filaments in 89% of eyes in one month (Hamilton et al, 2009).

DOI: 10.4018/978-1-7998-6937-5.ch006

Figure 1. The upper photo: filaments are seen at the superior peripheral cornea, note the postherpetic stromal scar. Below: the same eye after removal of filaments with a contact lens (left photo). The same eye after 1-month without a contact lens and with no recurrence of filaments (right photo)

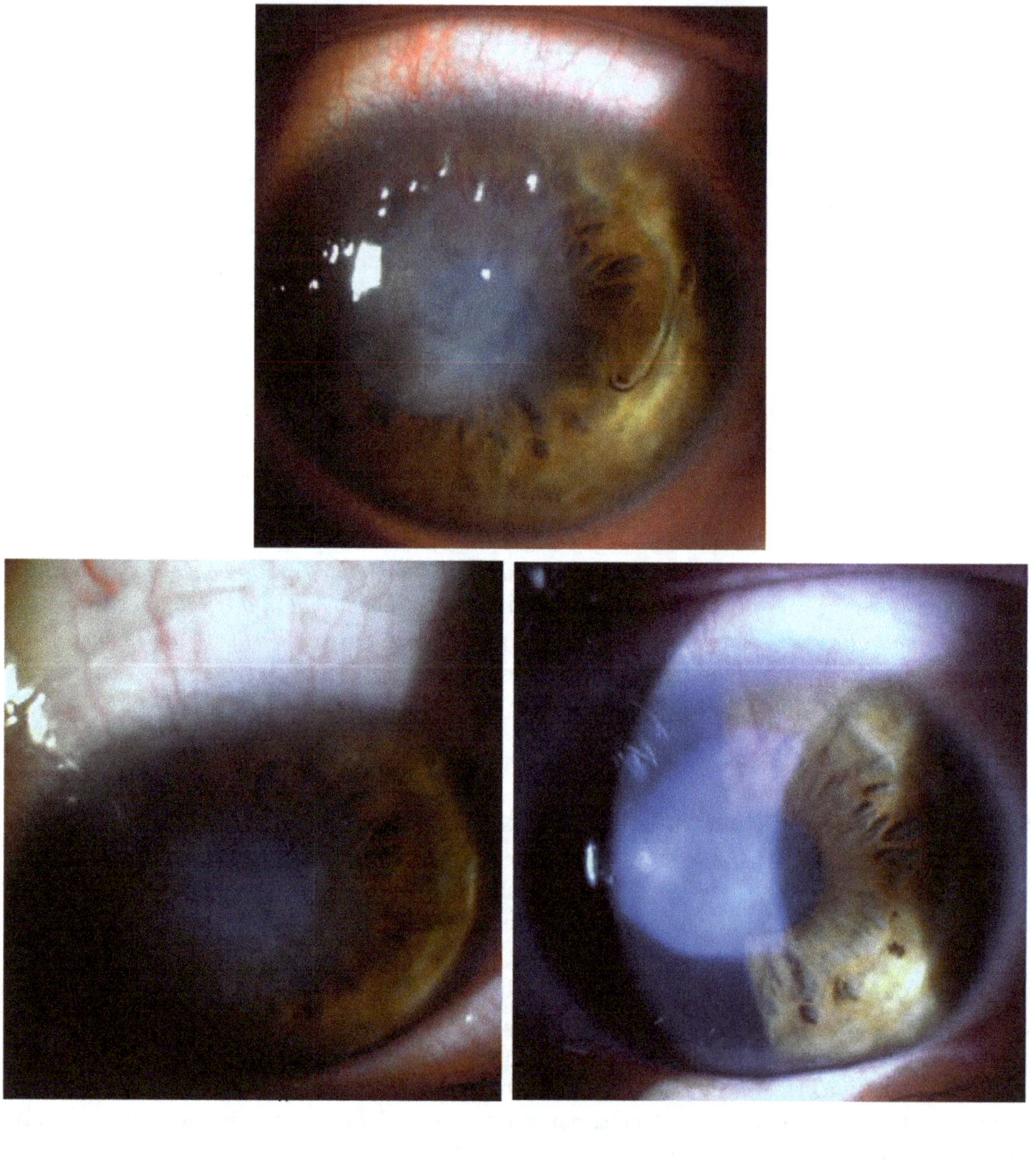

Figure 2. Patient with dry eye syndrome. Filaments are seen on the graft

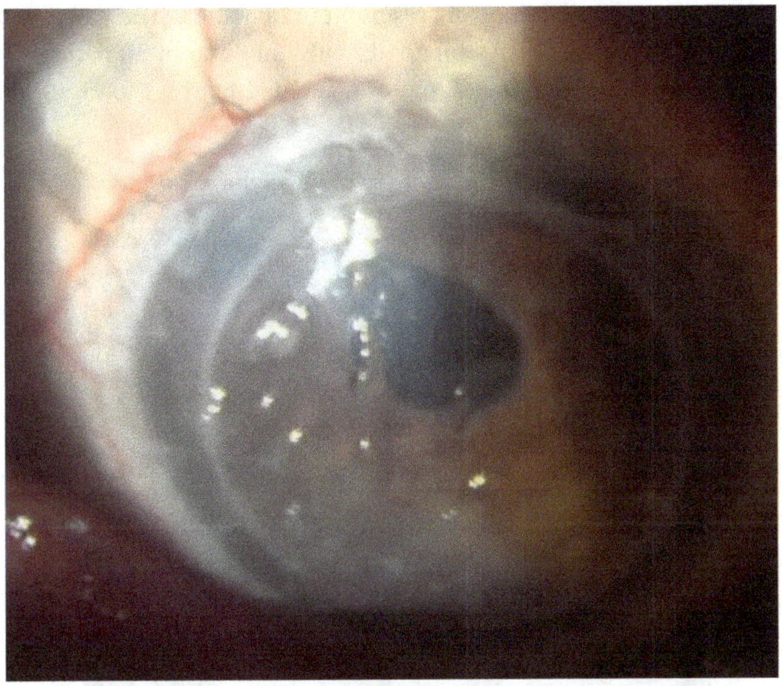

Figure 3. Long filaments, herpetic stromal scar with NV

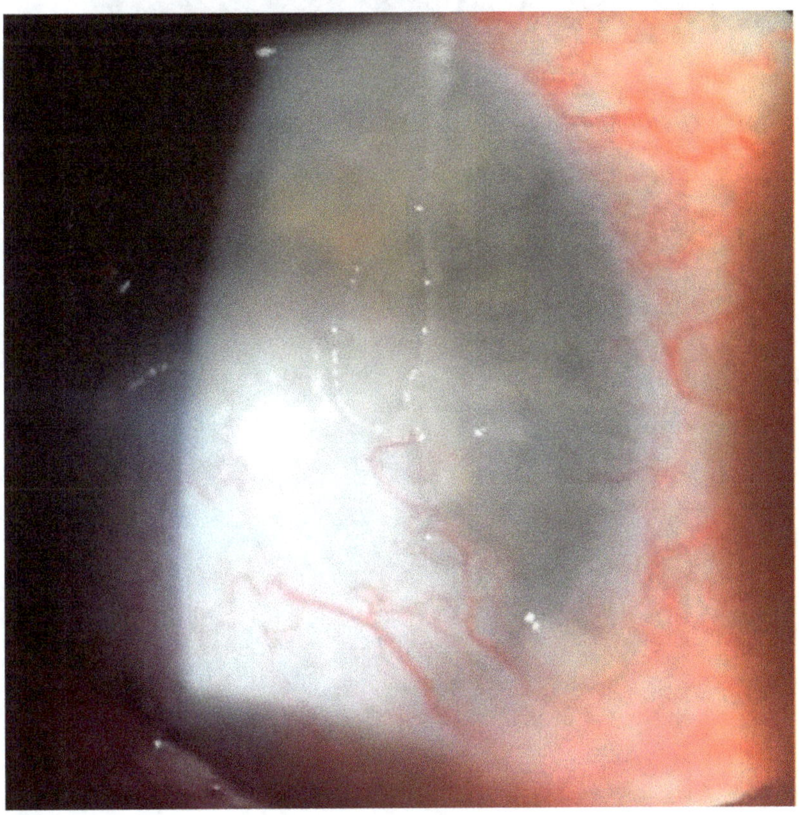

Superficial punctate keratitis of Thygeson is an epithelial keratopathy which clinically represents as oval or round punctate itraepithelial deposits resembling opacities. The cause of the disease is still unknown. The presentation is almost always bilateral, with only one in 20 patients having a unilateral disease (Fig 4, 5) (Nagra et al, 2004). Main symptoms include tearing, foreign-body sensation, pho-

Figure 4. Thygeson's superficial keratitis. The same eye. Intraepithelial location of lesions is seen

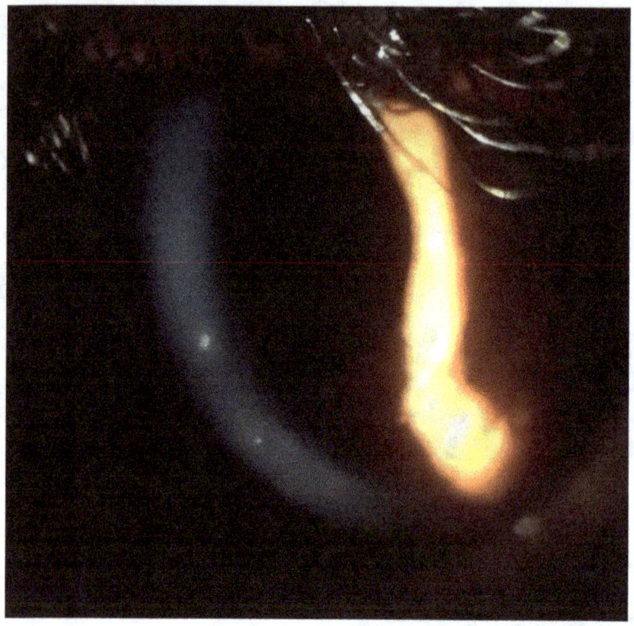

Figure 5. Thygeson's superficial keratitis. Small, round punctate lesions are seen

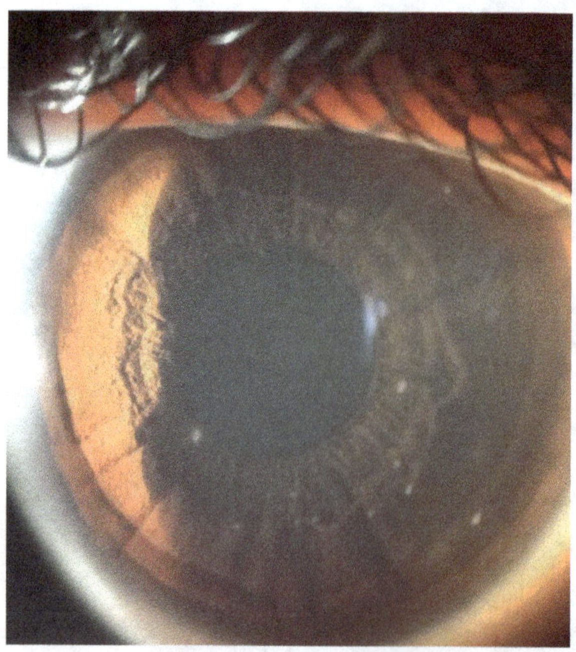

tophobia, and sometimes reduced vision. Artificial tears are often adequate for mild cases. Low-dose topical corticosteroids are commonly used during exacerbations of disease (e.g. Fluorometholone 0.1%) (Marquezan et al, 2015). Topical cyclosporine or tacrolimus can also be effective (Vieira et al, n.d.).

Phlyctenular keratoconjunctivitis and **marginal staphylococcal keratitis** (catarrhal ulcer) represent ocular surface noninfectious inflammatory processes (Mondino et al, 1982). Staphylococcal marginal keratitis usually presents with one or more peripheral stromal infiltrates, which usually localize where the lid margin crosses the limbus (4,8,10 o'clock). Classically, these lesions are parallel to the limbus and separated from the limbus by 1-2mm of the transparent cornea (Fig 6) (McCulley et al, 1982). Conjunctival phylctenules most commonly occur near the limbus but can be observed anywhere on the bulbar

Figure 6. Staphylococcal marginal keratitis. The clear corneal zone is seen between the lesion and the limbus (left photo). Multiple lesions (right photo)

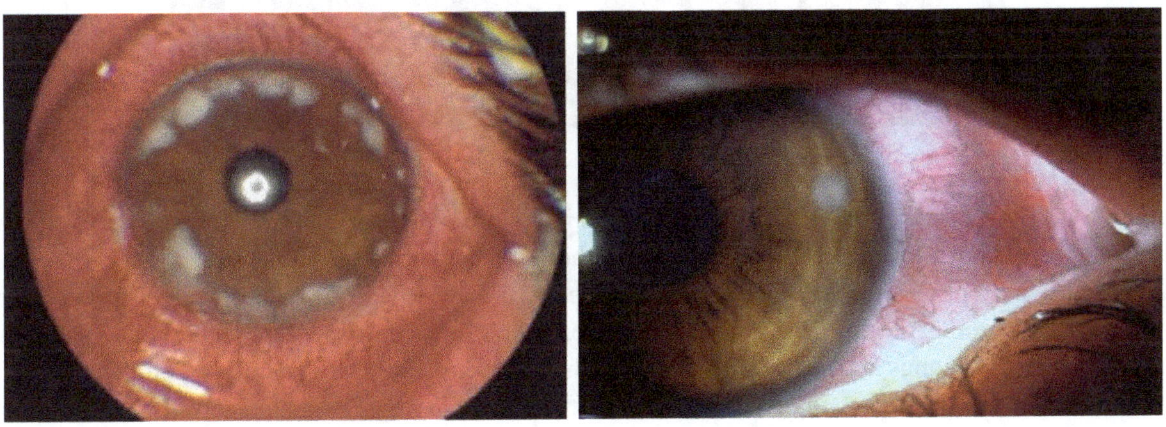

Figure 7. Corneal «wandering» phlyctenule. Small central lesion with mild pannus are seen

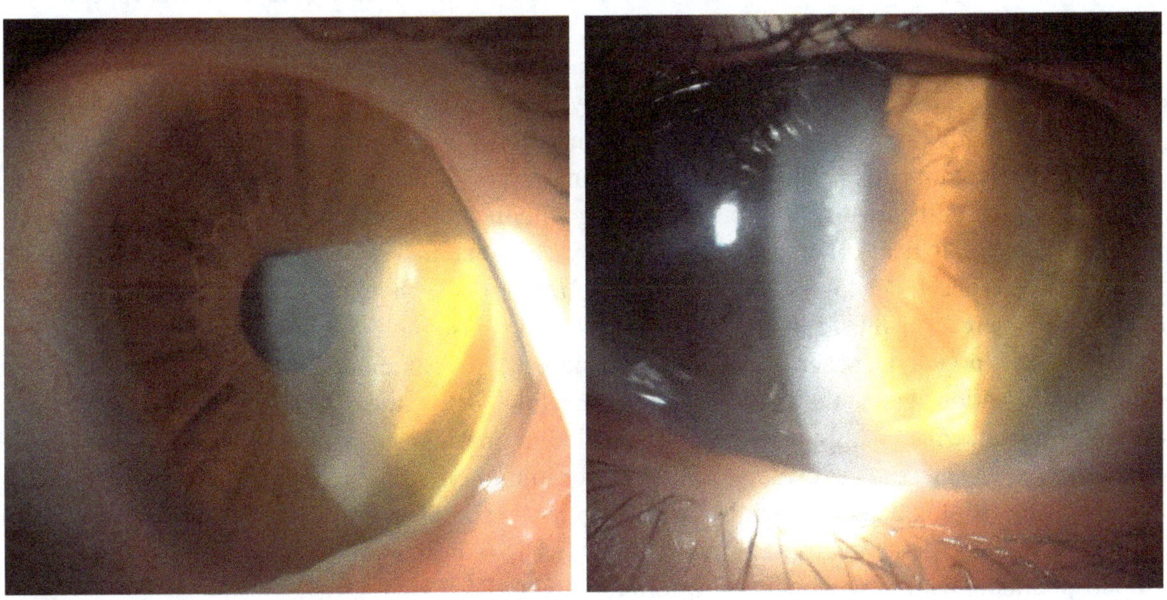

Figure 8. Conjunctival phlyctenule

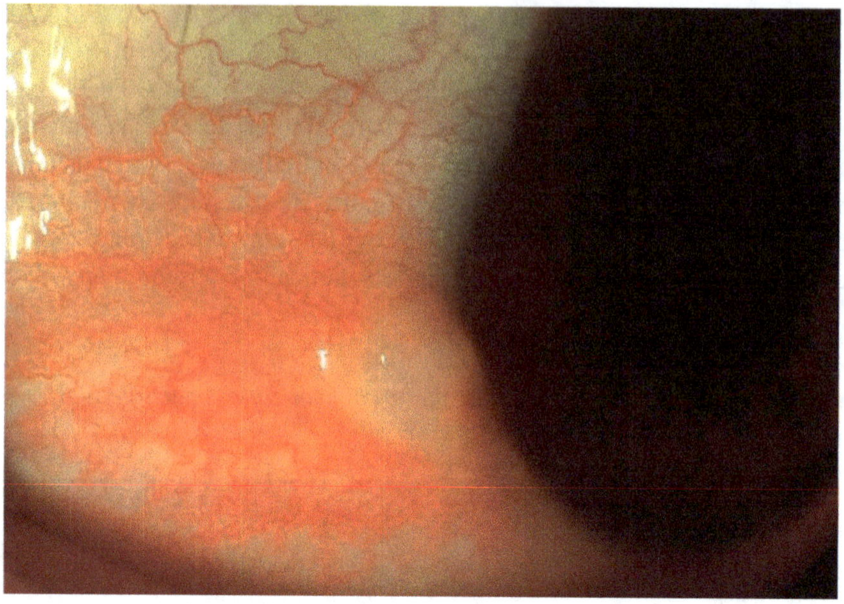

conjunctiva (Fig 8). In countries where tuberculosis is common, Mycobacterium tuberculosis remains the primary cause of PKC. In developed countries though, he most common pathogen associated with this disorder is Staphylococcus. Corneal phlyctenules typically appear at the limbus as a small white nodule and are accompanied by a conjunctival injection. Subsequent corneal phlyctenules can arise at the central edge of the pannus and cross the cornea, reaching the opposite side (wandering phlyctenule, Fig 7) (Beauchamp et al, n.d.). The treatment of this conditions includes topical corticosteroids. Prednisolone acetate 1% or other steroids given 4-6 times daily can be used as a starting dose. If the underlying disease is tuberculosis, systemic treatment must be initiated. In cases where conditions are related to blepharitis or meibomitis, lid hygiene and treatment with topical/systemic tetracyclines are effective, especially for cases with recurrences of diseases (Culbertson et al, 1993).

Peripheral ulcerative keratitis (PUK) presents as a crescent-shaped destructive lesion localized in the peripheral corneal stroma, usually with an overlying epithelial defect. About 1/3rd of patients also have scleritis. The disease may be complicated with corneal perforation due to progressive thinning. PUK is associated with autoimmune disorders, commonly with rheumatoid arthritis (9, 10) (Shiuey et al, 1998). The goal of the treatment is to stop melting with the help of lubricants, patching, or a bandage contact lens. Several topical collagenase inhibitors (ex, sodium citrate 10%, acetylcysteine solution 20%, medroxyprogesterone 1%) and systemic collagenase inhibitors such as tetracyclines (ex, doxycycline) should be considered as well. Topical corticosteroids, which also inhibit collagenase function, can have variable effects. In general, when steroids are considered, the clinician should weigh the benefits of treating inflammation against the risks of impaired healing. Oftentimes, definitive management can be achieved by enhancement of systemic treatment, including immunosuppression therapy with oral prednisone, cytotoxic agents such as cyclophosphamide, or immunomodulatory agents such as methotrexate or cyclosporine. Biologic agents such as infliximab have reportedly been used with some success in more severe cases. Patients with severe, rapid melting may require intravenous therapy with high-dose cyclophosphamide, with or without corticosteroid therapy (Bhat et al, 2015).

Figure 9. PUK associated with rheumatoid arthritis, crescent-shaped peripheral ulcer, pending perforation

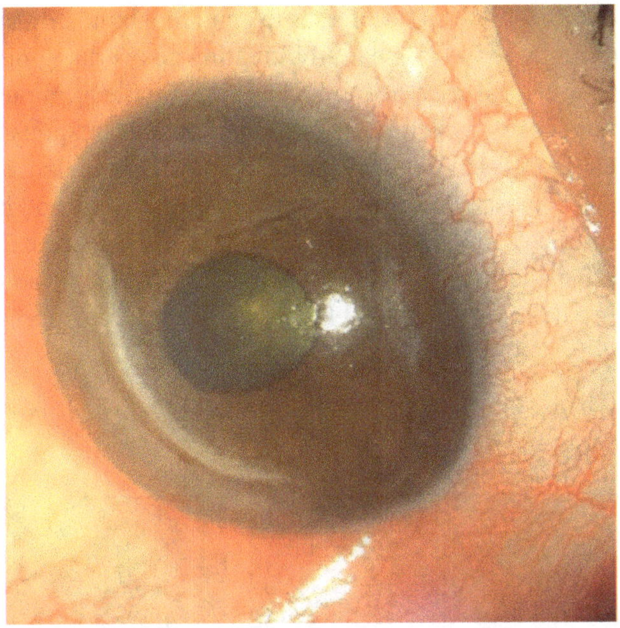

Figure 10. PUK. The crescent-shaped corneal ulcer is seen

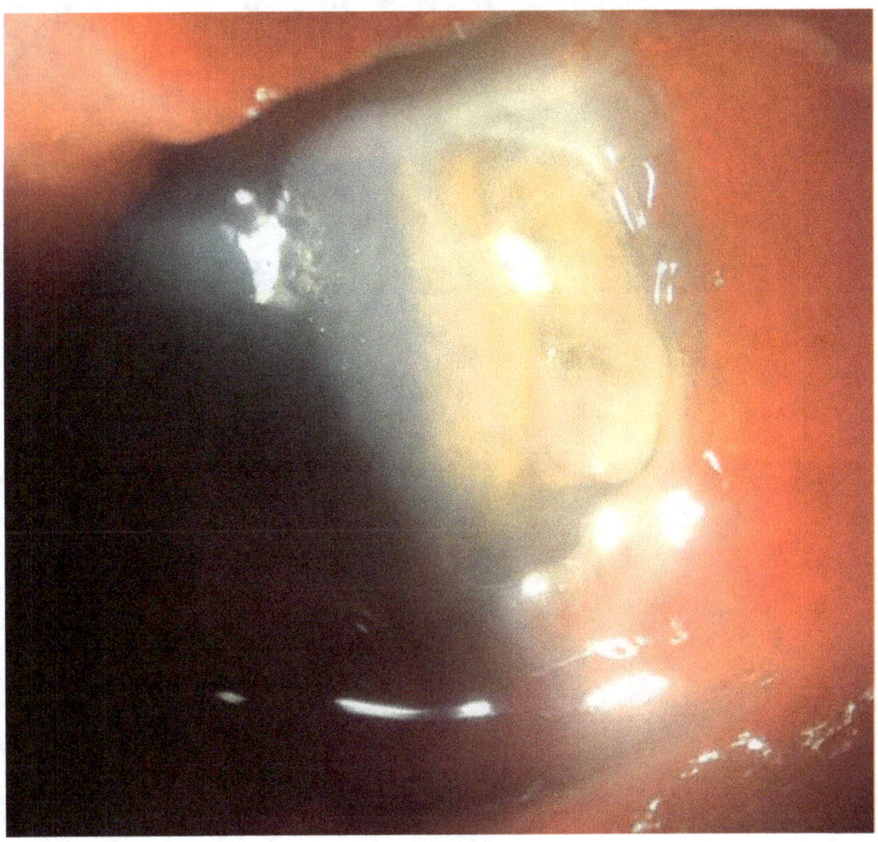

Mooren's ulcer is a disease of unknown etiology that starts as a crescent-shaped gray-white infiltrate in the peripheral cornea. Similar to PUK, it progresses to epithelial breakdown and stromal melting. The ulcer progresses circumferentially as well as centrally, creating an overhanging edge at its central border (Wood et al, 1971). Mooren's ulcer is assumed to be an idiopathic autoimmune disease occurring in a complete absence of any diagnosable systemic disorder that could be responsible for the ulceration and the destruction of the cornea (Fig 11-16). Topical corticosteroids, contact lenses, acetylcysteine 10% and l-cysteine (0.2 molar), topical cyclosporine, limbal conjunctival excision, and lamellar keratoplasty have variable success. Topical interferon-a2a (IFN-a2a) and topical cyclosporine 2%, as well as infliximab, have been reported as effective alternatives (Garg et al, 2017). Our case responded to topical lubricants, Betamethasone sub/tenon weekly injections, oral Prednisone and Cyclosporine.

Figure 11. Mooren's ulcer. Conjunctivolimbal ulcer, peripheral corneal melting (left photo), and the same eye stained with fluorescein (right photo)

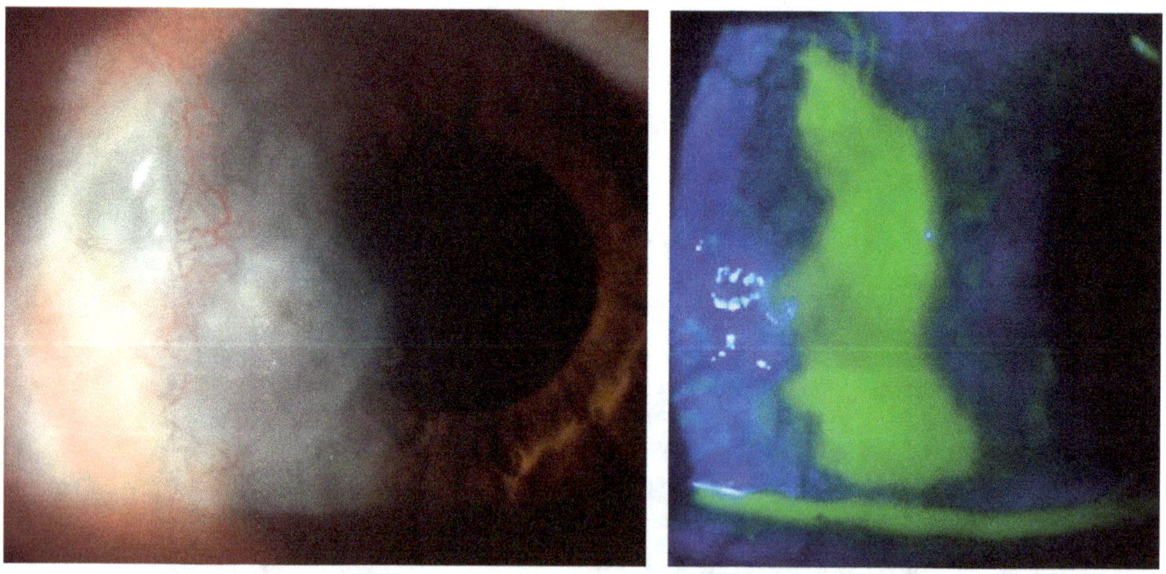

Figure 12. Mooren's ulcer. The right and left eyes of the same patient. Peripheral corneal perforation (left photo) and corneolimbal thining are seen

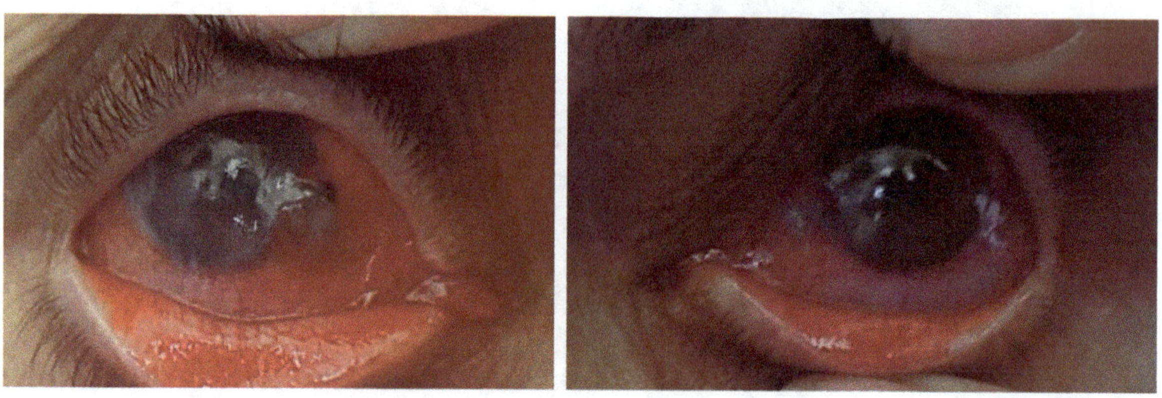

Figure 13. The same patient after 3 months of medical treatment

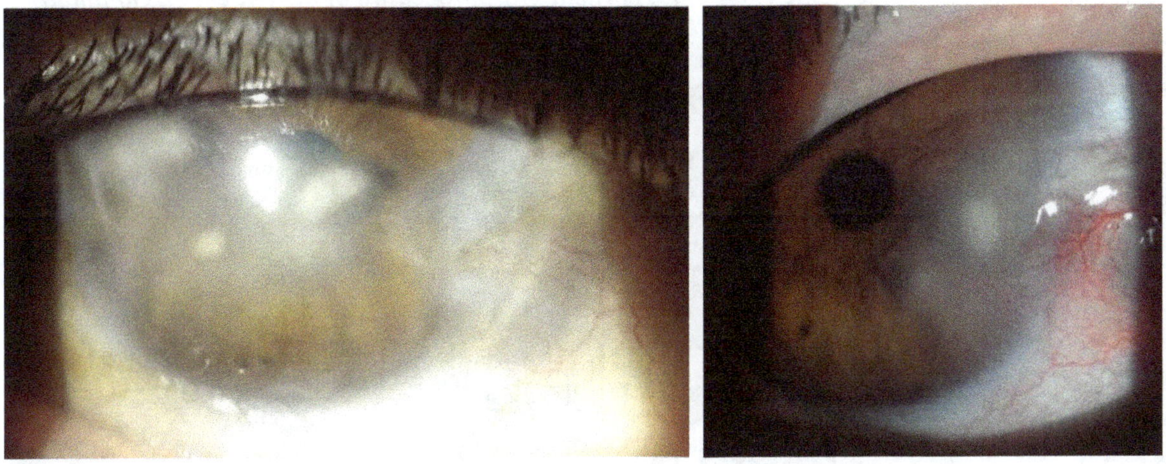

Figure 14. The same patient presented with scleritis 18 months later

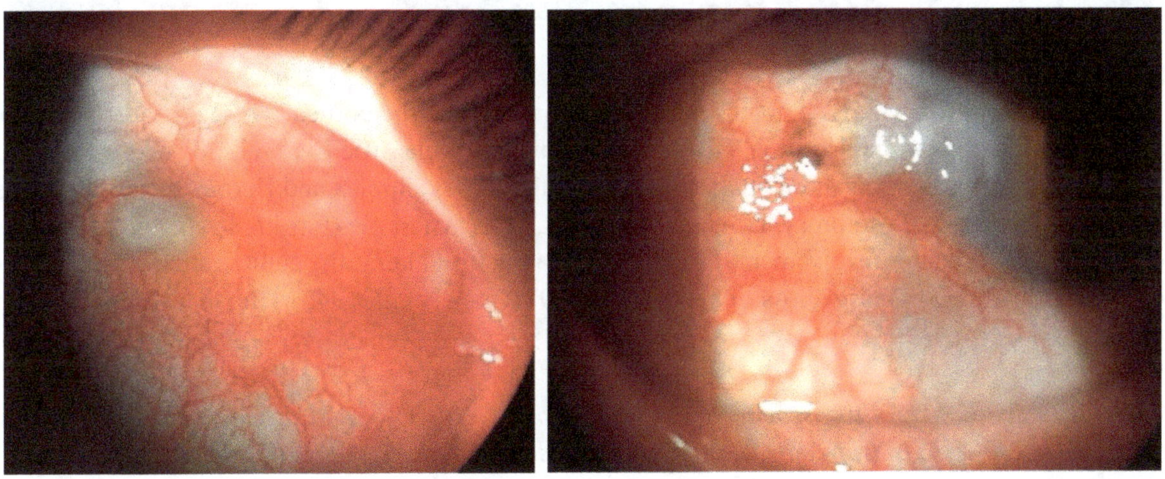

Figure 15. Same patient with Mooren's ulcer 3 years later presented with corneal perforation in the left eye

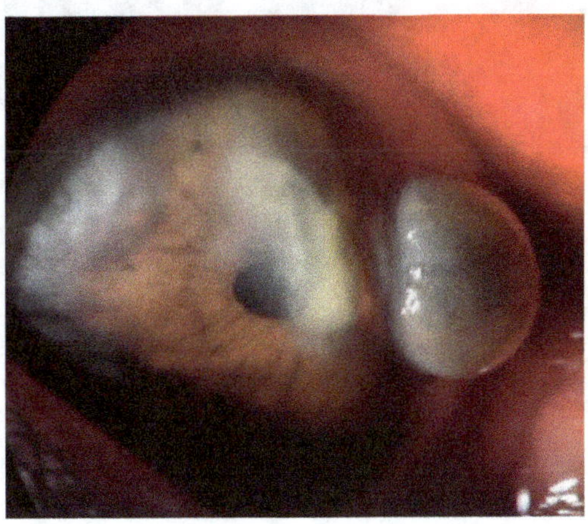

Figure 16. Mooren's ulcer. The same patient; right and left eyes. Note the sites of peripheral corneal perforation. 2 months post tectonic embryonal corneal graft procedure of the left eye (right photo)

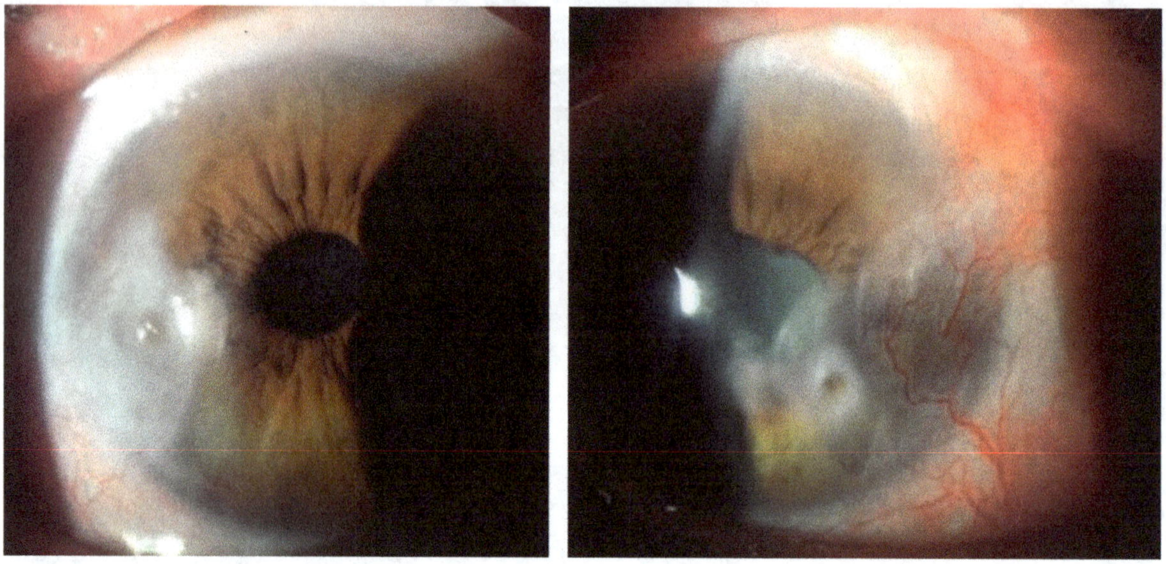

Interstitial keratitis (IK) is a nonulcerating inflammation of the corneal stroma, characterized by infiltration and farther vascularization. Historically, IK has been classified as syphilitic (Fig 20) or non-syphilitic. Nonsyphilitic IK is more often associated with Herpes simplex and Herpes zoster infections, Tuberculosis, Sarcoidosis, Leprosy, Lyme disease and Cogan syndrome (Fig 17, 18). Cogan syndrome is characterized by ocular involvement, primarily with interstitial keratitis, audiovestibular symptoms, accompanied with a progressive loss of hearing (Fig 19) (Cogan et al, 1945). The main complaints in-

Figure 17. Interstitial keratitis associated with sarcoidosis (left photo) and the same eye after 3 weeks of treatment with steroids drops started hourly and tapering within 6 weeks (right photo)

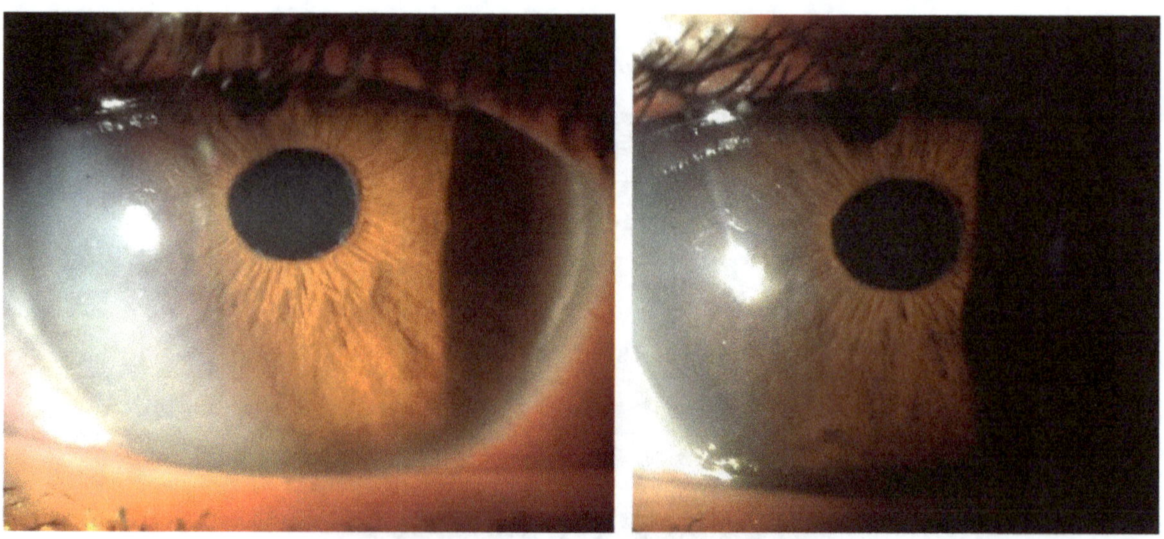

Figure 18. Interstitial keratitis associated with herpes simplex

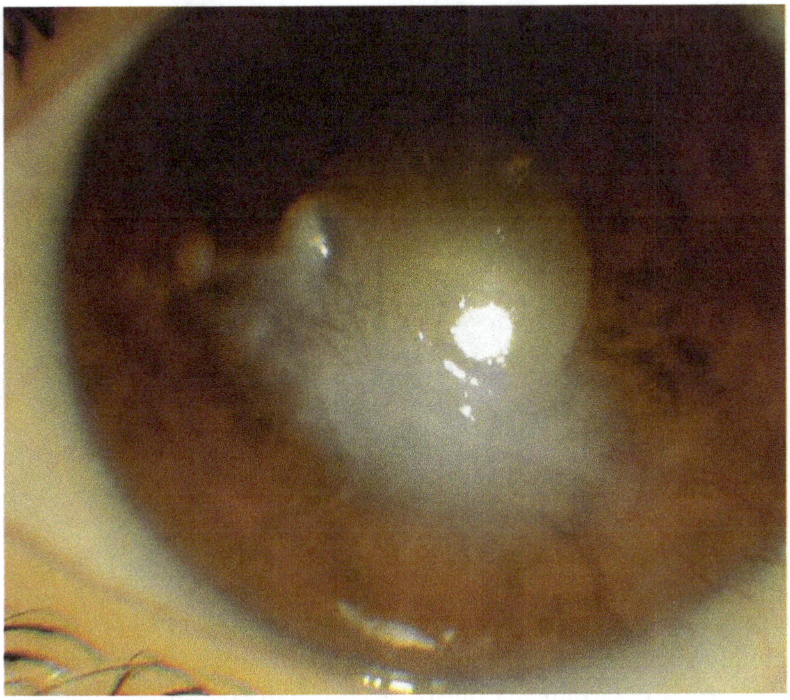

Figure 19. Interstitial keratitis associated with Cogan syndrome, superiotempoarlly active inflammation, inferionasally old anterior stromal scar

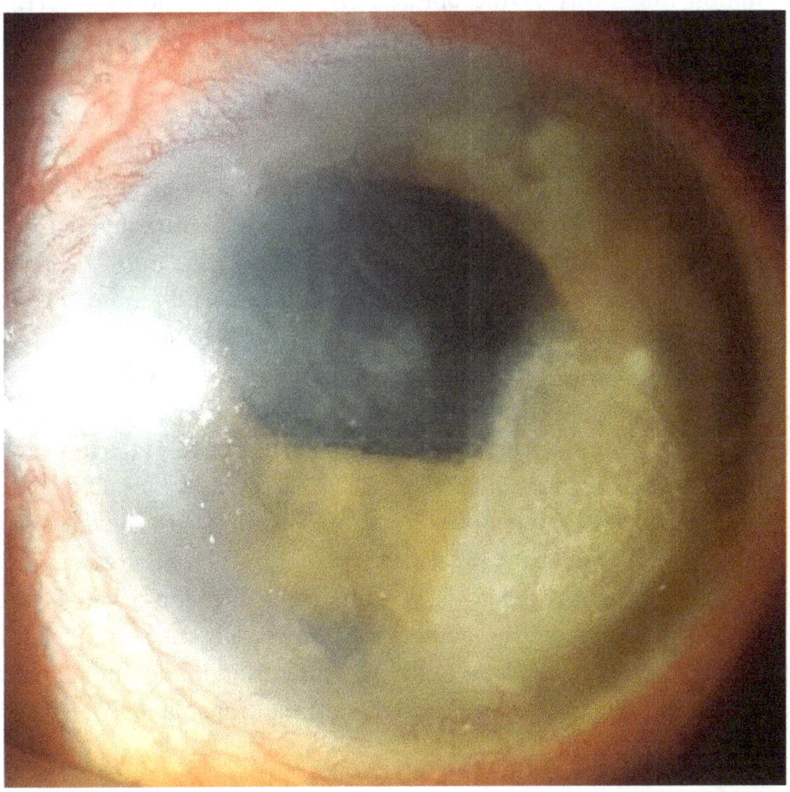

Figure 20. Interstitial bilateral syphilitic keratitis

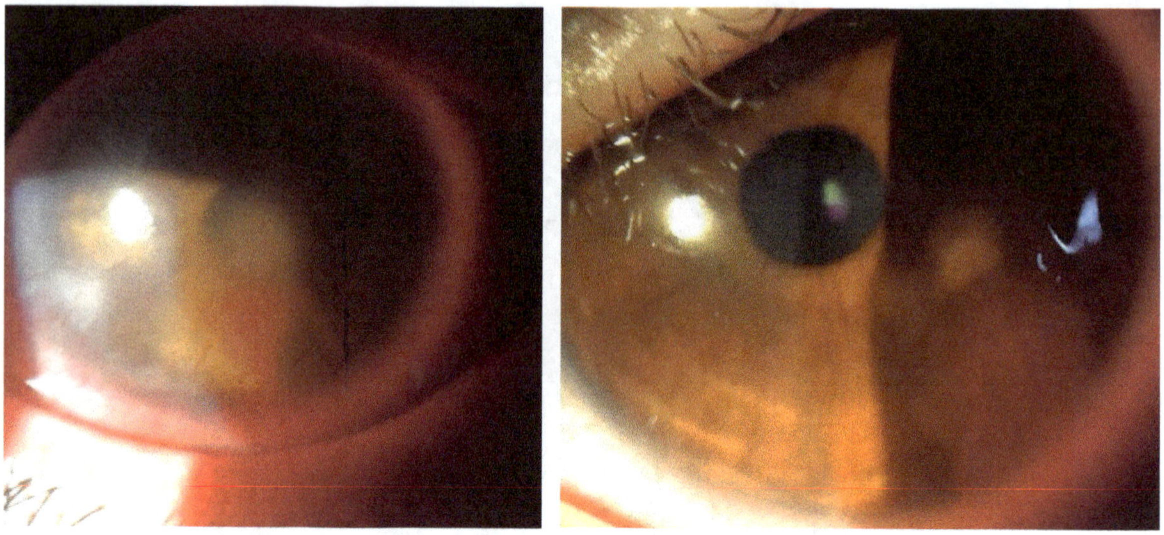

clude photophobia, mild to moderate redness, worsening of vision. Topical corticosteroid shortens the course of active syphilitic keratitis, reduces opacification. Usually the cornea clears completely. Topical steroids (eg, prednisolone 1% or dexamethasone 0.1%) is usually prescribed 4-8 times daily for stromal keratitis. Topical cyclosporine or tacrolimus may help patients not sufficiently responsive to topical corticosteroid treatment (Miserocchi et al, 2008).

Topical anesthetic abuse keratopathy is considered a self-induced ocular injury. The anesthetic ocular medications inhibit the ability of the epithelium to migrate and divide (Epstein et al, 1968; Rosenwasser et al, 1990; Mackie et al, 1978). As the patient continues to administer the anesthetic, the epithelial defect enlarges and becomes trophic. Typical findings include diffuse stromal edema, full-thickness stromal infiltration, keratic precipitates, and hypopyon (Fig 21, 22). Once the diagnosis is made, corneal healing usually occurs if anesthetic is removed. Oral analgesics or narcotics may be indicated for control of pain. Topical cycloplegics may help decrease inflammation and diminish pain. Use of topical corticosteroids is uncommon and may lead to corneal thinning. A mild topical antibiotic may help prevent secondary infection.

Neurotrophic keratitis is a degenerative disease of the corneal epithelium. The main characteristic feature is impaired healing. The hallmark of the condition is the absence of corneal sensitivity leading to stromal melting and perforation (Mackie et al, 1973). Herpes simplex (HSV) and zoster (HZV) virus infections of the ocular surface are considered the most common cause. Tumors and surgical procedures damaging the ophthalmic branch of the trigeminal nerve such as congenital syndromes, corneal dystrophies, local trauma to the corneal nerves, infections such as leprosy, systemic disease, topical medications, and exposure to toxins, constitute other possible causes leading to the development of neurotrophic keratitis (Mackie et al, 1978). Clinically, it presents as a round or oval defect, localized paracentrally (Fig 23). In mild cases the treatment requires lubrication, especially preservative-free, and therapeutic contact lenses. The neurotrophic ulcers respond very well to autologous serum tears (Jeng et al, 2009). Oral doxycycline prevents stromal necrosis, and helps with epithelial healing (Donzis et al, 1987). In severe cases surgical intervention such as amniotic membrane transplantation (Khokhar et la, 2005).,

Figure 21. Tetracaine abuse keratopathy. Epithelial defect stained with fluorescein, underlying stromal infiltrate, stromal edema, and mild hypopyon are seen. The same eye two weeks after treatment with mild steroids, oral Doxycycline, cycloplegic and removal of anesthetic drops. A sub/tenon Betamethasone Injection was given as well. Redness is decreased, hypopyon is resolved, stromal infiltrate with overlying defect is seen (left photo) and the same eye after 4 weeks of treatment, mild anterior scar is formed. (right photo)

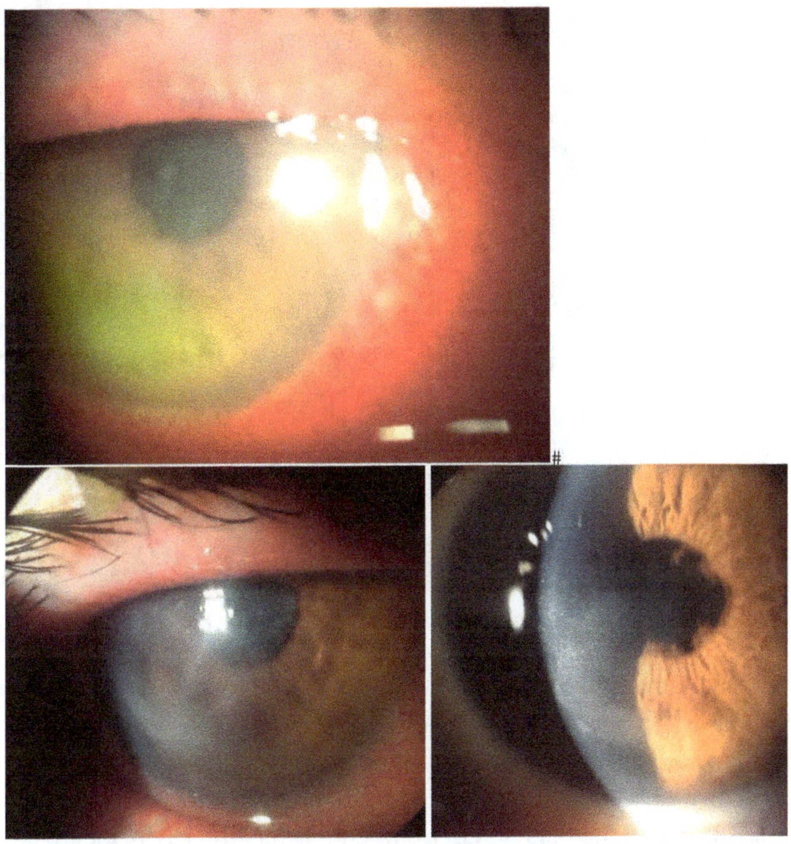

Figure 22. Tetracaine abuse keratopathy. Severe injection, epithelial defect, hyphema, and granuloma in the anterior chamber are seen (left photo), and the same eye after 8 weeks of treatment (right photo)

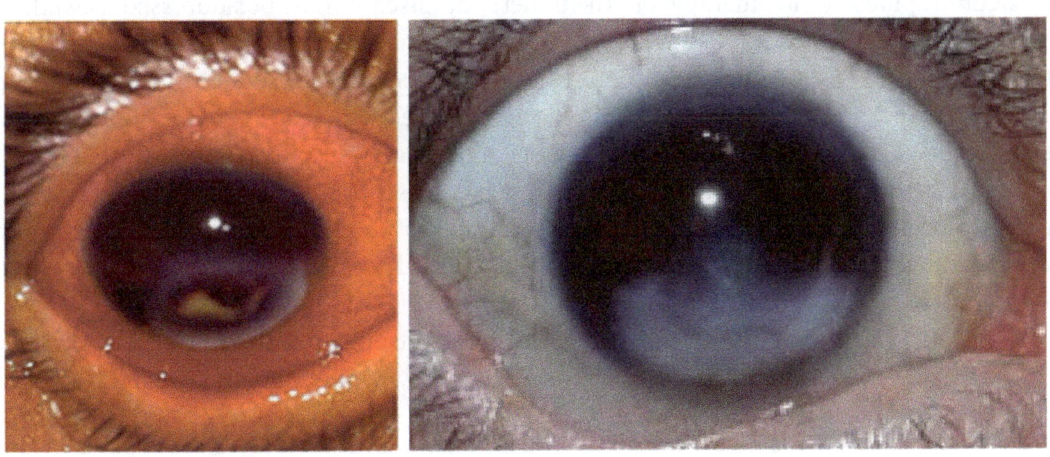

Figure 23. Neurotrophic ulcer due to Herpes simplex. The paracentral oval shaped ulcer is seen with enrolled margins

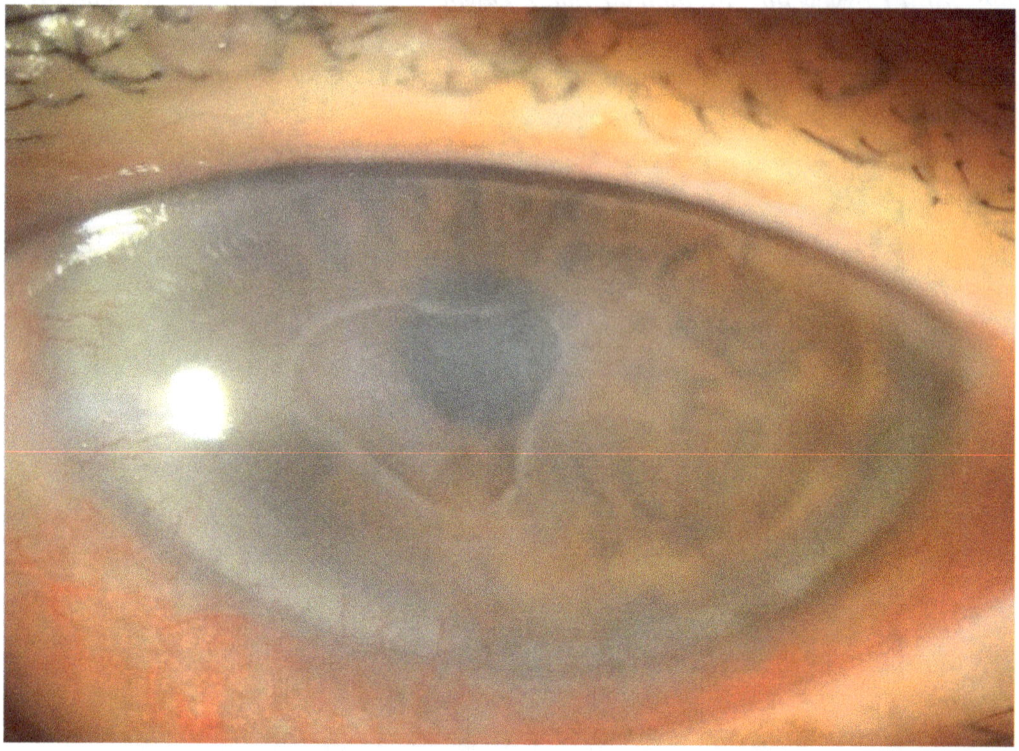

conjunctival flap, tectonic lamellar keratoplasty, tarsorrhaphy, application of cyanoacrylate glue (Hick et al, 2005) are required. New treatment options include Oxervate 0.002% ophthalmic solution, although it may cause mild to moderate eye discomfort/pain during treatment.

Exposure keratopathy (EK) is the damage to the cornea that occurs primarily from prolonged exposure of the ocular surface to the outside environment. Typically, EK is localized in the inferior peripheral cornea.[24] EK can lead to ulceration, perforation, secondary microbial invasion, and permanent vision loss from scarring. EK is associated with lagophthalmos (Fig 33), proptosis (particularly thyroid eye disease; Fig 24-29), neurologic diseases (Fig 30, 31), and lid malposition (Fig 32). The treatment is similar to neurotrophic keratitis therapy, but the underlying disease must be addressed as well.

Recurrent corneal erosion syndrome occurs due to weakly adherent corneal epithelium, which can lead to the development of spontaneous epithelial defects. Episodes have a sudden onset of pain, typically upon waking up in the morning or during the night, accompanied with tearing, redness and photophobia. Patients usually have a prior history of corneal trauma or corneal dystrophy (Fig 33) (Grixti et al, 2012). In the acute phase of this condition, traditional approach consists of frequent lubrication, patching with antibiotic ointments, cycloplegia, hypertonic saline solution (5% sodium chloride) during the day for at least 6 weeks to facilitate epithelial attachment[2] Low-dose oral doxycycline and short-term use of topical corticosteroids are effective[27]. Bandage contact lens may be helpful. Surgical management of recurrent corneal erosion includes epithelial debridement and anterior stromal puncture (Wong et al, 2009);. An alternative to these procedures is excimer laser ablation either with phototherapeutic keratectomy (PTK) or photorefractive keratectomy (PRK).

Figure 24. Exposure keratopathy associated with thyroid disease. Right and left eyes of the same patient. Ovoid-shaped inferior peripheral epithelial defect is seen in the right eye (left photo) and sterile hypopyon and stromal scar are seen in the left eye (right photo)

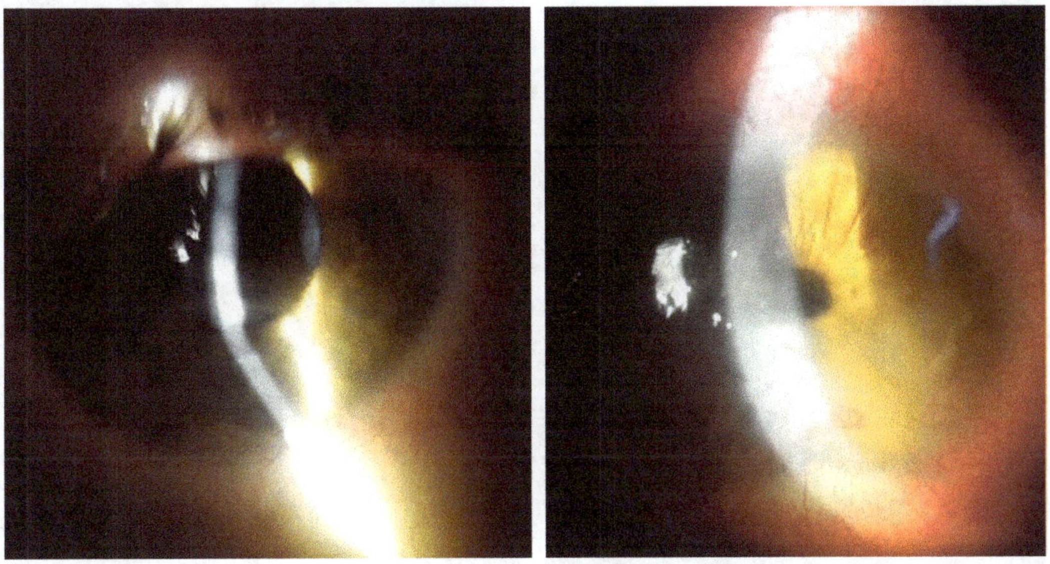

Figure 25. The same patient

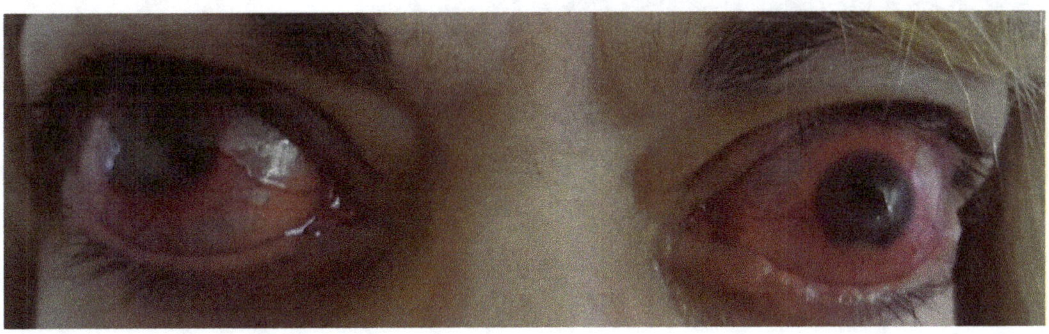

Figure 26. EK associated with thyroid eye disease. Inferiorly located ulcer is seen with underlying infiltrate and edema in the right eye, and the proptosis is seen in the left eye

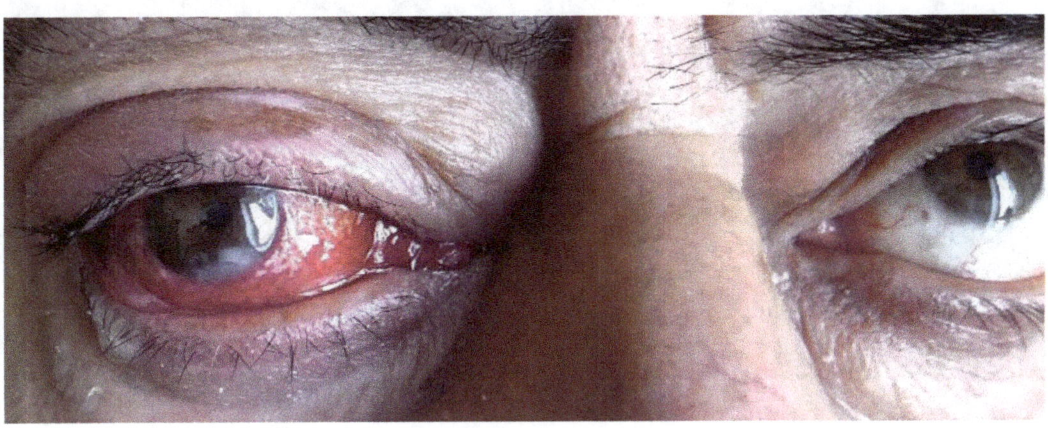

Figure 27. The same patient's right eye under a slit lamp

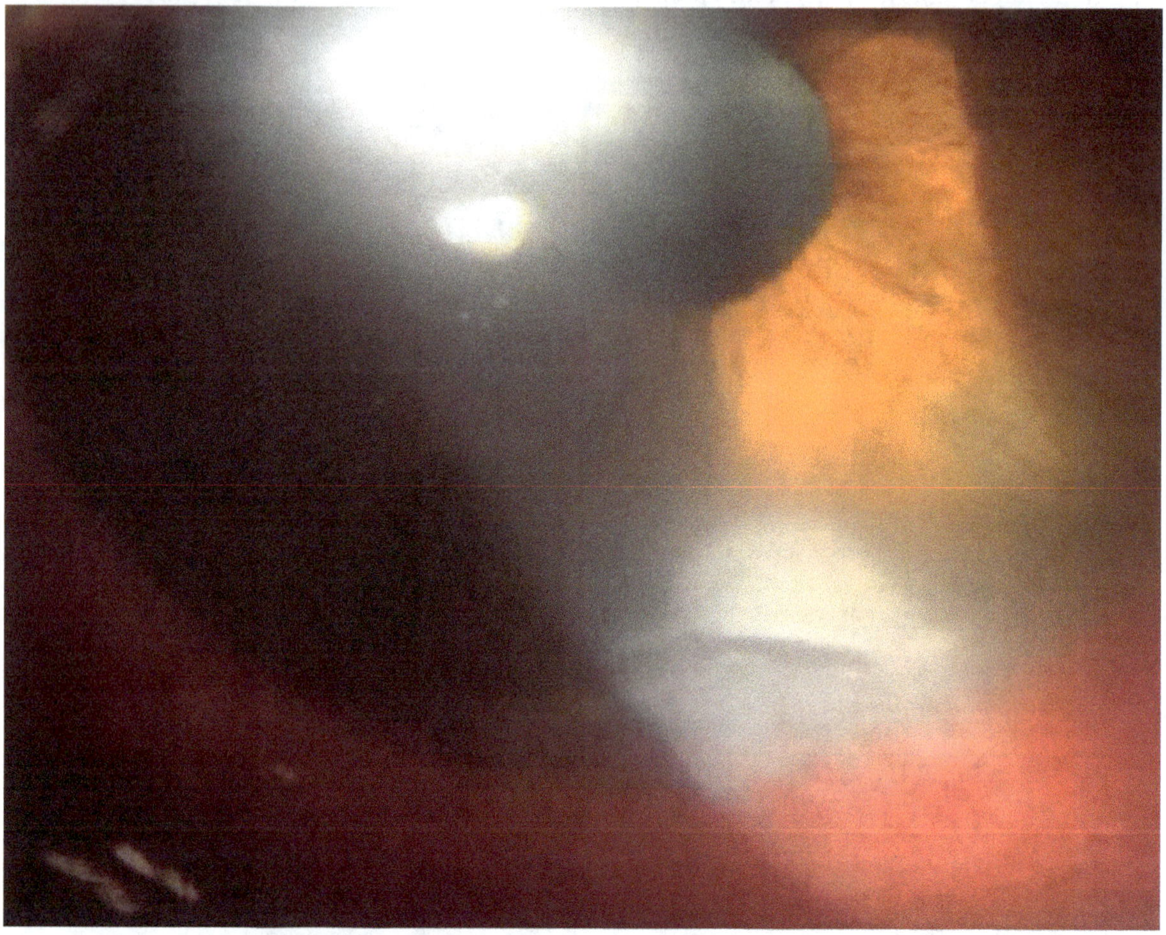

Figure 28. The same patient after 2 years with uncontrolled thyroid disease. The EK is seen in the fellow eye, the tarsorrhaphy is visible

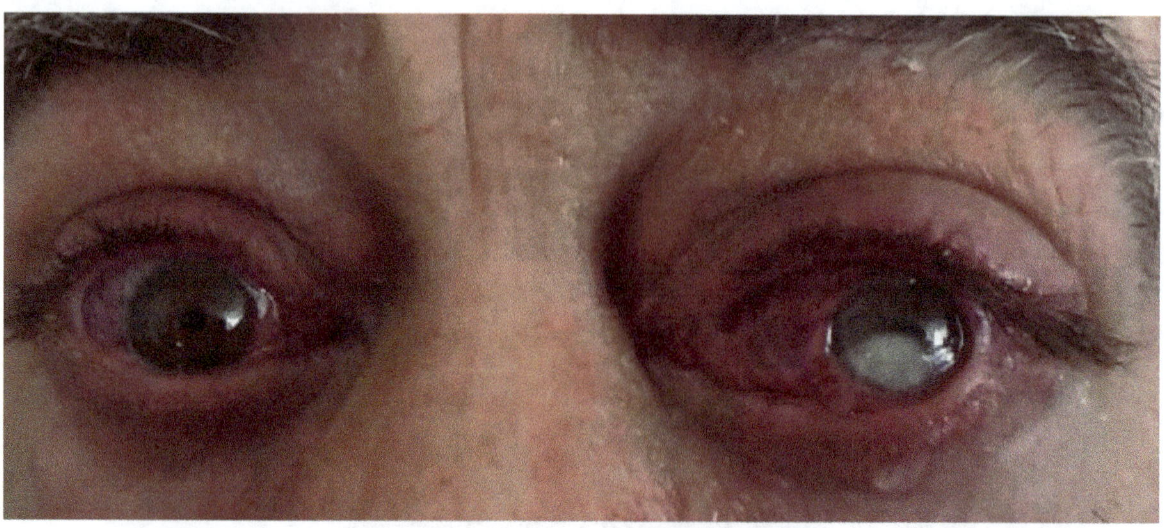

Figure 29. The same eye under slit lamp. The epithelial defect with underlying stromal infiltrate is seen

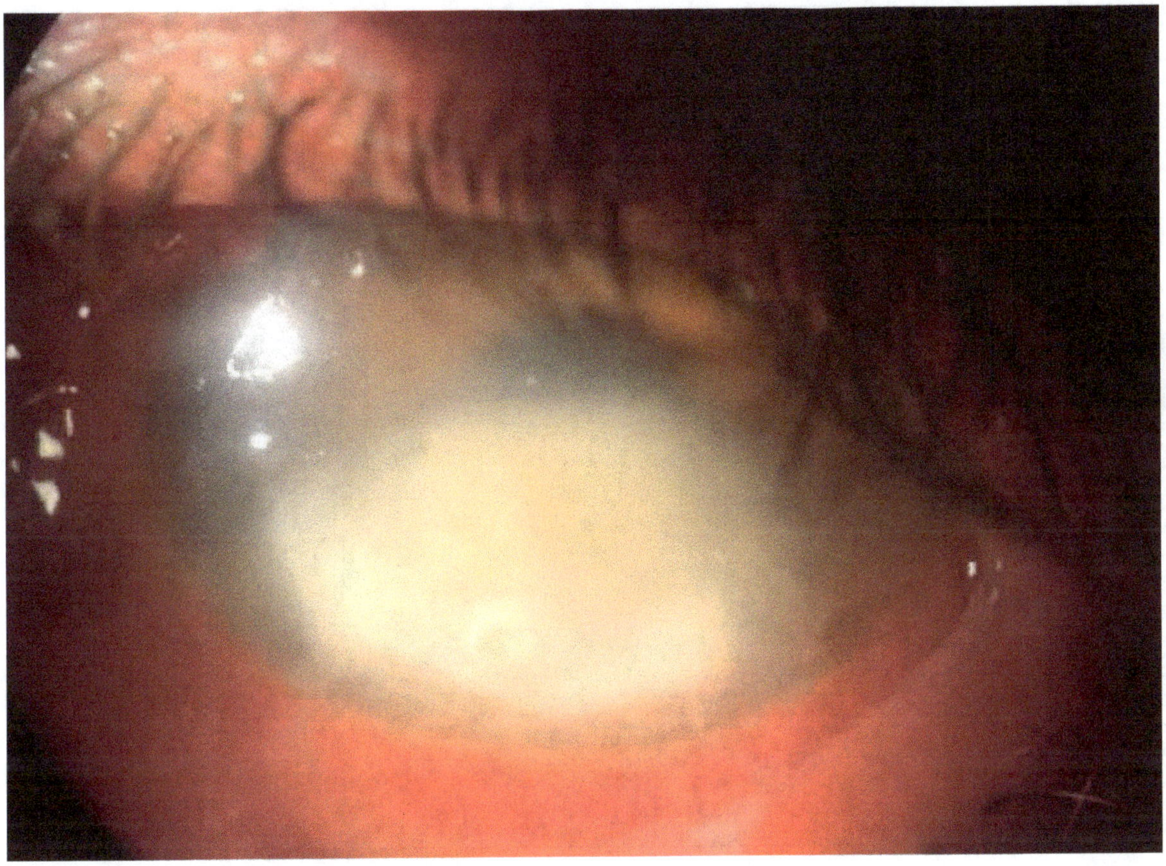

Figure 30. Exposure keratopathy associated with myasthenia gravis

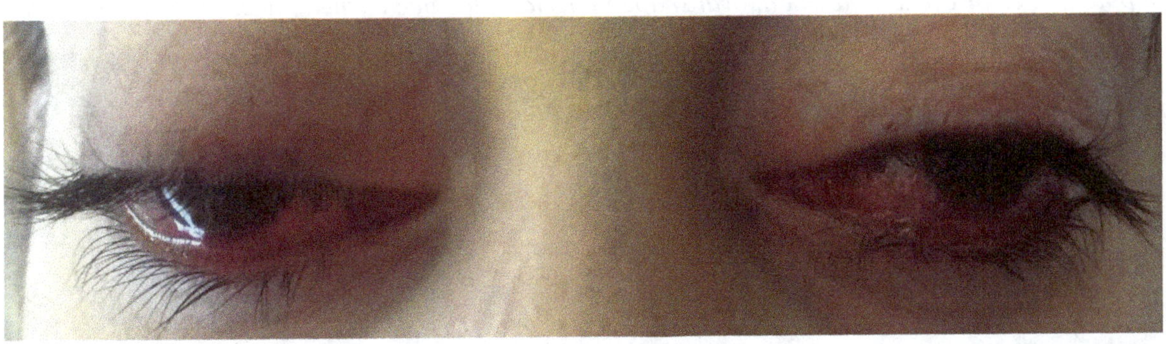

Figure 31. The same eye under slit lamp. Inferiorly located epithelial ulcer is seen with edematous margins

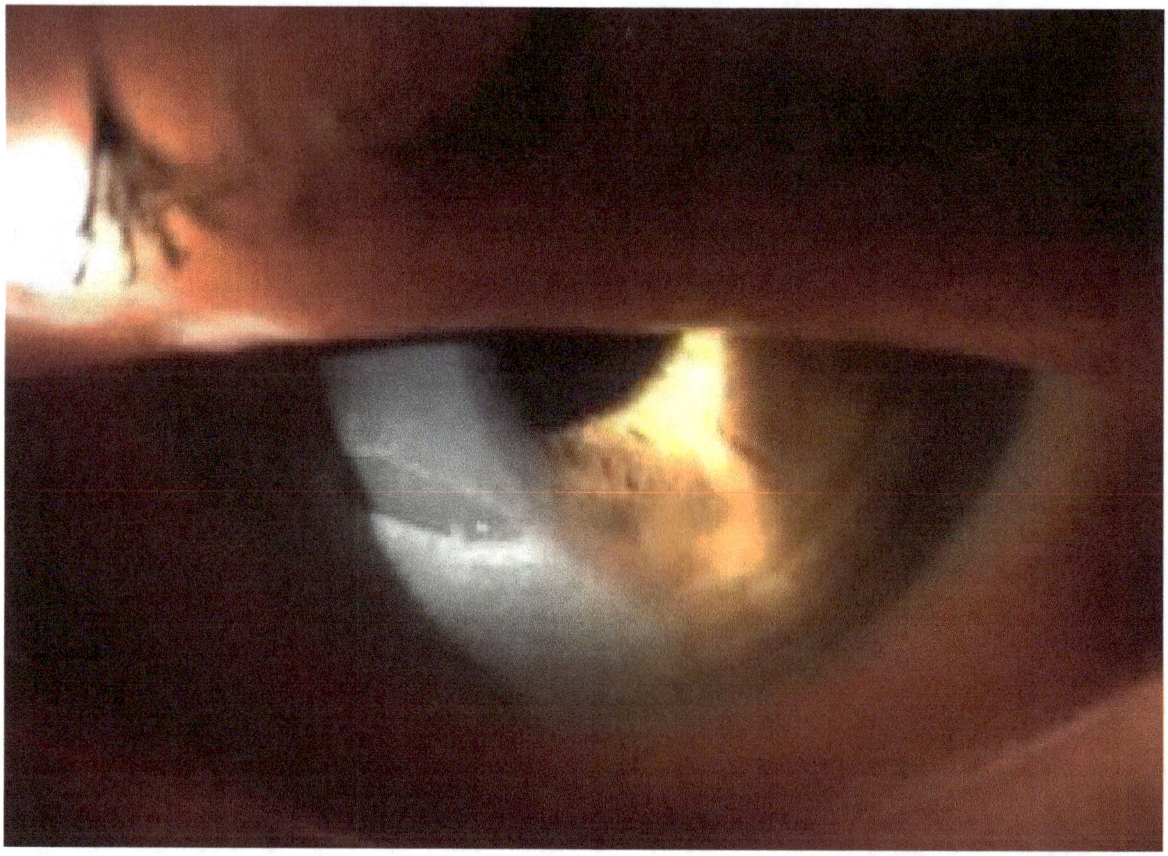

Figure 32. EK associated with entropion. The everted inward eyelid is seen (left photo), and the same eye with pulled inferior eyelid. The small, oval shaped inferiorly located corneal ulcer is seen (right photo)

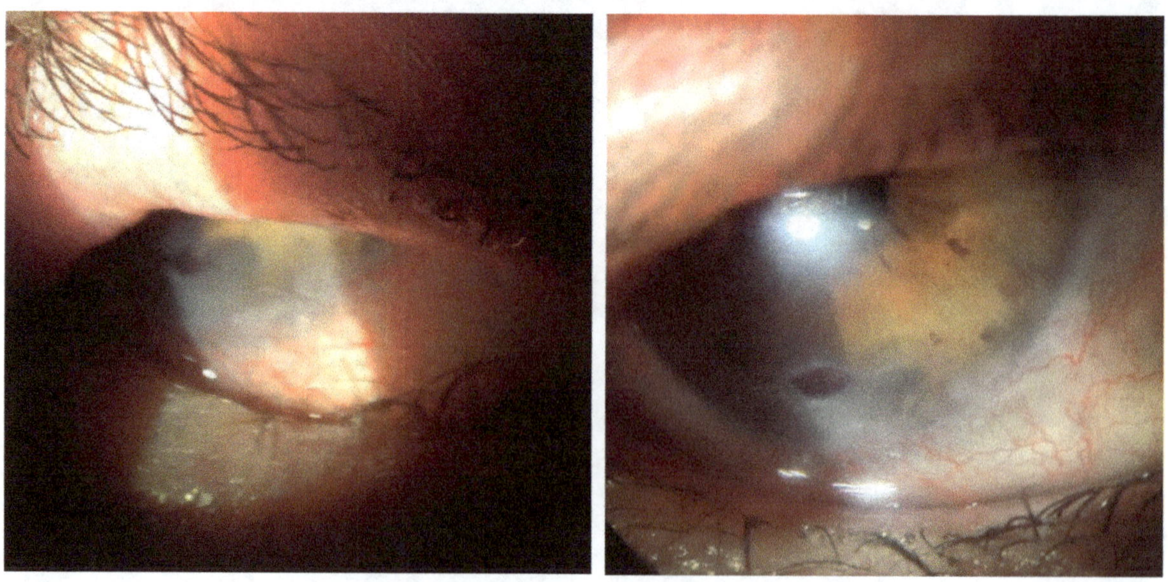

Figure 33. A) EK associated with lagophthalmos. Inferiorly located epithelial defect surrounded with edema is seen, b, c) Recurrent erosion syndrome

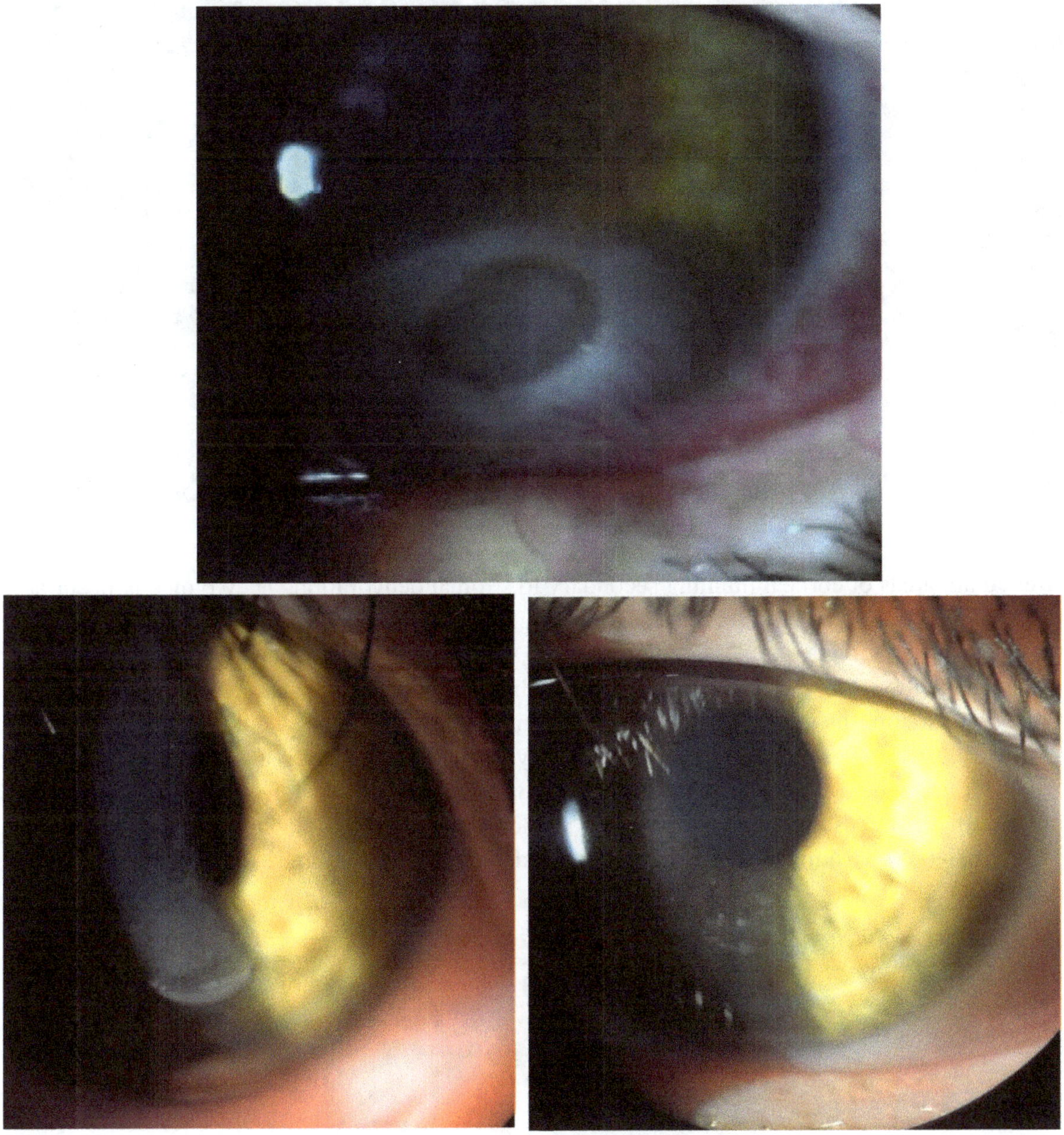

Figure 34. Dellen associated with inflamed pinguecula. The oval shaped thinning is noted adjacent to the limbus (left photo), and the thinning is shown by light beam narrowing (right photo)

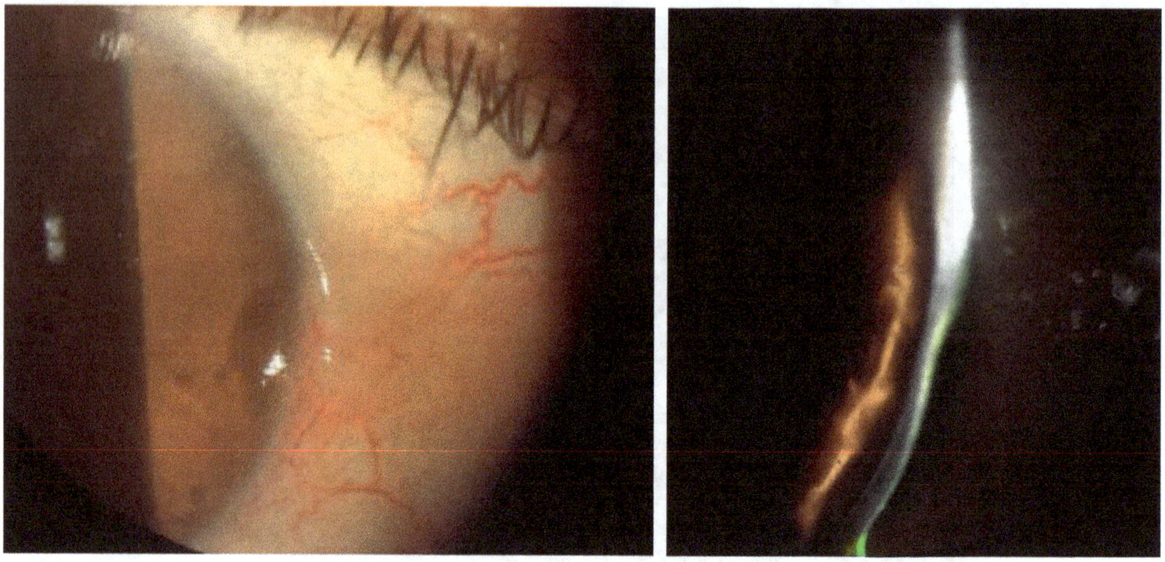

Dellen are areas of corneal thinning secondary to stromal dehydration. They typically occur at the corneal limbus near areas of adjacent elevation (Fig 34) (Mai et al, 1991). Dellen can be associated with pingueculae, pterygia, dermoids, filtering blebs, or any other elevated bulbar structure. Treatment includes rehydration, lubrication of the dellen, and elimination of the adjacent elevation.

Toxic epitheliopathy, due to the misuse or treatment of some topical medication, is a toxic effect that directly causes superficial punctate keratopathy, or indirectly causes inflammation (Burstein et al, 1980). It interferes with the migration of the limbal epithelial cells. Many agents are causing toxic epitheliopathy. The most known is benzalkonium chloride (BAK), which is highly toxic to the corneal epithelium (Fig 35). Treatment includes non-preserved lubricating drops, and elimination of toxic agents.

Figure 35. Toxic epitheliopathy is seen due to chronic use of topical Ganciclovir by patient

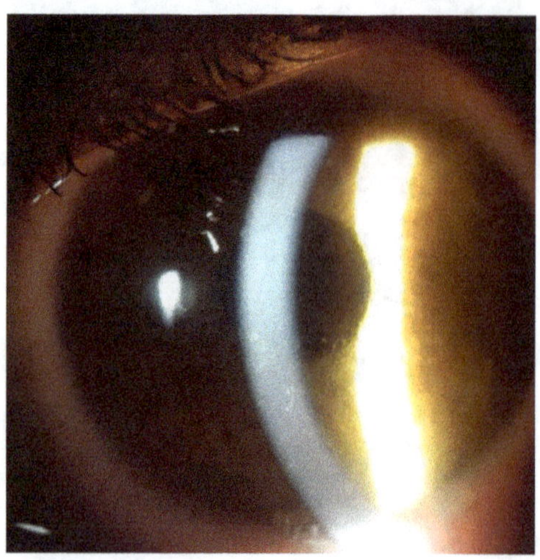

Bullous keratopathy is a pathological condition in which small vesicles, or bullae, are formed in the cornea when the endothelial function is impaired ('Ocular Pathology", 2018). Intraocular surgeries can lead to the loss of some corneal endothelial cells. In cases of extensive endothelial cell loss, the cornea may decompensate postoperatively. Clinically, it presents by Descemet folds and stromal edema, which farther lead to intracellular epithelial edema. Bullous keratopathy is more commonly seen after cataract surgery, followed by multiple glaucoma procedures or retinal detachment repair with silicone oil (Fig 36, 37). Fuchs endothelial dystrophy can be another cause of symptomatic bullous keratopathy. The treatment is surgical; endothelial replacement is required (DSAEK, DMEK, etc...)

Figure 36. Bullous keratopathy associated with pseudophakia. Bullae are seen paracentrally

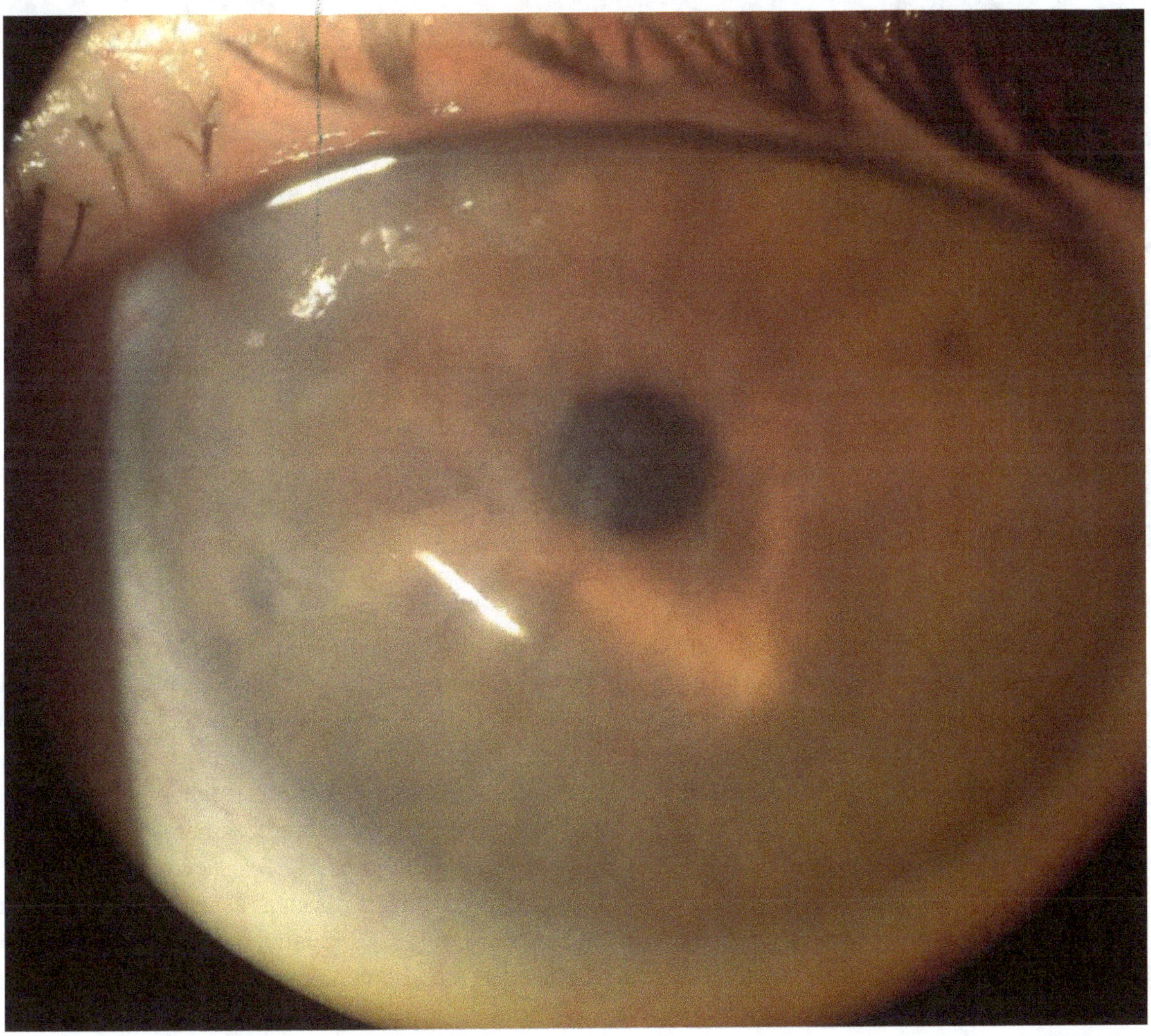

Figure 37. The same eye, the total edema is seen with Descemet folds

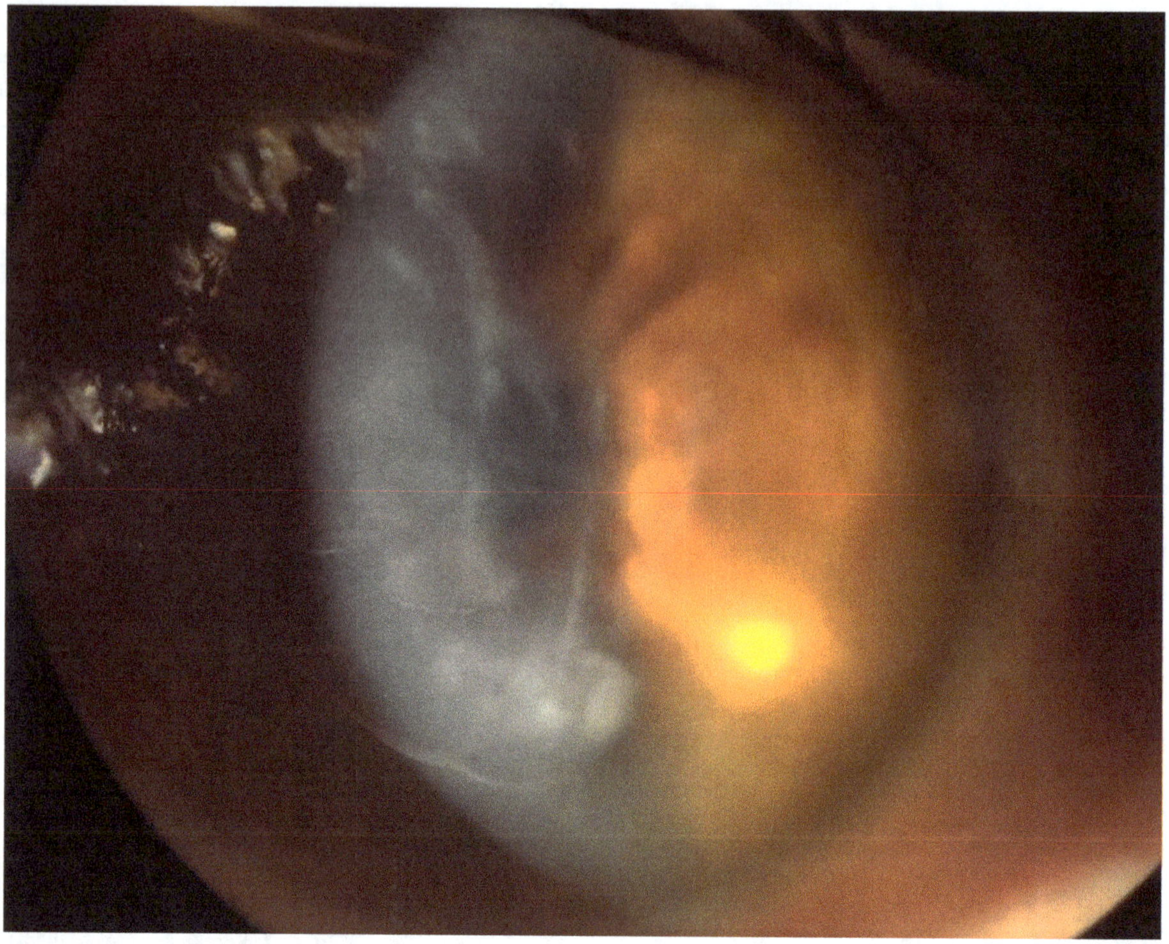

Descemetocele is a lesion where the epithelium and stroma are destructed, with only the Descemet membrane and endothelium remaining (Arentsen et al, 1985). Descemet membrane often bulges anteriorly and forms a dome-shaped, transparent membrane due to its high elasticity and intraocular pressure. At this stage, the cornea is in danger of perforation (Fig 38, 39). Corneal transplant surgery may be required.

Rosacea keratitis is seen in approximately 5-30% of patients with rosacea cutaneous (Starr et al, 1969). It occurs most commonly in middle-aged and older individuals, more common in women than men (James et al, 2011). The Demodicosis may play a role in pathogenesis of rosacea. The Demodex load is increased in individuals with rosacea. Patients with advanced rosacea, especially males, may develop rhinophyma (hypertrophy and hyperemia of the distal nose). Clinically, it represents by lesions that usually involve the inferior cornea but can advance toward the center (Vieira et al, 2013). Lids, conjunctiva, and rarely episclera may be involved. Ulceration, infrequently perforation can also occur (Fig 40-45). Symptoms of rosacea keratitis include burning, photophobia, and foreign body sensation. Topical steroids are effective for rosacea keratitis, but treatment should also include lids hygiene, topical antibiotics (e.g., Tetracycline), omega-3 fatty acid for relief of blepharitis, and systemic Doxycyline.

Figure 38. Descemetocele associated with necrotizing herpetic keratitis

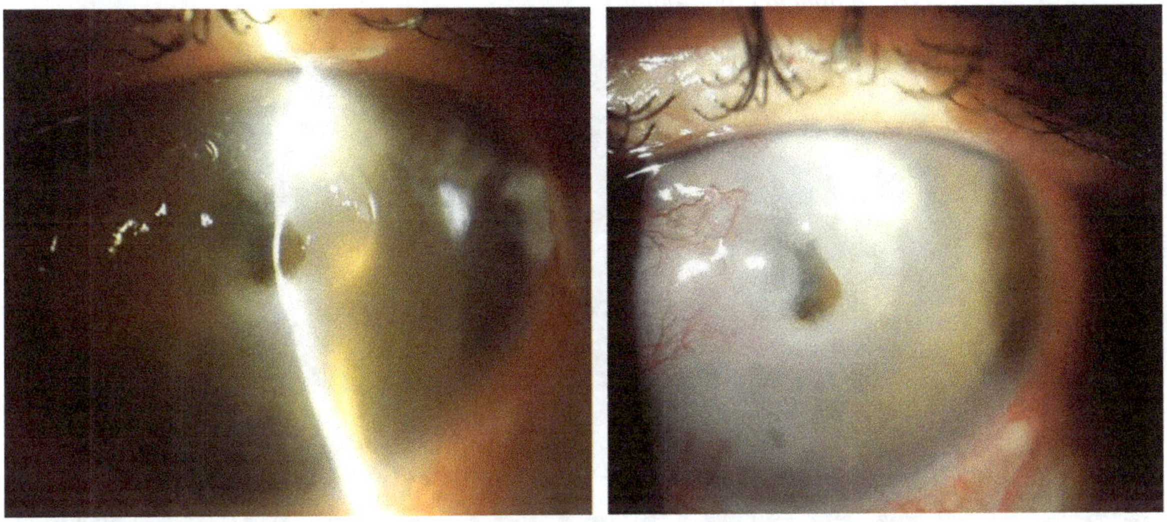

Figure 39. Postherpetic Descemetocele

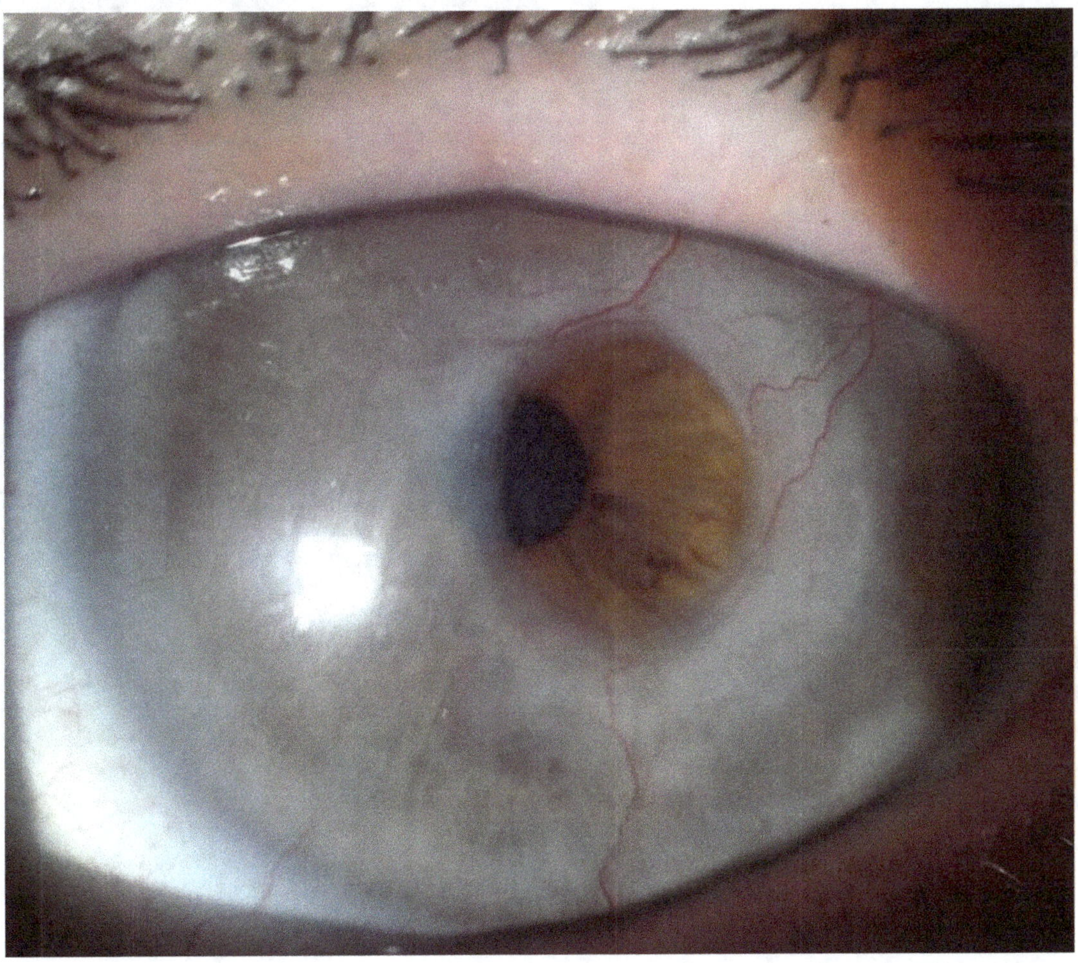

Figure 40. Rosacea keratitis. Superficial punctate lesions are seen with neovascularization (left photo). The same eye 3 weeks post treatment (right photo)

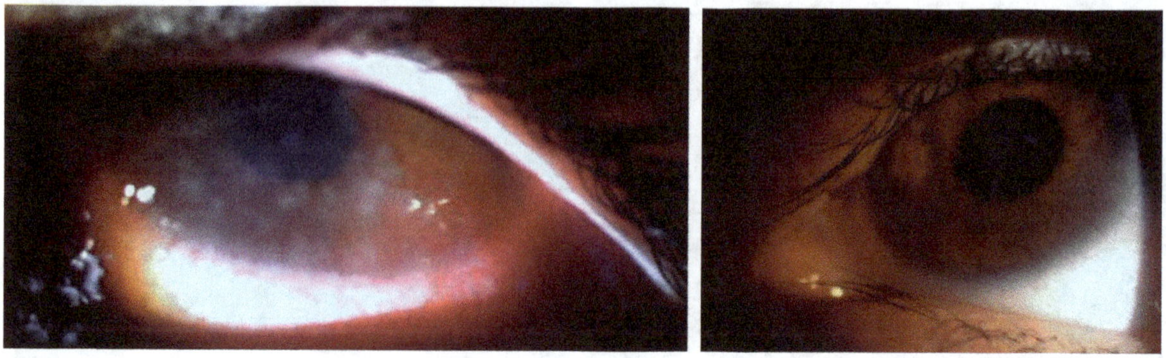

Figure 41. Rosacea keratitis, punctate lesions with atypical localization

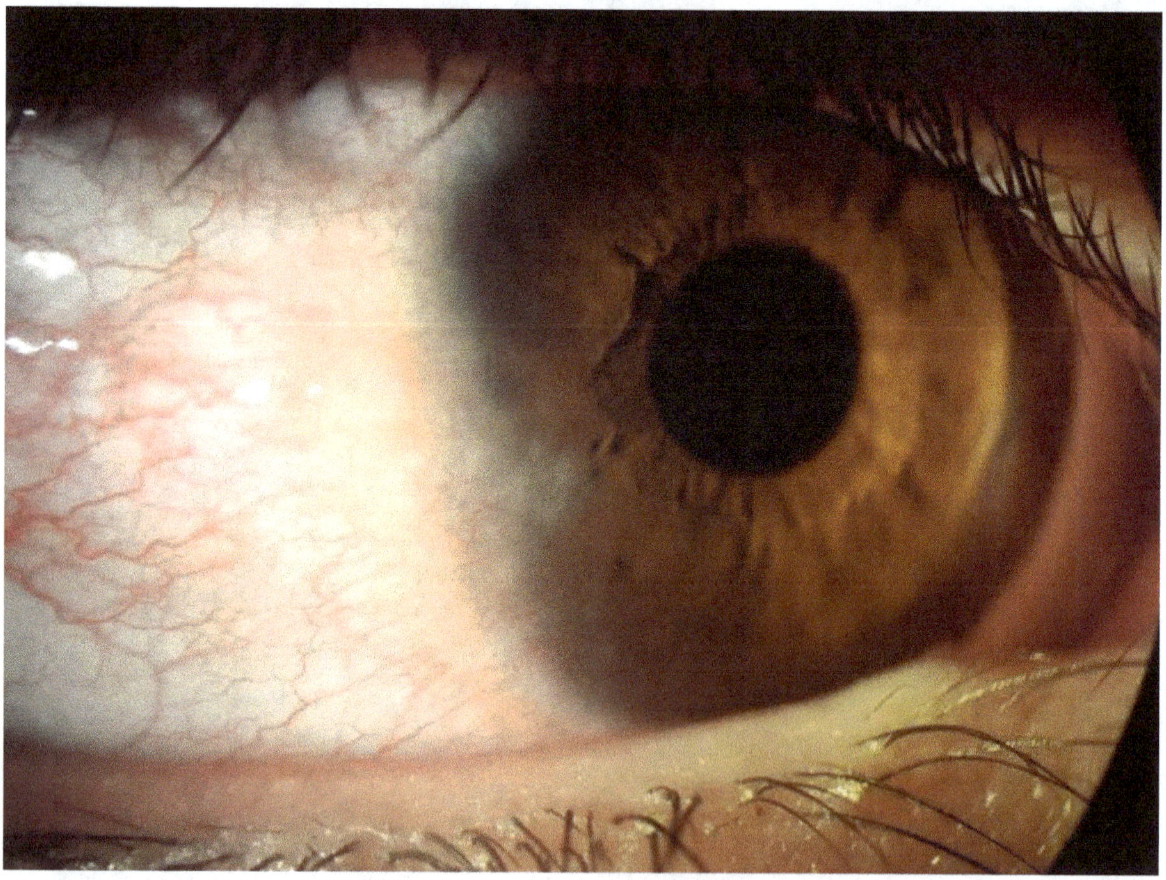

Figure 42. Patient with Rosacea keratitis, meibomitis, and rhinophyma

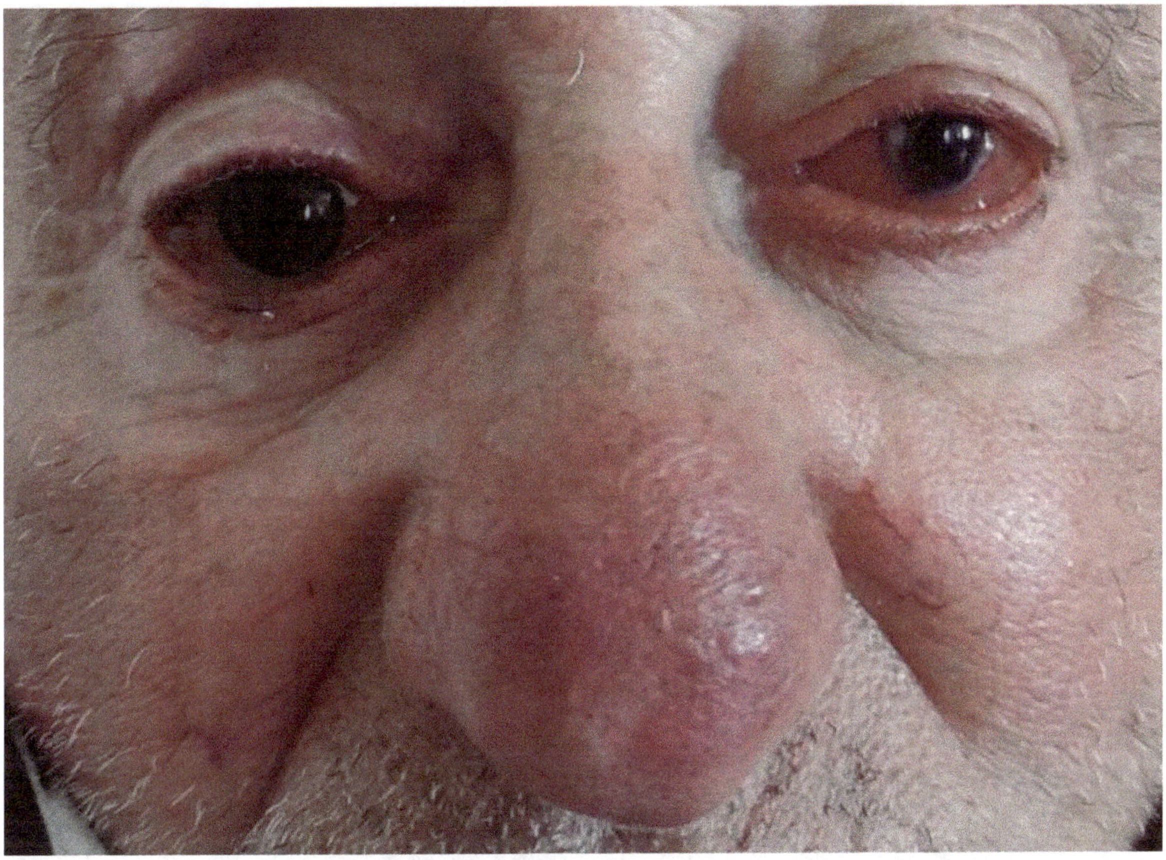

Figure 43. Advanced rosacea. 360 degrees of neovascularization with inferior stromal opacification are seen

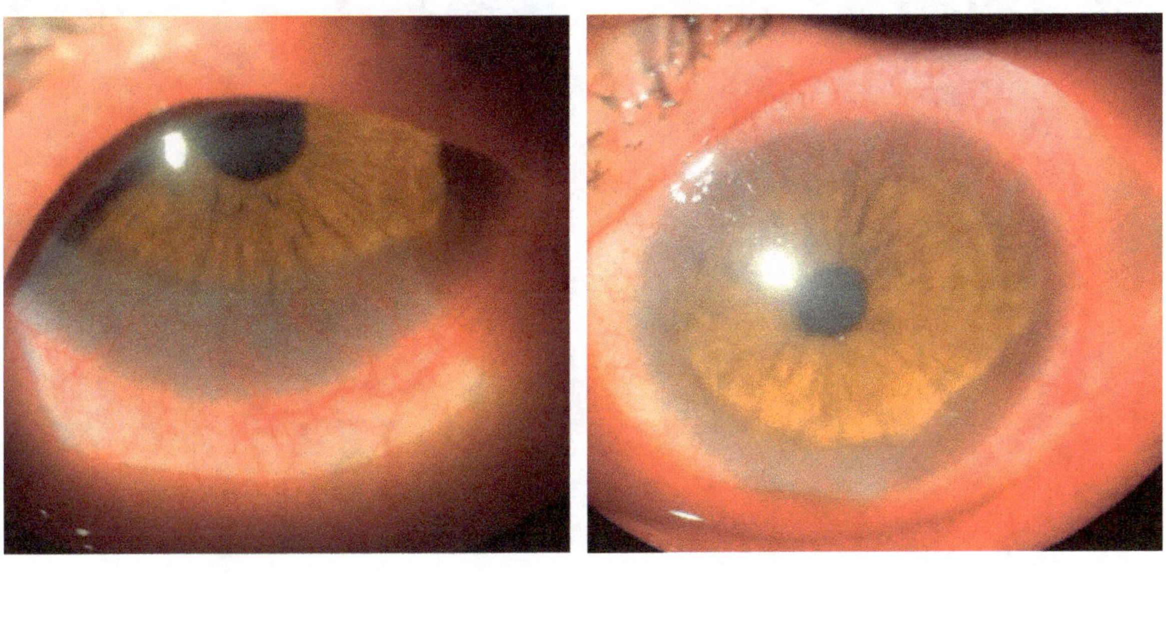

Figure 44. The same patient. The associated demodex blepharitis is seen

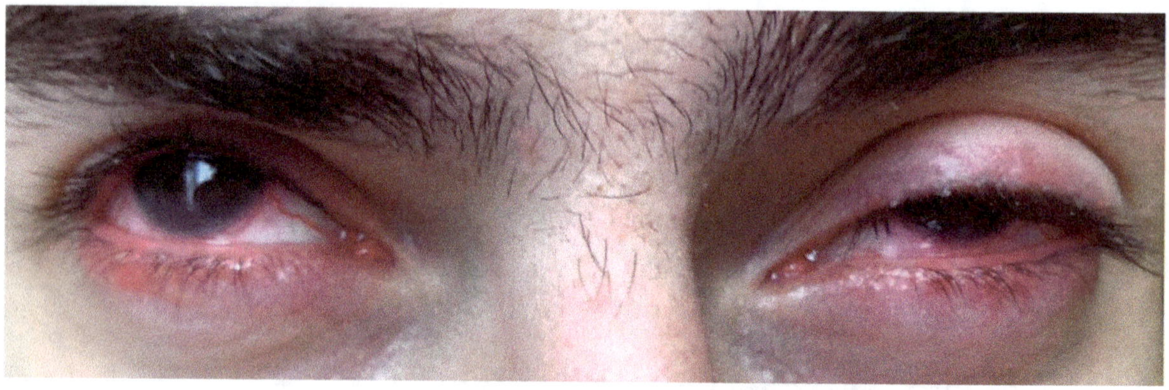

Figure 45. Recurrence of rosacea keratitis associated with iridocyclitis, posterior synechia are seen

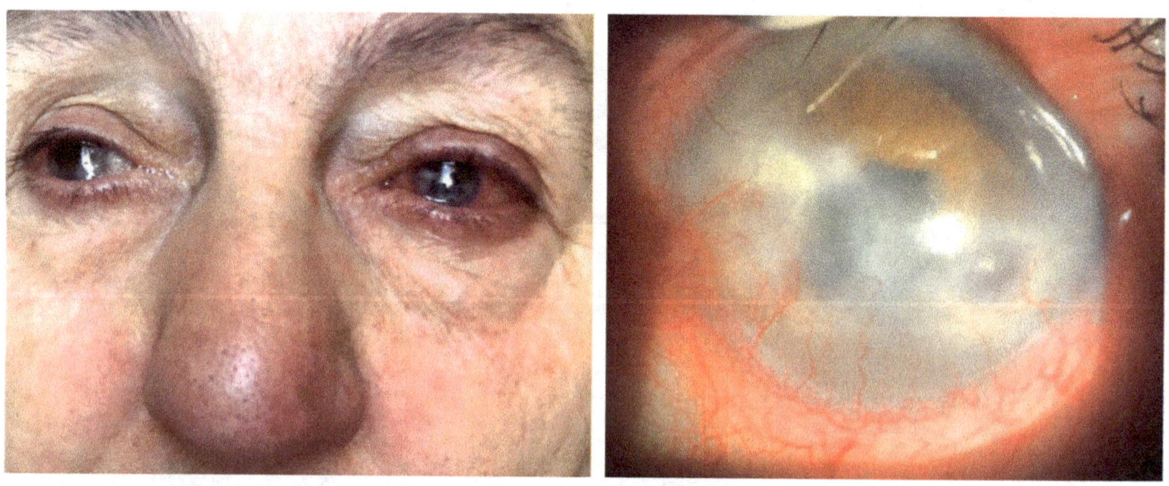

REFERENCES

Arentsen, J., Laibson, P. R., & Cohen, E. J. (1985). Management of corneal descemetoceles and perforations. *Ophthalmic Surgery*, *16*, 29–33.

Beauchamp, Gillette, & Friendly. (n.d.). Phlyctenular keratoconjunctivitis. *J Pediatr Ophthalmol Strabismus*.

Bhat, P., & Birnbaum, A. D. (2015). Diagnosis and management of noninfectious corneal ulceration and melting. In Focal Points: Clinical Modules for Ophthalmologists. American Academy of Ophthalmology.

Burstein, N. L. (1980). Corneal cytotoxicity of topically applied drugs, vehicles and preservatives. *Survey of Ophthalmology*, *25*(1), 15–30.

Cogan, D. G. (1945). Syndrome of nonsyphilitic interstitial keratitis and vestibuloauditory symptoms. *Archives of Ophthalmology*, *33*, 144–149.

Culbertson, W. W., Huang, A. J., Mandelbaum, S. H., Pflugfelder, S. C., Boozalis, G. T., & Miller, D. (1993). Effective treatment of phlyctenular keratoconjunctivitis with oral tetracycline. *Ophthalmology*, *100*(9), 1358–1366. doi:10.1016/S0161-6420(93)31475-2 PMID:8371924

Diez-Feijoo, E., Grau, A. E., & Abusleme, E. I. (2014). Clinical presentation and causes of recurrent corneal erosion syndrome: Review of 100 patients. *Cornea*, *33*(6), 571–575.

Donzis, P. B., & Mondino, B. J. (1987). Management of noninfectious corneal ulcers. *Survey of Ophthalmology*, *32*, 94.

Els Marquezan, M. C., Nascimento, H., & Vieira, L. A. (2015). Effect of topical tacrolimus in the treatment of Thygeson's superficial punctate keratitis. *American Journal of Ophthalmology*, *160*(4), 663–668. doi:10.1016/j.ajo.2015.06.019 PMID:26133248

Epstein, D. L., & Paton, D. (1968). Keratitis from misuse of corneal anesthetics. *The New England Journal of Medicine*, *279*(8), 396–399.

Ewald, M., & Hammersmith, K. M. (2009). Review of diagnosis and management of recurrent erosion syndrome. *Current Opinion in Ophthalmology*, *20*(4), 287–291.

Garg, P., Reddy, J. C., & Sangwan, V. S. (2017). Mooren ulcer. In M. J. Mannis & E. J. Holland (Eds.), *Cornea* (4th ed., Vol. 1, pp. 1082–1087). Elsevier.

Grixti, A., Sadri, M., Edgar, J., & Datta, A. V. (2012). Common ocular surface disorders in patients in intensive care units. *The Ocular Surface*, *10*, 26–42.

Hamilton, W., & Wood, T. O. (1982). Filamentary keratitis. *American Journal of Ophthalmology*, *93*(4), 466–469. doi:10.1016/0002-9394(82)90135-0 PMID:7072810

Hick, S., Demers, P. E., & Brunette, I. (2005). Amniotic membrane transplantation and fibrin glue in the management of corneal ulcers and perforations: A review of 33 cases. *Cornea*, *24*(4), 369–377.

James, W. D., Elston, D. M., & Berger, T. G. (2011). *Andrews' diseases of the skin: clinical dermatology* (11th ed.). Saunders London.

Jeng, B. H., & Dupps, W. J. Jr. (2009). Autologous serum 50% eyedrops in the treatment of persistent corneal epithelial defects. *Cornea*, *28*(10), 1104.

Khokhar, S., Natung, T., & Sony, P. (2005). Amniotic membrane transplantation in refractory neurotrophic corneal ulcers: A randomized, controlled clinical trial. *Cornea*, *24*(6), 654–660.

Mackie, I. A. (1978). Role of the corneal nerves in destructive disease of the cornea. *Transactions of the Ophthalmological Societies of the United Kingdom*, *93*, 373.

Mackie, I. A. (1973). Neuroparalytic (neurotrophic) keratitis. In *Symposium on contact lenses: Transactions of the New Orleans Academy of Ophthalmology*. Mosby.

Mai, G., & Yang, S. (1991). Relationship between corneal dellen and tearfilm breakup time. *Yan Ke Xue Bao*, *7*(1), 43–46.

McCulley, J. P., Dougherty, J. M., & Deneau, D. G. (1982). Classification of chronic blepharitis. *Ophthalmology*, *89*(10), 1173–1180. doi:10.1016/S0161-6420(82)34669-2 PMID:6218459

Miserocchi, E., Modorati, G., & Rama, P. (2008). Effective treatment with topical cyclosporine of a child with steroid-dependent interstitial keratitis. *European Journal of Ophthalmology*, *18*, 816–818.

Mondino, B. J., & Kowalski, R. P. (1982). Phlyctenulae and catarrhal infiltrates. Occurrence in rabbits immunized with staphylococcal cell walls. *Archives of Ophthalmology*, *100*(12), 1968–1971. doi:10.1001/archopht.1982.01030040948017 PMID:7150063

Nagra, P. K., Rapuano, C. J., Cohen, E. J., & Laibson, P. R. (2004). Thygeson's superficial punctate keratitis. Ten years' experience. *Ophthalmology*, *111*(1), 34–37. doi:10.1016/j.ophtha.2003.05.002 PMID:14711711

Ocular Pathology: Bullous Keratopathy of the Cornea. (2018). Missionforvisionusa.org

Rosenwasser, G. O., Holland, S., & Pflugfelder, S. C. (1990). Topical anesthetic abuse. *Ophthalmology*, *97*(8), 967–972.

Shiuey, Y., & Foster, C. S. (1998). Peripheral ulcerative keratitis and collagen vascular disease. *International Ophthalmology Clinics*, *38*(1), 21–32. doi:10.1097/00004397-199803810-00004 PMID:9532470

Sobolewska, B., Doycheva, D., & Deuter, C. (2014). Treatment of ocular rosacea with once-daily low-dose doxycycline. *Cornea*, *33*, 257–260.

Starr, P. A. J., & McDonald, A. (1969). Oculocutaneous aspects of rosacea. *Proceedings of the Royal Society of Medicine*, *62*, 9.

Tanioka, H., Yokoi, N., Komuro, A., Shimamoto, T., Kawasaki, S., Matsuda, A., & Kinoshita, S. (2009). Investigation of the corneal filament in filamentary keratitis. *Investigative Ophthalmology & Visual Science*, *50*(8), 3696–3702. doi:10.1167/iovs.08-2938 PMID:19443713

Vieira, A. C., & Mannis, M. J. (2013). Ocular rosacea: Common and commonly missed. *Journal of the American Academy of Dermatology*, *69*, 536.

Vieira, A. C., & Schwab, I. R. (n.d.). Superficial punctate keratitis of Thygeson. In M. J. Mannis & E. J. Holland (Eds.), Cornea (4th ed., Vol. 1). Academic Press.

Wang, L., Tsang, H., & Coroneo, M. (2008). Treatment of recurrent corneal erosion syndrome using the combination of oral doxycycline and topical corticosteroid. *Clinical & Experimental Ophthalmology, 36*(1), 8–12.

Wong, V. W., Chi, S. C., & Lam, D. S. (2009). Diamond burr polishing for recurrent corneal erosions: Results from a prospective randomized controlled trial. *Cornea, 28*(2), 152–156.

Wood, T., & Kaufman, H. (1971). Mooren's ulcer. *American Journal of Ophthalmology, 71*, 417–422.

Chapter 7
Corneal Degenerations and Ectasias

ABSTRACT

Degeneration of a tissue is defined as a deterioration that results in impaired structure and function. These changes occur at the cellular level and are caused by biomolecular alterations induced by aging, as well as a wide variety of adverse external and internal influences. Traditionally, degenerations have been classified as involutional (age-related) or non-involutional, depending on type of deposition (hyaline, amyloid, lipid, calcific), and by anatomic location (anterior, posterior, central or peripheral). Degenerations may be unilateral or bilateral, often with asymmetric involvement. Heredity does not play a direct role in these processes. The noninflammatory ectatic diseases of the cornea discussed in this chapter include keratoconus, pellucid marginal degeneration, keratoglobus, and posterior keratoconus. An exceptional degeneration unreported in literature (presumed alimentary cuprum keratopathy) is presented in this chapter. Pseudogerontoxon is one of the characteristic degenerations commonly seen in Middle Eastern populations.

CORNEAL DEGENERATIONS

Arcus senilis/Cornea senilis, after the fourth decade, and arcus juvenilis, before the fourth decade, represents a degenerative change resulting in lipid deposition in the peripheral cornea. Lipid deposition usually starts as a gray to yellow arc, firstly developing in the inferior, and then the superior cornea (Francois et al, 1973; Ritfkind et al, 1972). The deposition gradually progresses and forms a complete ring (Fig 1). Corneal arcus has no visual significance; thus, no treatment is required. Nevertheless, patients under the age of 40 with corneal arcus have an increased risk of coronary artery disease and should be evaluated for hyperlipoproteinemia.

The limbal girdle of Vogt is a symmetrical, yellowish-white band, which is located parallel to the interpalpebral limbus (Sugar et al, 1960). The depositions are located beneath the epithelial layer, adjacent to the Bowman's layer. Histologically, the deposits are calcific in nature, or they can represent a focal area of hyaline accumulation (Fig 2). This degeneration is an incidental finding and is asymptomatic. No treatment is required.

DOI: 10.4018/978-1-7998-6937-5.ch007

Figure 1. Arcus senilis. Dense, complete ring is seen

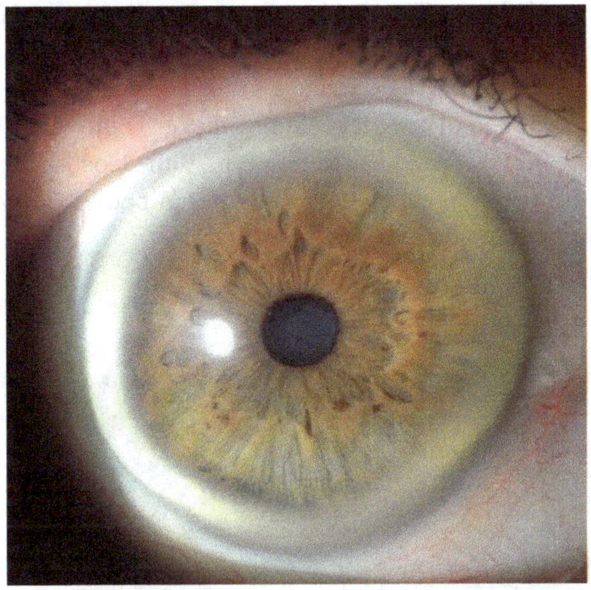

Figure 2. Vogt limbal girdle

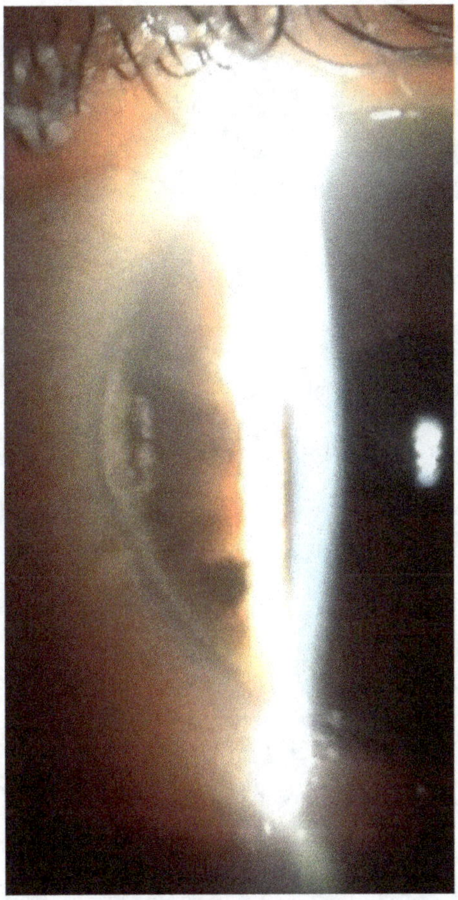

Iron lines can be found when there are alterations of the ocular surface that produce focal elevations and depressions (Loh et al, 2009). The most common iron line is the Hudson-Stahli line, usually located at the juncture of the lower and middle thirds of the cornea (Rose et al, 1968). Iron lines can be seen after glaucoma surgery (Ferry's line) (Ferry et al, 1968). located anterior to the filtering bleb. Iron lines have been observed at the edge of the pterygium (Stocker's line) and the base of the cone in the keratoconus (Fleischer's ring, Fig 3). The less common type is the Coat's ring, a circular or oval-shaped deposition associated with history of previous metallic foreign bodies (Fig 4). Iron lines represent an incidental finding and are asymptomatic.

Figure 3. Fleischer's ring is seen at the base of the cone

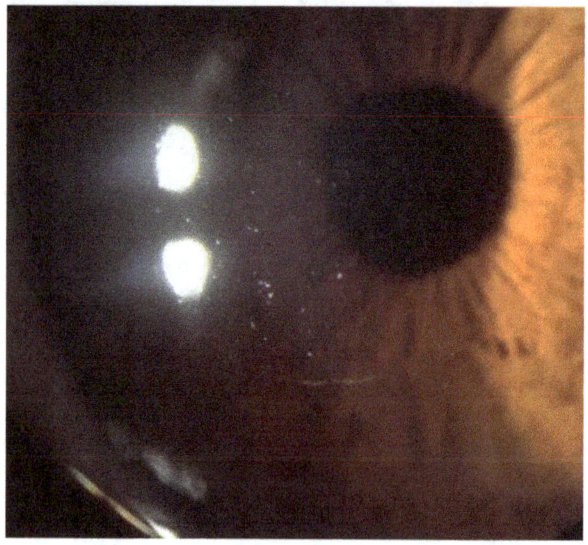

Figure 4. Coats ring after intracorneal foreign body removal

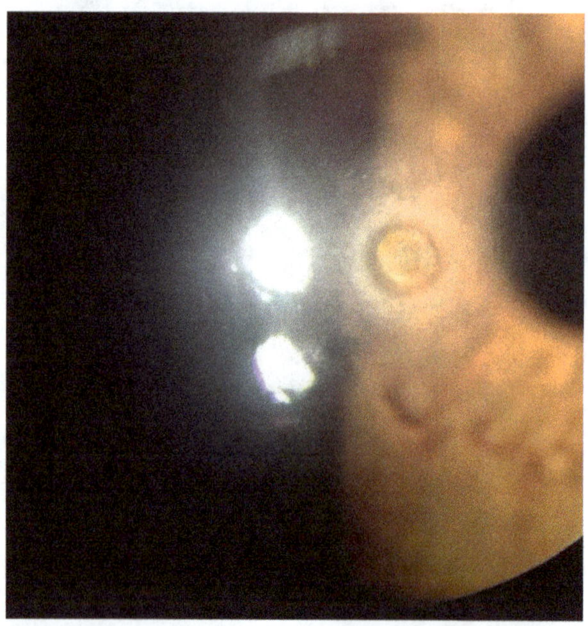

Band-keratopathy (Calcific degeneration) is usually associated with chronic inflammation, uveitis, absolute or chronic glaucoma, phthisis bulbi, etc (O'Connor et al, 1972). It can also be associated with systemic or hereditary diseases related with abnormalities in calcium metabolism (Sarcoidosis, Hyperparathyroidism, etc.) or topical/intraocular medications that can cause a local disturbance in calcium metabolism. It usually occurs in the interpalpebral zone, with a clear zone adjacent to the limbus. Clinically, small, dark, round holes are seen within the band and thought to represent corneal nerves passing through the Bowman's layer (Lemp et al, 1977). The band may progress and involve the visual axis (Fig 5, 6, 7, 8, 9). Early stages of band keratopathy are asymptomatic. These lesions progress slowly over months to years. Later stages can be symptomatic with signs and symptoms such as decreasing vision, foreign body sensation, tearing, or photophobia. If the patient becomes symptomatic, the favored initial treatment is the application of disodium ethylene diamine tetra-acetic acid (EDTA) (Bokosky et la, 1985). After the instillation of topical anesthetic, the overlying epithelium is debrided with a blade and 1.7% (0.05 molar) EDTA is applied to the calcific areas for 2–3 minutes, usually in a well (optical zone marker) or on saturated cellulose sponges. Phototherapeutic keratectomy is especially useful if Bowman's layer has been damaged or destroyed (Rapuano et al, 1997). Seldom, amniotic membrane might be required after primary surgical removal of band keratopathy in patients more prone to delayed epithelial healing (Anderson et al, 2001).

Figure 5. Band keratopathy. Small, dark, round holes are seen within the lesion. Patient with a history of chronic glaucoma

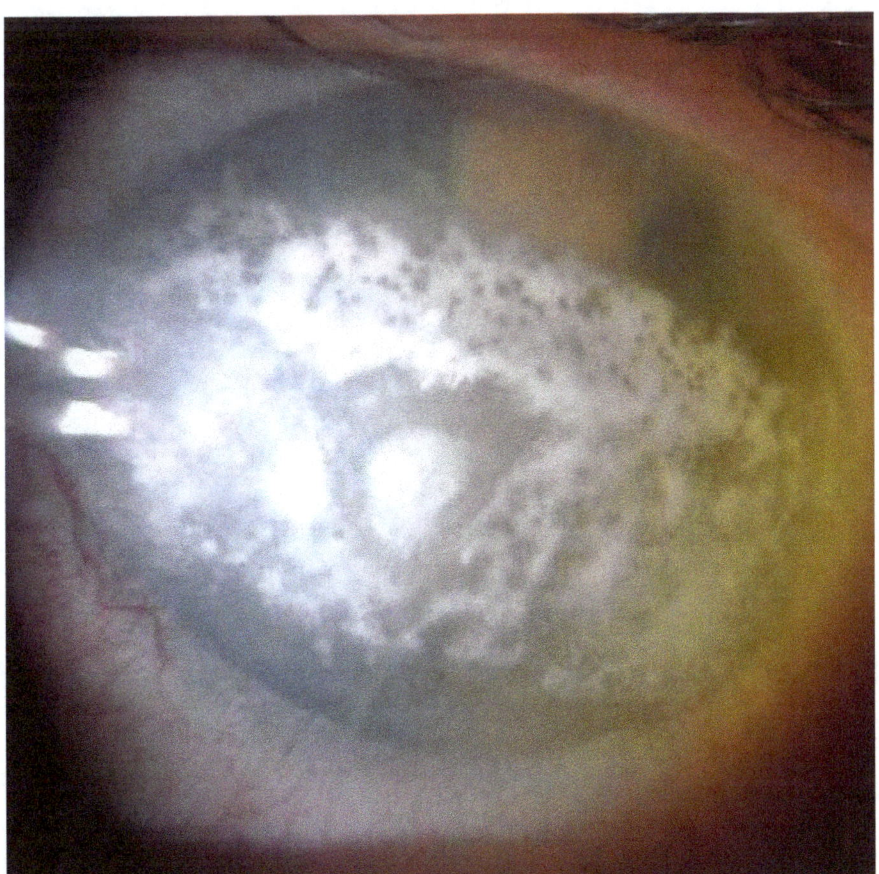

Figure 6. Band keratopathy associated with chronic uveitis. The transparent zone between the lesion and the limbus is seen. The second lesion in the darker field is also noted

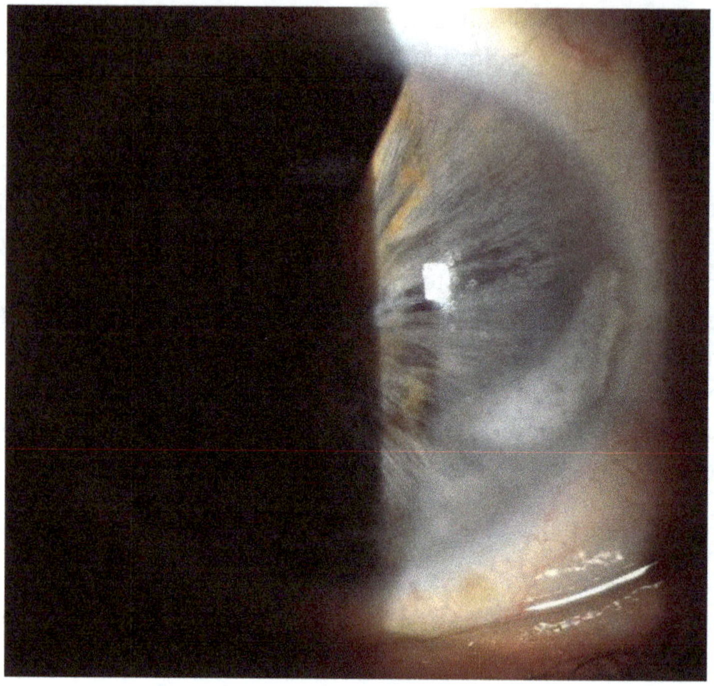

Figure 7. Band keratopathy associated with chronic glaucoma in OR before scraping/superficial keratectomy

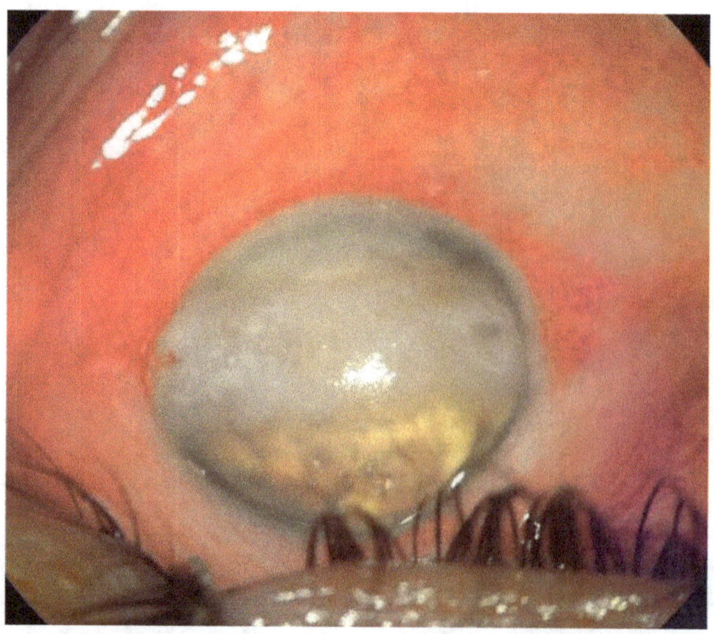

Figure 8. The same eye after scraping, covered with amniotic membrane

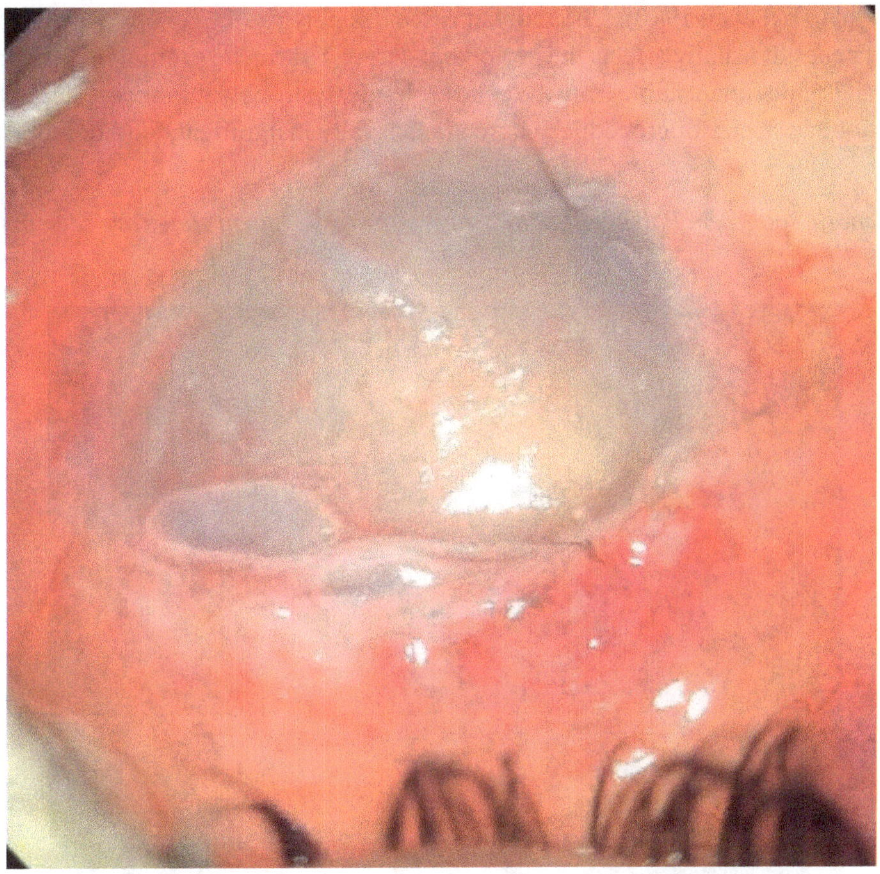

Figure 9. The same eye 40 days later

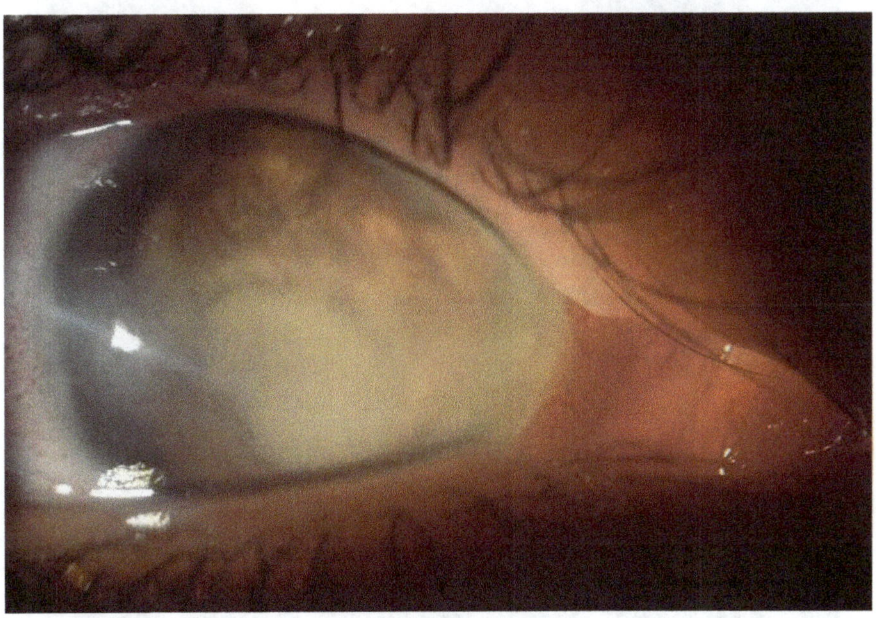

Crocodile shagreen is usually a bilateral, symmetric corneal opacity with a mosaic appearance looking like crocodile skin (Vogt et al, 1930). Clinically, it is seen as polygonal gray opacifications separated by thin transparent zones. It usually affects the peripheral cornea but can be prominent in the central cornea also. Clinically, it is indistinguishable from the central cloudy dystrophy of Francois (Fig 10). The opacity seen with anterior and posterior crocodile shagreen is visually insignificant and requires no treatment.

Figure 10. Crocodile shagreen. Polygonal opacities separated by lucent zones are seen in the peripheral cornea

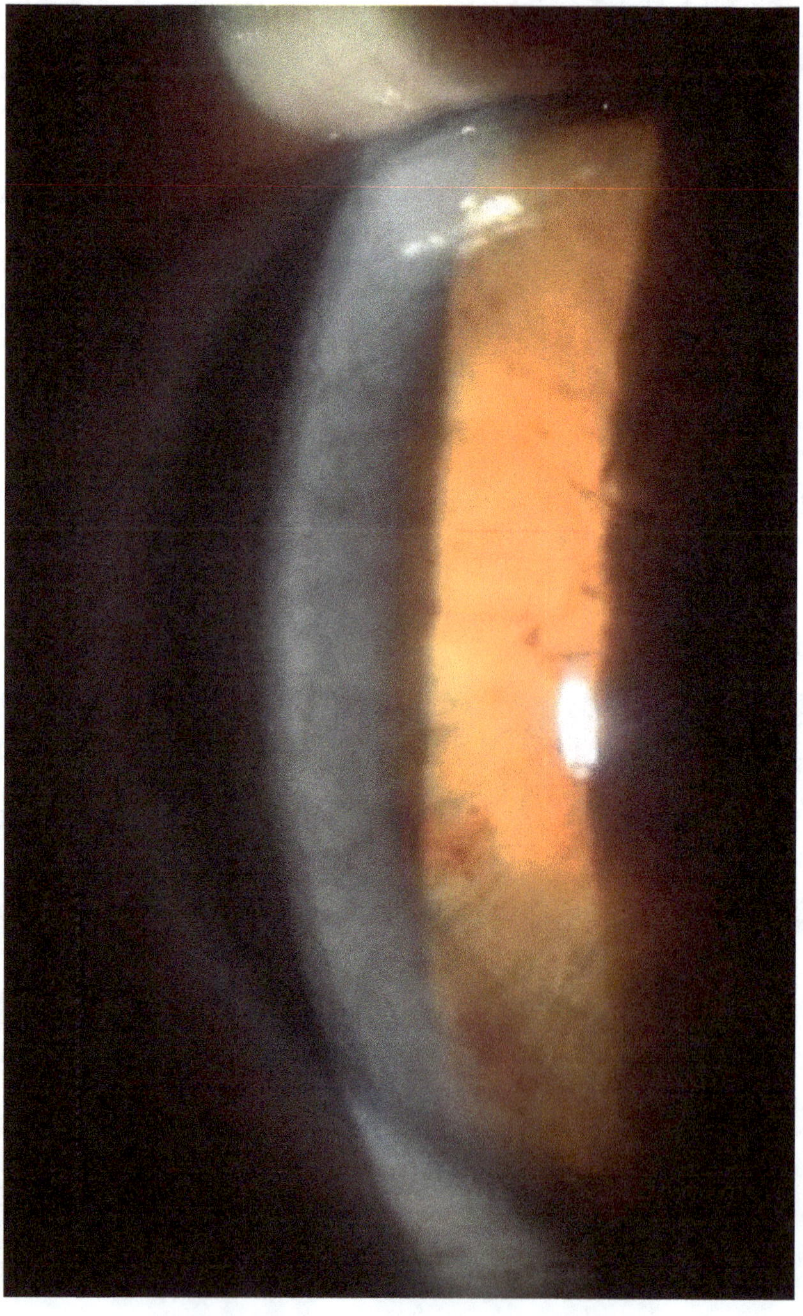

Senile furrow is a rare degeneration seen in elderly patients. Peripheral thinning is observed in the avascular zone between arcus senilis and the limbal vascular arcades. These lesions do not vascularize or perforate (Fig 11). The thinning is usually shallow and of no visual significance, thus, no treatment is required.

Figure 11. Senile furrow. Arcus senilis (left photo) associated with perilimbal thinning (right photo)

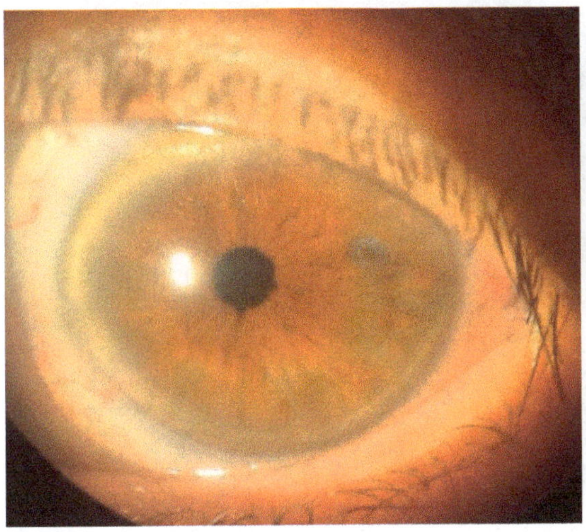

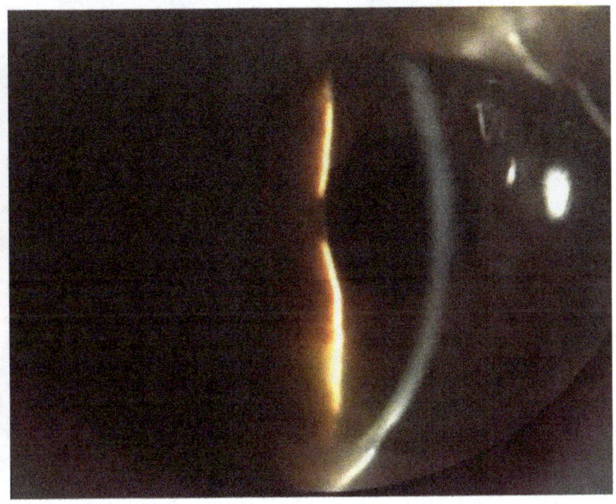

Lipid degeneration of the cornea can be primary and secondary. Primary lipid degeneration occurs without corneal inflammation and vascularization with no prior history of trauma or infection. Secondary lipid degeneration is related to **lipid keratopathy**, which is associated with corneal neovascularization,

Figure 12. Lipid keratopathy with neovascularization is seen

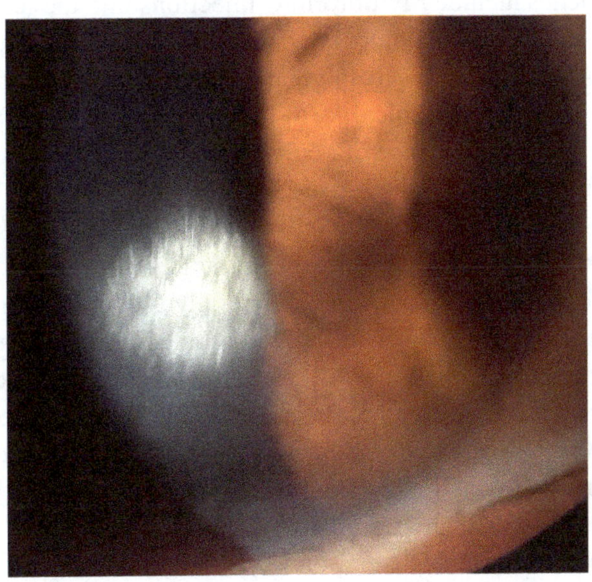

Figure 13. Lipid keratopathy. Dense yellow-white lesion is seen in front of the pupil (left photo), and the same eye after PK (right photo). Photos are taken in the OR

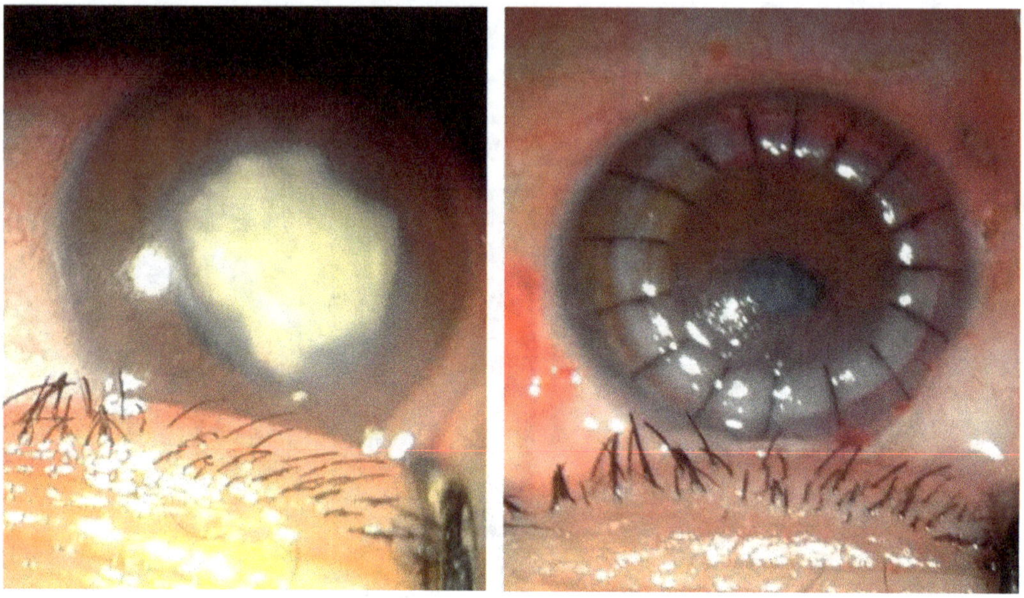

and most commonly occurs following herpetic infections, corneal ulceration, trauma, and interstitial keratitis (Cogane t al, 1958). Onset is usually gradual but may be sudden resulting in a rapid decrease in vision. The corneal opacity usually has a gray to yellow-white appearance; crystals may be seen at the edges of the lesions (Fig 12, 13). Treatment of feeder vessels with argon laser photocoagulation can decrease the density and extent of the lipid deposition (Marsh et al, 1982). Administration of topical, subconjunctival, and intrastromal VEGF inhibitors, alone or in combination, has been shown to induce regression of corneal neovascularization and decrease lipid deposition in some patients (Stevenson et al, 2012). The central vision-threatening lesions require lamellar or penetrating keratoplasty. Current promising treatment approaches include Mytomycin C injections into the feeding vessels.

Spheroidal degeneration (Labrador keratopathy, climatic droplet keratopathy, etc) is often seen in places where environmental conditions result in greater exposure to UV radiation, higher winds, and low humidity. There are three different clinical forms; (Ayres et al, 2006). Type 1 is the primary form and occurs in older patients with no evidence of ocular pathology. The depositions have a yellow-gold, small, droplet-like appearance, usually located in the intrapalpebral limbus. Type 2 is a secondary form and is associated with some type of ocular pathology (Fig 15-17). The deposits are usually seen in the lower two-thirds of the cornea. Type 3 represents the conjunctival form of the degeneration (Fig 14). Primary and conjunctival forms are often presented bilaterally. Accumulation of abnormal proteins associated with spheroidal degeneration may be associated with chronic inflammation caused by chronic exposure to harsh environmental conditions and ultraviolet irradiation. Spheroidal degeneration may be progressive if a patient remains exposed to the causative factors. Patients are asymptomatic unless the disease advances to the point of decreased vision. Treatment is instituted for the symptomatic stage. Conjunctival lesions are directly excised. Lamellar or penetrating keratoplasty is performed to treat the corneal form and restore vision. Excimer laser phototherapeutic keratectomy may also be beneficial for treating mild forms of climatic droplet degeneration (Ayres et al, 2006).

Figure 14. Spheroidal degeneration. Type 3 Conjunctival form

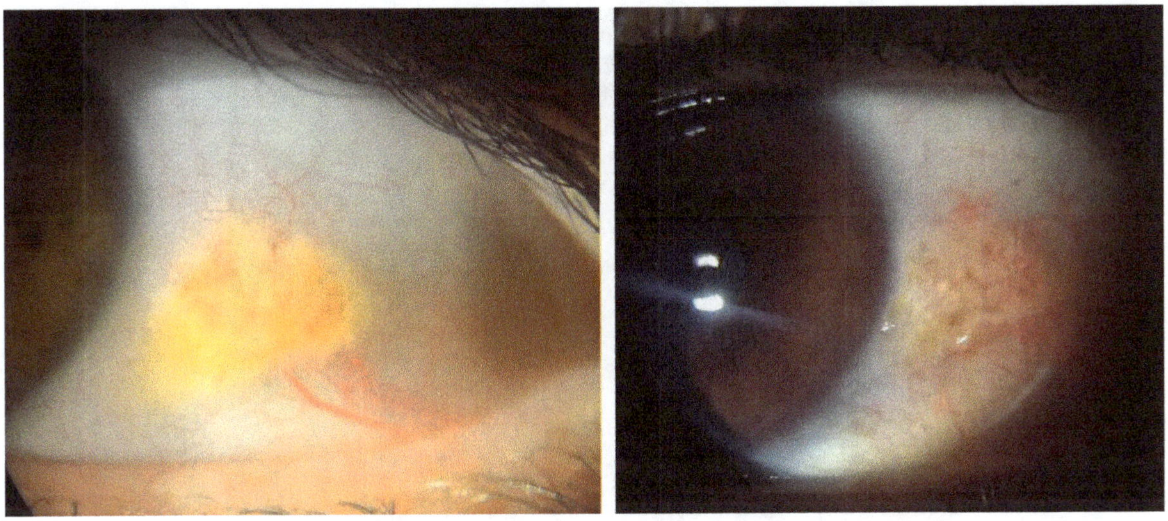

Figure 15. Secondary spheroidal degeneration associated with h/o trauma

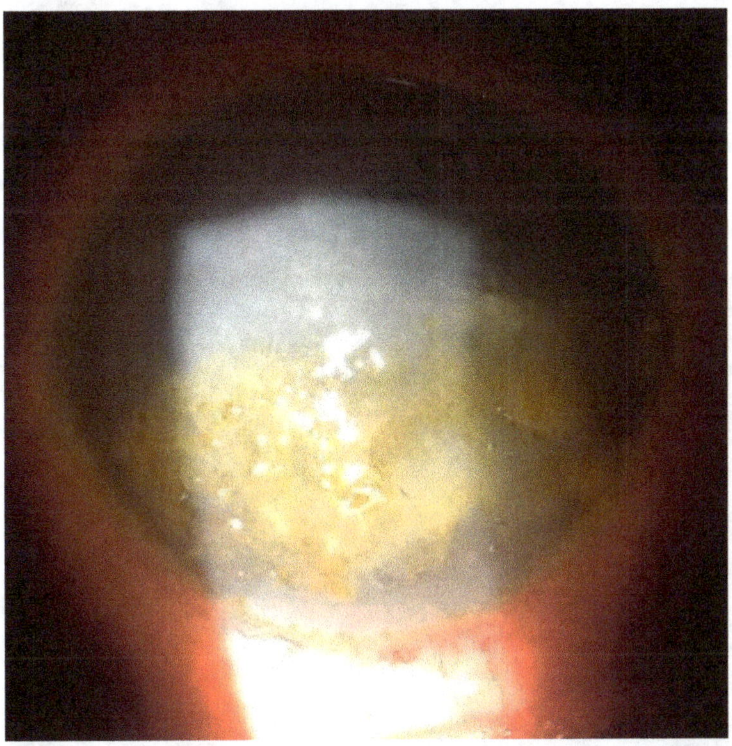

Figure 16. The same eye after superficial keratectomy covered with an amniotic membrane

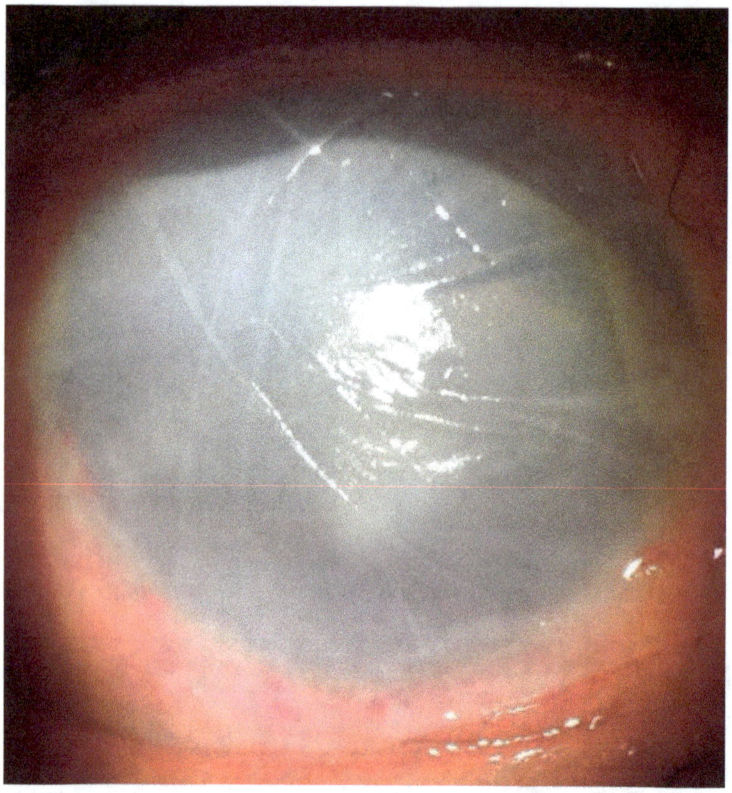

Figure 17. The same eye after 2 months of treatment

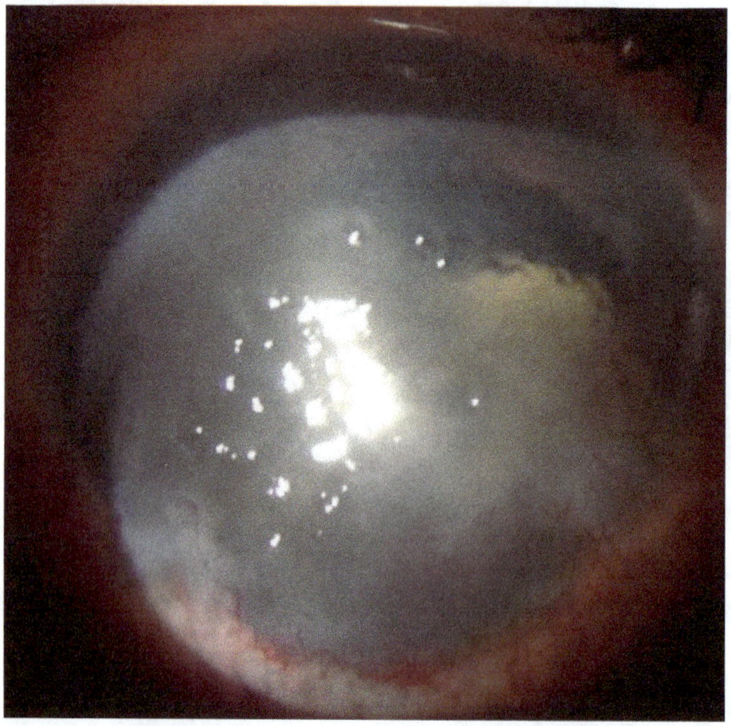

Salzman's nodular degeneration has primary and secondary forms. The primary form is the most common form without evidence of other ocular diseases and affects females most commonly (Wood et al, 1990). Progression of the lesions is slow. Vascularization may be seen adjacent to, but not as a main portion of the lesion. Most cases of secondary Salzman's degeneration are associated with phlyctenular disease. Moreover, Secondary Salzman's degeneration has also been noted after vernal keratoconjunctivitis, interstitial keratitis, trachoma, measles, and scarlet fever. Clinically, this degeneration represents as gray-white elevated nodular lesions usually located in the mid-peripheral cornea (Fig 18, 19). Salzmann's degeneration is usually asymptomatic. Epithelial erosions may occasionally overlie the lesion causing symptoms like lacrimation, photophobia, or irritation. Nodules that approach or involve the visual axis may cause irregular astigmatism, leading to decreased vision. Lubrication can be prescribed for mildly symptomatic lesions. Superficial keratectomy by manual dissection or with phototherapeutic keratectomy, may be performed for lesions close to or within the visual axis (Das et la, 2005). For lesions extending deeper into the stroma, lamellar keratoplasty may be necessary. Recurrence is possible after keratoplasty (Beauchamp et al, 1982).

Figure 18. Salzman's degeneration. Three elevated white nodules are seen

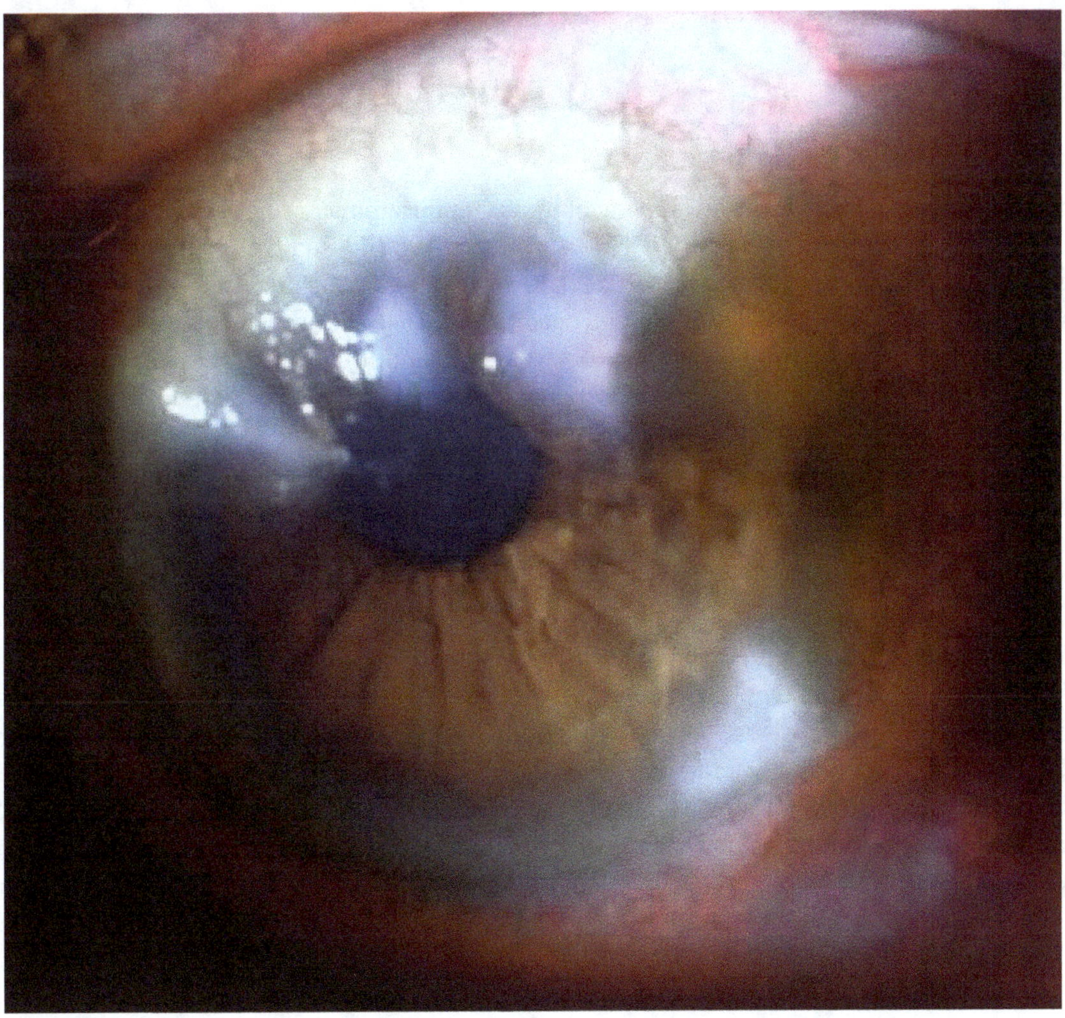

Figure 19. Salzman's nodular degeneration associated with phlyctenular disease (left photo). The elevated appearance of lesion is more relevant in the right photo

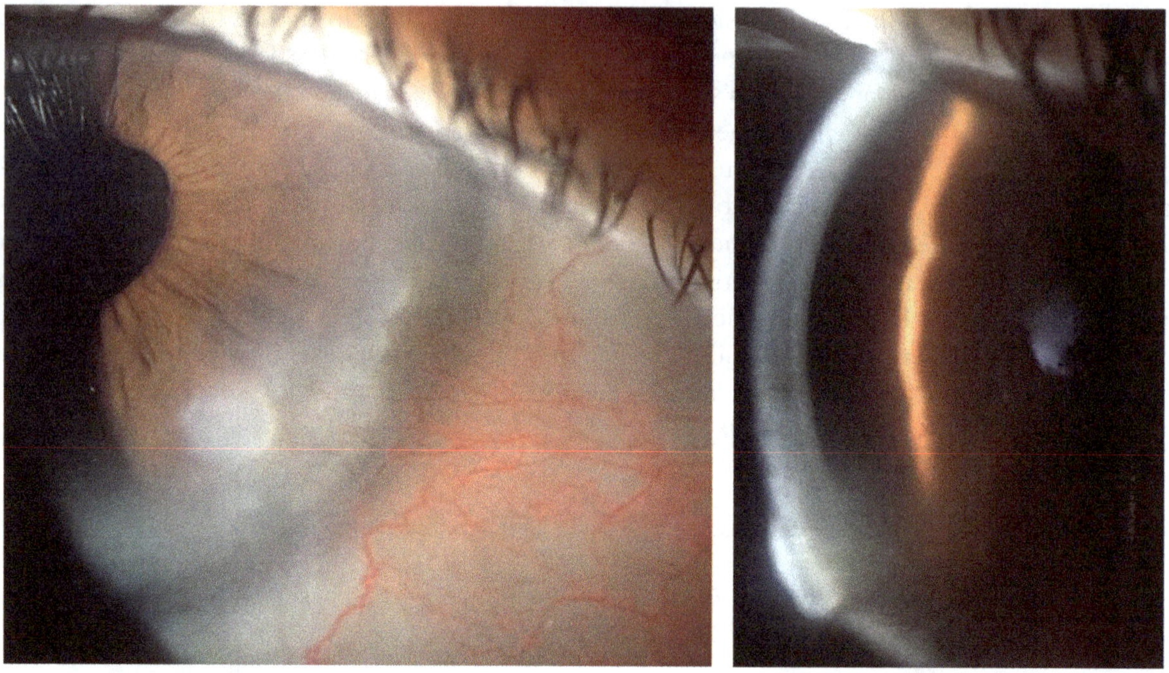

Terrien's Marginal Degeneration is an uncommon, noninflammatory marginal thinning disorder of the cornea, considered to be degenerativ (Beauchamp et al, 1982). Usually, the disease is bilateral and symmetric and is commonly seen between 20 and 40 years of age. Men are affected more than women. The lesion usually starts superonasally with mild opacification in the stroma and pure neovascularization. The stroma progressively thins with the intact overlying epithelium. This results in a characteristic horizontal or oblique "bow-tie" pattern observed with computerized corneal topographic analysis (Wilsone t al, 1990). It has a characteristic yellow-white coloring of lipid and is usually observed central to the advancing edge of the lesion (Fig 20). This condition can be associated with atypical pseudopterygium which usually grows onto the cornea at an oblique axis. Patients are usually asymptomatic but may complain of occasional mild irritation. Although there is no treatment to prevent the disease from advancing, progression is slow. Most patients can be safely observed If there is no serious visual disturbance. High astigmatic error that cannot be treated with spectacles may be treated with hybrid contact lenses, or specialized scleral lenses (Mahadevan et al, 2014).

PHSD (Peripheral hypertrophic subepithelial degeneration) is an elevated circumferential and perilimbal subepithelial fibrosis associated with focal superficial corneal neovascularization (Maust et al, 2003). PHSD is usually bilateral, occurring more often in females (93%). It can cause irregular astigmatism of two diopters or more. The pathogenesis of PHSD is unknown but is presumed to be a degeneration that resembles Salzmann's nodular degeneration to some extent, rather than dystrophy (Fig 22). The indication for keratectomy may be the progression of the fibrosis or substantial astigmatism associated with worsening of visual acuity or ocular surface disease.

Figure 20. Terrien's Marginal Degeneration. The lipid deposition with neovascularization is seen (right photo). The limbal thinning is seen on the left photo

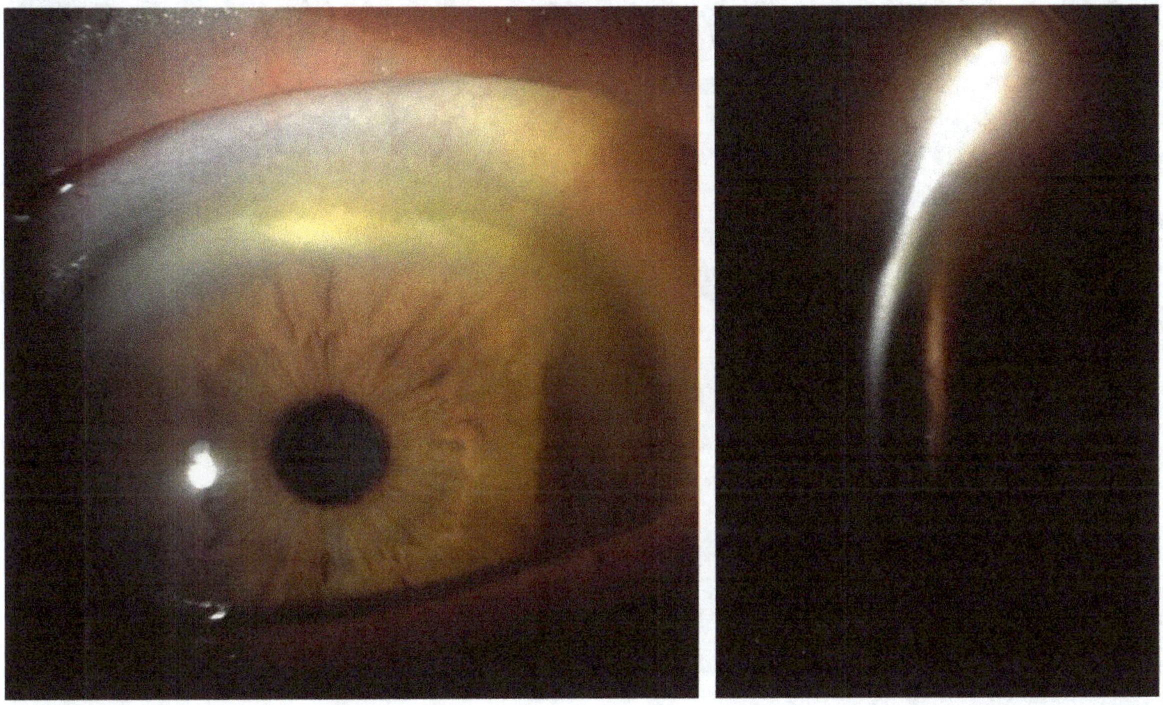

Figure 21. Presumed alimentary cuprum keratopathy due to excess use of sunflower seeds and excess intake of chlorophyll-containing herbal teas. Right and left eyes of the same patient. The patient is an otherwise healthy 72 yo female who reported overusing the above mentioned products for 15-20 years

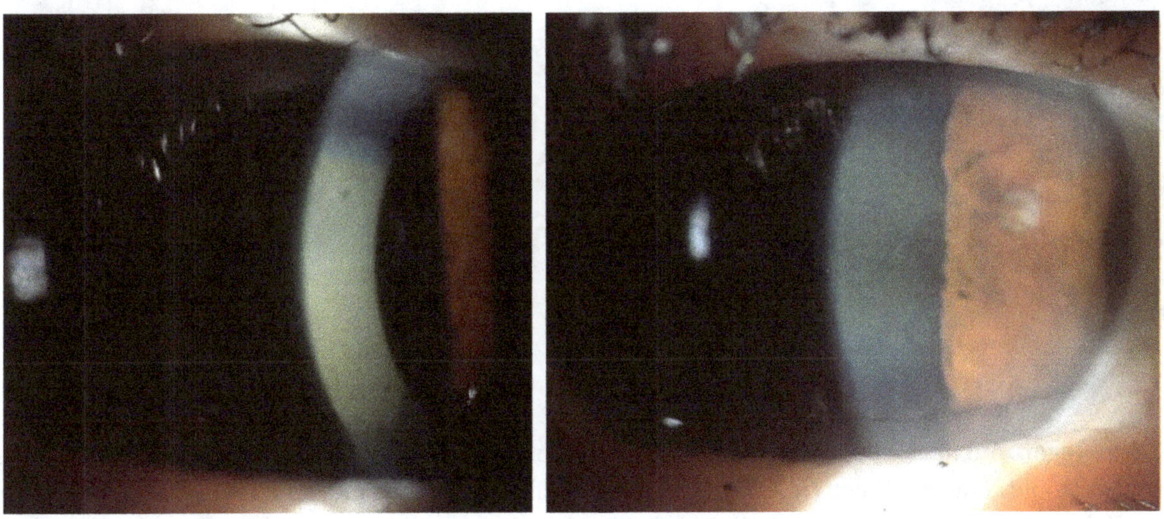

Figure 22. PHSD. Subepithelial fibrosis with focal neovascularization is seen

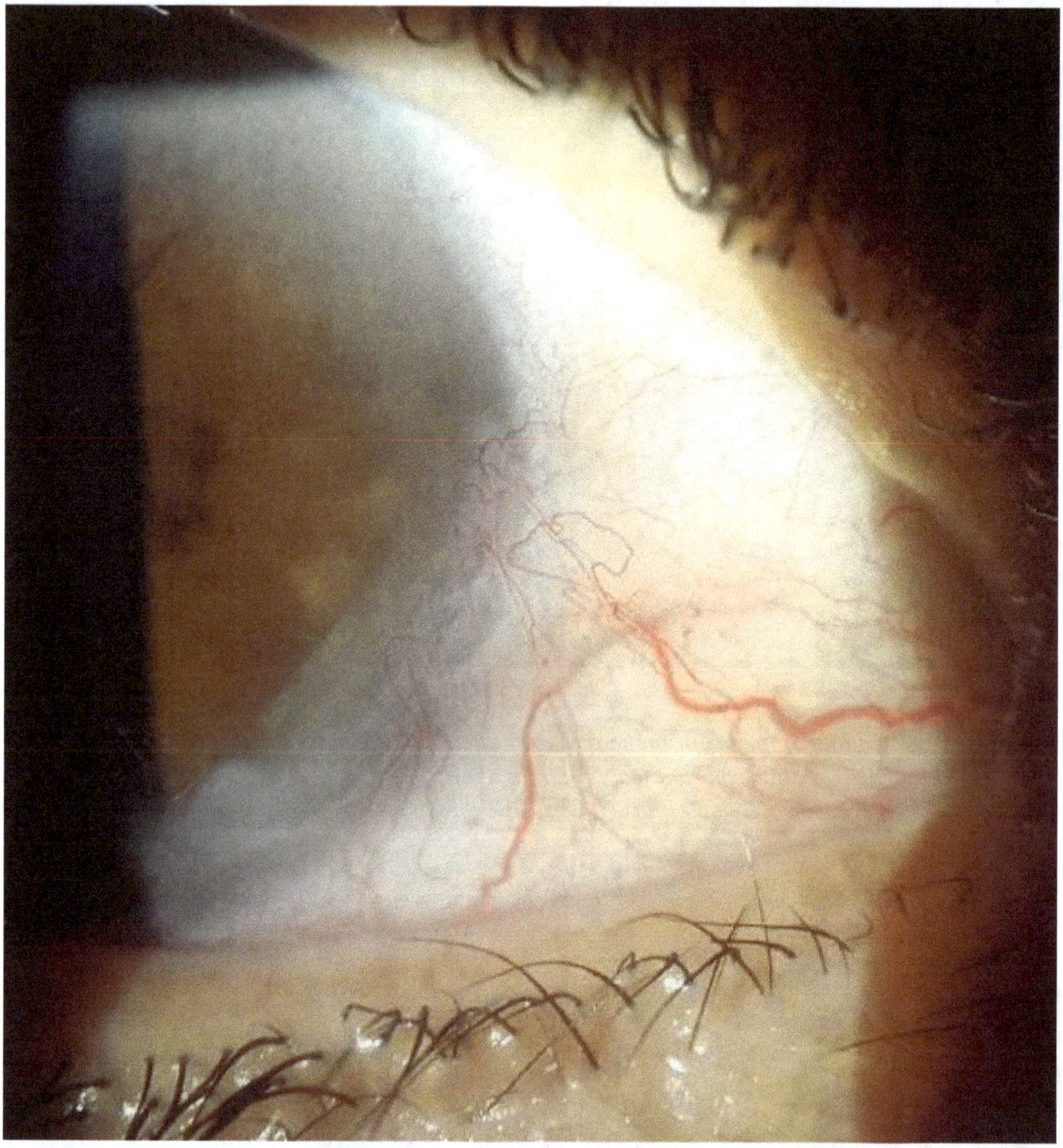

Psuedogerontoxon looks like a small segment of arcus senilis and is seen in many patients with limbal vernal or atopic keratoconjunctivitis. The lesions represent gray-white lipid deposits in the peripheral and superficial stroma. It is an essential clinical finding because pseudogerontoxon is sometimes the only clinical evidence of previous allergic eye disease (Fig 23). Pseudogerontoxon has no visual significance, and thus no necessary treatment is required.

Figure 23. Pseudogerontoxon after vernal keratoconjunctivitis. The right and left eyes of the same patient

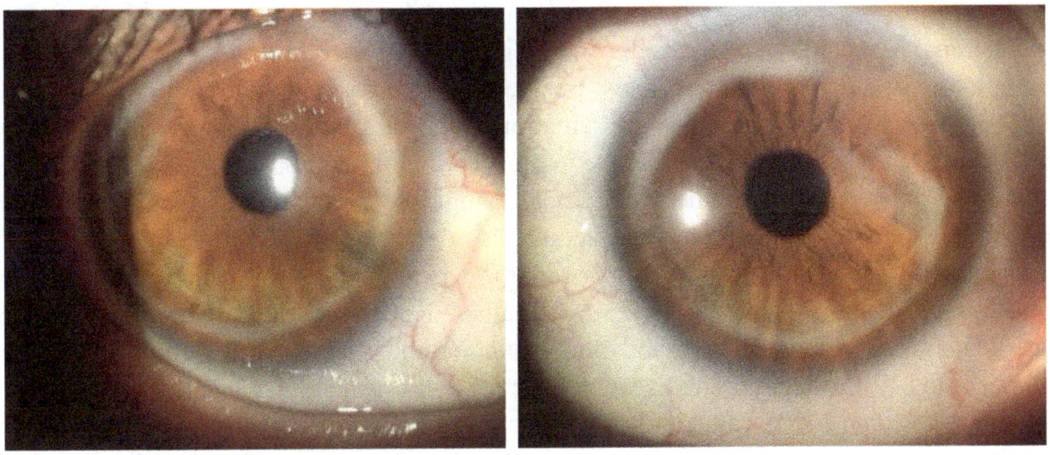

Vortex keratopathy (Drug-induced lipidoses) represents horizontal lines in a whorl-like pattern. Usually, the lines start from the inferior pupillary margin and extend toward the limbus.[28] The drug-induced verticillata was first associated with Amniodarone, Cordarone, and Chloroquine.[29] However, Tamoxifen, Sumarin, and Phenotiazines can also cause vortex keratopathy. This condition is typically bilateral and symmetric, related to both dosage and duration (Fig 24). Discontinuation or reduction of the medications can lead to regression of lesions. The differential diagnosis includes Fabrys' disease, which is an X-linked recessive disorder derived from the deficiency of the enzyme α-galactosidase A, with progressive deposition of sphingolipids within the lysosomes of most visceral tissues, blood vessels, and ocular tissues including the epithelium of conjunctiva, cornea, lens capsule, ciliary and iris sphincter muscle, and connective tissue fibroblasts. Cornea verticillata is visually insignificant but may represent a sign with high sensitivity and specificity for the early diagnosis of Fabry's disease[30].

Figure 24. Vortex keratopathy associated with Cordarone (right and left eyes of the same patient)

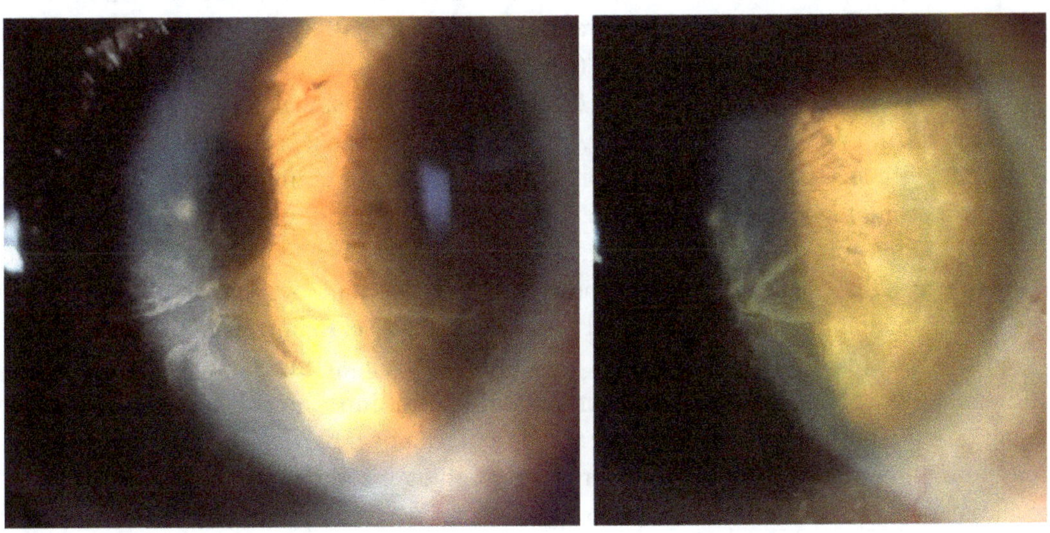

Corneal Ectasias

The noninflammatory ectatic diseases of the cornea include keratoconus, pellucid marginal degeneration, keratoglobus, and posterior keratoconus. Beside the similarities in their names, these conditions, to varying degrees, are similar in clinical presentation. Corneal thinning is a hallmark of these ectatic diseases. The area of maximal thinning relative to the location of maximal corneal protrusion, is useful in differentiating between these conditions. Corneal topography and corneal tomography have hugely improved the sensitivity of detection of these ectatic disorders, particularly in the case of keratoconus.

Keratoconus is the most common ectatic disorder in which the cornea assumes a conical shape due to thinning and protrusion that cause irregular astigmatism. Keratoconus usually presents alone but can also be associated with systemic disease and other ocular pathologies. The microtrauma associated with eye rubbing could be the etiologic link between the conical cornea and associated systemic and ocular diseases. (Bawazeer et al, 2000). Clinically, an eccentric, usually inferiorly located ecstatic protrusion of the cornea is noted. Superior keratoconus can also occur. A hallmark of keratoconus is corneal thinning occurring at the cone apex, which presents the point of the maximal protrusion. Typical clinical signs include Vogt's striae, Fleischer iron ring, Munson's and Rizutti's signs (Fig 25-28) (Iwamoto et al, n.d.) Acute keratoconus or corneal hydrops result from Descemet membrane ruptures with subsequent stromal imbibition of aqueous (Fig 29-33) (Margo et al, 1987). The management of keratoconus begins with spectacle correction. Once glasses fail to provide adequate visual function, contact lens fitting is required. Contact lens wear improves visual function by creating a new anterior refractive surface. Contact lenses do not prevent progression of corneal ectasia. Relatively flat-fitting, rigid gas-permeable (RGP), hard contact lenses with light apical corneal touch, the so-called three-point touch technique, is considered the mainstay of contact lens treatment for keratoconus(Szczotka et al, 2001). Contact lens-intolerant keratoconus patients without central scarring, who have mild or moderate disease, may benefit from intrastromal ring segment insertion (Siganos et al, 2002). The ideal candidates also have low spherical equivalents and average keratometry readings of less than 53 D.

Cornea cross-linking (CXL) is the most recent addition to the surgical armamentarium and may slow or stop the progression of keratoconus by using a photo-oxidative treatment to increase the rigidity of the corneal stroma. The procedure in its classic form, the Dresden protocol, begins with the removal of the central epithelium to enhance stromal saturation with the topically applied riboflavin (vitamin B2). The cornea is then irradiated with ultraviolet A (UVA) light at 370 nm for 30 minutes. The irradiation of the riboflavin results in chemical reactions that create covalent bonds, which bridge amino groups of the stromal collagen fibrils (Wollensak et al, 2006). An alternative treatment protocol in which the epithelium is left in place may reduce postoperative discomfort and the risk of complications. However, adequate stromal concentration of riboflavin may not be achieved and the long-term efficacy of CXL using the "epi-on" technique may be less than with the traditional approach. While penetrating keratoplasty (PK) has traditionally been the surgery of choice, lamellar surgery (deep anterior lamellar keatoplasty DALK) has become more popular for patients with mild to moderate disease. Recurrent keratoconus in the donor following cornea transplant has been reported; however, recurrent keratoconus is far more likely to be related to incomplete excision of the cone(Kremer et al, 1995). Intracameral air has been widely used in the management of corneal hydrops. The air acts as a mechanical barrier, reducing aqueous flow into the stroma through the rupture. Because the air is absorbed over a few days, the longer-lasting alternatives like intracameral gases sulfur hexafluoride (SF6) and perfluoropropane (C3F8), in isoexpansile concentrations, are more advantageous (Panda et al, 2007).

Figure 25. Rizutti's sign. Conical reflection on the nasal cornea is seen when light is shed from the temporal side

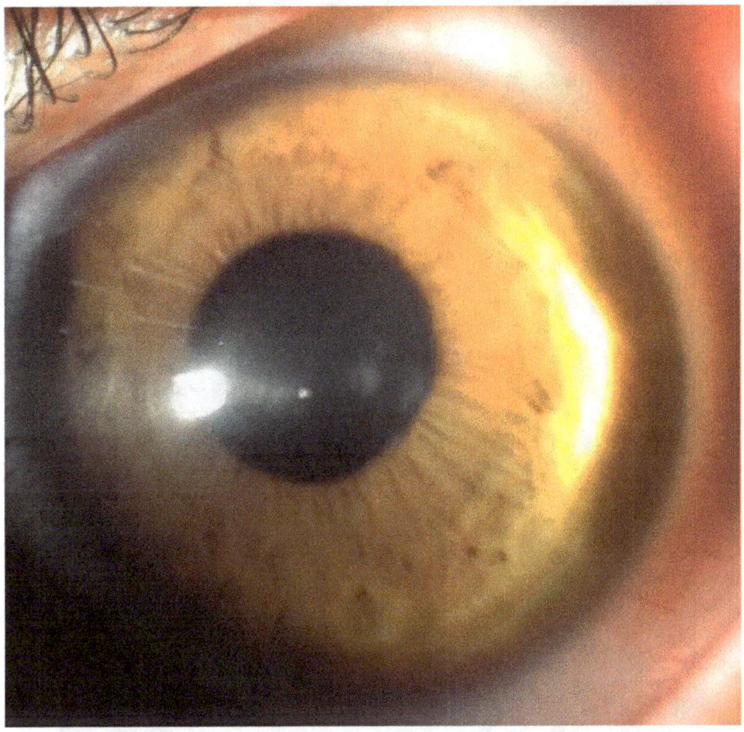

Figure 26. Munson's sign (V-shaped). Angulation of the lower lid on downgaze is seen

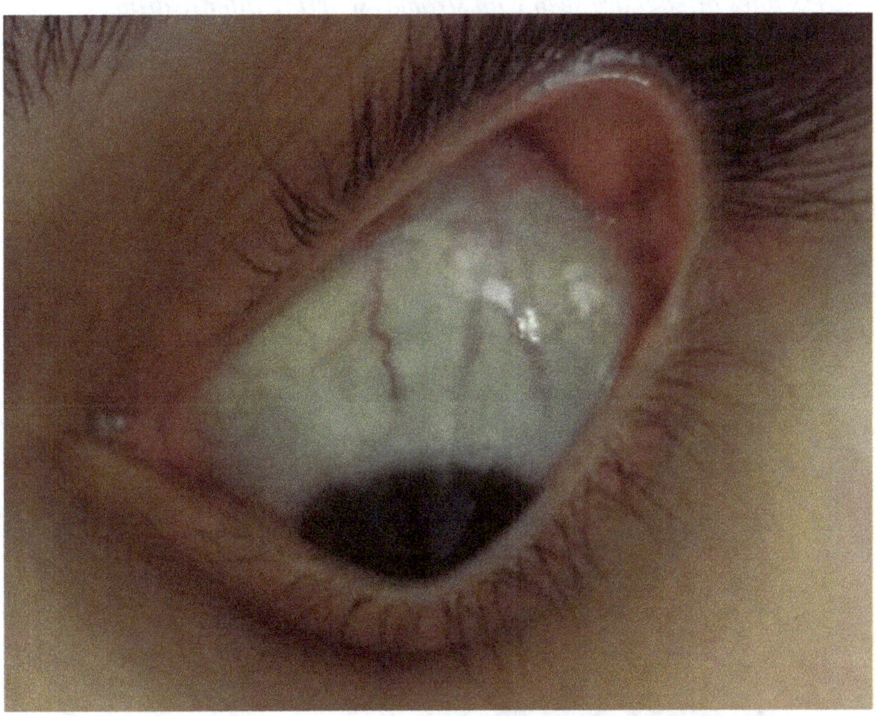

Figure 27. Vogt's stress line

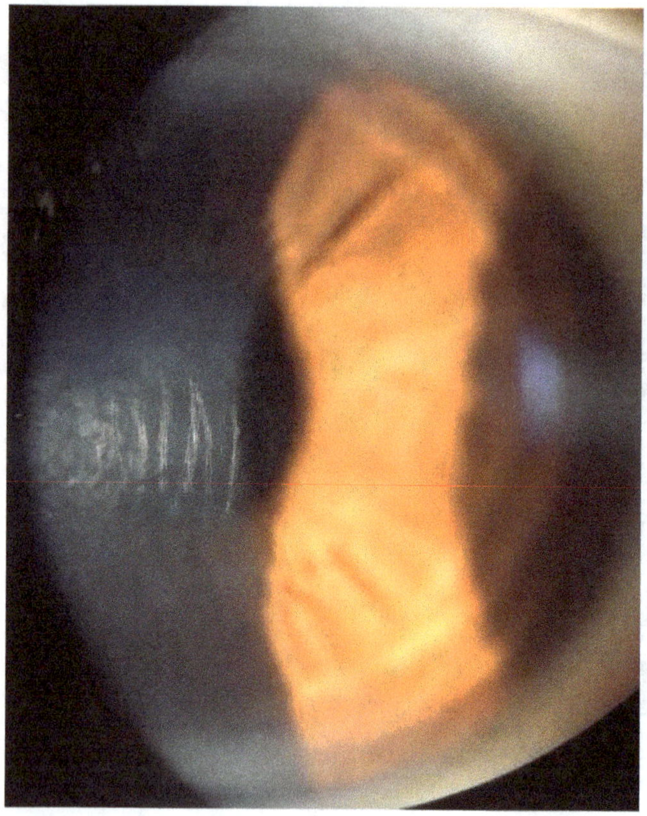

Figure 28. Fine stress lines of Vogt are seen with stromal scarring after hydrops

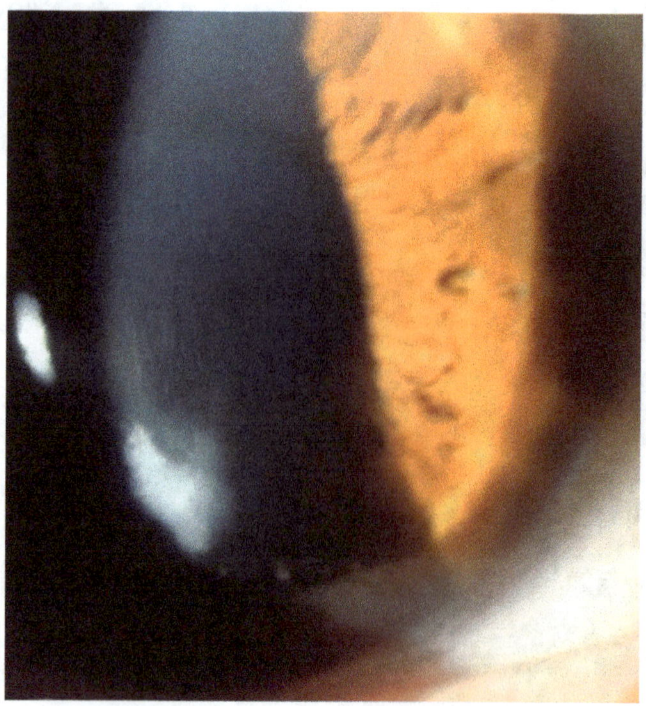

Figure 29. Acute keratoconus. Eccentric conical shaped corneal protrusion is seen inferiorly. The same patient with slit lamp (left photo) and without magnification (right photo)

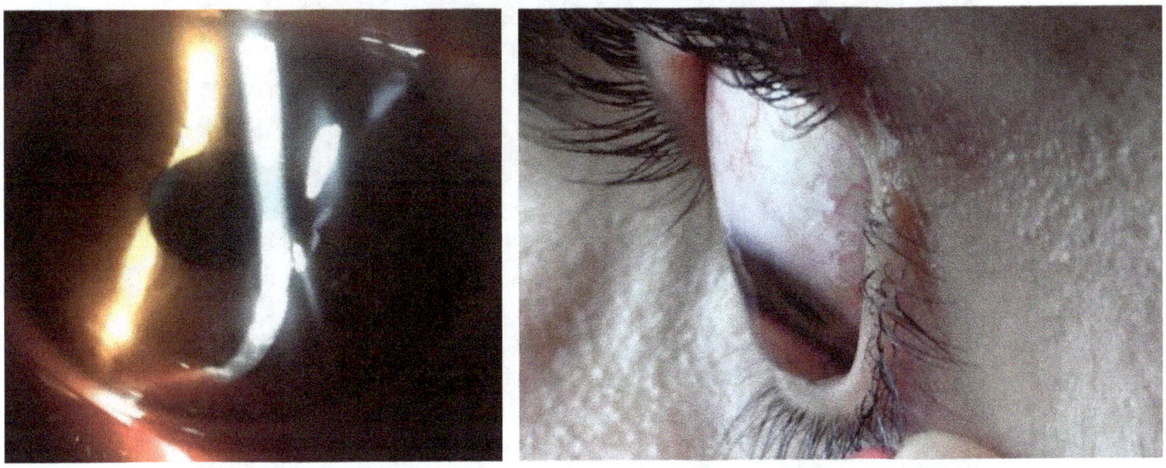

Figure 30. Bilateral acute keratoconus associated with hydrops in the right eye. The patient also has congenital nystagmus

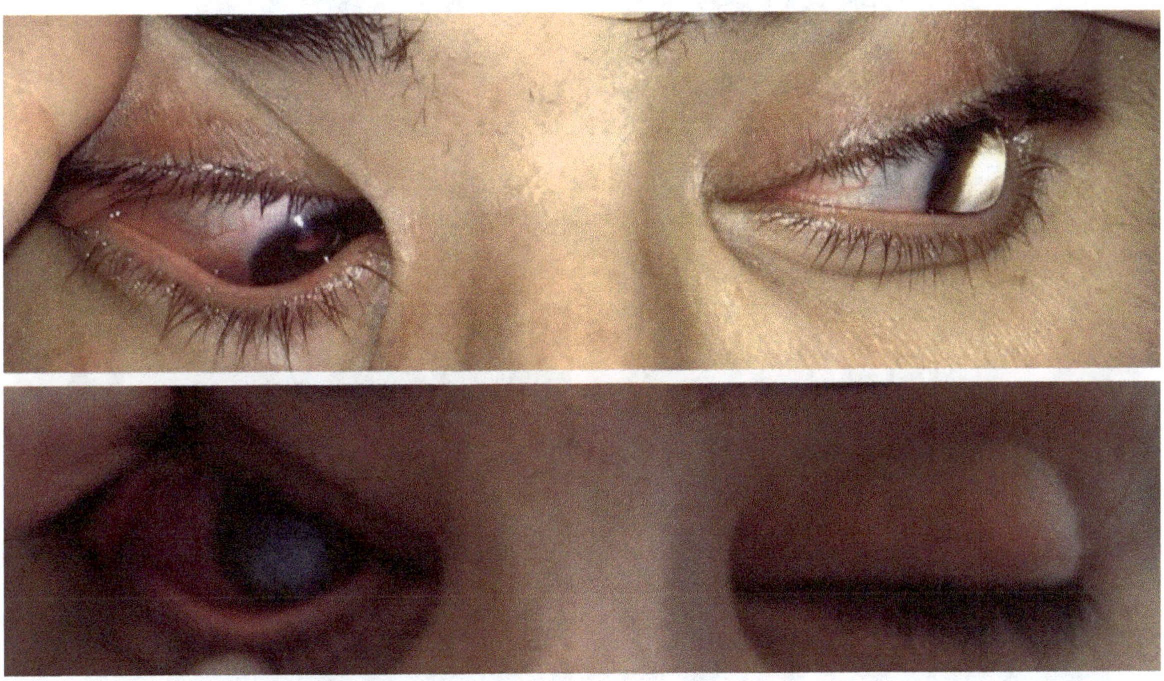

Figure 31. Hydrops. Paracentral edema is seen

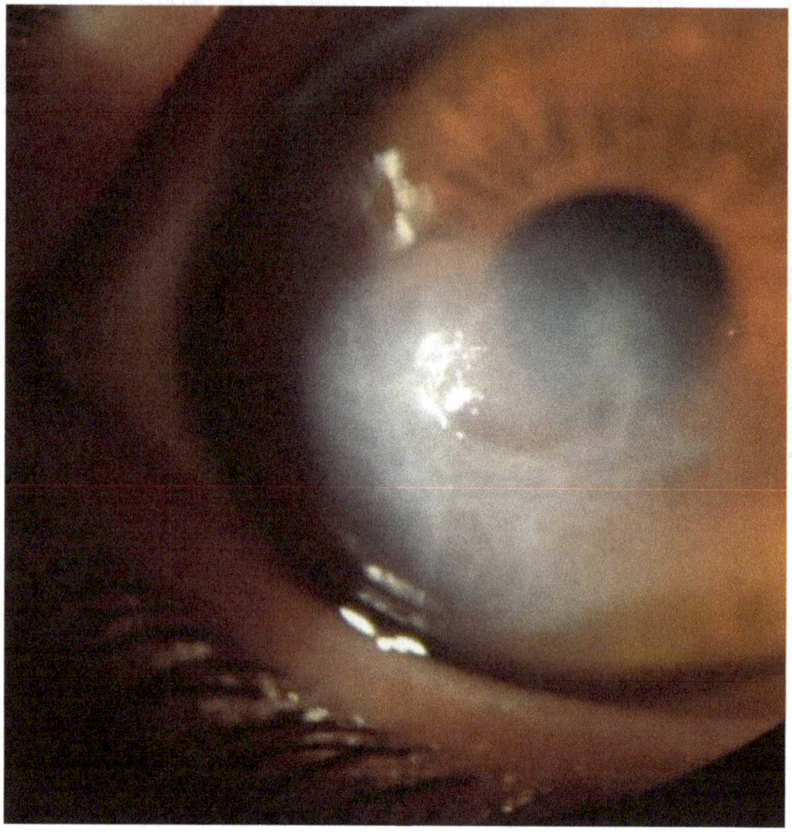

Figure 32. Hydrops (left photo) and the same eye after resolution three months later; corneal scarring is seen (right photo)

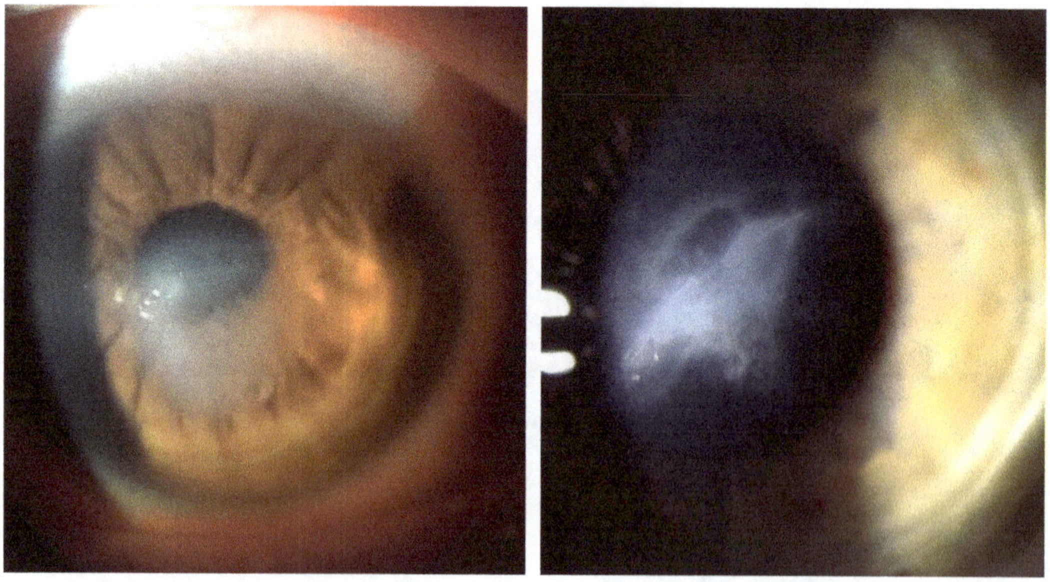

Figure 33. Severe hydrops in keratoconus and Pellucid marginal degeneration. The thinning located in the inferior cornea is seen

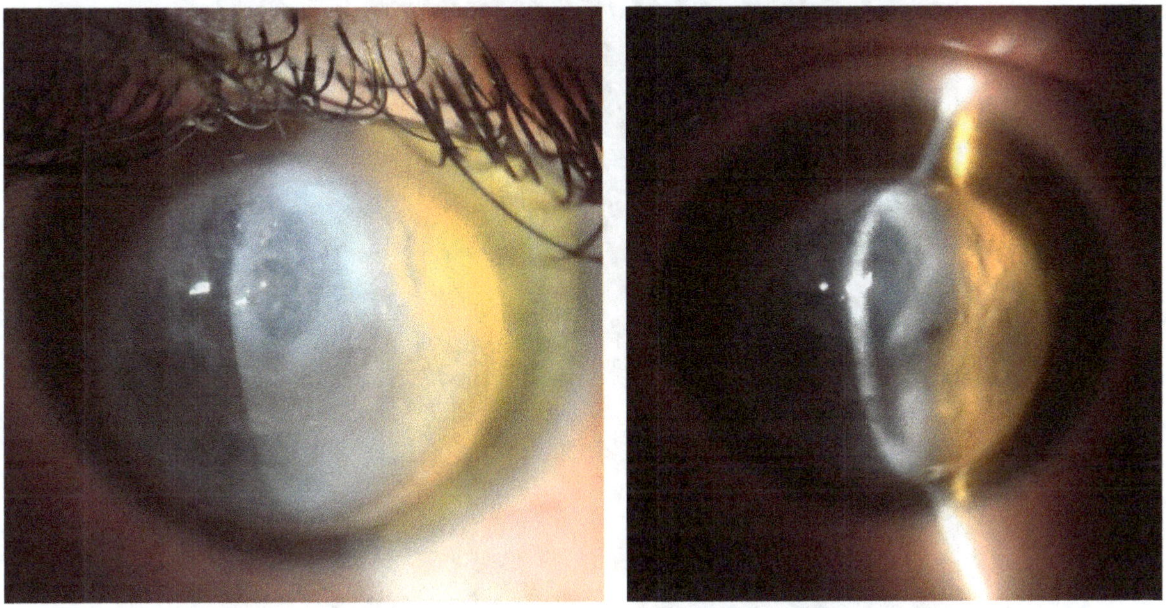

Figure 34. Pellucid marginal degeneration. The thinning located in the inferior cornea is seen

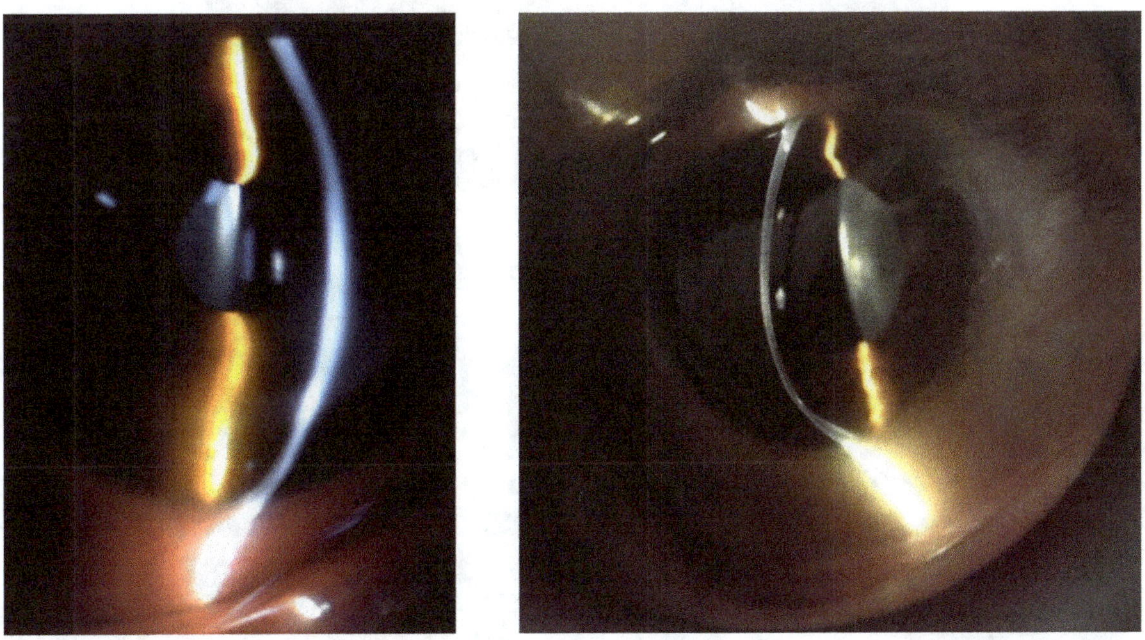

Figure 35. Superior pellucid marginal degeneration

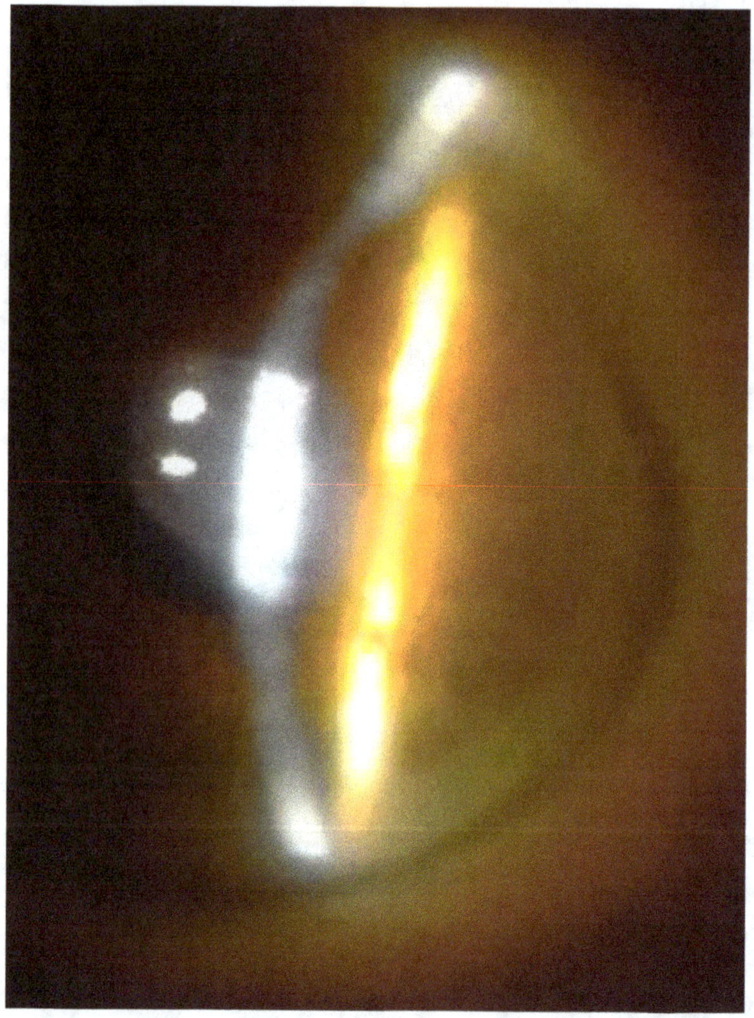

Figure 36. Keratoglobus and topography of the same patient (right photo)

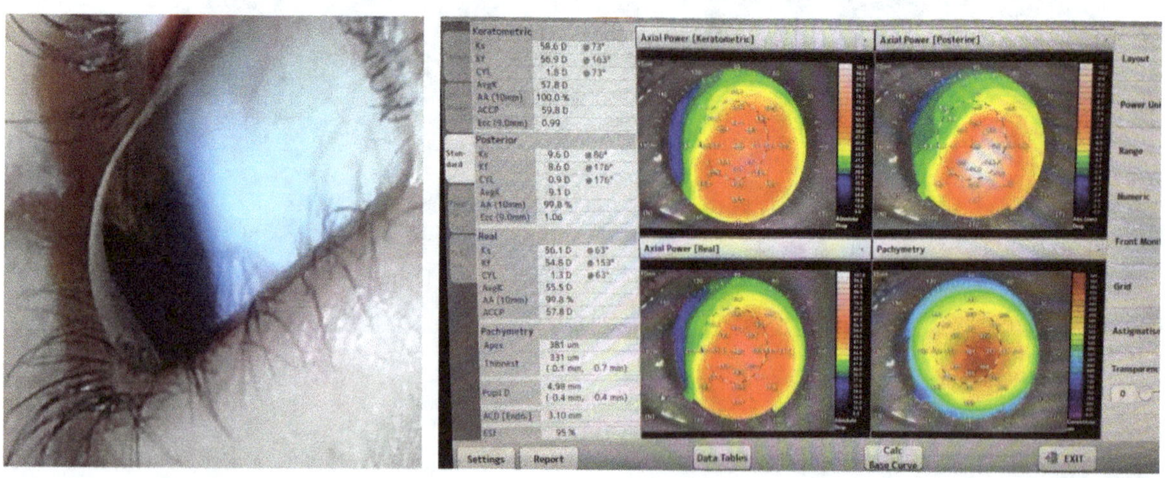

Figure 37. The same patient with associated posterior polymorphous dystrophy under slit lamp. Band shown by the arrow (right photo)

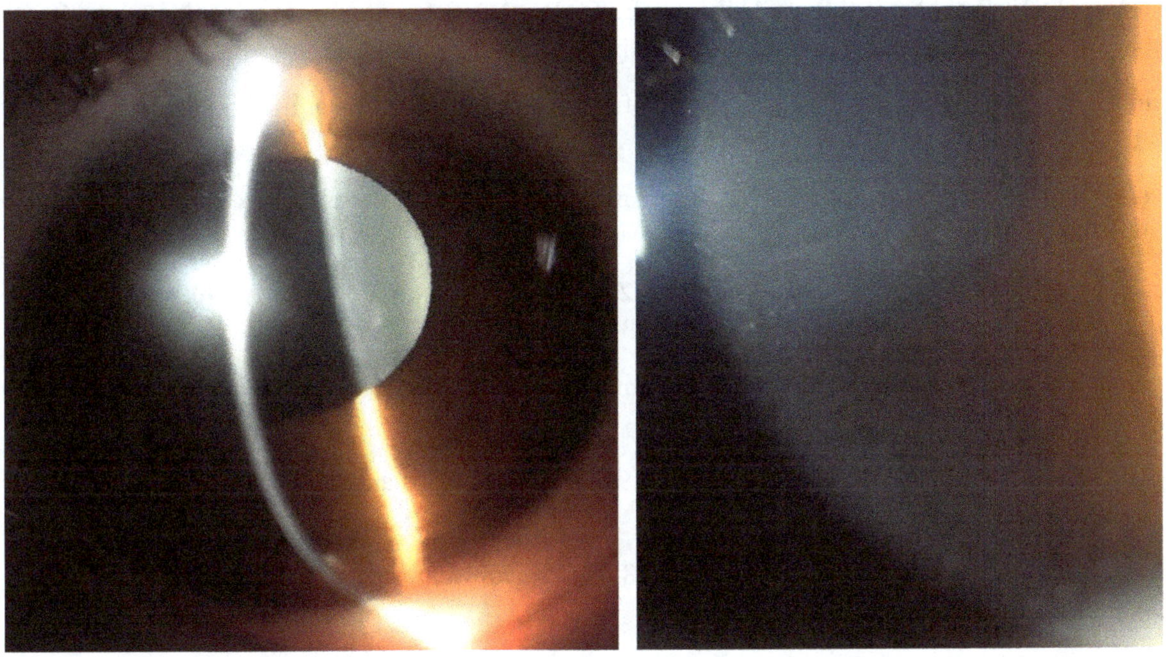

Pellucid marginal degeneration is a bilateral, peripheral corneal ecstatic disorder, although unilateral cases have also been described. Pellucid marginal degeneration is characterized by a 1-2mm band of thinning in width, typically in the inferior cornea that usually extends from 4 to 8 o'clock (Rao et al, 1999). The zone of thinning is usually located around 1-2mm central to the inferior limbus (Fig 33). It can be a cause of irregular astigmatism. The cornea often remains clear and avascular. Superior pellucid marginal degeneration has been described as well (Fig 34). (Bower et al, 1997) Spectacles usually fail to adequately correct the high irregular astigmatism associated with typical cases of PMD. Large-diameter, rigid gas-permeable contact lenses can be tried. However, a stable long-term fit can be difficult to achieve. The hybrid lenses have been used successfully in PMD (Astin et al, 1994) A surgical approach may be required for visual rehabilitation. Large-diameter or eccentric penetrating keratoplasty may be necessary to encircle the area of peripheral thinning.

Keratoglobus is a bilateral ecstatic disorder, usually nonprogressive. The typical globular protrusion of the cornea develops from generalized thinning, often most remarkable in the periphery (Fig 35, 36). Associated scleral thinning has also been described (Biglan et al, 1977). Acute hydrops occurs less frequently as opposed to keratoconus. Patients with keratoglobus may get corneal rupture after minimal trauma (Gupta et al, 1985) Spectacle correction is the first step in the management of keratoglobus. Functional vision can sometimes be obtained with glasses. Spectacles also provide the patient some protection from corneal rupture associated with trauma. A stable contact lens fit is difficult to achieve due to the abnormal corneal contour, however, scleral lenses are considered better options that provide a comfortable stable fit. Surgical intervention should be considered when functional vision cannot otherwise be attained. As in pellucid marginal degeneration, a large diameter penetrating keratoplasty may be required to encompass the considerably thin peripheral pathology.

REFERENCES

Anderson, D. F., Prabhasawat, P., & Alphonso, E. (2001). Amniotic membrane transplantation after the primary surgical management of band keratopathy. *Cornea*, *20*, 354–361.

Astin, C. L. (1994). The long-term use of the SoftPerm lens on pellucid marginal corneal degeneration. *The CLAO Journal*, *20*(4), 258–260.

Ayres, B. D., & Rapuano, C. J. (2006). Excimer laser phototherapeutic keratectomy. *The Ocular Surface*, *4*, 196–206.

Bawazeer, A. M., Hodge, W. G., & Lorimer, B. (2000). Atopy and keratoconus: A multivariate analysis. *The British Journal of Ophthalmology*, *84*(8), 834–836.

Beauchamp, G. R. (1982). Terrien's marginal corneal degeneration. *Journal of Pediatric Ophthalmology and Strabismus*, *19*, 97–99.

Biglan, A. W., Brown, S. I., & Johnson, B. L. (1977). Keratoglobus and blue sclera. *American Journal of Ophthalmology*, *83*(2), 225–233.

Bokosky, J. E., Meyer, R. F., & Sugar, A. (1985). Surgical treatment of calcified band keratopathy. *Ophthalmic Research*, *16*, 645–647.

Bower, K. S., Dhaliwal, D. K., & Barnhorst, D. A. Jr. (1997). Pellucid marginal degeneration with superior corneal thinning. *Cornea*, *16*(4), 483–485.

Caporossi, A., Mazzotta, C., & Paradiso, A. L. (2013). Transepithelial corneal collagen crosslinking for progressive keratoconus: 24-month clinical results. *Journal of Cataract and Refractive Surgery*, *39*(8), 1157–1163.

Cogan, D. G., & Kuwabara, T. (1958). Lipid keratopathy and atheroma. *Transactions of the American Ophthalmological Society*, *56*, 109–122.

Das, S., Link, B., & Seitz, B. (2005). Salzmann's nodular degeneration of the cornea. *Cornea*, *24*, 772–777.

Ferry, A. P. (1968). A 'new' iron line in the cornea. *Archives of Ophthalmology*, *79*(2), 142–145. doi:10.1001/archopht.1968.03850040144005 PMID:5635336

François, J., & Feher, J. (1973). Arcus senilis. *Documenta Ophthalmologica. Advances in Ophthalmology*, *34*, 165–182. doi:10.1007/BF00151805 PMID:4122363

Fraunfelder, F. T., Hanna, C., & Parker, J. M. (1972). Spheroid degeneration of the cornea and conjunctiva. *American Journal of Ophthalmology*, *74*, 821–828.

Gupta, V. P., Jain, R. K., & Angra, S. K. (1985). Acute hydrops in keratoglobus with vernal keratoconjunctivitis. *Indian Journal of Ophthalmology*, *33*(2), 121–123.

Hollander, D. A., & Aldave, A. J. (2004). Drug-induced corneal complications. *Current Opinion in Ophthalmology*, *15*(6), 541–548.

Iwamoto, T., & DeVoe, A. G. (n.d.). Electron microscopical study of the Fleischer ring. *Archives of Ophthalmology*, *94*(9), 1579–1584.

Jeng, Whitcher, & Margolis. (2004). Pseudogerontoxon. *Clin Exp Ophthalmol, 32*(4), 433-4.

Kaufman, Baron, & McDonald. (1988). Sugar: Corneal and conjunctival degenerations. In *The cornea*. Churchill Livingstone.

Kremer, I., Eagle, R. C., & Rapuano, C. J. (1995). Histologic evidence of recurrent keratoconus seven years after keratoplasty. *American Journal of Ophthalmology*, *119*(4), 511–512.

Lemp, M. A., & Ralph, R. A. (1977). Rapid development of band keratopathy in dry eyes. *American Journal of Ophthalmology*, *83*(5), 657–659. doi:10.1016/0002-9394(77)90131-3 PMID:868965

Linke, S., Kugu, C., & Gisbert, R. (2009). An in vivo confocal microscopic analysis of Salzmann's nodular degeneration: Pre and post surgical intervention. *Acta Ophthalmologica*, *87*, 233–234.

Loh, A., Hadziahmetovic, M., & Dunaief, J. L. (2009). Iron homeostasis and eye disease. *Biochimica et Biophysica Acta*, *1790*(7), 637–649. doi:10.1016/j.bbagen.2008.11.001 PMID:19059309

Mahadevan, R., Fathima, A., & Rajan, R. (2014). An ocular surface prosthesis for keratoglobus and Terrien's marginal degeneration. *Optometry and Vision Science*, *91*, S34–S39.

Margo, C. E., & Mosteller, M. W. (1987). Corneal pseudocyst following acute hydrops. *The British Journal of Ophthalmology*, *71*(5), 359–360.

Marsh, R. J., & Marshall, J. (1982). Treatment of lipid keratopathy with the argon laser. *The British Journal of Ophthalmology*, *66*, 127–135.

Maust, H. A., & Raber, I. M. (2003). Peripheral hypertrophic subepithelial corneal degeneration. *Eye & Contact Lens*, *29*, 266–269.

O'Connor, G. R. (1972). Calcific band keratopathy. *Transactions of the American Ophthalmological Society*, *70*, 58–81. PMID:4677022

Oh, J. Y., Kim, M. K., & Wee, W. R. (2009). Subconjunctival and intracorneal bevacizumab injection for corneal neovascularization in lipid keratopathy. *Cornea*, *28*, 1070–1073.

Orlando, R. G., Dangel, M. E., & Schaal, S. F. (1984). Clinical experience and grading of amiodarone keratopathy. *Ophthalmology*, *91*, 1184–1187.

Panda, A., Aggarwal, A., & Madhavi, P. (2007). Management of acute corneal hydrops secondary to keratoconus with intracameral injection of sulfur hexafluoride (SF6). *Cornea*, *26*(9), 1067–1069.

Rao, S. K., Fogla, R., & Padmanabhan, P. (1999). Corneal topography in atypical pellucid marginal degeneration. *Cornea*, *18*(3), 265–272.

Rapuano, C. J. (1997). Excimer laser phototherapeutic keratectomy: Long-term results and practical considerations. *Cornea*, *16*, 151–157.

Rifkind, B. M. (1972). Corneal arcus and hyperlipoproteinemia. *Survey of Ophthalmology*, *16*, 295–304. PMID:4620953

Rose, G. E., & Lavin, M. J. (1987). The Hudson-Stähli line. I: An epidemiological study. *Eye (London, England)*, *1*(4), 466–470. doi:10.1038/eye.1987.69 PMID:3443199

Siganos, D., Ferrara, P., & Chatzinikolas, K. (2002). Ferrara intrastromal corneal rings for the correction of keratoconus. *Journal of Cataract and Refractive Surgery*, *28*(11), 1947–1951.

Sodi, A., Ioannidis, A. S., & Mehta, A. (2007). Ocular manifestations of Fabry's disease: Data from the Fabry Outcome Survey. *The British Journal of Ophthalmology*, *91*(2), 210–214.

Stevenson, Ching, & Dastjerdi. (2012). Corneal neovascularization and the utility of topical VEGF inhibition: ranibizumab (Lucentis) vs bevacizumab (Avastin). *Ocul Surf.*, *10*, 67-83.

Sugar, H. S., & Kobernick, S. (1960). The white limbus girdle of Vogt. *American Journal of Ophthalmology*, *50*(1), 101–107. doi:10.1016/0002-9394(60)90843-6 PMID:13835558

Szczotka, L. B., Barr, J. T., & Zadnik, K. (2001). A summary of the findings from the Collaborative Longitudinal Evaluation of Keratoconus (CLEK) Study. CLEK Study Group. *Optometry (St. Louis, Mo.)*, *72*(9), 574–584.

Vogt, A. (1930). *Lehrbuch und atlas der Spaltlampenmikroscopie des lebenden Auges*. Springer Berlin.

Wilson, S. E., Lin, D. T., & Klyce, S. E. (1990). Terrien's marginal degeneration: Corneal topography. *Refractive & Corneal Surgery*, *6*, 15–20.

Wollensak, G. (2006). Crosslinking treatment of progressive keratoconus: New hope. *Current Opinion in Ophthalmology*, *17*(4), 356–360.

Wood, T. O. (1990). Salzmann's nodular degeneration. *Cornea*, *9*, 17–22.

Chapter 8
Corneal Dystrophies

ABSTRACT

Corneal dystrophies have classically referred to inherited, bilateral disease without systemic findings, although there are several exceptions to this definition. Hereditary pattern is not present in most patients with epithelial basement membrane dystrophy (EBMD). Unilateral corneal changes may be found in some patients with posterior polymorphous corneal dystrophy (PPCD). TGFBI gene mutation (p.His572del) is associated with a unilateral, late-onset variant of lattice corneal dystrophy. Among all dystrophies, macular corneal dystrophy and posterior amorphous corneal dystrophy are associated with decreased corneal thickness. The International Committee for Classification of Corneal Dystrophies (IC3D) was created in 2005 to revise the corneal dystrophy nomenclature and create a current and accurate corneal dystrophy classification system. Evidential categories were created in the IC3D classification for reflecting the natural evolution of a corneal dystrophy and indicate the level of evidence supporting the existence of a given dystrophy.

INTRODUCTION

Evidential categories for IC3D classification from: Weiss JS, Møller H, Lisch W, et al. The IC3D classification of the corneal dystrophies. Cornea 2008; 27: S1–S42, S4.

Category 1. A well-defined corneal dystrophy in which the gene has been mapped and identified and specific mutations are known.

Category 2. A well-defined corneal dystrophy that has been mapped to one or more specific chromosomal loci, but the gene(s) remains to be identified.

Category 3. A clinically well-defined corneal dystrophy in which the disorder has not yet been mapped to a chromosomal locus.

Category 4. This category is reserved for a suspected new, or previously documented, corneal dystrophy, where the evidence for it being a distinct entity is not yet convincing.

DOI: 10.4018/978-1-7998-6937-5.ch008

Corneal dystrophies are divided by anatomy and genetics into categories of epithelial and subepithelial, epithelial-stromal TGFBI, stromal, and endothelial corneal dystrophies.

The IC3D classification from: Weiss JS, Møller H, Aldave, A, et al. The IC3D classification of the corneal dystrophies-edition 2. Cornea 2015; 34:117–159.

Epithelial and subepithelial dystrophies

- Epithelial basement membrane dystrophy (EBMD) – majority degenerative, some C1
- Epithelial recurrent erosion dystrophies (EREDs) C4 (Franceschetti corneal dystrophy (FRCD) C3, Dystrophia Smolandiensis (DS) C3 and Dystrophia Helsinglandica (DH) C3)
- Subepithelial mucinous corneal dystrophy (SMCD) C4
- Meesmann corneal dystrophy (MECD) C1
- Lisch epithelial corneal dystrophy (LECD) C2
- Gelatinous drop-like corneal dystrophy (GDLD) C1

Epithelial-stromal TGFBI dystrophies

- Reis–Bücklers corneal dystrophy (RBCD) – granular corneal dystrophy type 3 C1
- Thiel–Behnke corneal dystrophy (TBCD) C1
- Lattice corneal dystrophy, type 1 (LCD1) C1-variants (III, IIIA, I/IIIA, IV) of lattice corneal dystrophy C1
- Granular corneal dystrophy, type 1 (GCD1) C1
- Granular corneal dystrophy, type 2 (GCD2) C1

Stromal dystrophies

- Macular corneal dystrophy (MCD) C1
- Schnyder corneal dystrophy (SCD) C1
- Congenital stromal corneal dystrophy (CSCD) C1
- Fleck corneal dystrophy (FCD) C1
- Posterior amorphous corneal dystrophy (PACD) C1
- Central cloudy dystrophy of François (CCDF) C4
- Pre-Descemet corneal dystrophy (PDCD) C1 or C4

Endothelial dystrophies

- Fuchs endothelial corneal dystrophy (FECD) C1, C2 or C3
- Posterior polymorphous corneal dystrophy (PPCD) C1 or C2
- Congenital hereditary endothelial dystrophy (CHED) C1
- X-linked endothelial corneal dystrophy (XECD) C2

Meesmann Juvenile Epithelial Dystrophy (IC3D, MECD, Category 1) is an autosomal, dominant, bilaterally symmetric epithelial dystrophy.[2] The dystrophy is observed in the first few years of life. It clinically represents as intraepithelial small microcysts or vesicles (Fig 1). Patients usually don't complain of visual disturbances.[3] It is mostly an incidental finding. Usually no treatment is required.

Figure 1. Meesmann Epithelial Dystrophy. The small intraepithelial vesicles are seen

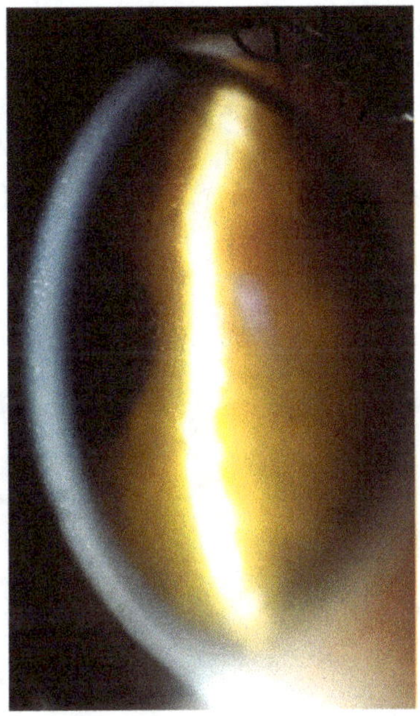

Lisch epithelial corneal dystrophy (IC3D LECD Category 2) has X-chromosomal dominant inheritance.[4] Clinically, it represents with a band-shaped and whorl microcystic pattern (Fig 2). Recurrent erosions appear infrequently. Blurred vision is observed if the cornea over the pupil is involved. Lubricating drops and bandage contact lens may occasionally be required.

Figure 2. Lisch epithelial corneal dystrophy. The whorl-like lesion is seen

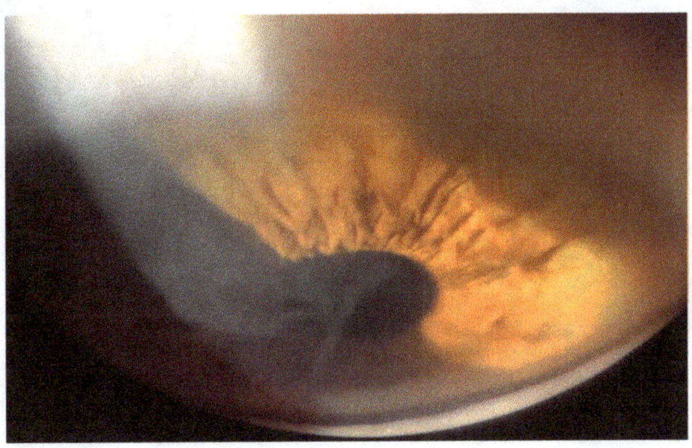

Epithelial Basement Membrane Dystrophy (IC3D, EMBD, Category 1), also known as Cogan or map-dot-fingerprint dystrophy, is nowadays considered an epithelial basement membrane degeneration. However, hereditary familial cases have also been reported. Clinically, microcystic changes[5] are in the epithelium surrounded by map-like changes (Vogt et al, 1930). (Fig 3-5). The third characteristic sign is fingerprint lines in the corneal epithelium (Guerry et al, 1950). This is a bilateral asymmetric dystrophy, and not all characteristic features can be revealed in the same eye. The main reason for visiting a doctor is a complaint due to recurrent erosion syndrome. The therapeutic treatment includes lubricating drops, ointments at bedtime, bandage contact lenses, hypertonic saline drops/ointment. Treatment of recalcitrant recurrent corneal erosions with topical corticosteroids and doxycycline, inhibitors of matrix metalloproteinase-9, has been effective in a small nonprospective study (Wood et al, 1988). Bent needle micropuncture of anterior storma (Rubinfeld et al, 1990)., Nd: YAG laser micropuncture (Geggel et al, 1990). and excimer laser phototherapeutic keratectomy (PTK) (Orndahl et al, 1998) are applied in severe cases.

Figure 3. Epithelial Basement Membrane Dystrophy. Map-like lesion with microcystic changes is seen

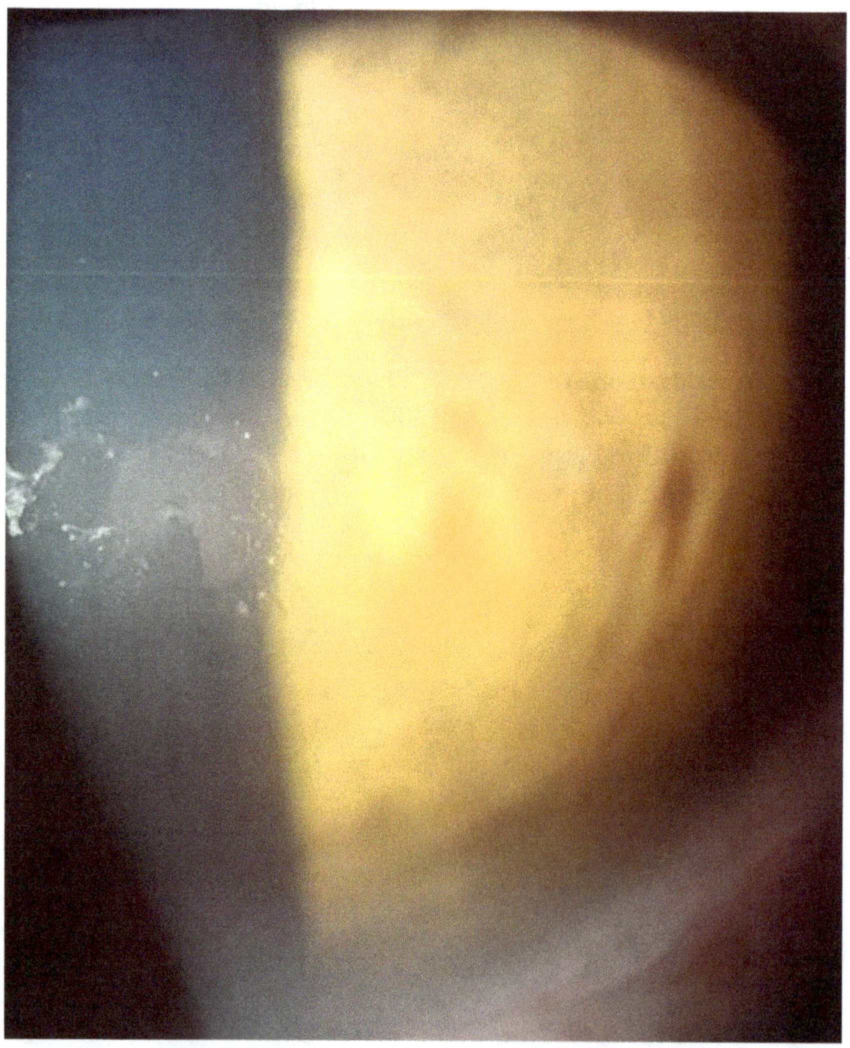

Figure 4. Epithelial Basement Membrane Dystrophy. The right and left eyes of the same patient. Map-like changes are seen

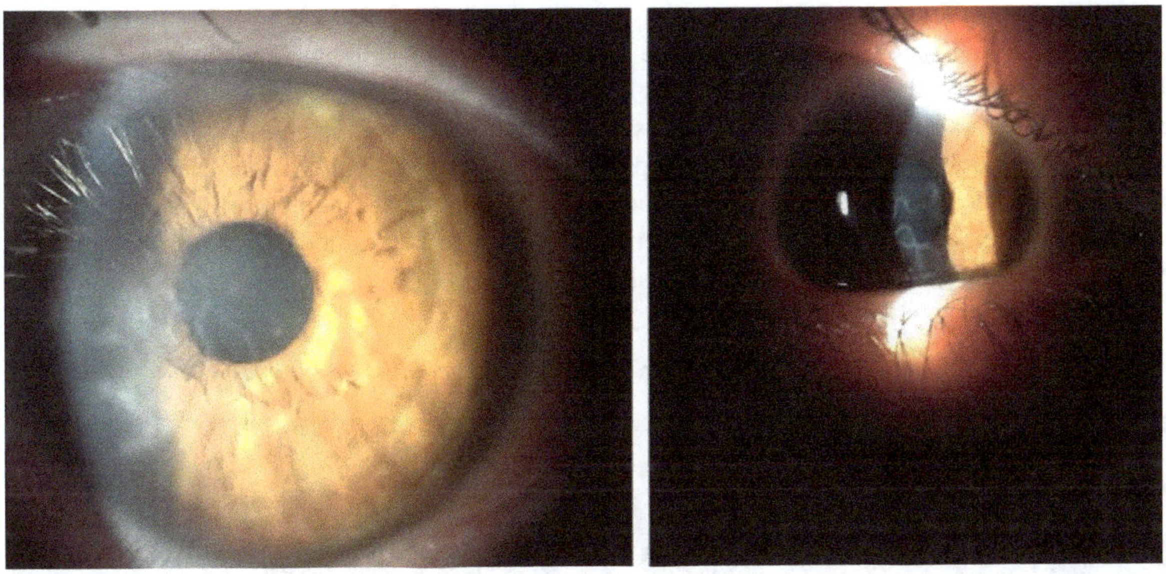

Figure 5. Epithelial Basement Membrane Dystrophy. Epithelial defect looking like dendrite stained with Fluorescein

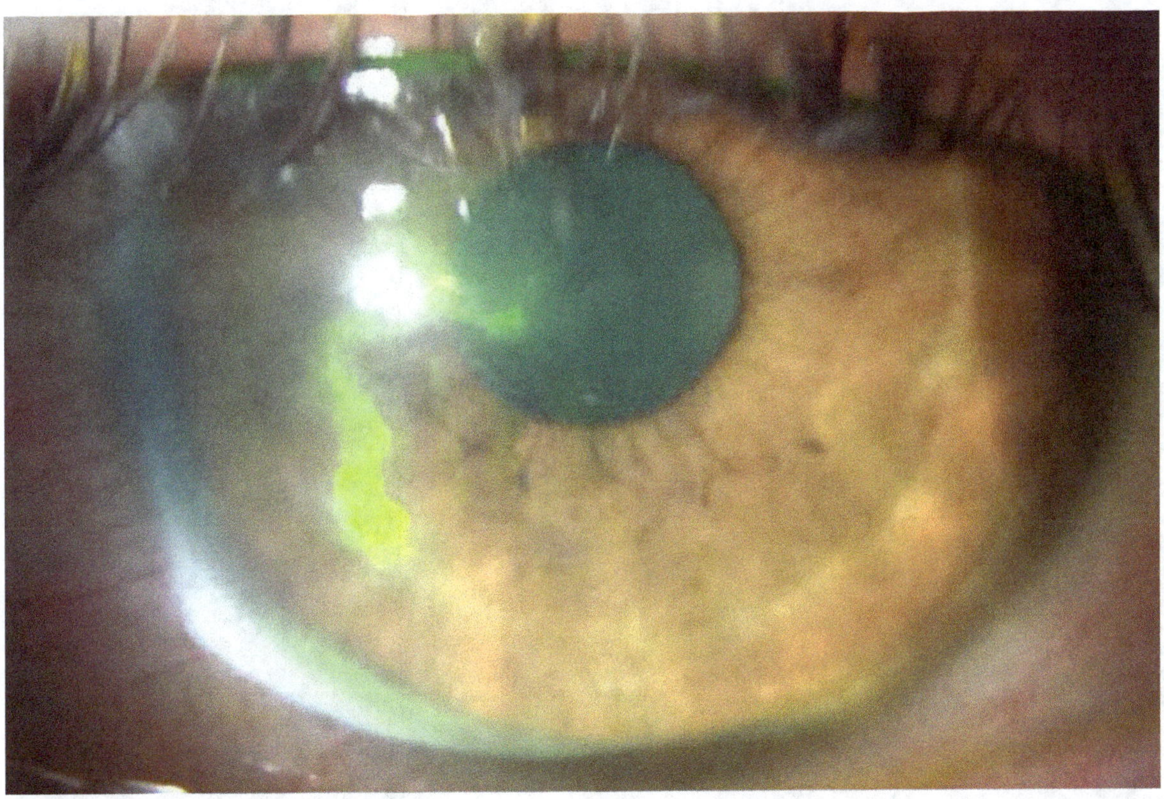

There are two types of Bowman's layer dystrophies; **corneal dystrophy of Bowman's layer** type I (CDB-I) and type II (CDB-II). Type I is synonymous with **Reis-Bucklers' original dystrophy** and has been called the superficial variant of granular dystrophy (Kuchle et al, 1995). Type II is honeycomb-shaped and should be known as **Theil-Behnke corneal dystrophy** (Fig 6). The inheritance of 2 types is dominant with a similar clinical appearance. Usually, only genetic analysis can differentiate the two types. They are characterized by a recurrent erosion syndrome starting from childhood, but visual acuity is reduced later in life in type II dystrophy, as opposed to type I. Recurrent erosions can be managed the same way as the therapy of recurrent erosion due to epithelial basement membrane dystrophy. If deeper scarring and opacities present, lamellar and penetrating keratoplasty can be performed. Recurrence of the dystrophy in the graft is frequent (Chan et al, 1993).

Figure 6. Presumed Type II Theil-Behnke dystrophy. The honeycomb-shaped opacification is seen

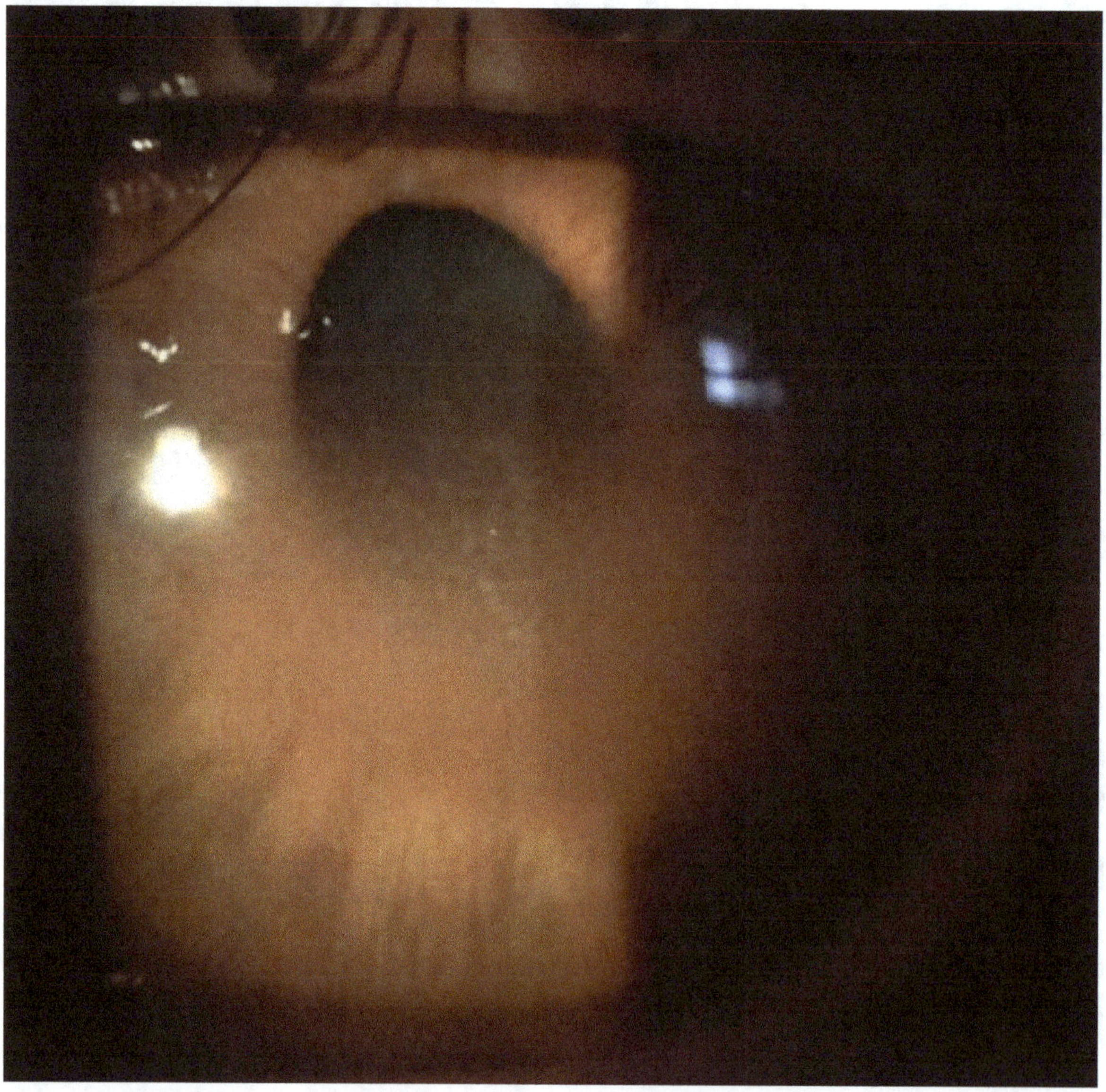

Granular corneal dystrophy type 1 (classic) (GCB1) is a bilateral, autosomal, dominant corneal disorder characterized by the accumulation of hyaline deposits in the anterior stroma (Weiss et al, Groenouw et al, 1890). Clinically, deposits appear as small, discrete, sharply demarcated, grayish-white opacities in the central stroma. Meanwhile, around 2-3mm of the peripheral cornea remains free of deposits (Fig 7, 8). Recurrent erosive syndrome can occur, but not commonly. The vision may be dramatically reduced between the 4th-5th decades of life. Recurrent erosions are managed as presented above. If vision is markedly reduced, surgical management may be considered (lamellar or penetrating keratoplasty). Granular dystrophy can recur in the grafts as early as one year after surgery, and the recurrence-free interval seems to be independent of size and type of graft performed (Stuart et al, 1975).

Lattice corneal dystrophy (LCD) is an autosomal dominant, bilateral dystrophy. Clinically, amyloid accumulation appears as small nodules, dots or thicker, radially oriented lines (Fig 6). The lines can extend into the deep stroma and superficially into epithelium and may become opacified. The stroma between the lines and dots is clear initially, however, the opacities coalesce with time, and a diffuse ground-glass haze may develop in the anterior and mid-stroma (Rodrigues eet al, 1929; Dubord et al, 1982). Recurrent erosions are frequently seen. Lattice corneal dystrophy recurs on the graft earlier compared to granular or macular dystrophies. Treatment of recurrent erosions are treated in a routine fashion. In patients with visually significant stromal opacification lamellar or penetrating keratoplasty is indicated.

Macular corneal dystrophy (MCD) is characterized by corneal opacification due to the deposition of unsulfated keratan sulfate within the cornel stroma (SundarRaj et al, 1987; Klintworth et al, 1986). Of the three classic stromal dystrophies, macular dystrophy is the least common and the most visually disabling. The opacifications extend to the corneal periphery and progress to involve the entire thickness of the cornea (Fig 10). The inheritance is autosomal recessive. Recurrent erosions are frequently seen. Lattice corneal dystrophy recurs on the graft earlier compared to granular or macular dystrophies. Treatment of recurrent erosions are treated in a routine fashion. In patients with visually significant stromal opacification lamellar or penetrating keratoplasty is indicated.

Central Cloudy Dystrophy of Francois (CCDF) is a Category 4 dystrophy, which means that it was previously considered corneal dystrophy (Weiss et al, 2015). However, the evidence for it being a distinct entity is not yet convincing. It is characterized by polygonal, gray, posterior stromal opacities separated by clear, crisscrossing lines. It is an asymptomatic and nonprogressive condition (Fig 11). Histopathologic examination reveals glycosaminoglycan depositions (Francois et al, 1956).No treatment is required.

Fleck corneal dystrophy is an autosomal dominant, bilateral, but often asymmetric condition. Clinically, gray-white, discrete, dandruff-like opacities are seen throughout the stroma in one or both eyes and are present from limbus to limbus, sparing the Bowman's layer (Fig 12). Usually, visual acuity is not affected. It is mostly an incidental finding (Purcell et al, 1977). No treatment is required.

Congenital hereditary stromal dystrophy (CHSD) (C1) is associated with bilateral, congenital corneal opacification due to disordered stromal fibrogenesis, either nonprogressive or slowly progressive. (Witschel et al, 1978; jing et al, 2014). The inheritance is autosomal dominant (Weiss et al, 2015). PKP is often indicted at an early age to prevent irreversible amblyopia.

Posterior polymorphous corneal dystrophy (PPCD) is an autosomal dominant disorder with varying clinical features, even within the same family. One family member may be asymptomatic with only a single band-like endothelial lesion, while a sibling may have corneal decompensation, broad peripheral synechiae, and advanced glaucoma. This dystrophy is usually bilateral, but unilateral cases have been reported as well. Cases associated with keratoconus and keratoglobus (photo is shown in Chapter 7) have been reported (Aldave et al, 2013). In the majority of patients PPCD is stable and asymptomatic.

Figure 7. Granular corneal dystrophy type 1. Discrete, small opacities are seen with an uninvolved peripheral cornea

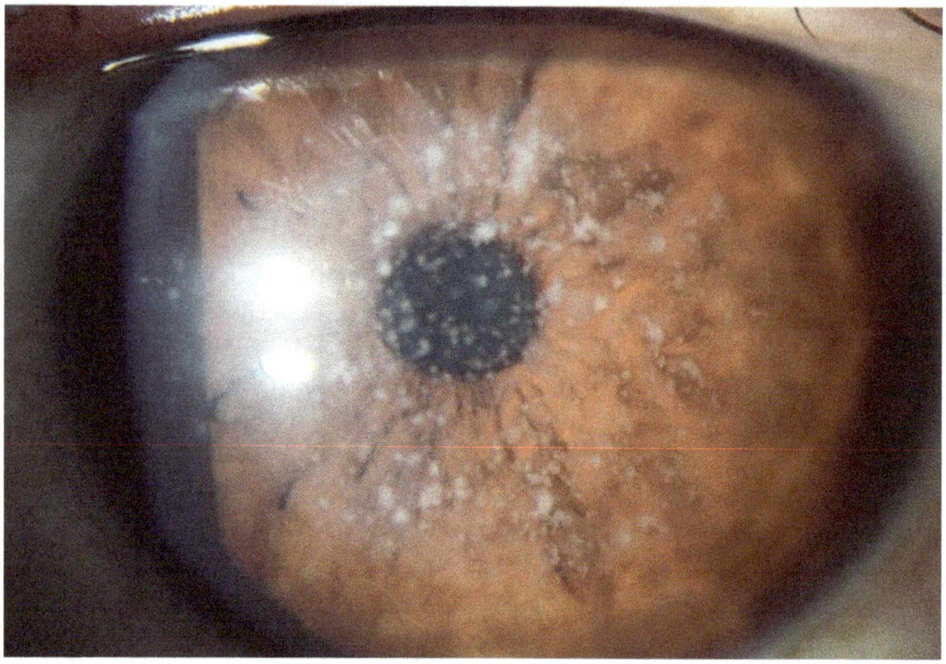

Figure 8. Presumed Granular corneal dystrophy type 1. Small stellate opacities are seen

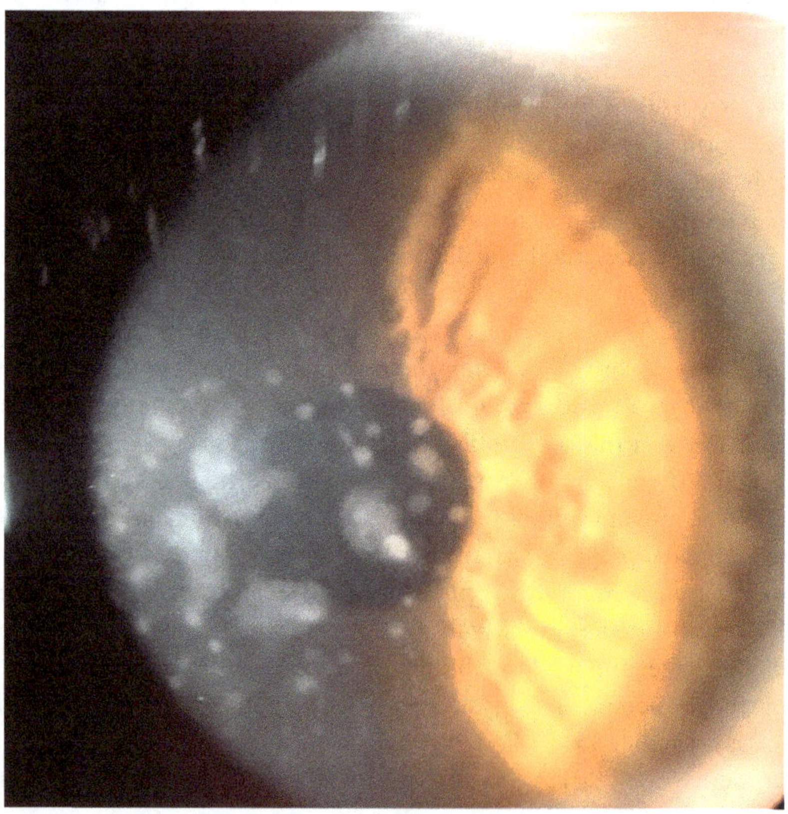

Figure 9. Lattice corneal dystrophy. The linear, branch-like lesions are seen

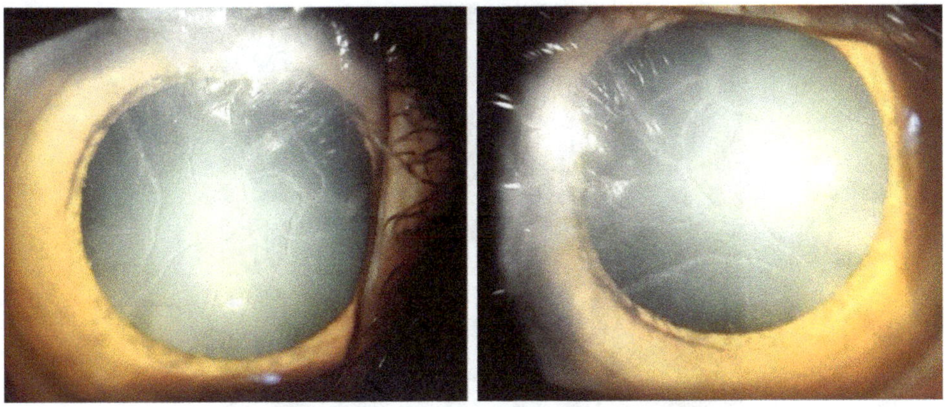

Figure 10. Macular corneal dystrophy. The entire cornea is opacified

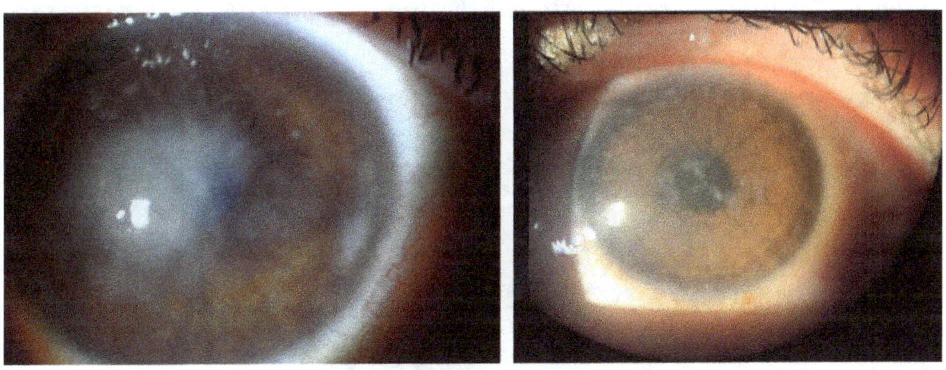

Figure 11. Central corneal dystrophy of Francois. The polygonal opacities are seen

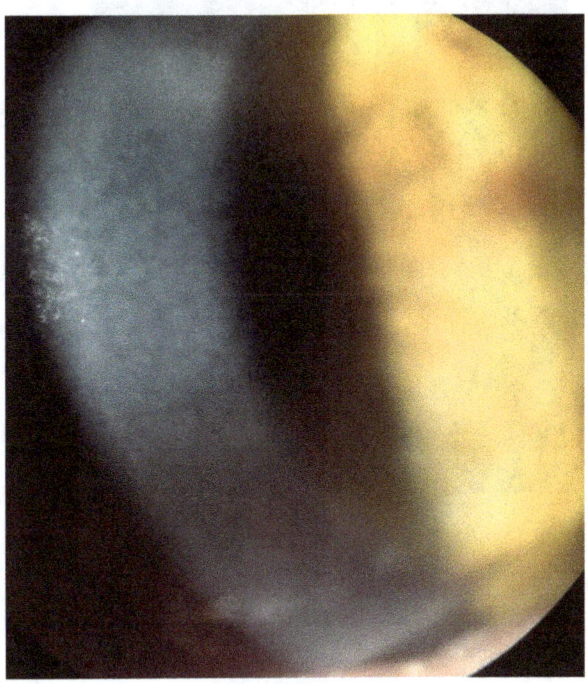

Figure 12. Fleck corneal dystrophy. The small dandruff like opacities are seen from limbus to limbus

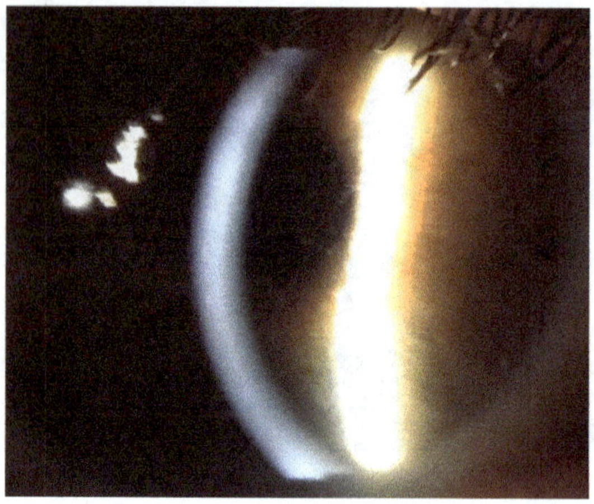

Figure 13. Presumed Congenital hereditary stromal dystrophy. Mother and sun, and the same eye under a slit lamp

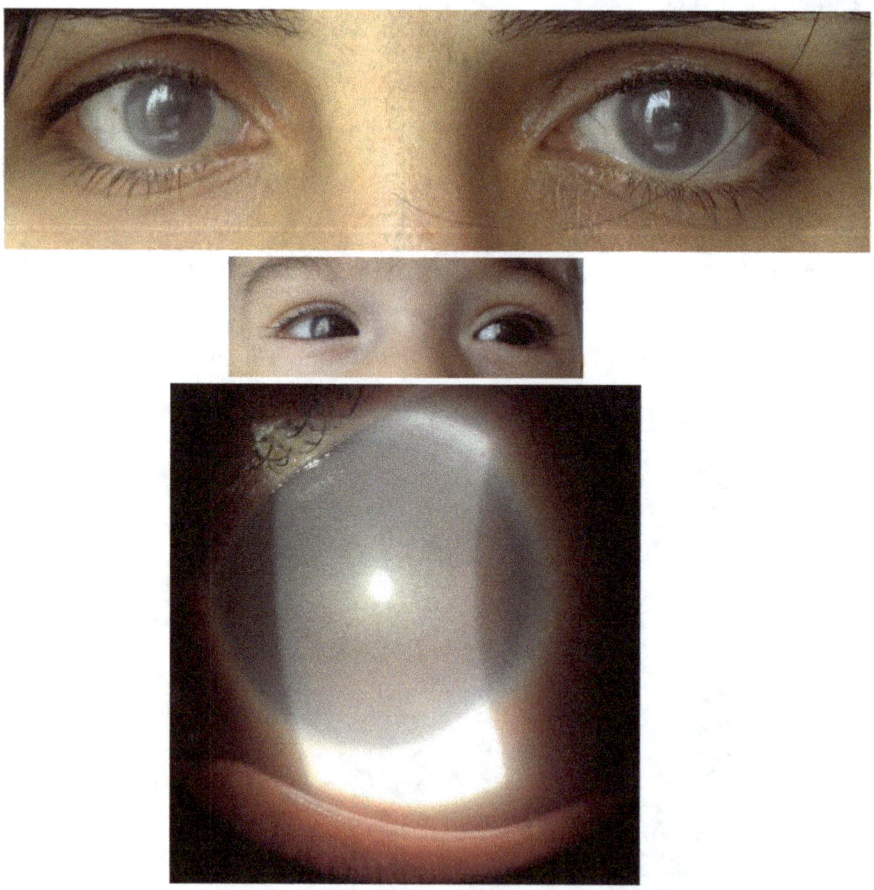

Figure 14. Posterior polymorphous corneal dystrophy. The vertical band shaped lesion is noted (shown by arrow)

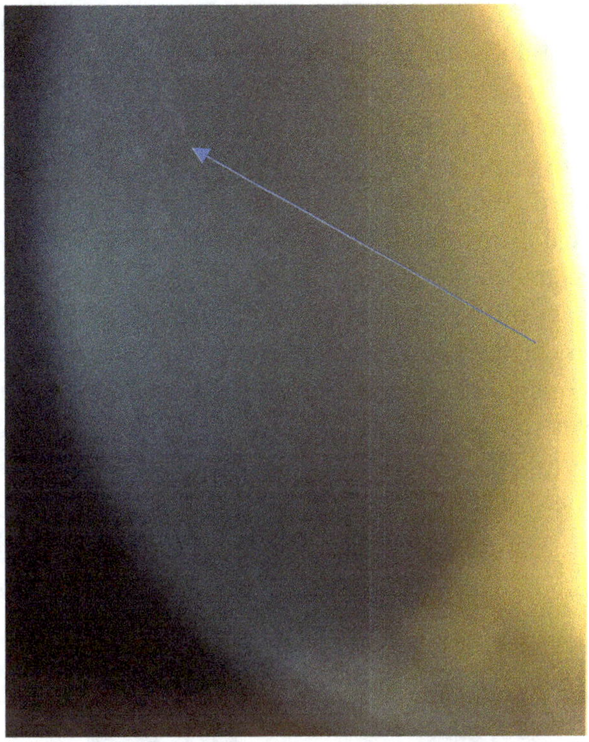

Figure 15. Presumed CHED. The ground-glass haze is seen

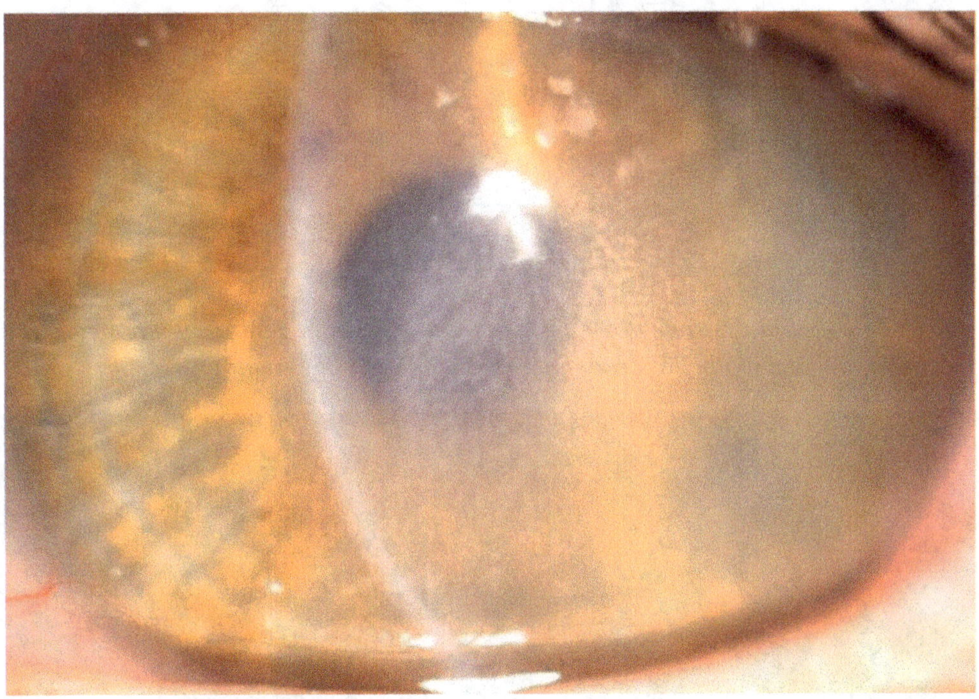

Risk factors for severe disease included the presence of PAS and increased intraocular pressure (IOP). Very extensive and progressive cases require corneal transplantation surgery and control of IOP with antiglaucoma medications.

Congenital Hereditary Endothelial Dystrophy (CHED, formerly referred to as CHED2), is an autosomal recessive disorder characterized by corneal clouding (Weiss et al, 2015). CHED usually presents from birth and doesn't progress. Clinically, stroma appears two to three times thicker than normal, and has a diffuse blue-gray, ground-glass haze (Fig 15). CHED requires corneal transplantation in early childhood to avoid amblyopia development.

Fuchs endothelial corneal dystrophy (FECD) is a slow progressive disease (Adamis et al, 1993). Its initial manifestation is central corneal guttae. The guttae appear as dark spots on the posterior corneal surface and can be seen by direct illumination. Many patients in this stage are asymptomatic. The progression of the disorder is characterized by endothelial decompensation and development of stromal edema. Once epithelial bullae or recurrent erosion develop, pain may be alleviated with use of lubricating drops, hypertonic saline solution, bandage contact lenses. Endothelial keratoplasty (DSAEK, DMEK, etc) is considered the mainstay of treatment. The prognosis for transplant surgery in FECD has been reported to be excellent in many studies.

Figure 16. Fuchs endothelial dystrophy. Corneal guttae are seen centrally with the stromal edema

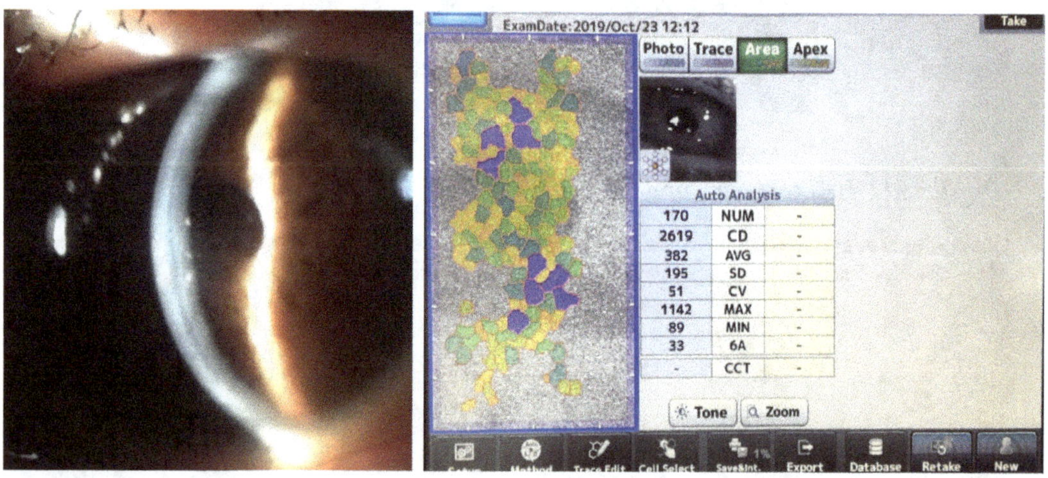

Figure 17. Fuchs endothelial dystrophy. The central thickening with central guttae in seen (left photo) and epithelial bulla due to endothelial decompensation is noted (right photo)

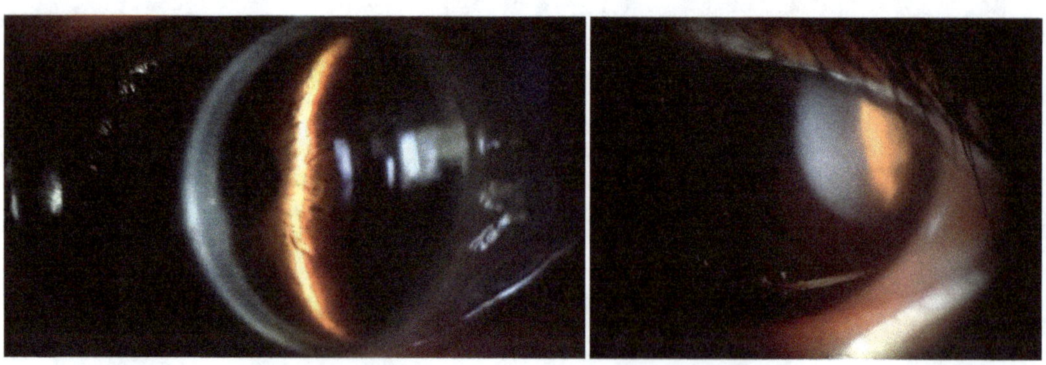

REFERENCES

Adamis, A. P., Filatov, V., Tripathi, B. J., & Tripathi, R. A. C. (1993). Fuchs' endothelial dystrophy of the cornea. *Survey of Ophthalmology, 38*(2), 149–168. doi:10.1016/0039-6257(93)90099-S PMID:8235998

Aldave, A. J., Ann, L. B., Frausto, R. F., Nguyen, C. K., Yu, F., & Raber, I. M. (2013). Classification of posterior polymorphous corneal dystrophy as a corneal ectatic disorder following confirmation of associated significant corneal steepening. *JAMA Ophthalmology, 131*(12), 1583–1590. doi:10.1001/jamaophthalmol.2013.5036 PMID:24113819

Aldave, Rayner, Kim, Prechanond, & Yellore. (2006, February 27). Unilateral lattice corneal dystrophy associated with the novel His572del mutation in the TGFBI gene. *Molecular Vision, 12*, 142–146.

Burns, R. P. (1968). Meesmann's corneal dystrophy. *Transactions of the American Ophthalmological Society, 66*, 530–636. PMID:4181022

Chan, C. C., Cogan, D. G., Bucci, F. S., Barsky, D., Li, Q., & Crawford, M.-A. (1993). Anterior corneal dystrophy with dyscollagenosis (Reis–Bücklers' type?). *Cornea, 12*(5), 451–460. doi:10.1097/00003226-199309000-00013 PMID:8306668

Dubord, P. J., & Krachmer, J. H. (1982). Diagnosis of early lattice corneal dystrophy. *Archives of Ophthalmology, 100*(5), 788–790. doi:10.1001/archopht.1982.01030030792013 PMID:6979328

François, J. (1956). A new hereditofamilial dystrophy of the cornea. *Journal de Genetique Humaine, 5*(3–4), 189–196. PMID:13398589

François, J., & Neetens, A. (1957). New hereditary-familial dystrophy of the corneal parenchyma (spotted hereditary dystrophy). *Bulletin de la Société Belge d'Ophtalmologie, 114*, 641–646. PMID:13446668

Geggel, H. S. (1990). Successful treatment of recurrent corneal erosion with Nd:YAG anterior stromal puncture. *American Journal of Ophthalmology, 110*(4), 404–407. doi:10.1016/S0002-9394(14)77021-7 PMID:2220975

Groenouw, A. (1890). Knotchenformige Hornhauttrubungen (noduli corneae). *Arch Augenheilkd., 21*, 281.

Guerry, D. III. (1950). Fingerprint lines in the cornea. *American Journal of Ophthalmology, 33*(5), 724–726. doi:10.1016/0002-9394(50)90194-2 PMID:15413672

Guerry, D. (1965). Observations on Cogan's microcystic dystrophy of the corneal epithelium. *Transactions of the American Ophthalmological Society, 63*, 320–334. PMID:5295319

Jing, Y., Kumar, P. R., Zhu, L., Edward, D. P., Tao, S., Wang, L., Chuck, R., & Zhang, C. (2014). Novel decorin mutation in a Chinese family with congenital stromal corneal dystrophy. *Cornea, 33*(3), 288–293. doi:10.1097/ICO.0000000000000055 PMID:24413633

Klintworth, G. K., Meyer, R., Dennis, R., Hewitt, A. T., Stock, E. L., Lenz, M. E., Hassell, J. R., Stark, W. J., Kuettner, K. E., & Thonar, E. J.-M. A. (1986). Macular corneal dystrophy. Lack of keratan sulfate in serum and cornea. *Ophthalmic Paediatrics and Genetics, 7*(3), 139–143. doi:10.3109/13816818609004130 PMID:2951638

Lisch, W. B., Buttner, A., & Offner, F. (2000). Lisch corneal dystrophy is genetically distinct from Meesman corneal dystrophy and maps to xp22.3. *American Journal of Ophthalmology, 130*(4), 461–468. doi:10.1016/S0002-9394(00)00494-3 PMID:11024418

Meesmann, A., & Wilke, F. (1939). Klinische und anatomische Untersuchungen uber eine bisher unbekannte, dominant verebte Epitheldystrophie der Hornhaut. *Klinische Monatsblätter für Augenheilkunde, 103*, 361–391.

Orndahl, M. J., & Fagerholm, P. P. (1998). Phototherapeutic keratectomy for map-dot-fingerprint corneal dystrophy. *Cornea, 17*(6), 595–599. doi:10.1097/00003226-199811000-00004 PMID:9820937

Purcell, J. J. Jr, Krachmer, J. H., & Weingeist, T. A. (1977). Fleck corneal dystrophy. *Archives of Ophthalmology, 95*(3), 440–444. doi:10.1001/archopht.1977.04450030082009 PMID:139144

Rodrigues & Krachmer. (1988). Recent advances in corneal stromal dystrophies. *Cornea, 7*(1), 19-29.

Rubinfeld, R. S., Laibson, P. R., & Cohen, E. J. (1990). Anterior stromal puncture for recurrent erosion: Further experience and new instrumentation. *Ophthalmic Surgery, 21*, 318–326. PMID:2199877

Stuart, J. C., Mund, M. L., Iwamoto, T., Troutman, R. C., White, H., & DeVoe, A. G. (1975). Recurrent granular corneal dystrophy. *American Journal of Ophthalmology, 79*(1), 18–24. doi:10.1016/0002-9394(75)90451-1 PMID:45922

SundarRaj, Barbacci-Tobin, & Howe. (1987). Macular corneal dystrophy: immunochemical characterization using monoclonal antibodies. *Invest Ophthalmol Vis Sci., 28*(10), 1678-1686.

Vogt. (1930). Lehrbuch und Atlas Spaltlampenmikroskopie des Lebenden Auges. *Julius Spring, 1*, 264-265.

Weiss, J. S., Moller, H. U., Aldave, A. J., Seitz, B., Bredrup, C., Kivelä, T., Munier, F. L., Rapuano, C. J., Nischal, K. K., Kim, E. K., Sutphin, J., Busin, M., Labbé, A., Kenyon, K. R., Kinoshita, S., & Lisch, W. (2015). IC3D classification of corneal dystrophies–edition 2. *Cornea, 34*(2), 117–159. doi:10.1097/ICO.0000000000000307 PMID:25564336

Witschel, H., Fine, B. S., Grutzner, P., & McTigue, J. W. (1978). Congenital hereditary stromal dystrophy of the cornea. *Archives of Ophthalmology, 96*(6), 1043–1051. doi:10.1001/archopht.1978.03910050563015 PMID:350201

Wood, T. O., & Griffith, M. E. (1988). Surgery for corneal epithelial basement membrane dystrophy. *Ophthalmic Surgery, 19*, 20–24. PMID:3257554

Chapter 9
Disorders of the Sclera

ABSTRACT

Episcleritis and scleritis are the most common diseases among disorders of sclera. Episcleritis is a relatively common condition in the Middle Eastern population. The true incidence is difficult to determine, as episcleritis are self-limited conditions and patients generally do not seek professional advice. Scleritis is characterized by a chronic inflammatory response located in the sclera, which can spillover and involve adjacent ocular structures, mainly the cornea and the uvea. Scleritis can be seen at any age, but most commonly occurs in the fourth to sixth decades. It has a small female preponderance (1.6:1), and the condition is bilateral in 52% of cases· This chapter includes a severe infectious scleritis case with before and after treatment photos. The disease responded to antibiotic treatment, but later the patient presented with immune disease recurrence which responded to oral immunosuppressive treatment. Treatment photos are shown chronologically.

EPISCLERITIS

Episcleritis is a relatively benign, self-limiting condition affecting the outer layer of the eye. The condition can be unilateral or bilateral. The adult groups found either no significant sex predilection or a predominance of women affected. However, the pediatric group showed mostly male involvement[1]. Episcleritis can be simple (**diffuse** and **sectoral**) and **nodular** (Watson et al, 1976). Clinically, episcleritis represents with a fiery or brick bulbar injection, which can be diffuse or sectoral (Fig 1, 2). Nodular episcleritis has a well-demarcated and elevated area of episcleral tissue. The majority of cases are idiopathic; however, episcleritis can be associated with systemic (vascular disease and vasculitis, rheumatoid arthritis) and ocular diseases (ocular rosacea, keratoconjunctivitis sicca) (Watson et al, 1992). The natural history of simple episcleritis treatment is usually not necessary, especially when the disease is asymptomatic, nevertheless, in moderate to severe cases, topical nonsteroidal anti-inflammatory drops (NSAIDs), topical steroids, topical artificial tears can help to resolve the disease in 3-4 weeks. The cases associated with systemic disease can take on a more prolonged course with further recurrences.

DOI: 10.4018/978-1-7998-6937-5.ch009

Figure 1. Diffuse episcleritis

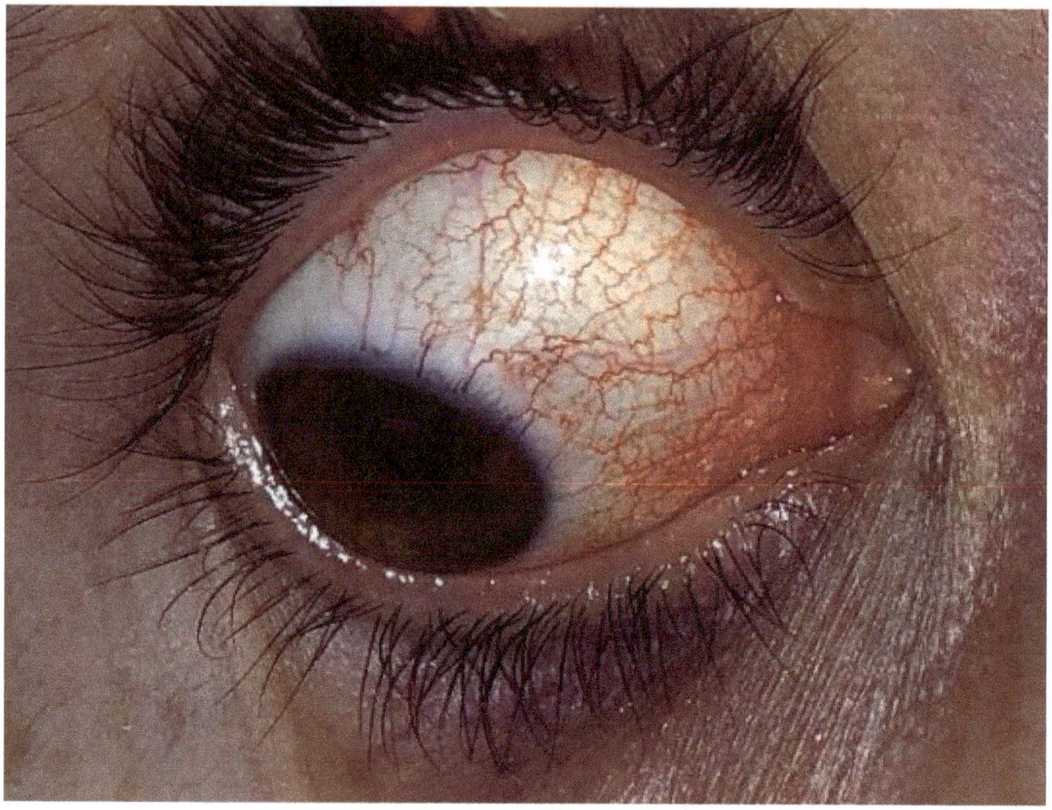

Figure 2. Sectoral episcleritis in both eyes associated with scleritis on the left eye in the same patient

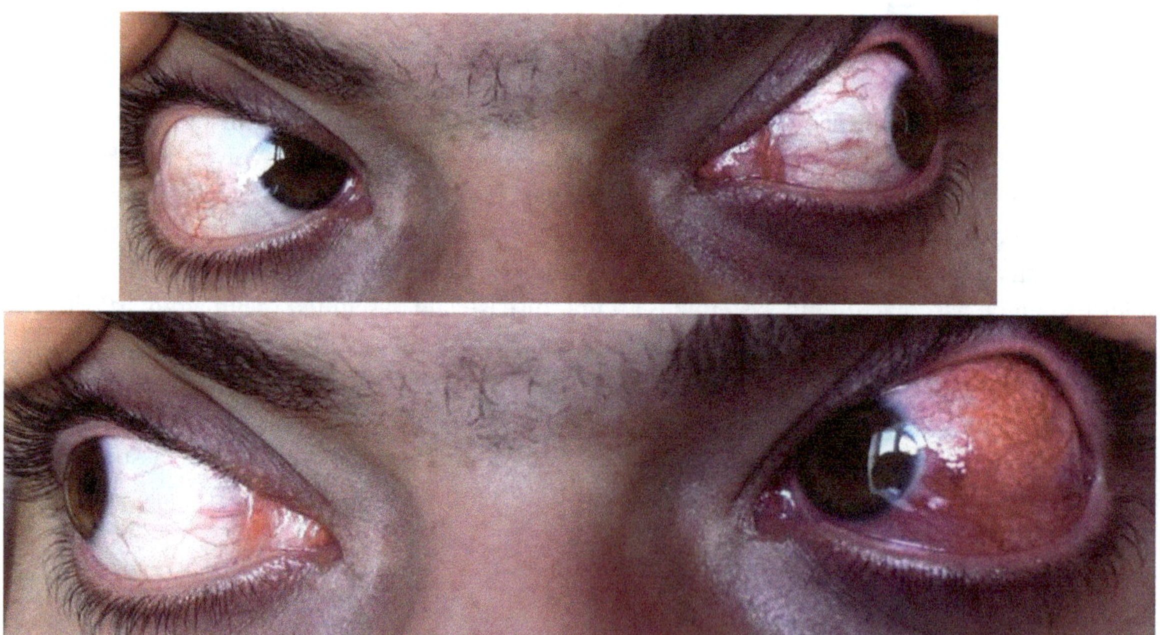

Scleritis

Scleritis can be divided into two groups: **noninfectious** and infectious. Noninfectious scleritis is most commonly caused by immune-mediated disorders, especially vasculitis (Fig 3, 4, 5, 8, 9). The second group, infectious scleritis, can be caused due to surgery or local extension from adjacent ocular tissues (McGavin et al, 1976; Akpek et al, 2004).

Immune-mediated scleritis is divided into two types: **anterior** and **posterior**. Anterior scleritis can be **diffuse**, **nodular**, **necrotizing with inflammation**, and **necrotizing without inflammation** (slceromalacia perforans) (Watson et al, 1976). Diffuse anterior scleritis is the most common clinical presentation. Clinically, distortion and tortuosity of the superficial and deep vascular networks with loss of the normal radial pattern are detected. Progression to either nodular or, less commonly, necrotizing scleritis is possible, but usually, most cases do not progress. Most infections of scleritis have a noninfectious origin. Corticosteroid are considered the mainstay of short-term treatment. In cases with a weak

Figure 3. Diffuse scleritis associated with Sjogren syndrome

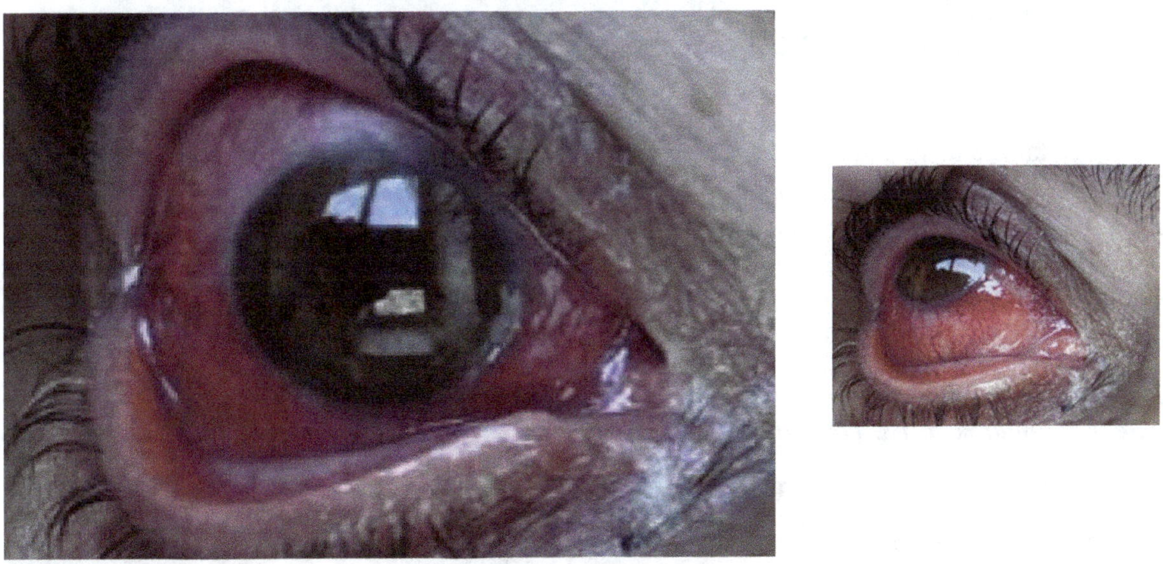

Figure 4. Sectorial scleritis associated with rheumatoid arthritis

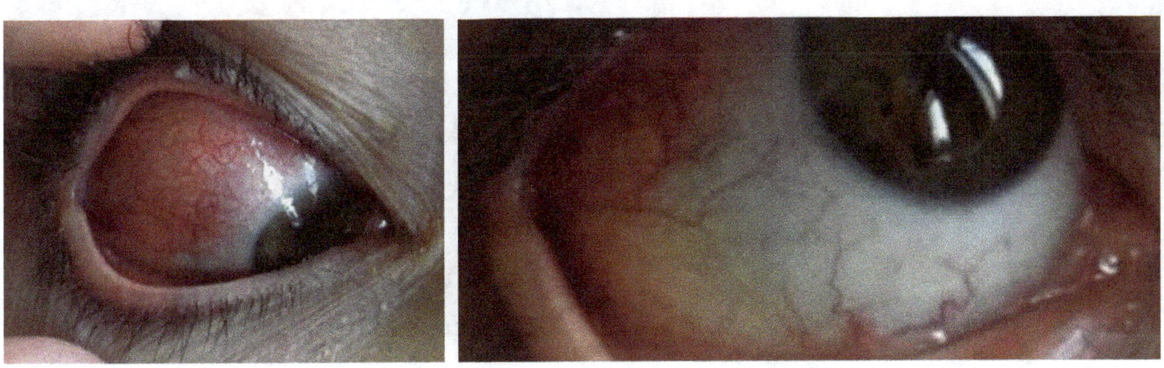

Figure 5. The hands of the same patient

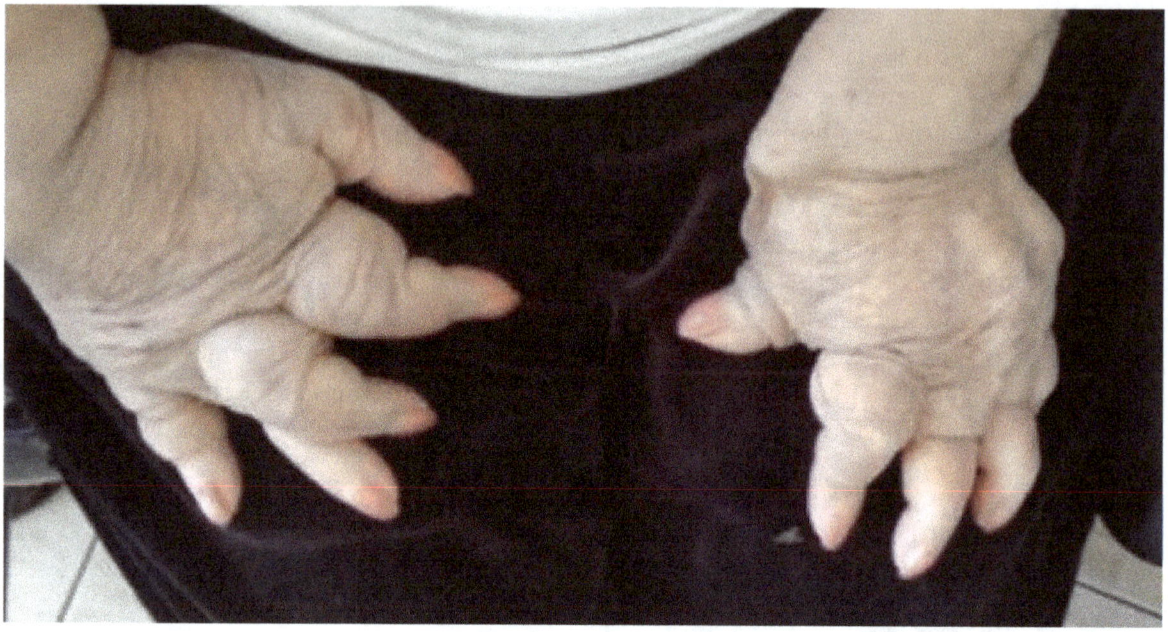

response or failure to steroids, corticosteroid-sparing immunosuppressive medications are considered (Azathioprine, Cyclosporine, Mycophenolate mofetil, etc.) Nowadays, biologic agents are progressively used in the management of scleritis, irresponsive to conventional therapies.

Nodular anterior scleritis appears as a firm, immobile, from yellow to deep red nodule. The nodule is usually localized in the interpalpebral zone, close to the limbus. The underlying sclera may become transparent, but not necrotic (Fig 6, 7) (Tuft et al, 1991).

Figure 6. Nodular scleritis. The red nodule is seen

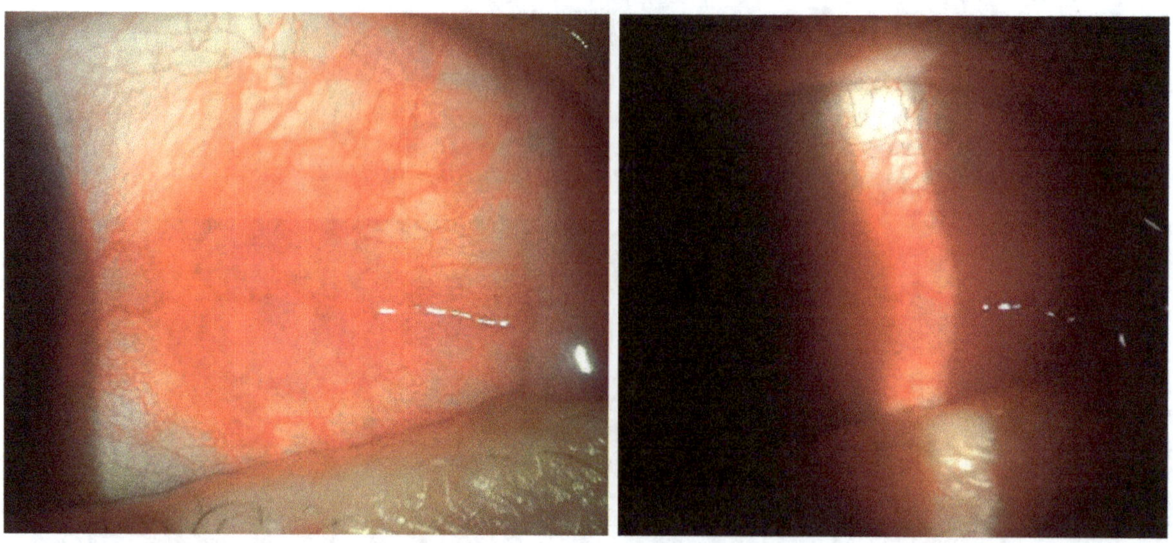

Figure 7. Nodular scleritis. The red nodule is seen near the limbus

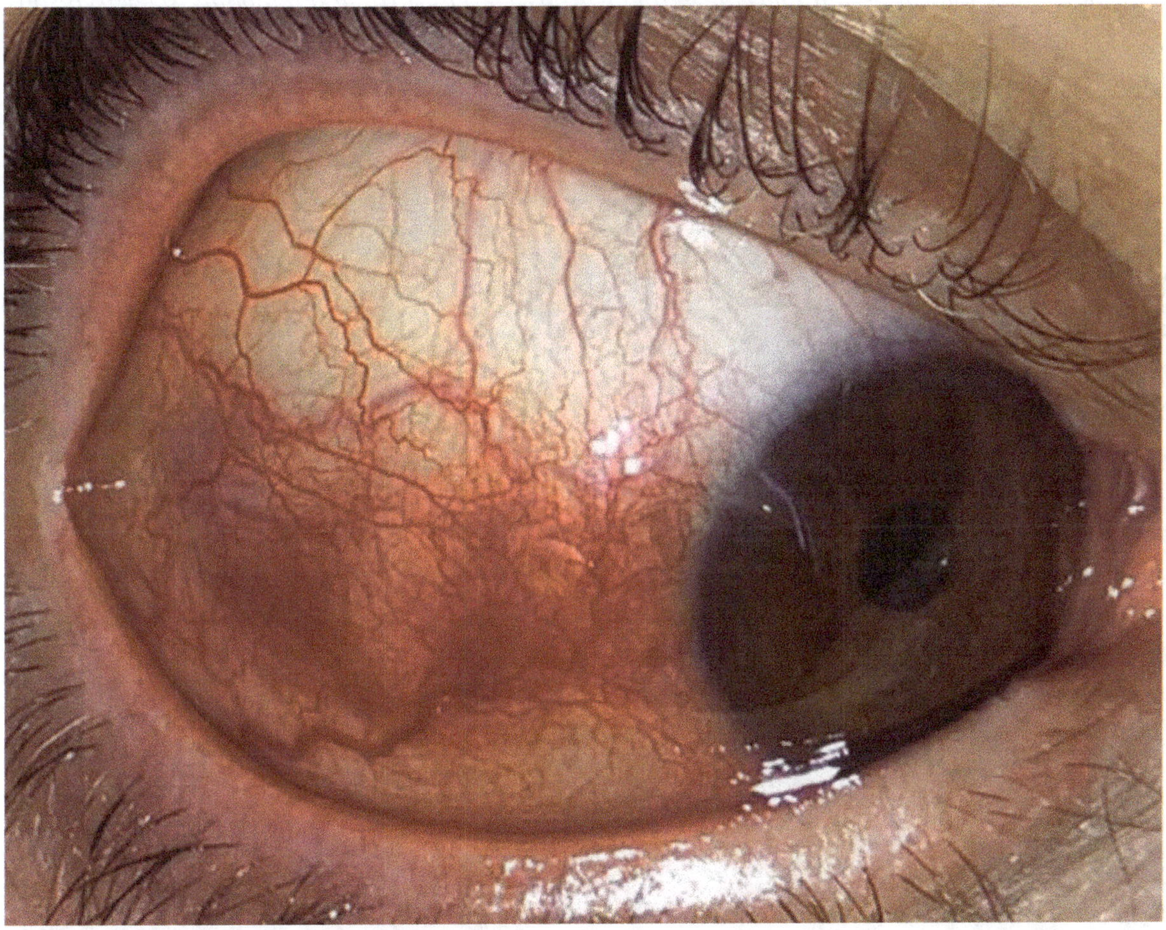

Figure 8. **Sectoral scleritis** *with peripheral corneal involvement. The edematous peripheral cornea is seen in the right photo*

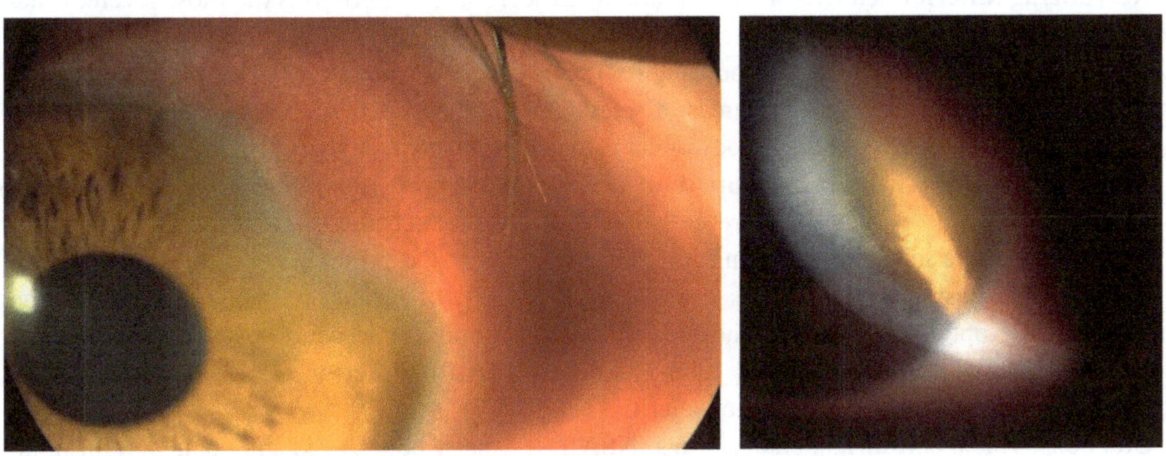

Figure 9. The same patient after 3 months of treatment with weekly injections of sub-Tenon Betamethasone, oral Azathioprine, topical steroid, and non-steroidal drops. Developed lipid keratopathy, scleritis resolved

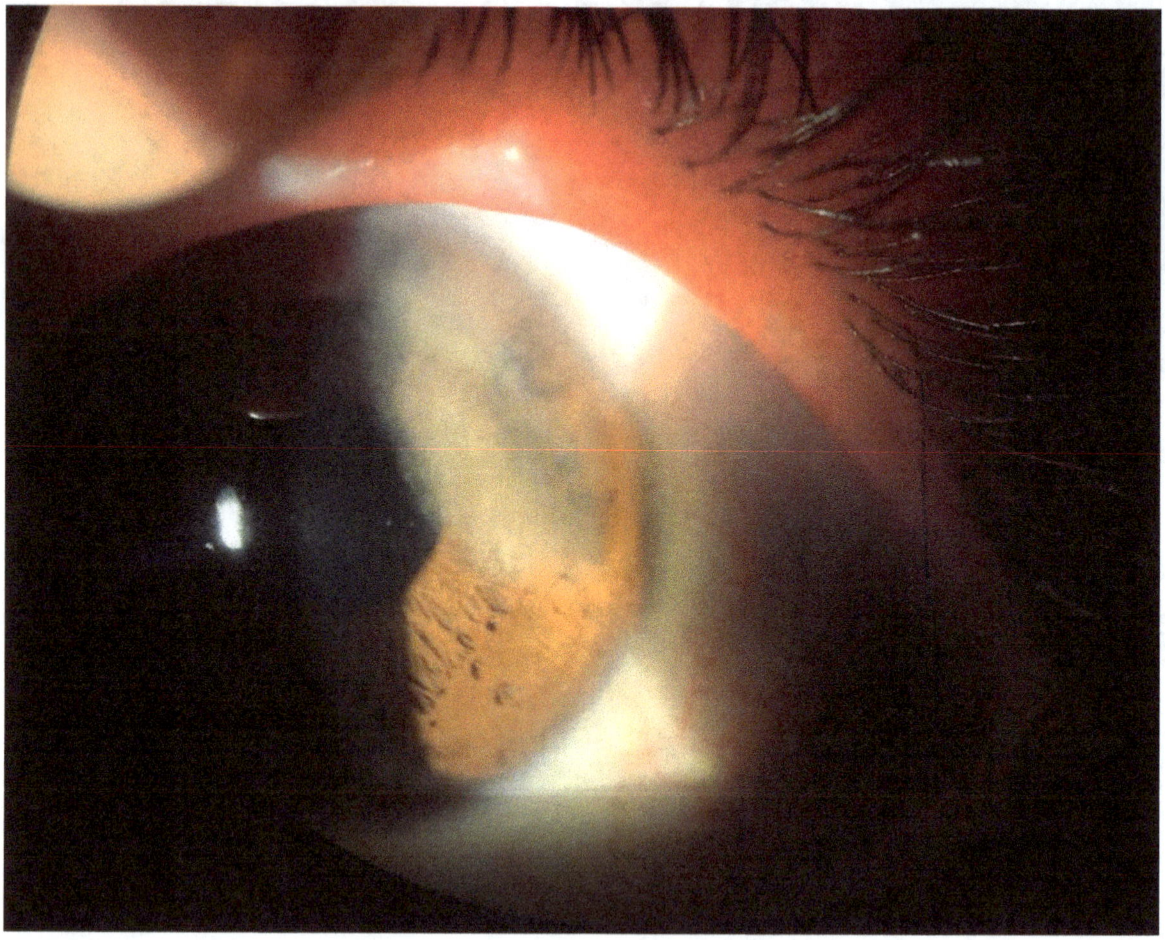

Necrotizing anterior scleritis with inflammation (necrotizing scleritis) is the most severe, usually bilateral scleritis. It is generally associated with systemic vasculitis (Fig 14), particularly with Wegener's granulomatosis (granulomatosis with polyangiitis) (Fig 10-12) (Hakine t al, 1991; Sainz et al, 2012). Examination reveals white, avascular areas of sclera and conjunctiva, with surrounding scleral edema and congestion. Some areas of ciliary body or choroid may remain covered only by conjunctiva (Fig 13).

Necrotizing scleritis without inflammation (**scleromalacia perforans**) is characterized by an almost total lack of symptoms. Patients may present with blurred vision because of astigmatism or may notice a discoloration of the sclera (15) (Hakin et al, 1991).

Patients with **posterior scleritis** may complain about loss of vision and pain. Posterior segment findings include optic nerve edema, choroidal folds, thickening, optic neuritis, serous and exudative retinal detachment, etc (Calthrope et al, 1988; Ronfas et al, 2010). Posterior scleritis may be difficult to diagnose unless accompanied by anterior scleritis (Fig 16, 17).

Oral nonsteroidal anti-inflammatory drugs (NSAIDs) usually help by reducing pain and inflammation in non-necrotizing scleritis. Topical corticosteroids and topical NSAIDs are generally inadequate in

Figure 10. Necrotizing scleritis with inflammation associated with granulomatosis with polyangiitis (Wegener's disease). Nasal deformity (saddle nose) is seen

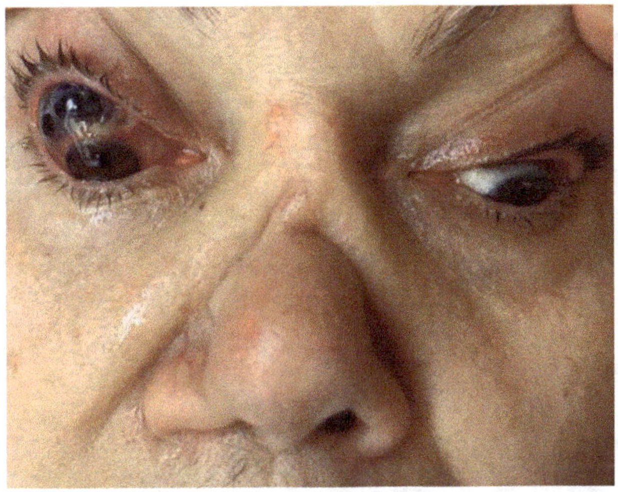

Figure 11. The same patient under a slit lamp. The scleral necrosis/thinning with uveal ectasia (right photo) and peripheral keratitis (left photo) are seen

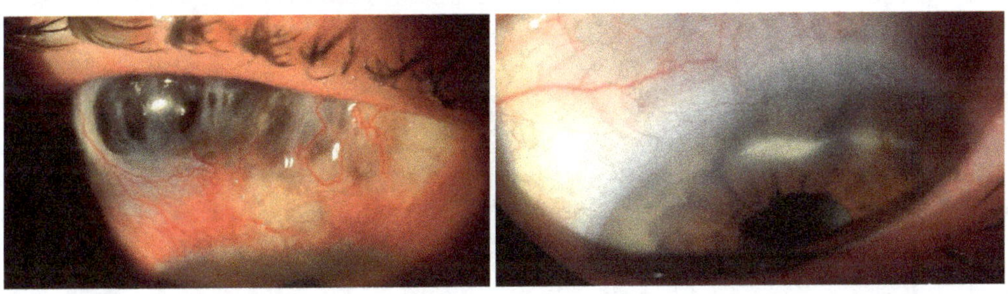

Figure 12. The same patient after 2 months of treatment with oral Cytoxan, Azathioprine, and lubricating drops. The inflammation has subsided

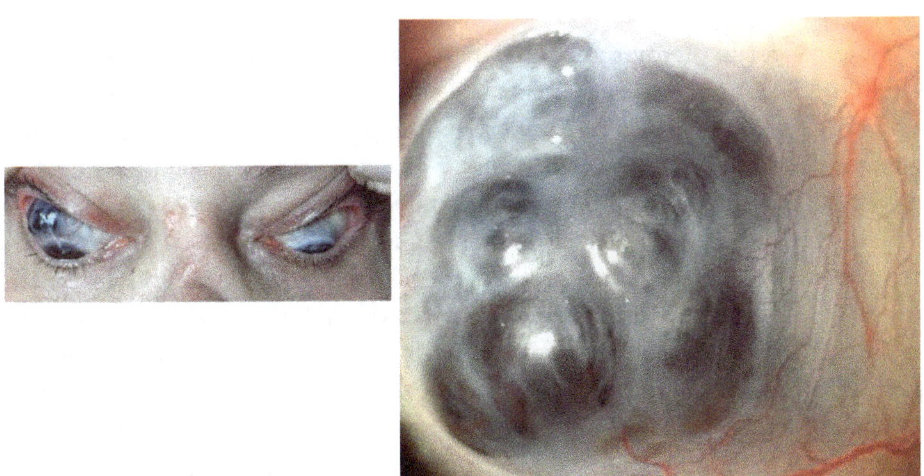

Figure 13. Bilateral necrotizing scleritis associated with RA in remission. The choroidal tissue is seen through the thin sclera

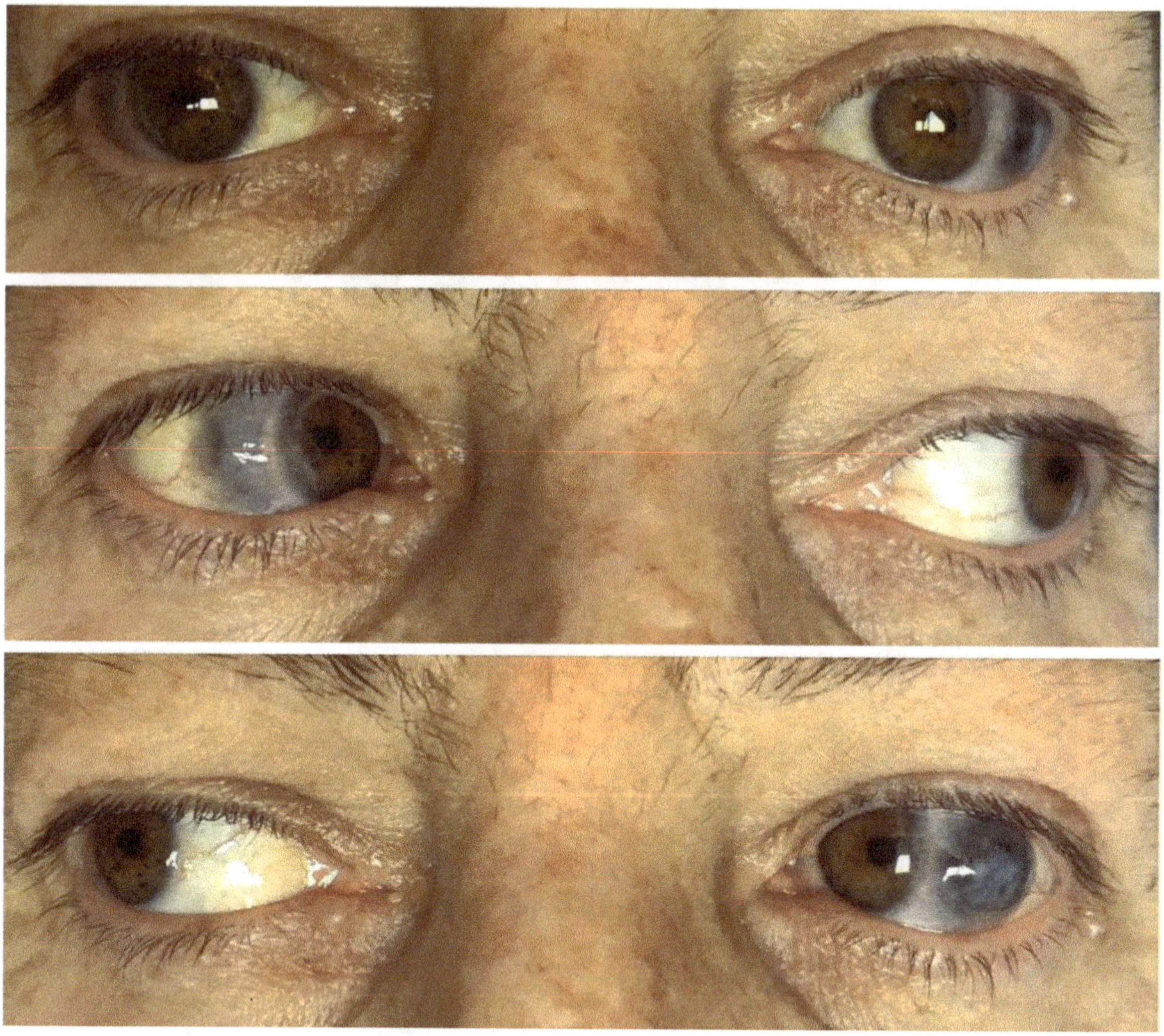

scleritis cases. Systemic corticosteroids are prescribed in some cases of severe non-necrotizing scleritis unresponsive to oral NSAIDs, and in necrotizing scleritis. Oral prednisone at a starting dose of 1 mg/kg per day is appropriate, followed by a slow taper according to response. Subconjunctival injections of triamcinolone may be a safe and effective treatment for resistant, non-necrotizing noninfectious anterior scleritis (Roufas et al, 2010). Systemic immunosuppressive agents are applied in cases of severe necrotizing scleritis, and scleritis of any type in the setting of GPA or polyarteritis nodosa (Sainz et al, 2012). Systemic immunosuppression may be required in over 25% of scleritis cases[14]. Use of methotrexate (up to 20–25 mg/week), azathioprine (starting dose of approximately 2.5 mg/kg/day and mycophenolate mofetil (2–3 g/day) in the therapy of scleritis is well documented (Jachens et al, 2008; Larkin et al, 1999). Biologic agents are now more widely utilized for their safety and efficacy in controlling chronic scleritis. These agents include the tumor necrosis factor inhibitors, etanercept, infliximab, adalimumab, and certolizumab pegol, the antilymphocyte medications; rituximab and alemtuzumab, and the inter-

Figure 14. Bilateral necrotizing scleritis in remission associated with scleroderma

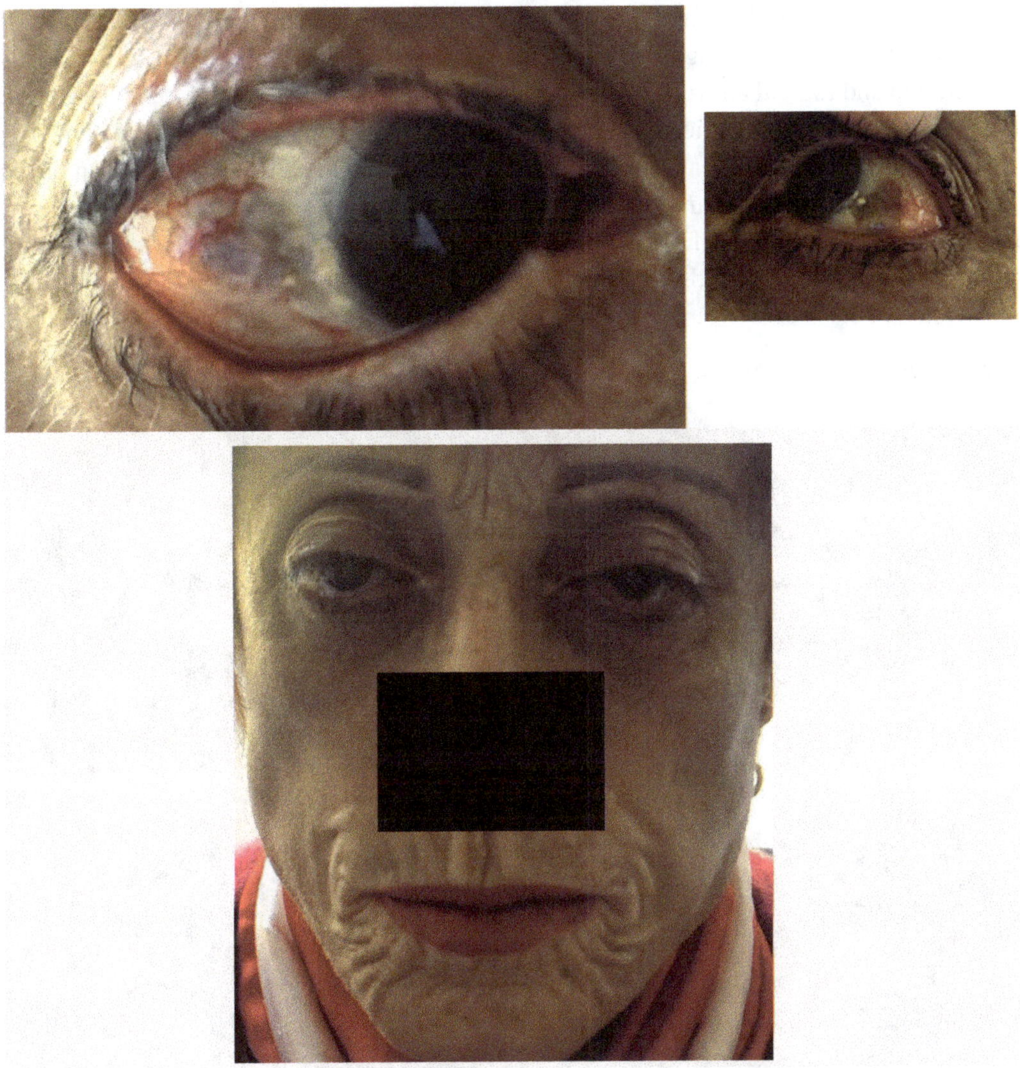

leukin-1 receptor antagonist; anakinra (Sainz et al, 2012). The management of posterior scleritis is controversial. Oral NSAIDs, oral corticosteroids, immunosuppressive agents, and some biologic agents have all been documented to be successful. In cases of necrotizing scleritis and scleromalacia perforans, surgical management may rarely be necessary. Tectonic scleral and peripheral corneal patch grafting can be performed with autologous or homologous sclera, fascia lata, dermis, periostium, aortic tissue, and synthetic material (Gore-Tex).

Infections of the sclera are rare. The most likely source of scleral infection is spread from contiguous ocular structures. Most cases of **infectious scleritis** result from severe bacterial infections of the cornea; however, viral, fungal, and parasitic keratitis may also evolve into sclerokeratitis. Gram-negative bacteria, most commonly Pseudomonas aeruginosa, can spread from the cornea to the sclera (Raber et al, 1981; Lebensohn et al, 1974; Cobo et al, 1983). Infectious scleritis caused by Staphylococcus aureus, Streptococcus pneumoniae has also been reported (Fig 18-22). Rarely, viruses, fungi, and parasites can cause scleritis. Effective treatment of infectious scleritis usually requires culture or pathologic evidence of a causative organism. Usually, clinicians add intravenous antibiotics when infection of the sclera is associated with keratitis. The management of fungal scleritis is exceptionally difficult in most cases. Prolonged systemic and topical antifungal therapy such as oral itraconazole and topical amphotericin B should be initiated but may not eradicate the infection. A combination of voriconazole and caspofungin has been used to treat Aspergillus flavus scleritis (Howell et al, 2005). Severe destruction of the cornea or scleral perforation may require lamellar or full thickness grafting (Huang et al, 2000) Despite these aggressive treatments, around 60% of eyes with infectious scleritis may require evisceration, enucleation, or have no light perception (Reynolds et al, 1991).

Figure 15. Scleromalacia perforans. Scleral thinning with underlying choroidea is seen

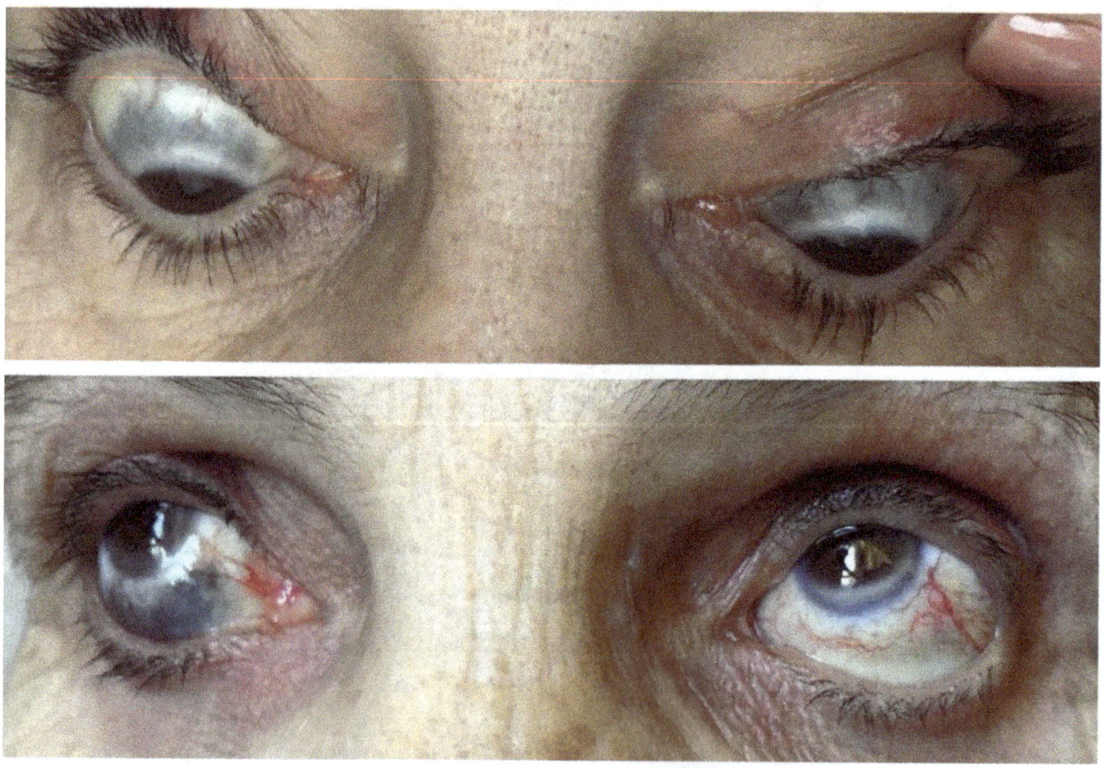

Figure 16. B-scan of a patient with bilateral posterior scleritis. The choroidal thickening is shown

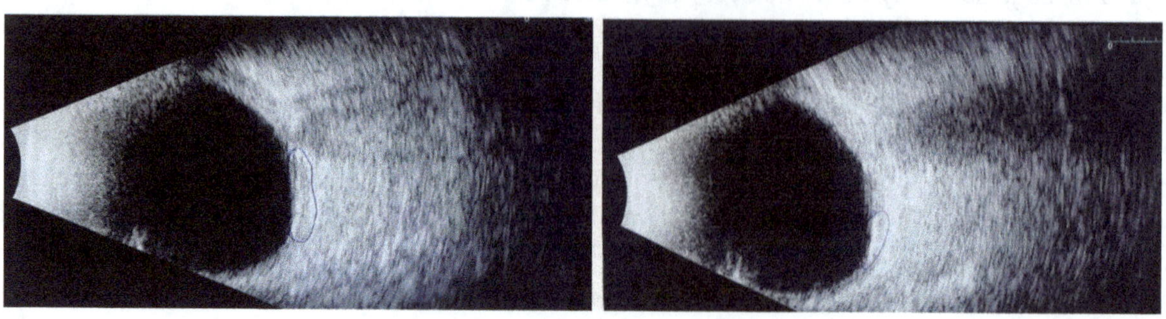

Figure 17. The fundus photography of the same patient. The optic disc edema and choroidal folds are present in both eyes

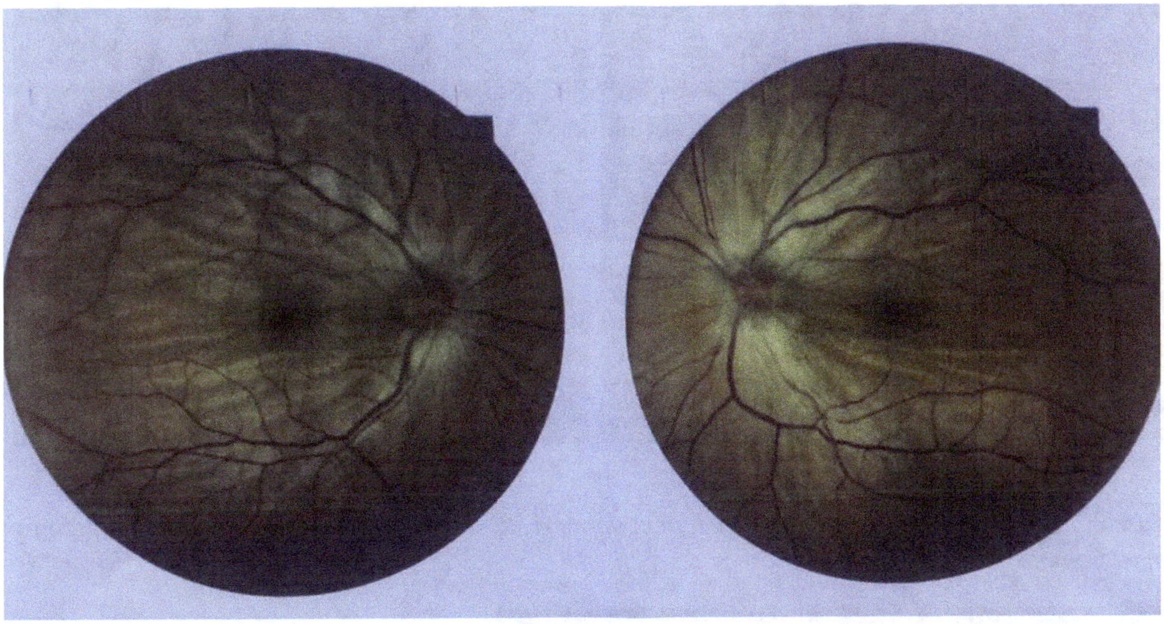

Figure 18. Infectious scleritis caused by Streptococcus pneumoniae in patient with h/o bilateral immune-mediated scleritis. Mucopurulent discharge, scleral melt and peripheral corneal ulceration are seen

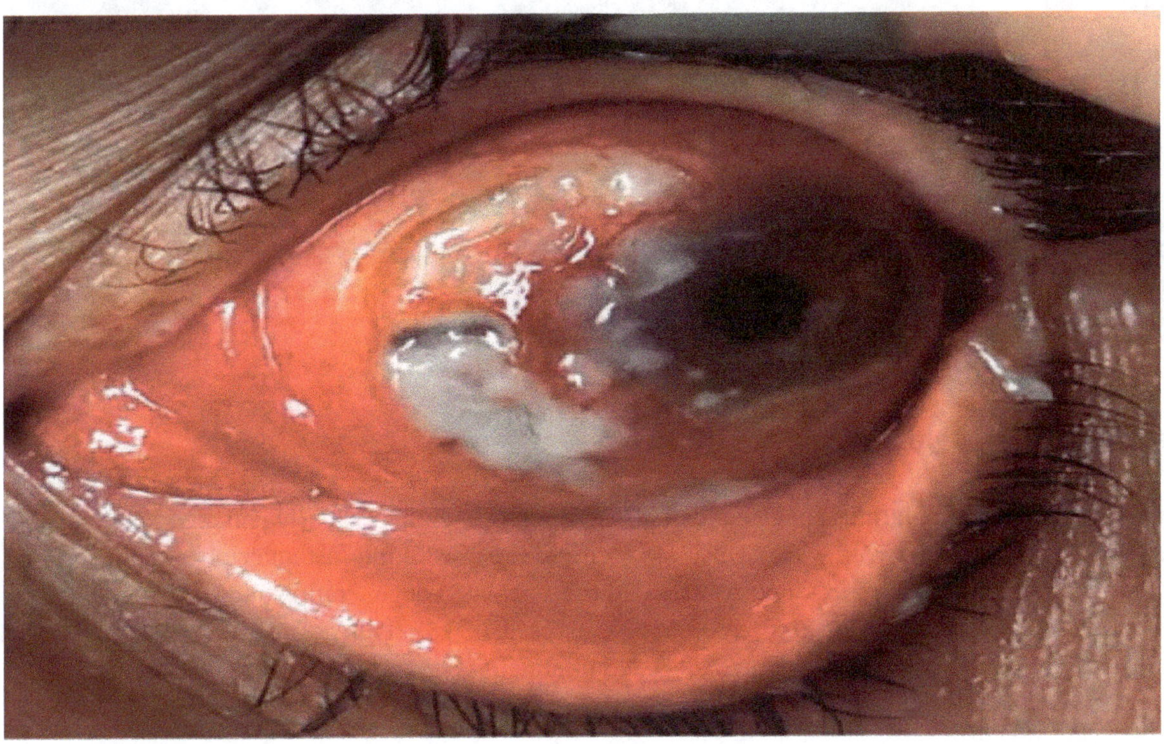

Figure 19. the same eye 7 days after antibiotic treatment with topical Tobramycin, cycloplegics, lubricants, intravenous Ciprofloxacin, oral Doxycycline, and Erythromycin eye ointment before sleep

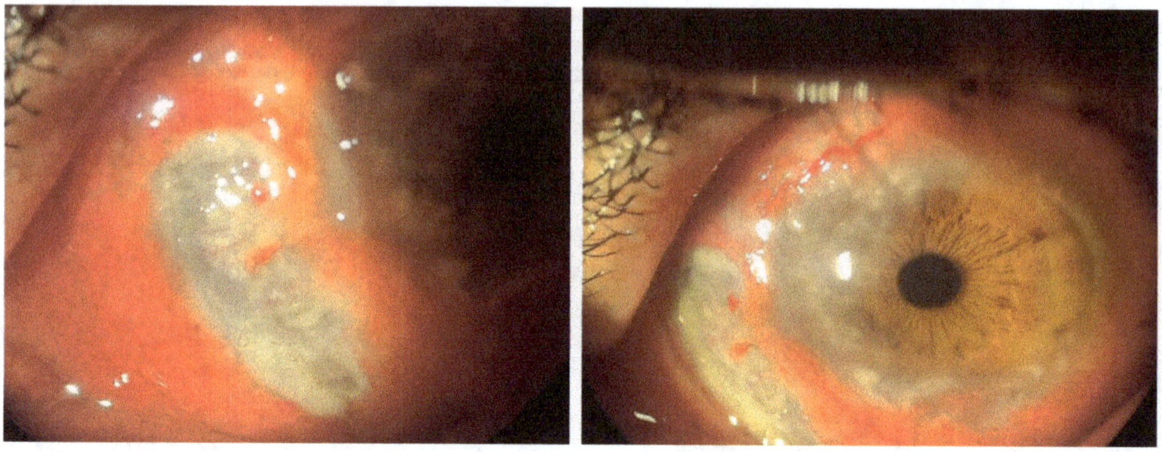

Figure 20. The same eye 6 weeks after treatment under a slit lamp (right photo) and without magnification (left photo)

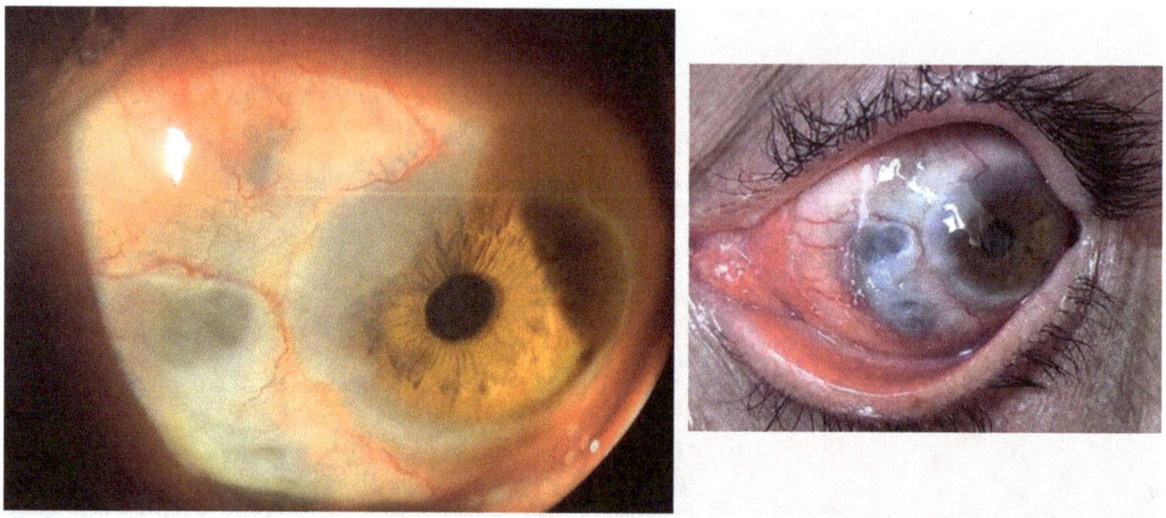

Senile Scleral Calcific Plaques

Senile scleral calcific plaques are an incidental finding in the sclera of elderly patients. Scleral plaques are usually described as ovoid, well-demarcated, greyish lesions found just anterior to the insertion of the horizontal recti. Their appearance is attributed to age-related degeneration and further calcification of the scleral hyaline (Alorainy et al, 2000 Manschot et al, 1978). This degeneration does not lead to structural weakening of the globe (Fig 23, 24). No treatment is required.

Figure 21. The same patient. Recurrence of immune scleritis after 3 months. Scleral melting is seen

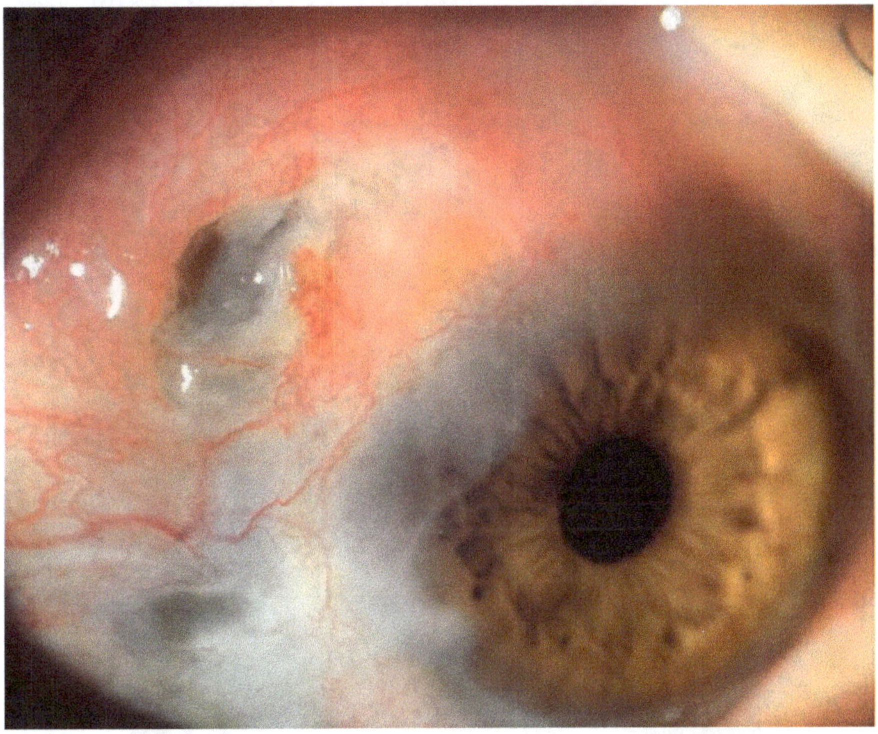

Figure 22. The same eye after 1 month of immunosuppressive treatment with Azathioprine 50mg bid

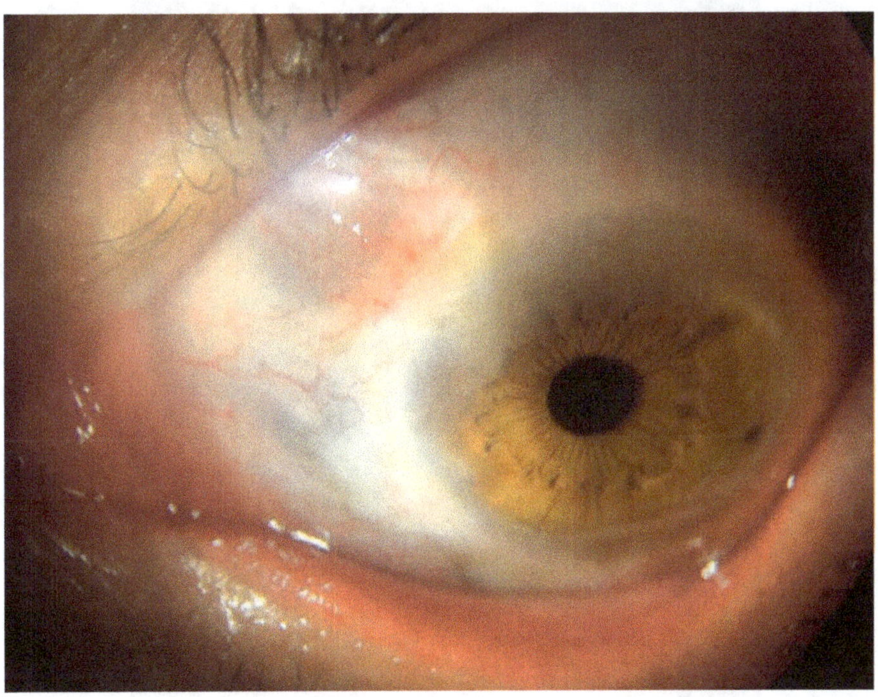

Figure 23. Senile scleral plaques are seen bilaterally, nasally, and temporally

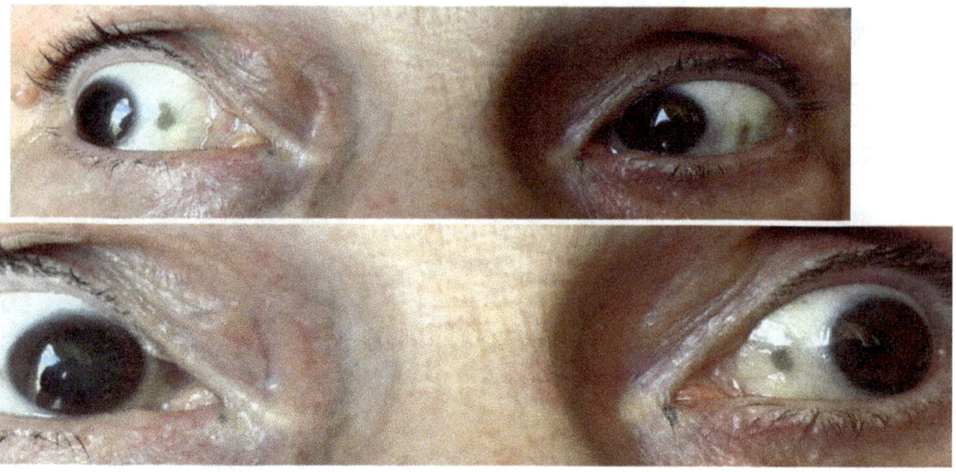

Figure 24. The same patient. Slit lamp view of calcific plaque

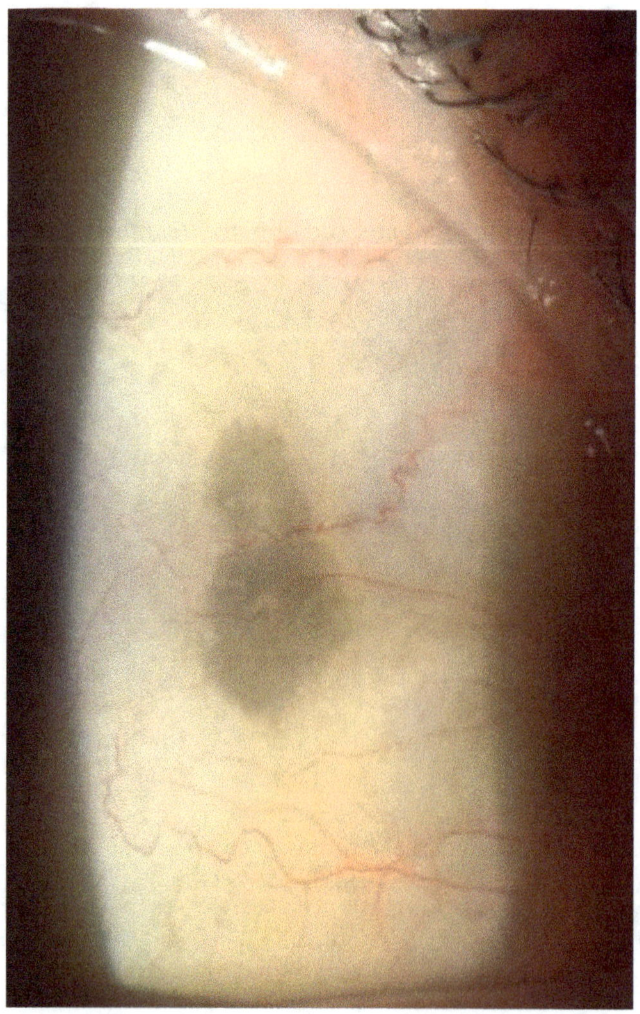

REFERENCES

Akpek, E. K., Thorne, J. E., & Qazi, F. A. (2004). Evaluation of patients with scleritis for systemic disease. *Ophthalmology, 111*, 501–506.

Alorainy. (2000). Senile scleral plaques: CT. *Neuroradiology, 42*, 145–148.

Benson, W. E. (1988). Posterior scleritis. *Survey of Ophthalmology, 32*, 297–316.

Calthorpe, C. M., Watson, P. G., & McCartney, A. C. E. (1988). Posterior scleritis: A clinical and histopathological survey. *Eye, 2*, 267–277.

Cobo, M. (1983). Inflammation of the sclera. *International Ophthalmology Clinics, 23*, 159–171.

Hakin, K. M., & Watson, P. G. (1991). Systemic associations of scleritis. *International Ophthalmology Clinics, 31*, 111–129.

Howell, A., Midturi, J., & Sierra-Hoffman, M. (2005). Aspergillus flavus scleritis: Successful treatment with voriconazole and caspofungin. *Medical Mycology, 43*, 651–655.

Huang, F. C., Huang, S. P., & Tseng, S. H. (2000). Management of infectious scleritis after pterygium excision. *Cornea, 19*, 34–39.

Jabs, D. A., Mudun, A., & Dunn, J. P. (2000). Episcleritis and scleritis: Clinical features and treatment results. *American Journal of Ophthalmology, 130*, 469–476.

Jachens & Chu. (2008). Retrospective review of methotrexate therapy in the treatment of chronic, noninfectious, nonnecrotizing scleritis. *Am J Ophthalmol., 145*, 487-492.

Larkin & Lightman. (1999). Mycophenolate mofetil. A useful immunosuppressive in inflammatory eye disease. *Ophthalmology, 106*, 370-374.

Lebensohn, J. E. (1974). Suppurative conjunctivitis with scleral involvement. *American Journal of Ophthalmology, 78*, 856–857.

Manschot, W. A. (1978). Senile scleral plaques and senile scleromalacia. *The British Journal of Ophthalmology, 62*, 376–380.

McGavin, D. D., Williamson, J., & Forrester, J. V. (1976). Episcleritis and scleritis: A study of their clinical manifestations and association with rheumatoid arthritis. *The British Journal of Ophthalmology, 60*, 192–226.

Nguyen, Q. D., & Foster, C. S. (1999). Scleral patch graft in the management of necrotizing scleritis. *International Ophthalmology Clinics, 39*, 109–131.

Raber, I. M., Laibson, P. R., & Kurz, G. H. (1981). Pseudomonas corneoscleral ulcers. *American Journal of Ophthalmology, 92*, 353–362.

Reynolds, M. G., & Alfonso, E. (1991). Treatment of infectious scleritis and keratoscleritis. *American Journal of Ophthalmology, 112*, 543–547.

Roufas, A., Jalaludin, B., & Gaskin, C. (2010). Subconjunctival triamcinolone treatment for non-necrotizing anterior scleritis. *The British Journal of Ophthalmology*, *94*, 743–747.

Sainz de la Maza, M., Molina, N., & Gonzalez-Gonzalez, L. A. (2012). Clinical characteristics of a large cohort of patients with scleritis and episcleritis. *Ophthalmology*, *119*, 43–50.

Sainz de la Maza, M., Molina, N., & Gonzalez-Gonzalez, L. A. (2012). Scleritis therapy. *Ophthalmology*, *119*, 51–58.

Sainz de la Maza, M., Molina, N., & Gonzalez-Gonzalez, L. A. (2012). Scleritis therapy. *Ophthalmology*, *119*, 51–58.

Sainz de la Maza, M., Tauber, J., & Foster, C. S. (2012). *The Sclera*. Springer-Verlag.

Sainz de la Maza, N. S. (1994). Severity of scleritis and episcleritis. *Ophthalmology*, *101*(2), 389–396. doi:10.1016/S0161-6420(94)31325-X PMID:8115160

Thorne, J. E., Jabs, D. A., & Qazi, F. A. (2005). Mycophenolate mofetil therapy for inflammatory eye disease. *Ophthalmology*, *112*, 1472–1477.

Tuft, S. J., & Watson, P. G. (1991). Progression of scleral disease. *Ophthalmology*, *98*, 467.

Watson, P. G. (1992). *Diseases of the sclera and episclera. In Clinical ophthalmology* (rev ed). Lippincott Philadelphia.

Watson, P. G., & Hayreh, S. S. (1976). Scleritis and episcleritis. *The British Journal of Ophthalmology*, *60*, 163.

Chapter 10
Lens and Anterior Uvea

ABSTRACT

This chapter illustrates photos of clinical signs seen in uveitis and interesting cases of lens pathologies. Anterior uveitis is the inflammation of the iris and the ciliary body. Anterior uveitis can be idiopathic, isolated, or associated with systemic diseases. The clinical findings observed in anterior uveitis include keratic precipitates, inflammatory cells and flare in anterior chamber, hypopyon, rarely hyphema, miosis, iris nodules and atrophy, synechiae, and band keratopathy in chronic cases (shown in corneal degenerations chapter). The inflammation in anterior uveitis is almost always immune. Treatment includes steroid eye drops, cycloplegic drops, sub-Tenon steroid injections when cystoid macular edema is present. Chronic macular edema can be treated with intravitreal Triamcinolone injection and Dexamethasone implants. In cases of refractory anterior uveitis or associated immune systemic diseases, immunomodulatory treatment or biologic agents are prescribed.

ANTERIOR UVEITIS

The term **anterior uveitis** is used to describe inflammation confined to the iris (iritis), or ciliary body (cyclitis), or both (iridocyclitis) (Jabs et al, 2005). Characteristic symptoms of acute anterior uveitis include pain, redness, and photophobia. Blurred vision may be seen in cases of severe inflammation with fibrin or with reactive cystoid macular edema (CME) (Hogan et al, 1959).

Keratic precipitates (KPs) are the most common corneal findings in anterior uveitis. They consist of inflammatory cells that accumulate on the corneal endothelium. Usually, they have a triangular configuration (Arlt's triangle) with the base down. Two types of KPs have been described; nongranulomatous and granulomatous (Fig 1). Small to medium-sized KPs are usually composed of lymphocytes and have white or slightly pigmented, round appearance, or stellate with fine filaments seen adjacent to the precipitates (Fig 2). Mutton-fat or granulomatous KPs are large collections of macrophages. Clinically, KPs are large with greasy appearance, and they may increase in size by coalescence. The presence of mutton-fat KPs and iris nodules is strong evidence of a granulomatous inflammatory response (Fig 3).

DOI: 10.4018/978-1-7998-6937-5.ch010

Figure 1. Nongranulomatous and granulomatous KPs are seen

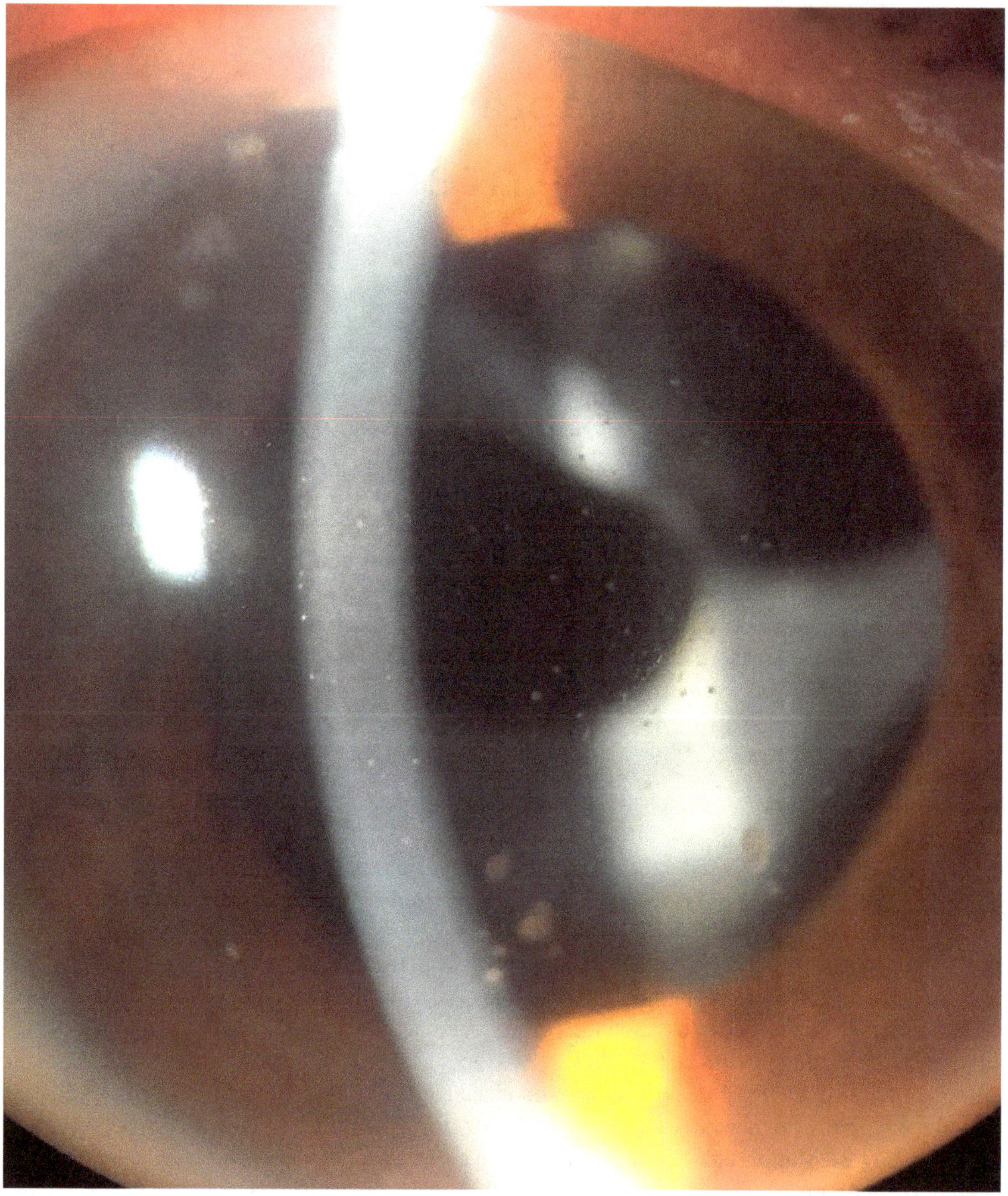

The presence of **inflammatory cells and flare** in the anterior chamber is a hallmark of anterior uveitis (Fig 4, 5). In severe cases inflammatory cells may collect in the inferior portion of the anterior chamber to form a **hypopyon** (Fig 6) (Jabs et al, 2005). HLA-B27, Behcet's disease, and endophthalmitis are the most common causes of hypopyon uveitis.

Figure 2. Stellate KPs associated with Fuchs uveitis syndrome. Small, diffusely localized KPs on endothelium with fine filaments are seen

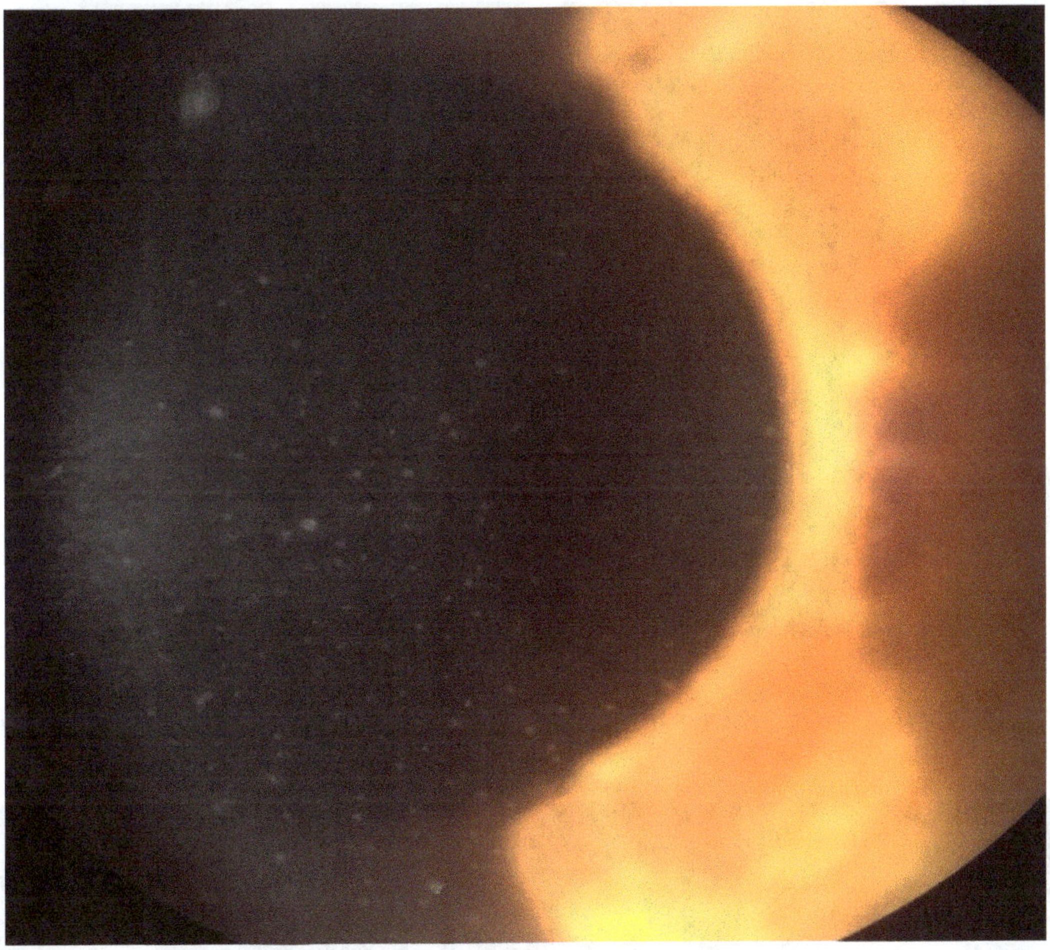

Figure 3. GKPs associated with sarcoidosis. Right and left eyes of the same patient

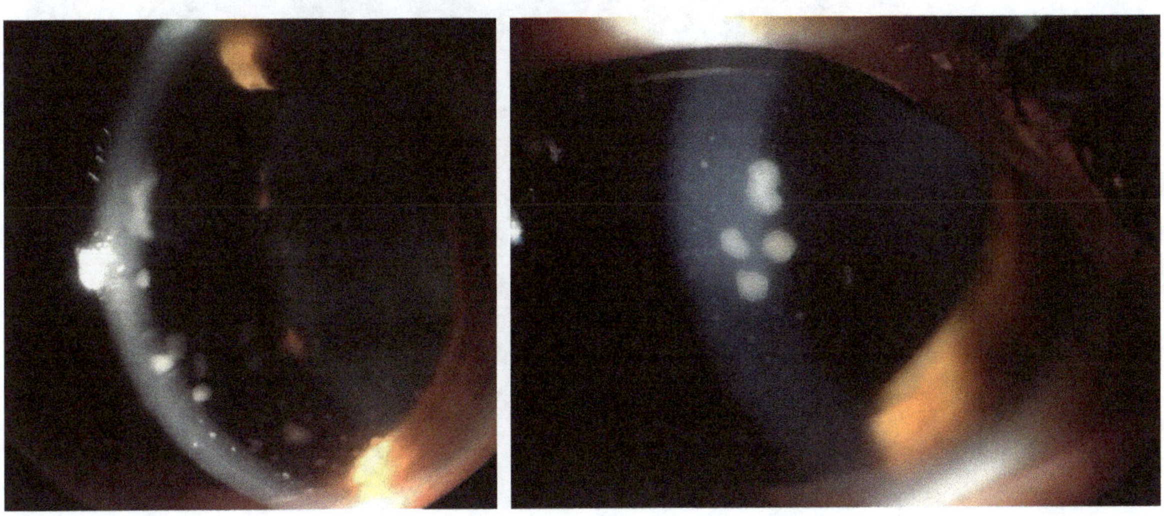

Figure 4. Moderate inflammatory reaction in the anterior chamber in a patient with idiopathic anterior uveitis

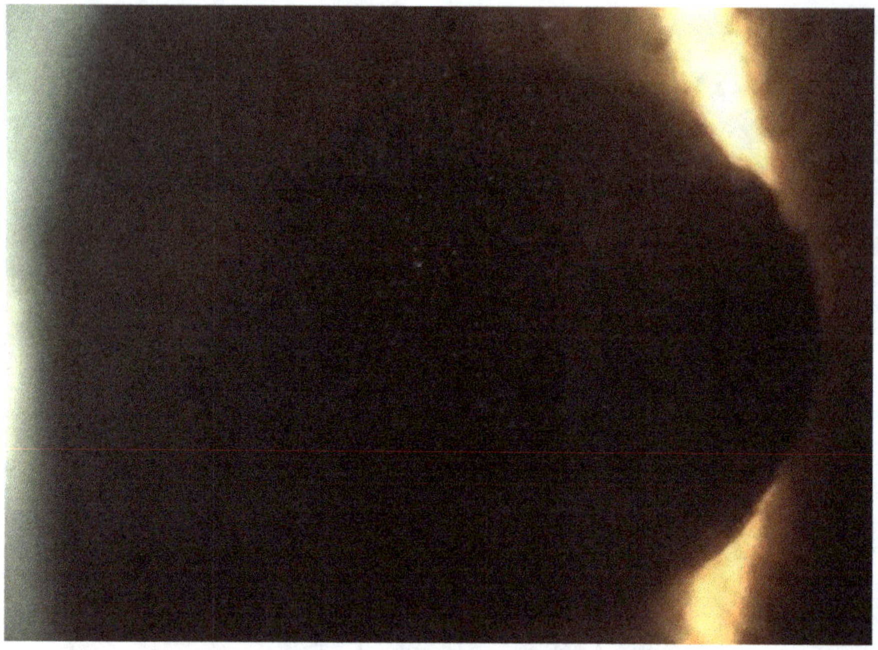

Figure 5. Severe inflammatory reaction in the anterior chamber in a patient with HLA-B27 associated uveitis

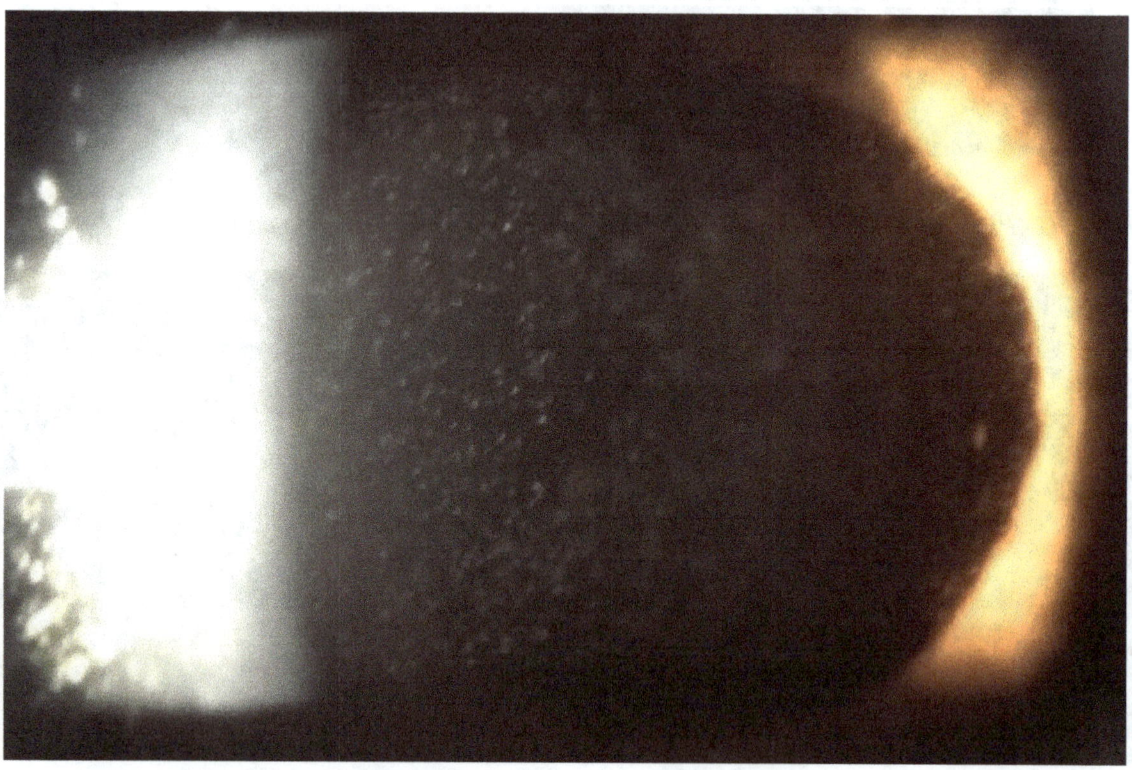

Figure 6. Patient with Behcet's disease; hypopyon with fibrin, aphthous stomatitis, and erythema nodosum skin changes are seen as well as Sectoral iris atrophy associated with herpes simplex uveitis

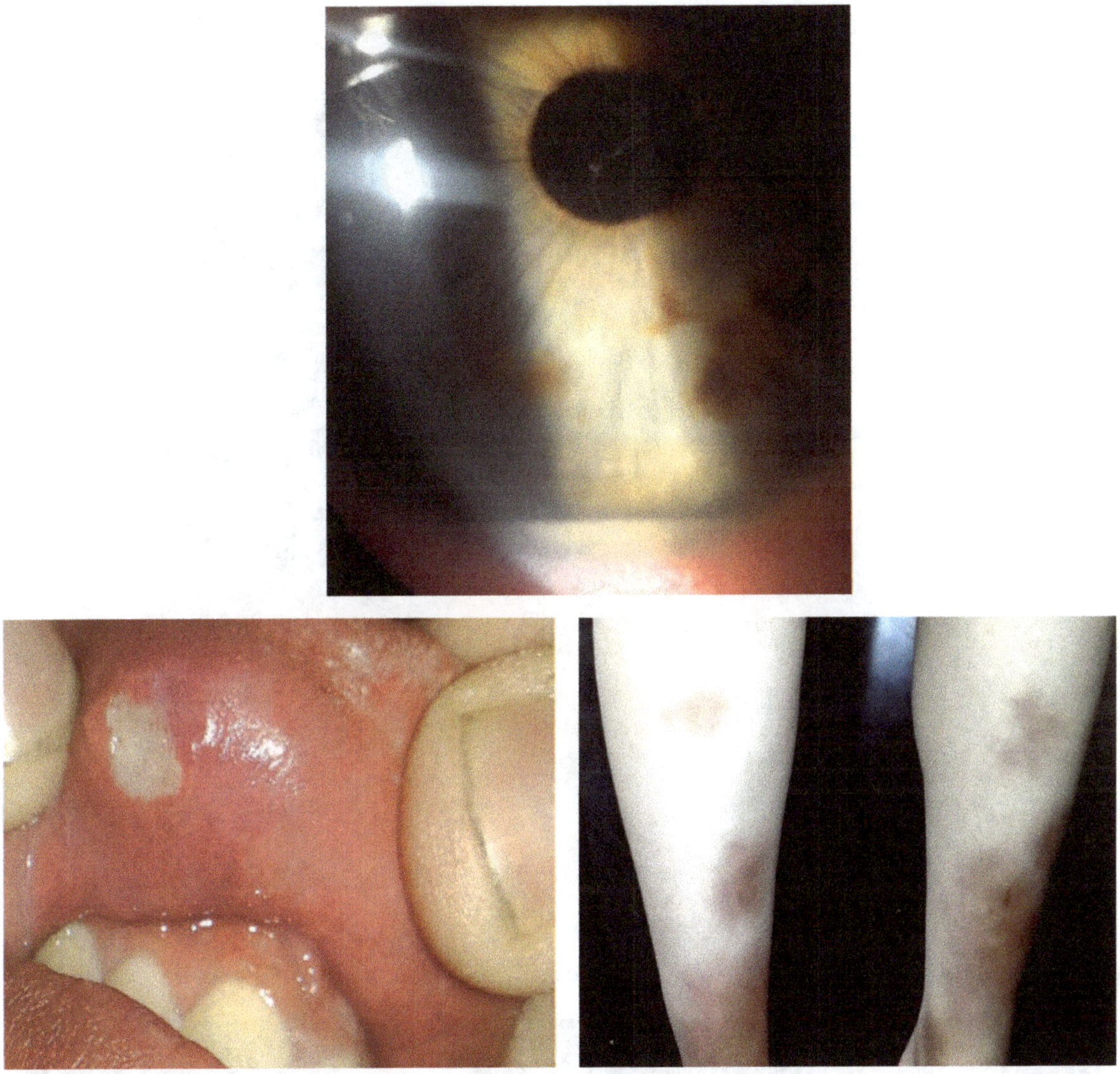

Another sign of anterior uveitis is **iris atrophy**. Diffuse stromal or pigment epithelial atrophy is a characteristic of chronic inflammation (Fig 9). Sectoral iris atrophy is most commonly seen in uveitis associated with herpes zoster or herpes simplex virus (Fig 6, 7) (Sugita et al, 2008). Patchy atrophy typically develops after the resolution of iris nodules (Fig 8). Atrophy of anterior iris stroma with loss of the normal pattern of iris crypts is typical for Fuchs uveitis syndrome (Fig 10-14).

Iris nodules are focal collections of inflammatory cells located in the iris stroma. They are commonly seen in granulomatous forms of uveitis. Koeppe nodules are located on the pupillary margin. They can be present in both granulomatous and nongranulomatous uveitis, whereas Busacca nodules are pathognomonic of granulomatous disease and are found throughout the iris. Iris nodules may also be present during the early stages of Fuchs heterochromic iridocyclitis, common in the Asian population (Fig 15, 16) (Rothova et al, 1994).

Figure 7. Iris atrophy associated with herpes simplex uveitis. The local atrophy is seen at the peripupillary dark zone. The moderate mydriasis is noted

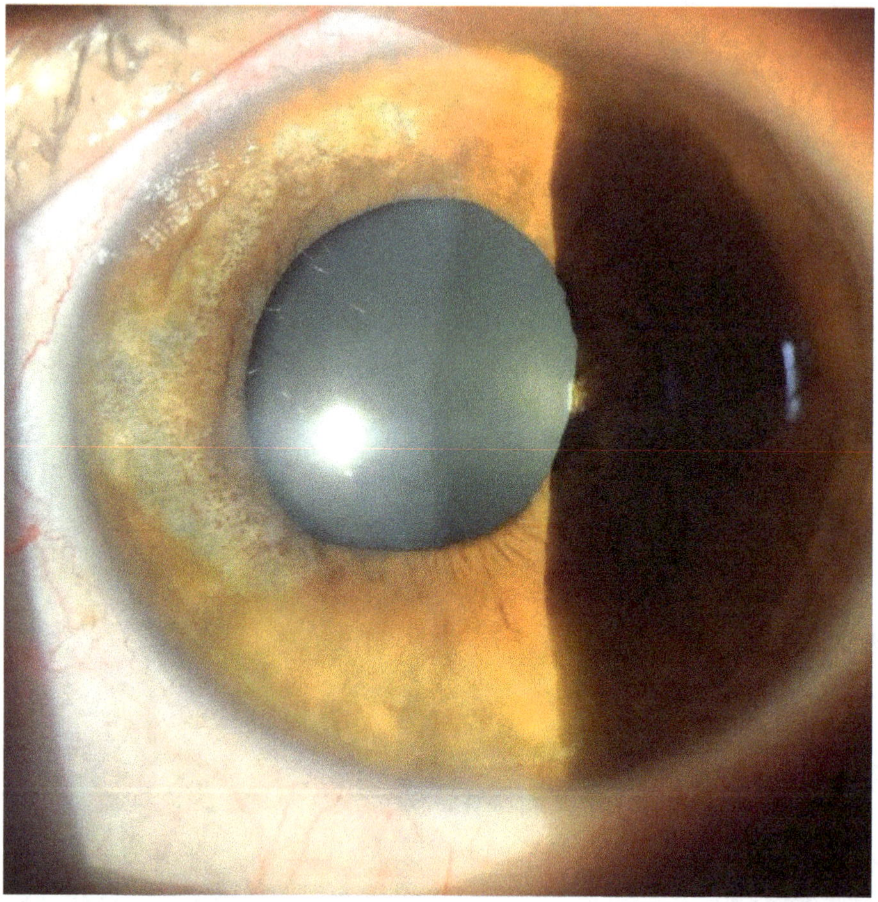

Figure 8. Patchy iris atrophy associated with herpes zoster uveitis. Stellate KPs are noted

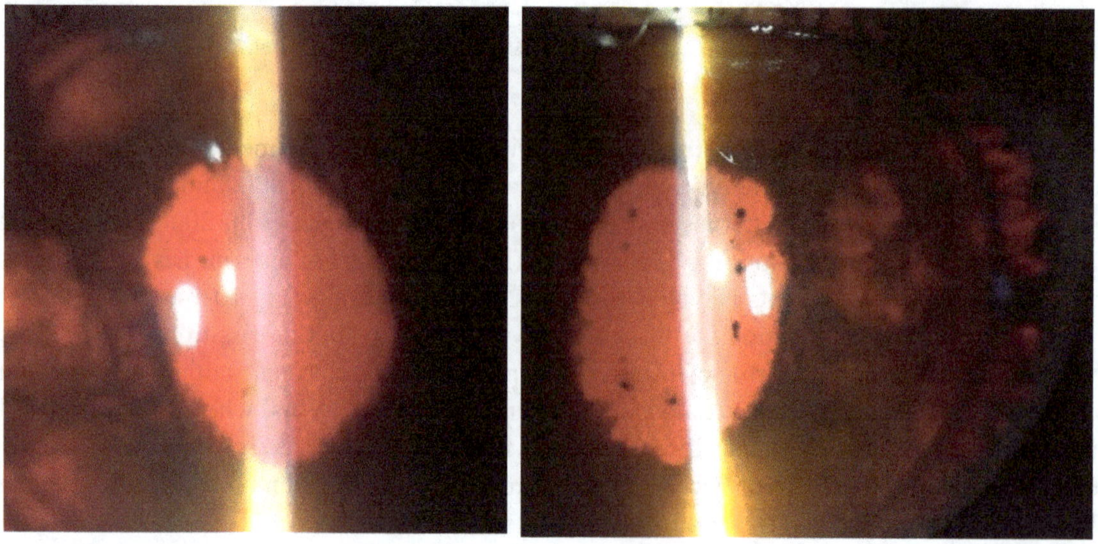

Figure 9. Iris pigment epithelium atrophy caused by herpes simplex uveitis

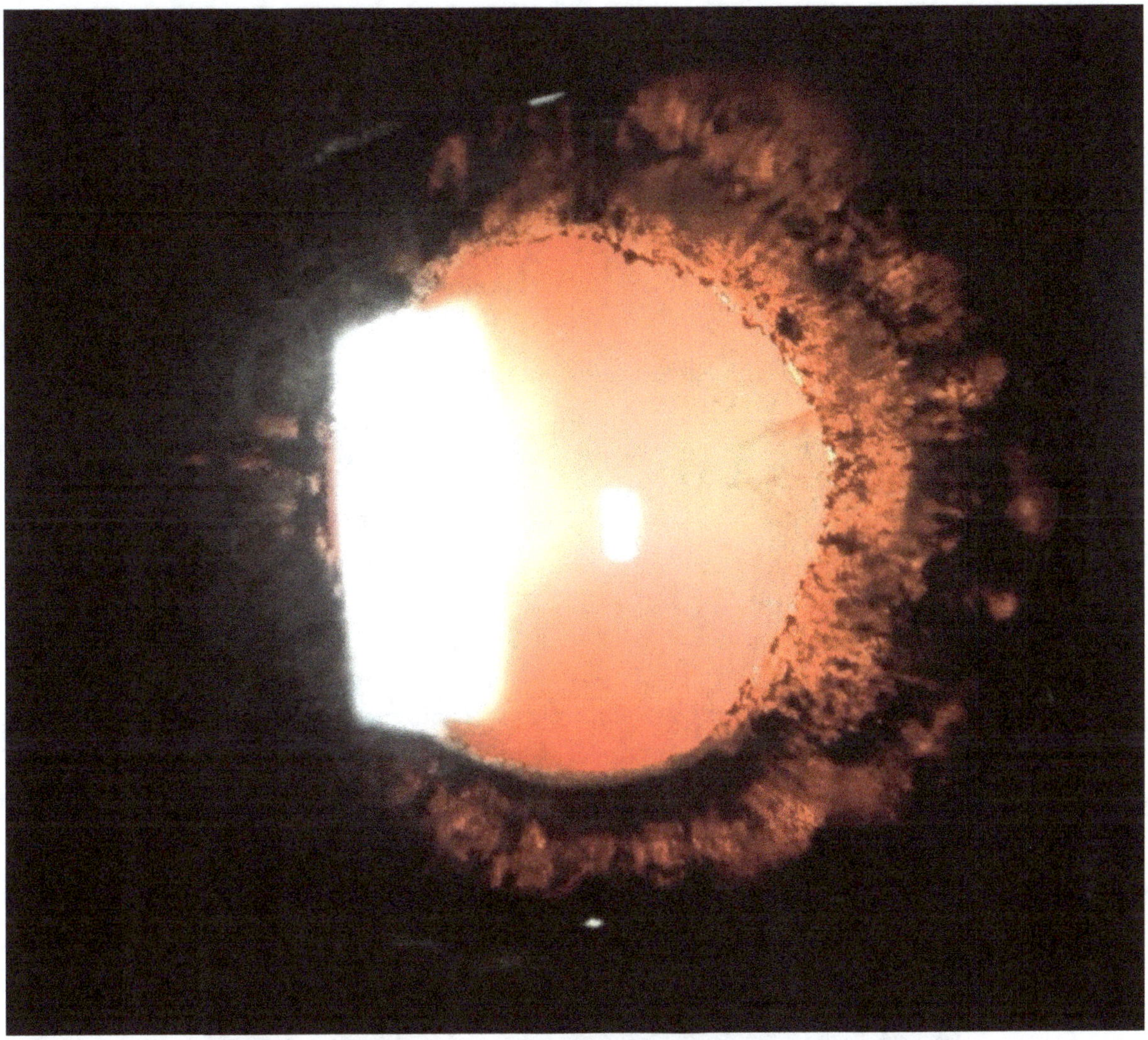

Figure 10. Iris atrophy associated with Fuchs uveitis syndrome. Mature cataract is seen in the affected left eye

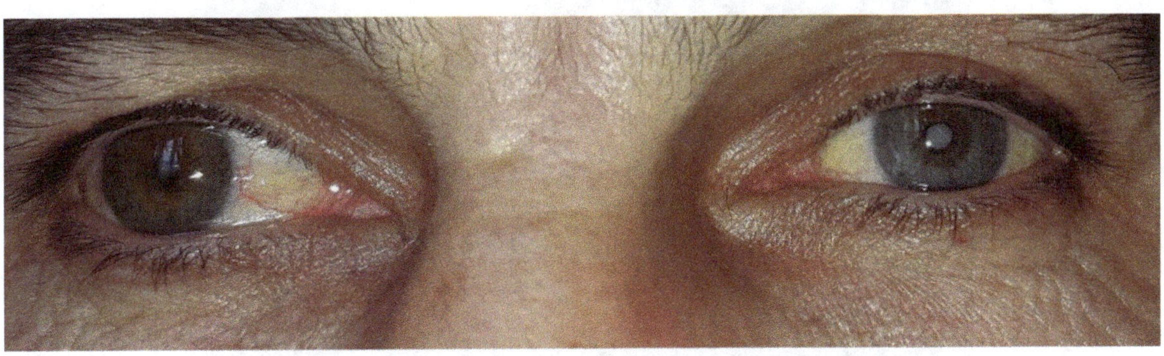

Figure 11. Heterochromia associated with Fuchs uveitis syndrome. Affected eye is light brown

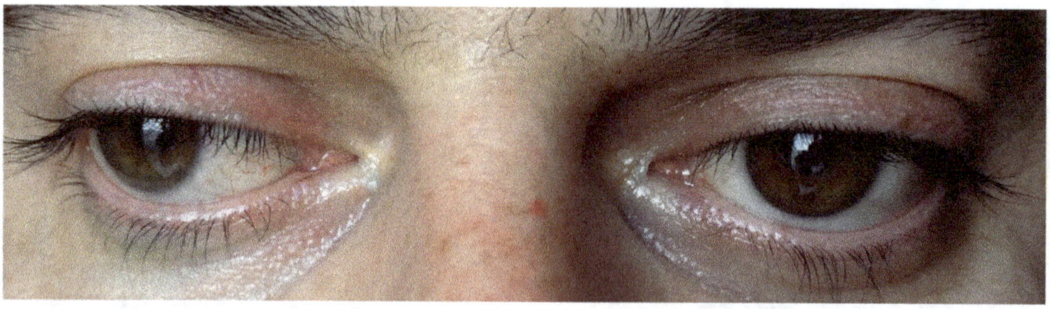

Figure 12. Iris atrophy associated with Fuchs uveitis syndrome (the affected right eye is darker)

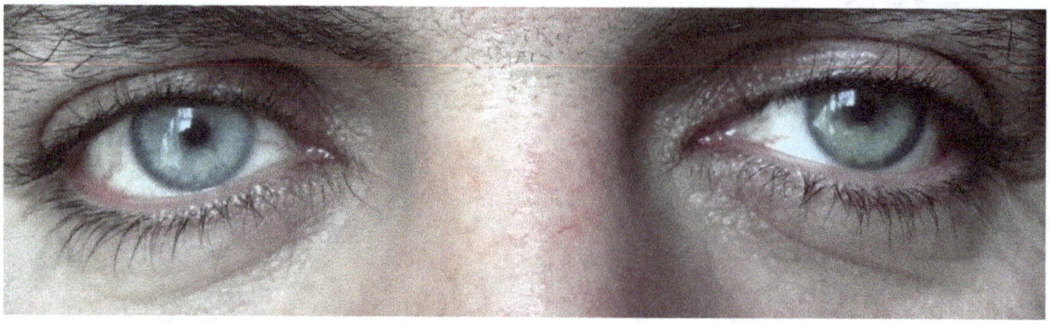

Figure 13. The same eye under a slit lamp. The small stellate KPs are seen

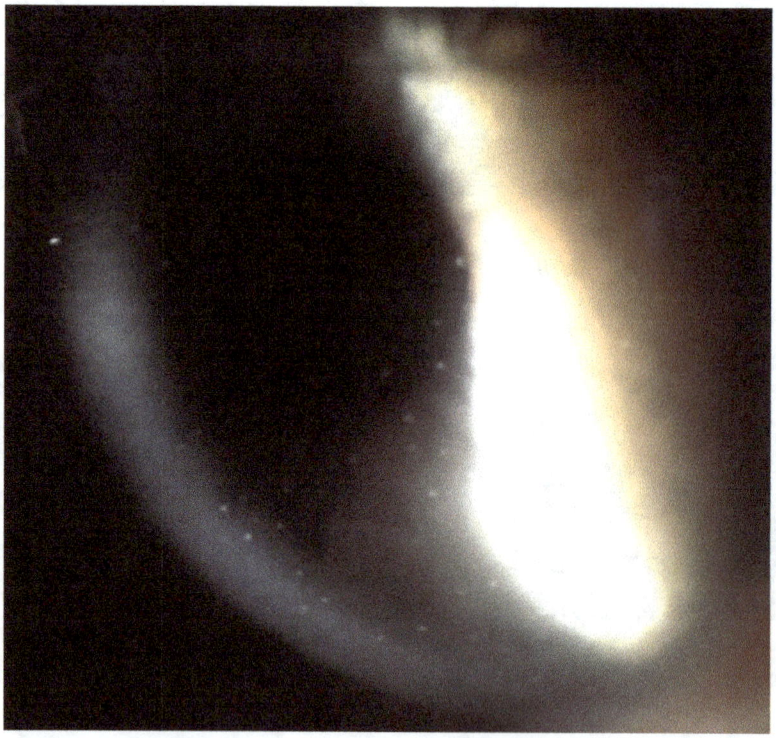

Figure 14. Iris atrophy associated with Fuchs uveal syndrome. The mild heterochromia due to peripupillary atrophy is seen on the left photo

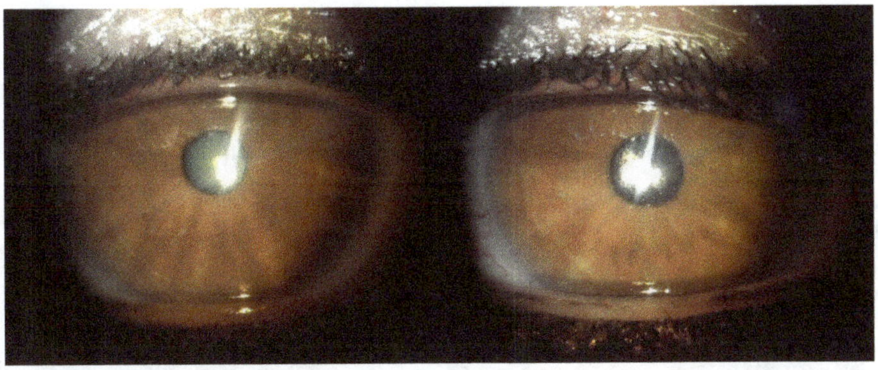

Figure 15. KPs stellate, Koeppe and Busacca nodules associated with Fuchs uveal syndrome are seen

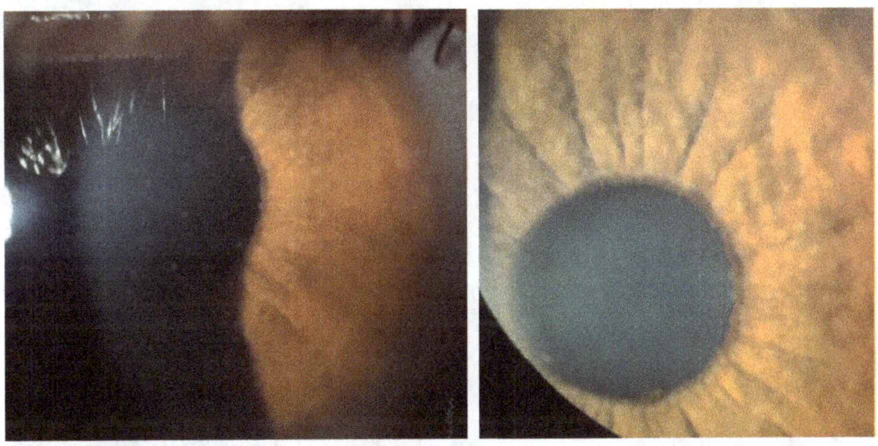

Figure 16. Koeppe nodules

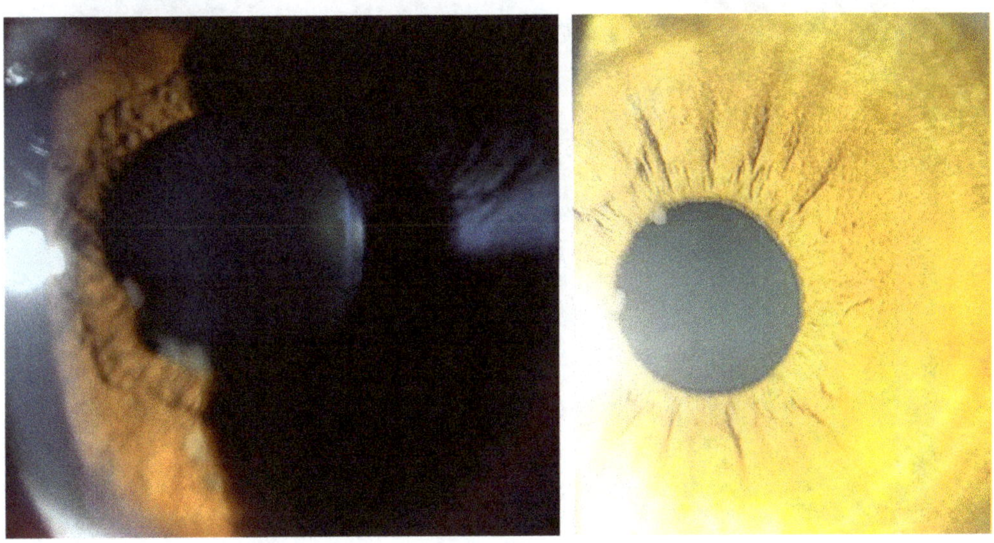

In many cases of anterior uveitis, the pupil may have decreased reactivity, or be nonreactive because of **posterior synechiae** or seclusion of the pupil. In patients with herpetic uveitis the pupil may be dilated in the absence of dilating drops or posterior synechiae. Posterior synechiae represent areas of adhesion between the iris and the anterior lens capsule (Fig 17, 18).

Figure 17. Posterior synechiae associated with Behçet's disease. Right and left eyes of the same patient

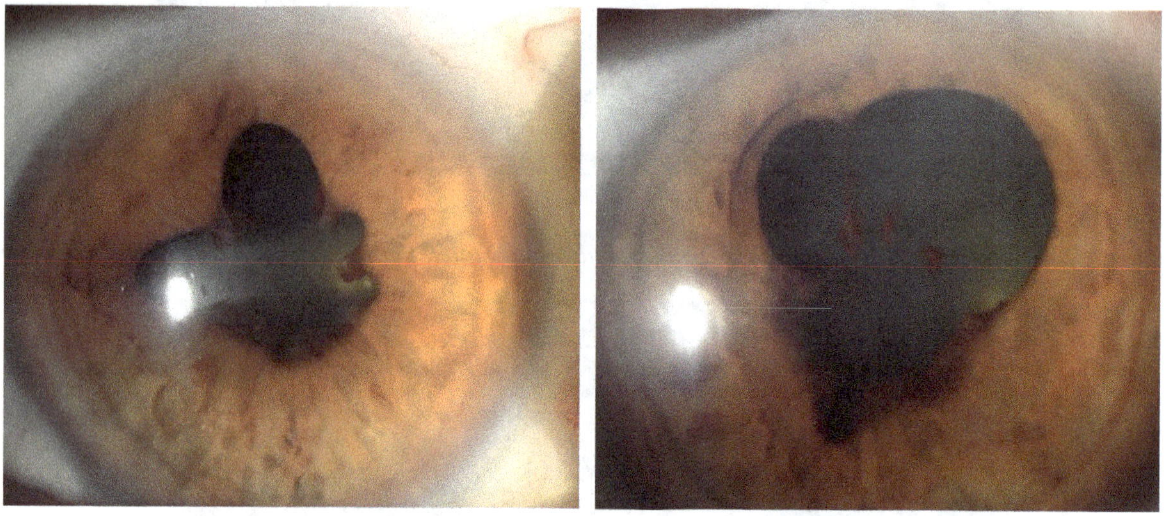

Figure 18. Mydriasis associated with herpetic uveitis. The superiorly located iris sectorial atrophy is noted

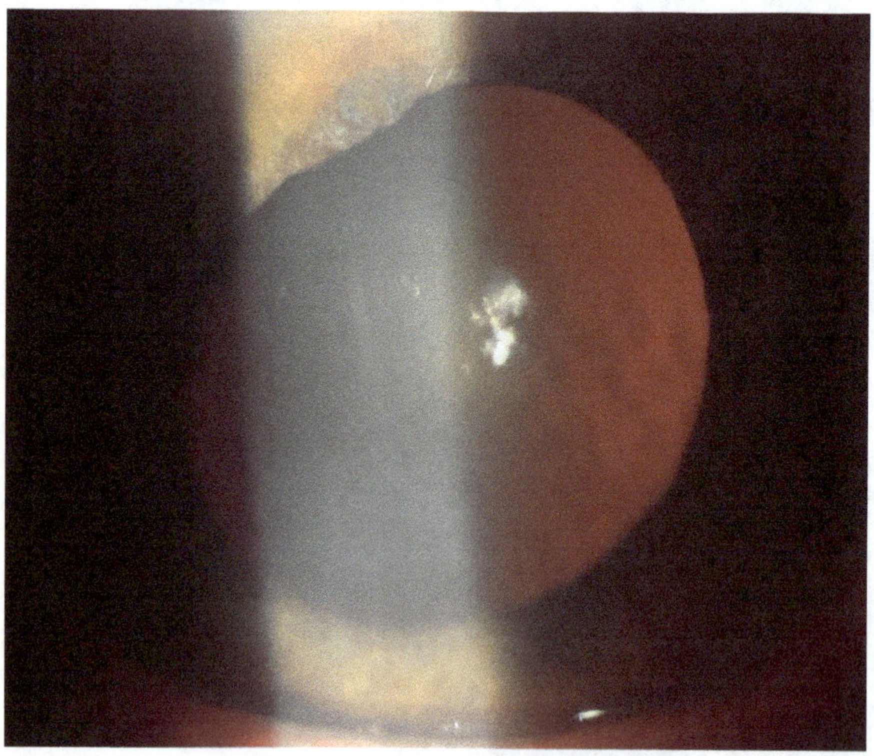

Clumped pigment deposits due to posterior synechiae are usually seen on the anterior capsule. They are a common sequela of chronic anterior uveitis, and may develop after a severe inflammation (Fog 19, 20, 21).

Figure 19. Patient with ankylosing spondylitis and associated HLA-B27 uveitis

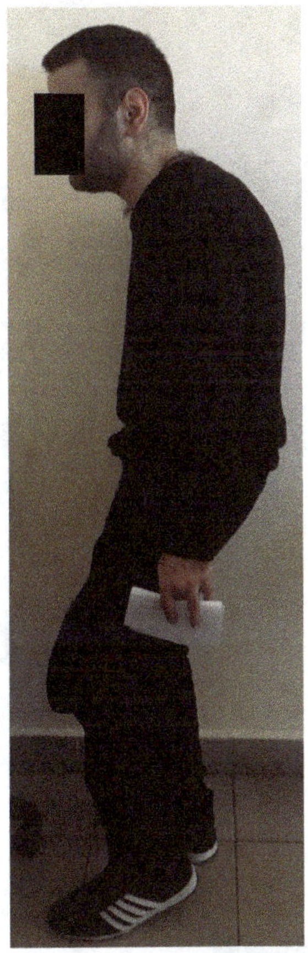

Figure 20. Same patient. Posterior synechiae with pigments on the anterior capsule. The cortical cataract is noted on the left photo

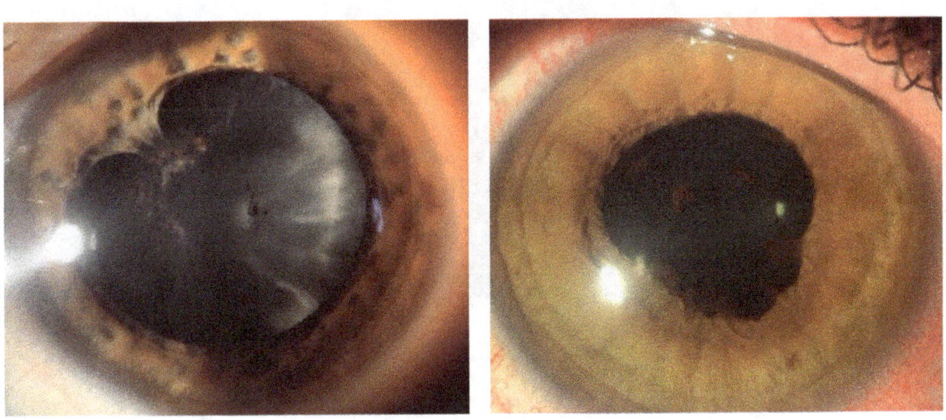

Figure 21. Posterior synechiae with band keratopathy (seen in the left dark zone) in a patient with Juvenile idiopathic arthritis (JIA)

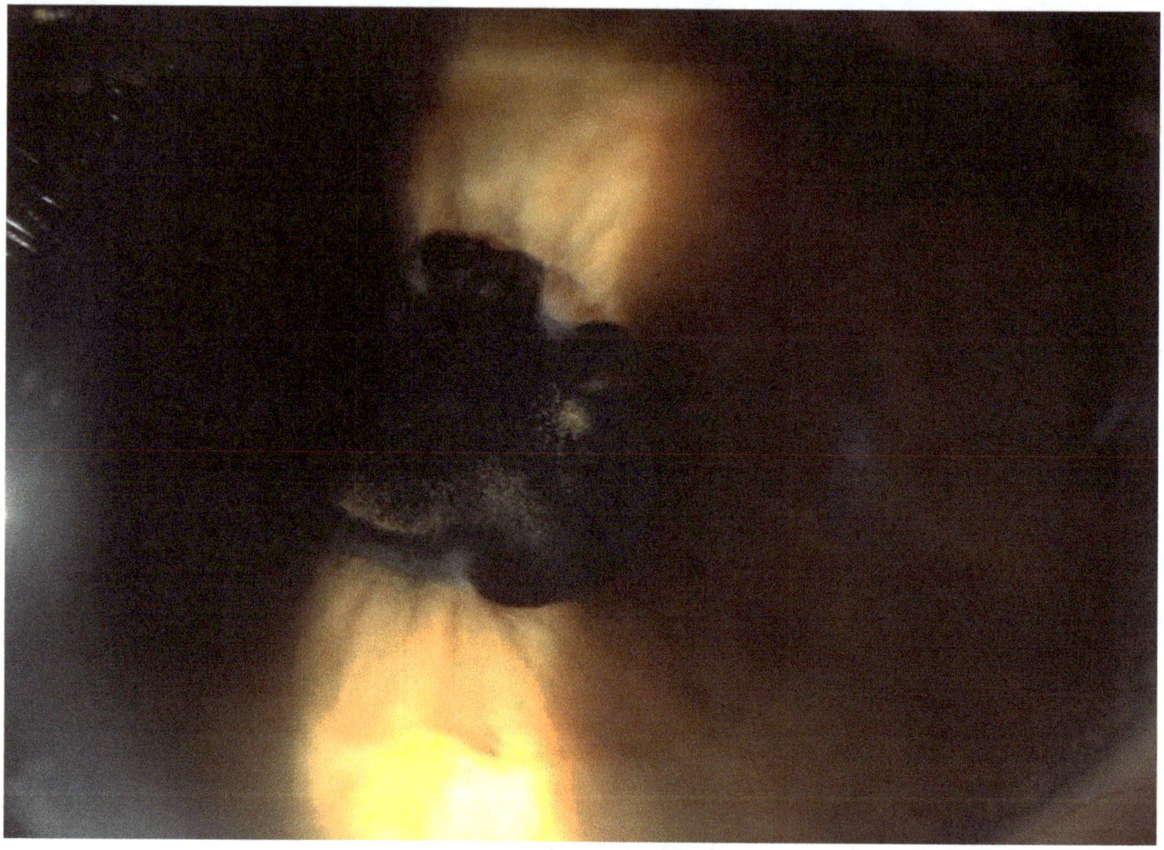

Figure 22. fine (right photo) and severe (left photo) rubeosis due to chronic uveitis

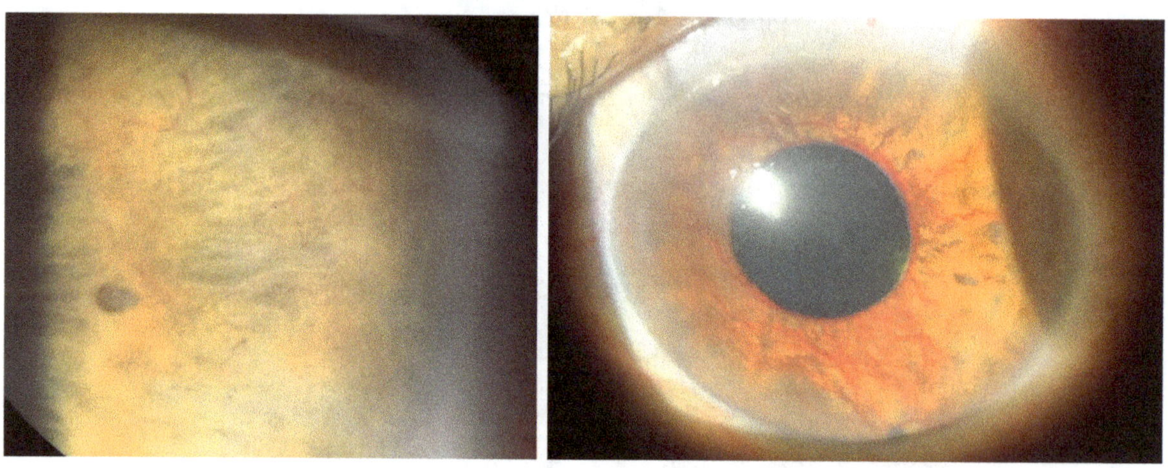

Iris Nevi

Iris nevi are pigmented or unpigmented spots on the iris with minimal disruption of the normal iris architecture. Occasionally, they can be associated with ectropion uveae (Fig 23). There are 2 types of iris nevi: circumscribed (discrete and nodular, Fig 24) and diffuse with sectoral or rarely entire iris involvement (Yanoff et al, 2009).

Figure 23. Iris nevus associated with ectropion uveae

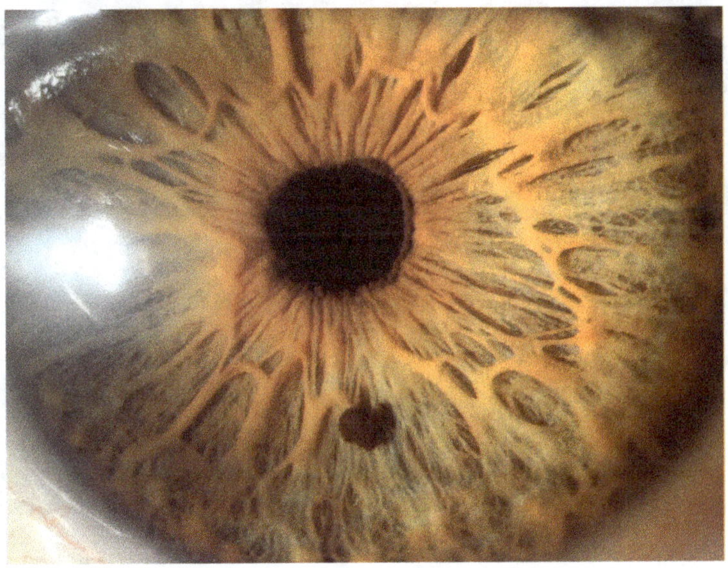

Figure 24. Iris nevus

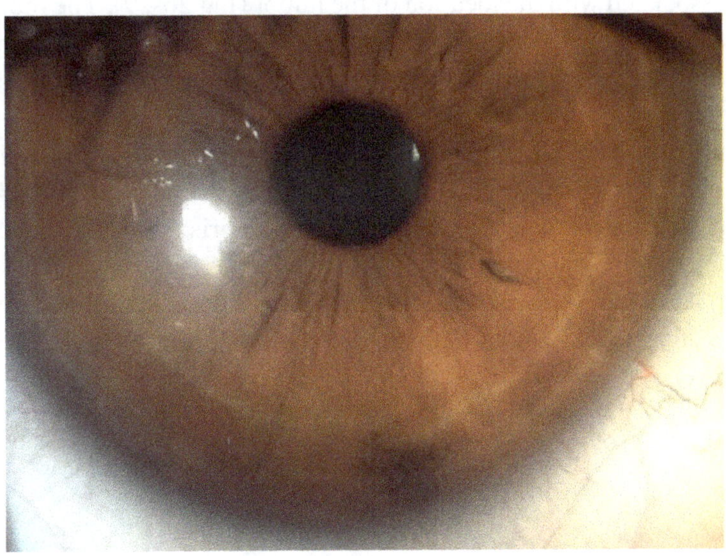

Figure 25. Diffuse iris nevus involving almost the entire iris

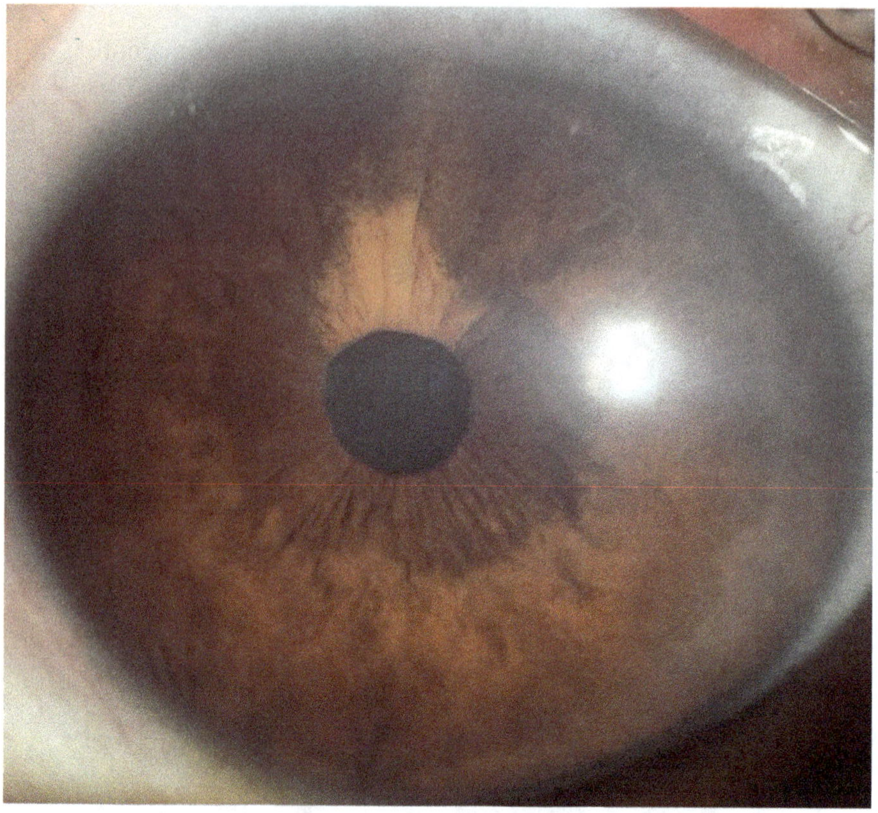

Uveal melanoma is the most common primary malignancy. It can arise from melanocytes in the choroid, ciliary body, or iris. The clinical presentation of malignant uveal melanoma is characterized by nonspecific findings associated with the location of the tumor (Fig 26-29). The more common posterior choroidal tumors have been shown to present with decreased visual acuity, floaters, photopsia, and visual field defects. Tumors involving the iris often present with the patient complaining of iris color changes or other externally observed iris abnormalities (Shields et al, 2001).

Iridocorneal Syndrome (ICE) is a disorder of the corneal endothelium. It presents by abnormal endothelial cell formation and changes of the anterior chamber angle, and iris. The etiology of ICE syndrome is unknown. ICE syndrome has three clinical forms: iris nodules (iris nevus and Cogan–Reese syndromes, Fig 32), corneal endothelial abnormality, or edema (Chandler syndrome, Fig 30), and essential (progressive) iris atrophy (Fig 31). ICE syndrome is a unilateral disorder without a hereditary pattern. Glaucoma is a significant issue of ICE (Scheie et al 1975; Eagle et al, 1979).

Figure 26. Iris dark brown circumscribed melanoma (arising from ciliary body by UBM)

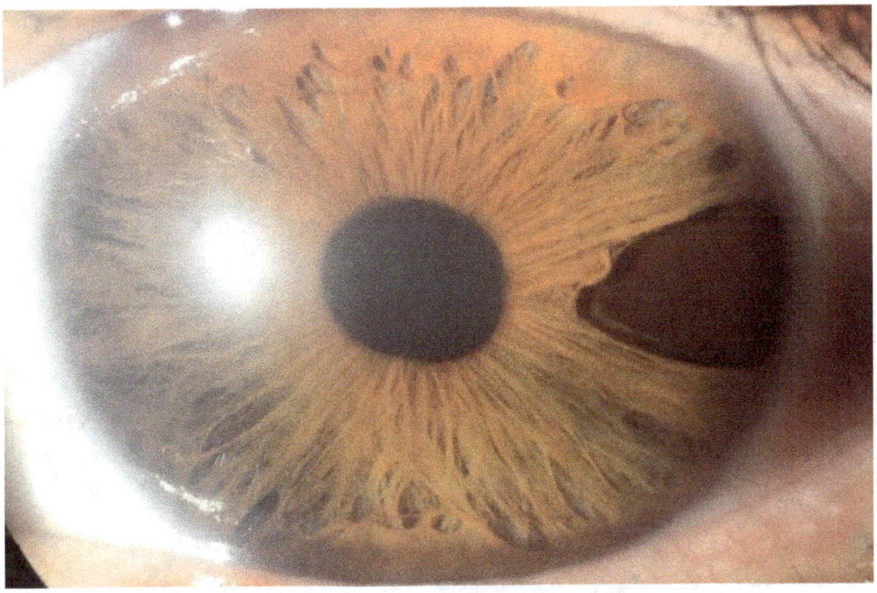

Figure 27. Choroidal melanoma, melanoma is seen through the pupil

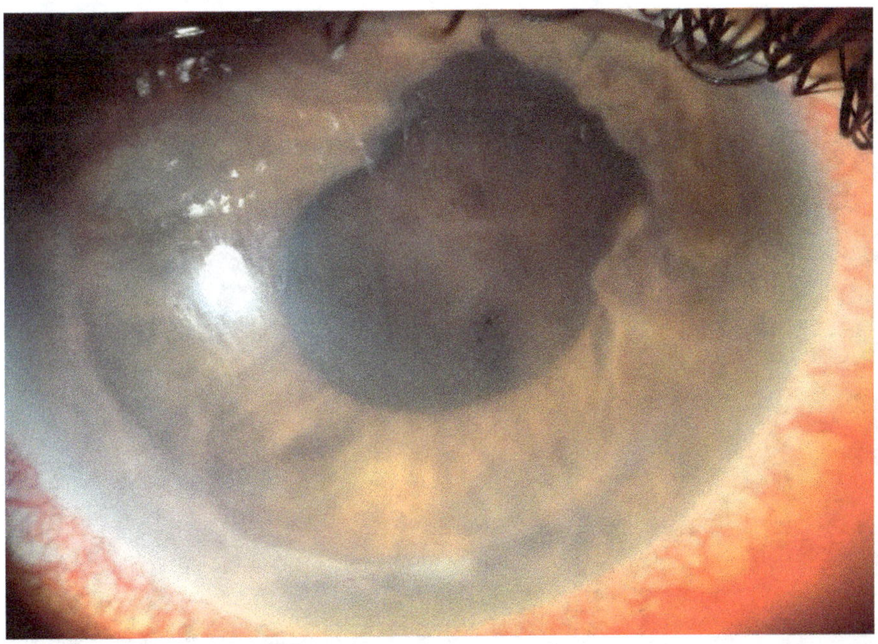

Figure 28. The B-scan of the same patient showing ciliary or choroidal melanoma

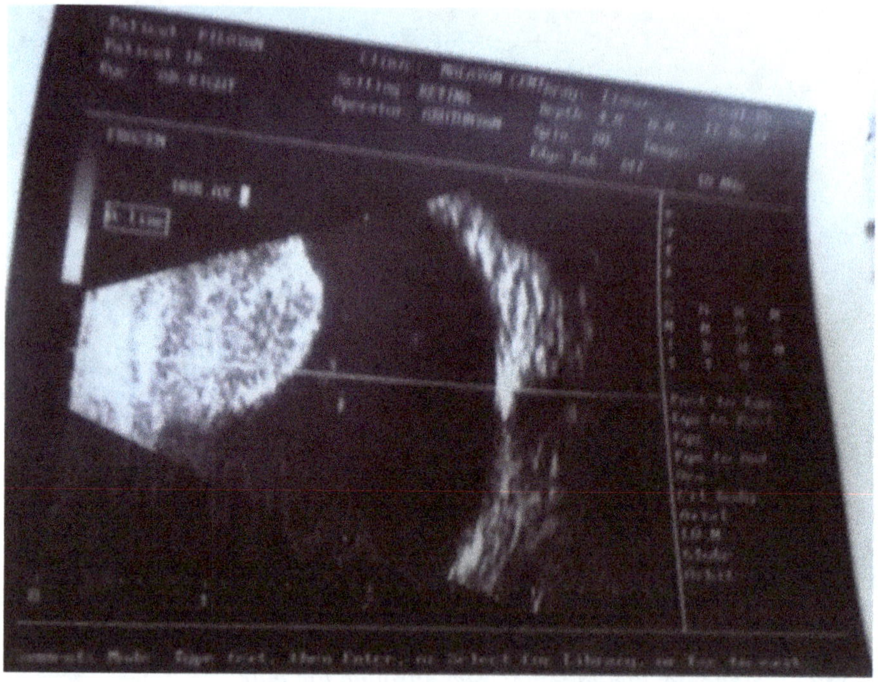

Figure 29. Choroidal melanoma. The lesion is seen through the pupil

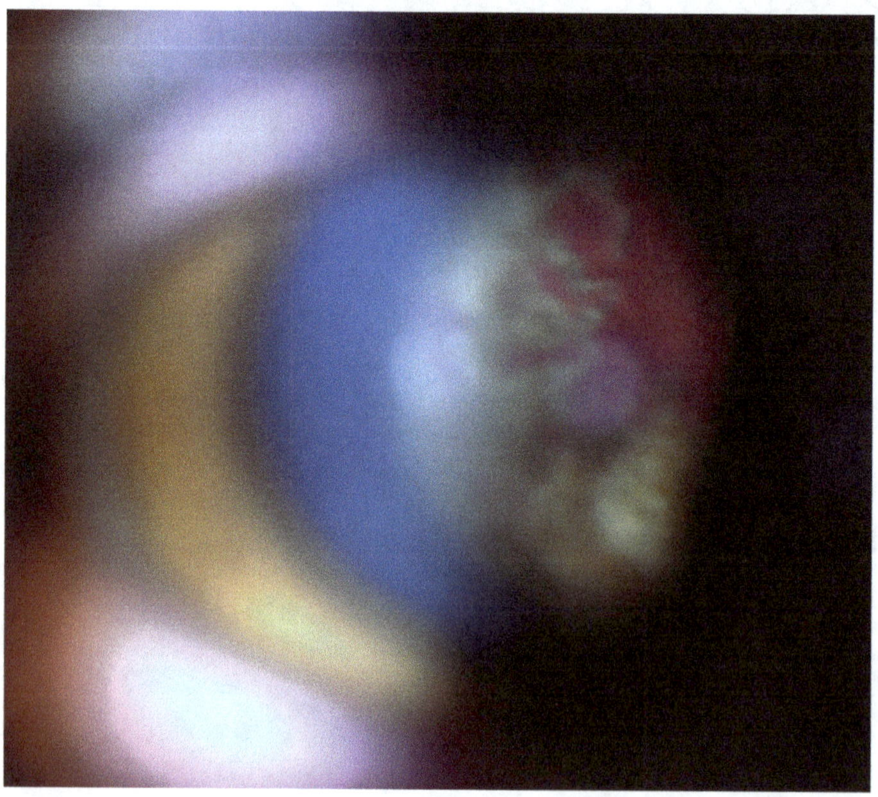

Figure 30. ICE associated with Chandler syndrome. Ectocoria with iris atrophy is noted

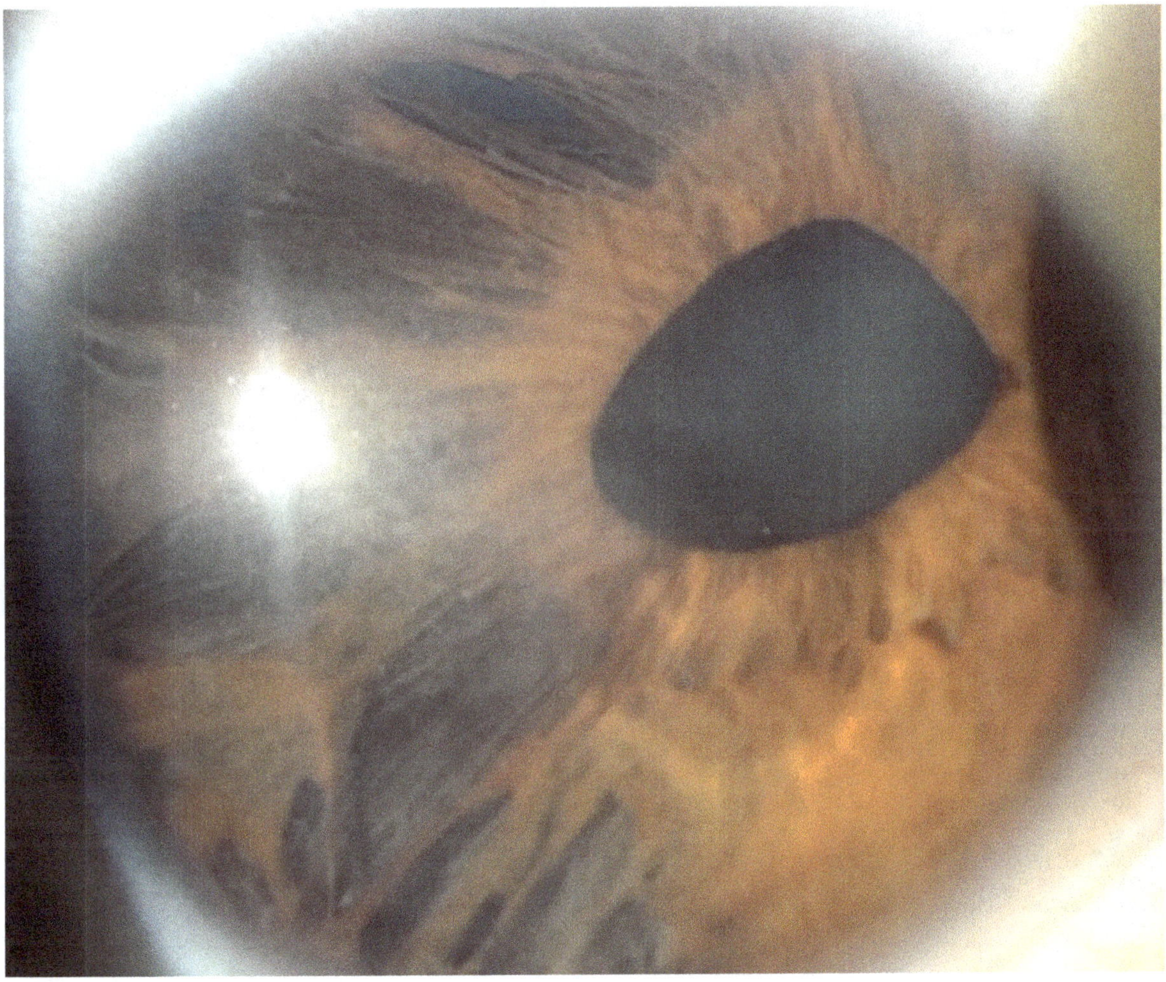

Figure 31. ICE associated with essential iris atrophy. The right and left eyes of the same patient; unilateral involvement is noted

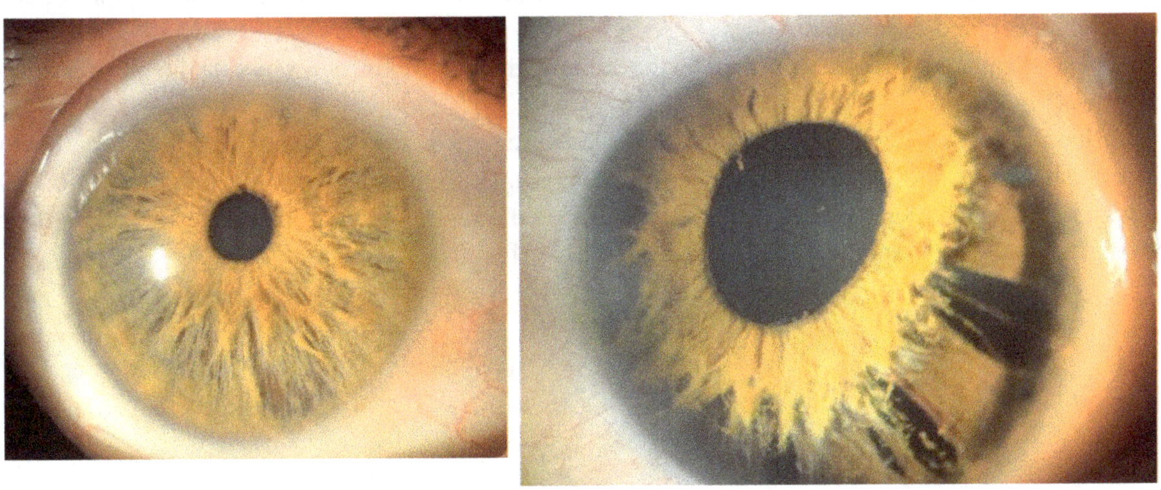

Figure 32. Cogan-Reese or iris nevus syndrome

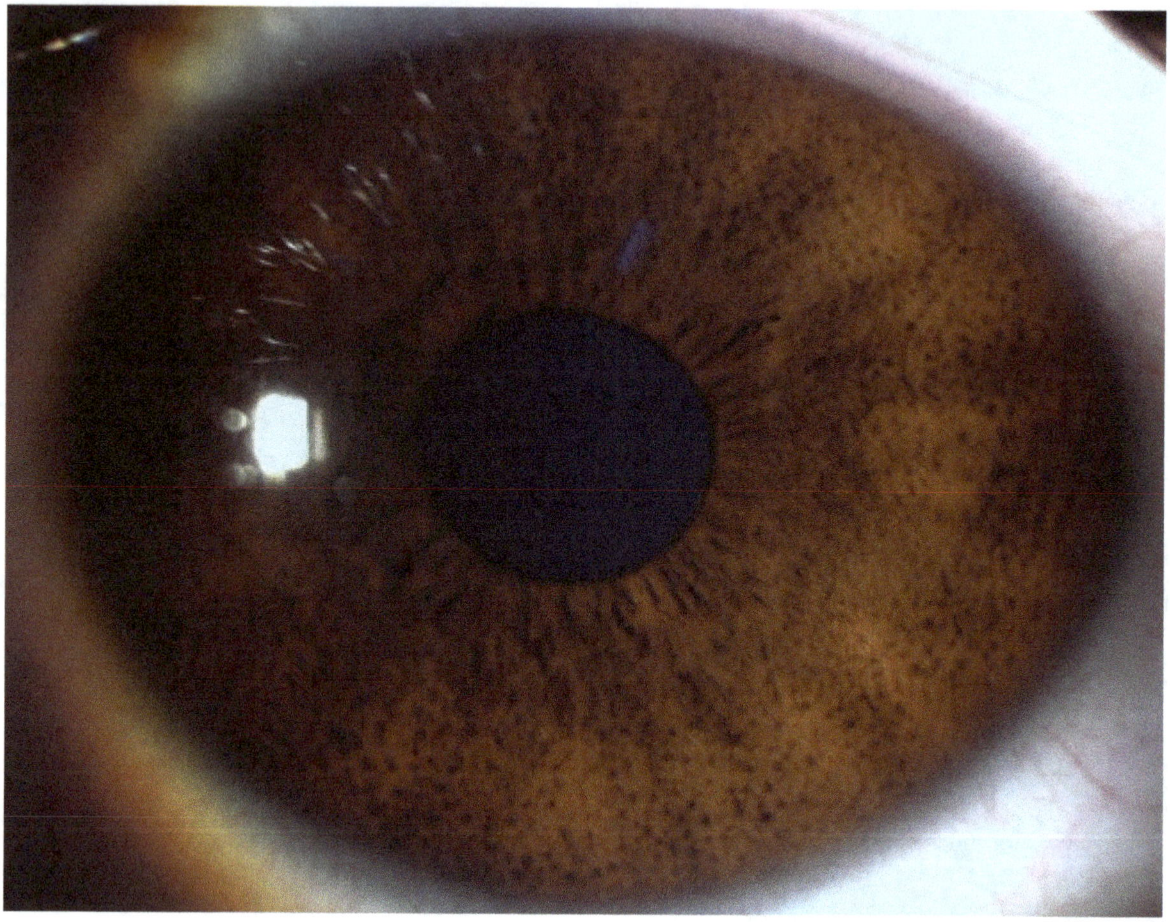

Cataract

Cataract is a clouding of the crystalline lens, which can cause decreased vision and lead to blindness if left untreated. Cataract can be acquired or congenital. Acquired cataract can be age-related or secondary to trauma, ocular, and systemic diseases (Fig 33-36).

Congenital cataracts are present from birth. Usually, they are nonprogressive or the progression is very slow. (Fig 37-39)

Lenticonus is a rare congenital anomaly of the eye characterized by a conical protrusion on the crystalline lens capsule and the underlying cortex (Fig 40). Lenticonus can be anterior or posterior. The posterior lenticonus is more common and can be associated with Lowe syndrome. Anterior and posterior lenticonus can also be associated with Alport syndrome (Jacobs et al, 2000).

Figure 33. Mature age-related cataract. Totally opacified lens is seen

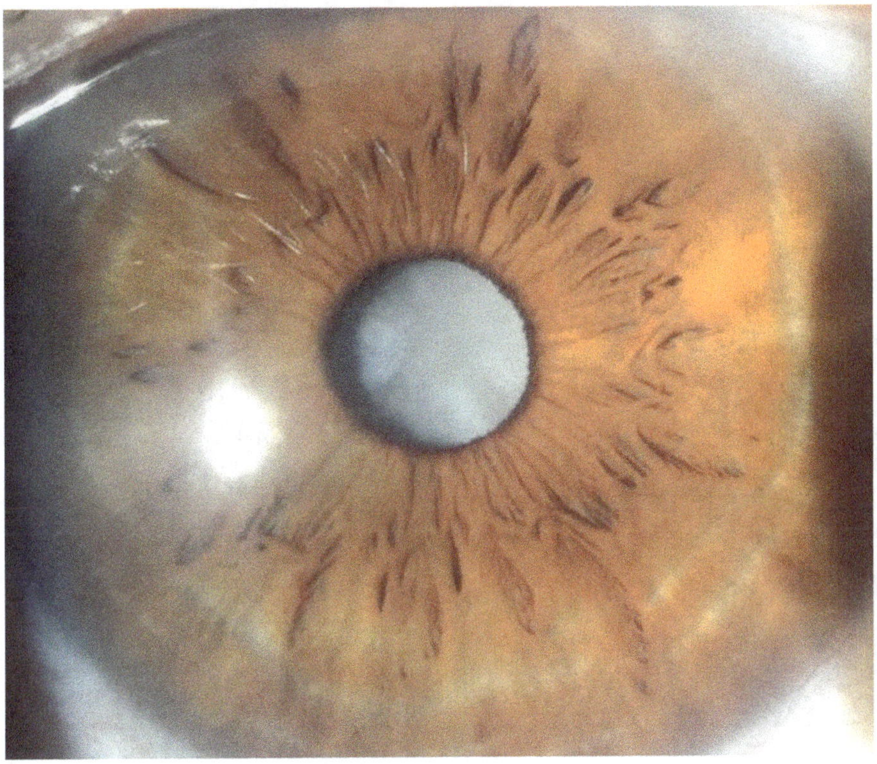

Figure 34. Polychromatic (Christmas tree) cataract. The red-blue-green dots opacification is noted. Cataract is caused by long term topical steroids use

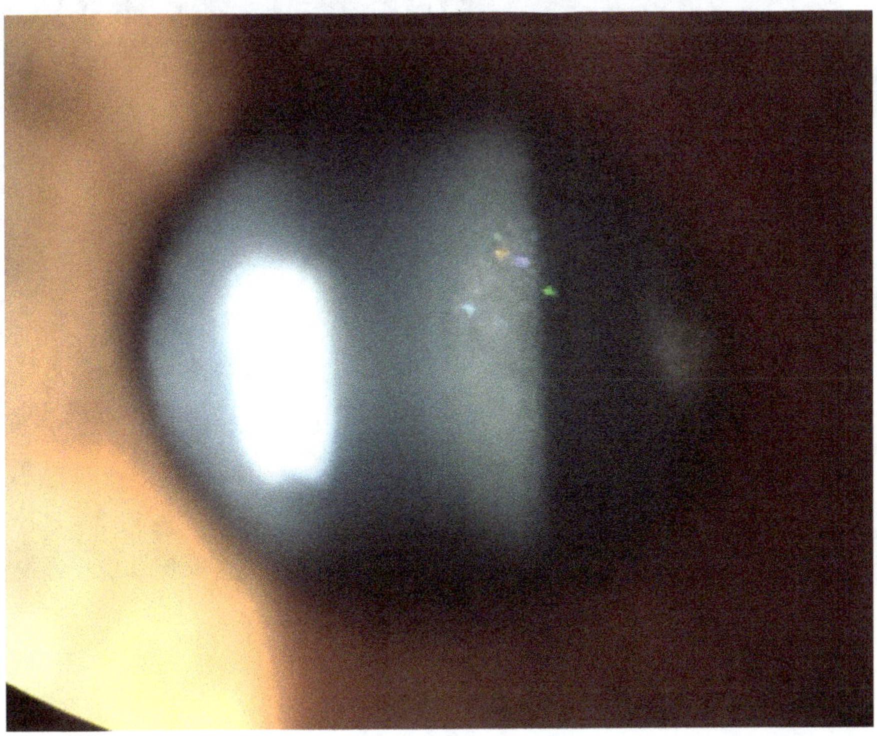

Figure 35. Rosette cataract due to blunt trauma

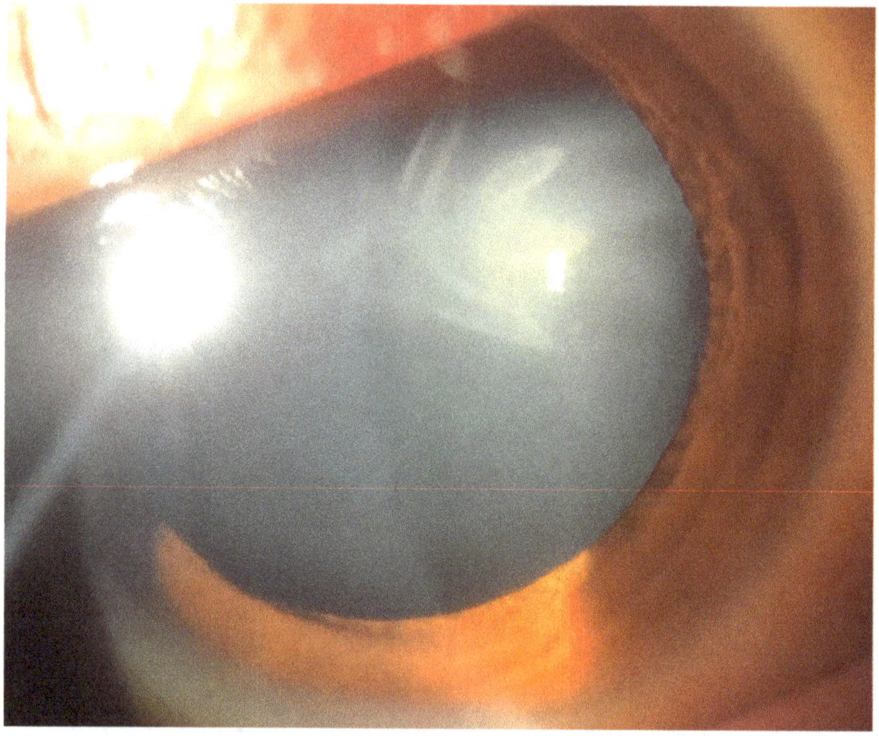

Figure 36. Mature cataract, dislocated lens associated with Marfan syndrome. The zonules are seen

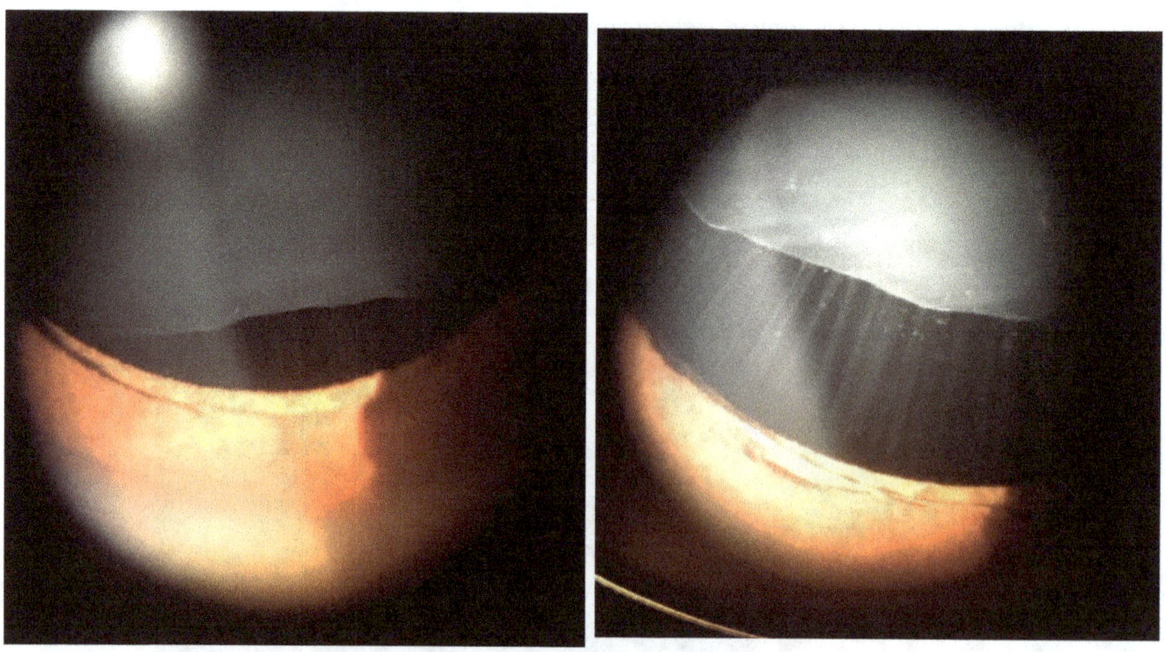

Figure 37. Congenital cataract

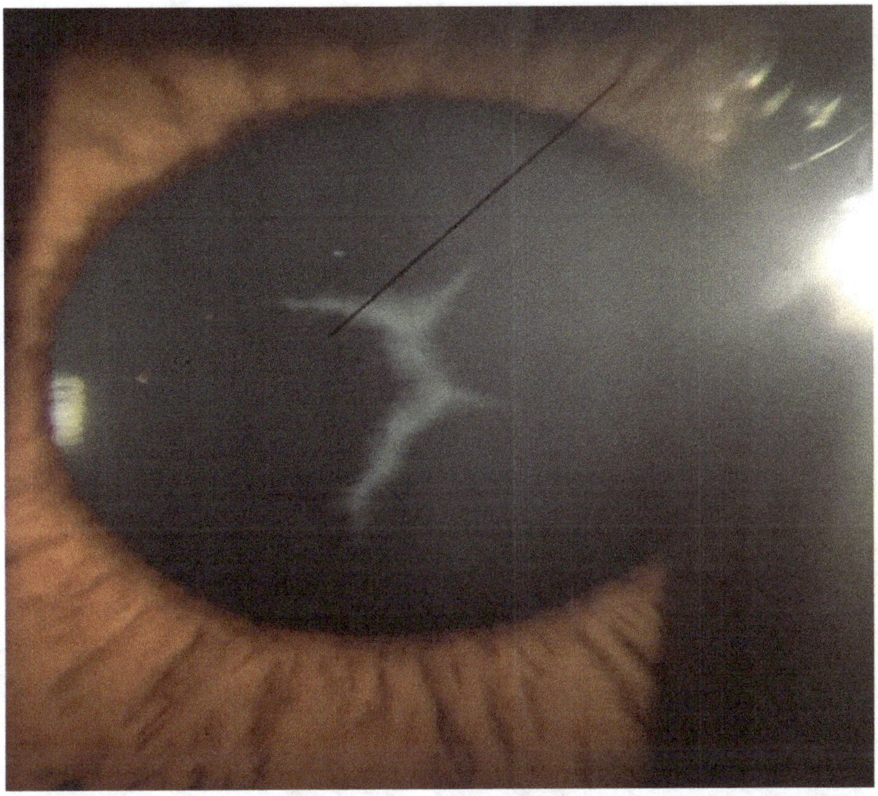

Figure 38. Congenital snowflake cataract

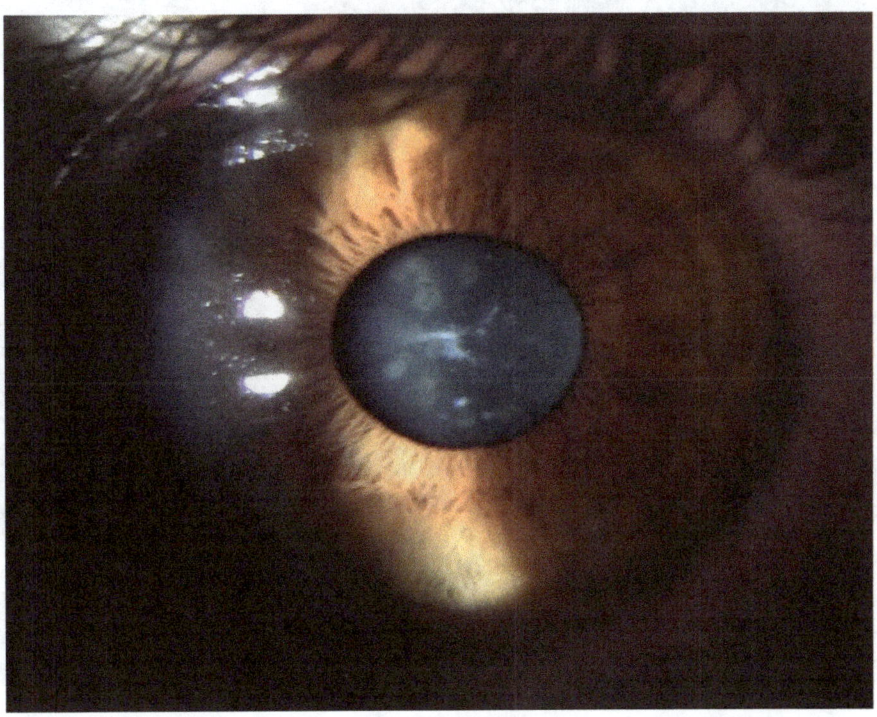

Figure 39. Congenital blue-dots cataract

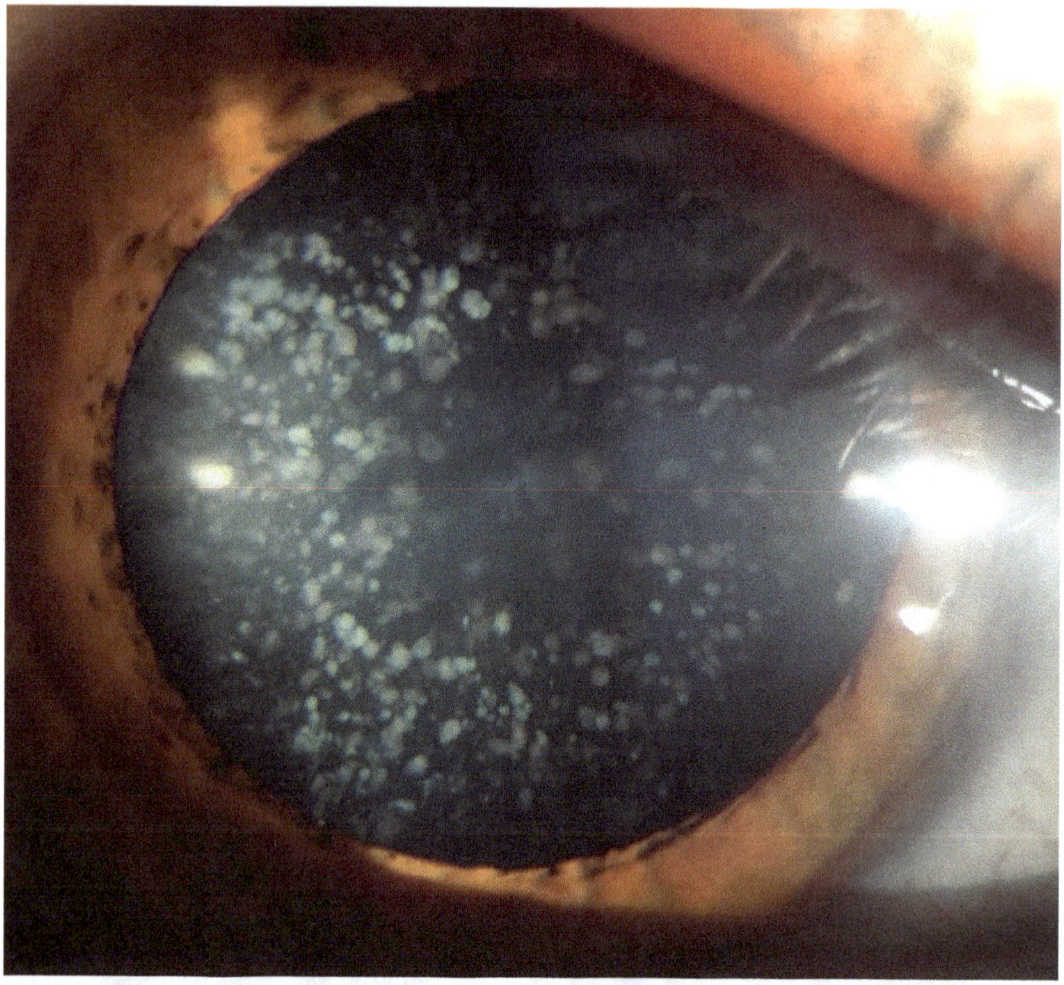

Figure 40. Anterior and posterior lenticonus associated with Alport syndrome. The right and left eyes of the same patient

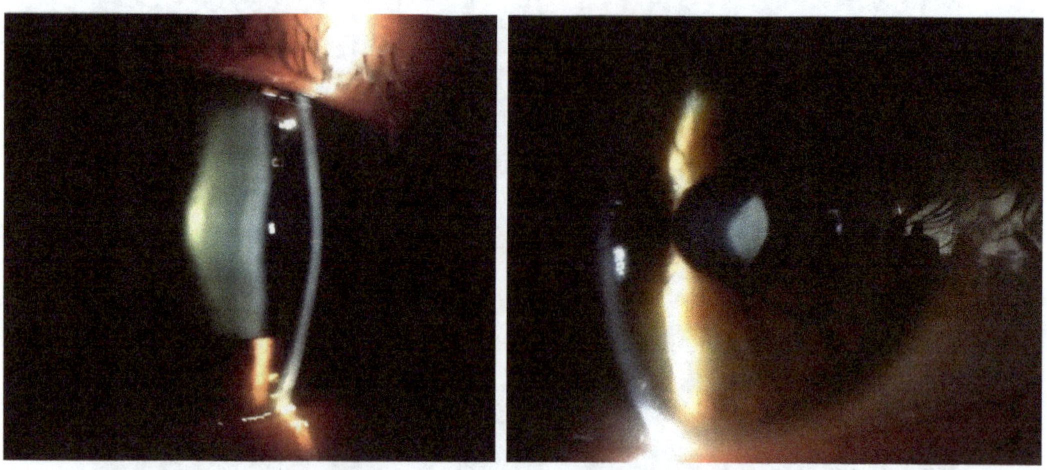

REFERENCES

Douglas, A. (2018, February). Immunosuppression For The Uveitides. *Ophthalmology*, *125*(2), 193–202. doi:10.1016/j.ophtha.2017.08.007 PMID:28942074

Eagle, R. C., Font, R. L., Yanoff, M., & Fine, B. S. (1979). Proliferative endotheliopathy with iris abnormalities: The iridocorneal endothelial syndrome. *Archives of Ophthalmology*, *97*, 2104–2111.

Habot-Wilner, Z., Sallam, A., Pacheco, P. A., Do, H. H., McCluskey, P., & Lightman, S. (2011). Intravitreal Triamcinolone Acetonide As Adjunctive Treatment With Systemic Therapy For Uveitic Macular Edema. *European Journal of Ophthalmology*, *21*(Suppl 6), S56–S61. doi:10.5301/EJO.2010.6062 PMID:23264330

Hogan, M. J., Kimura, S. J., & Thygeson, P. (1959). Signs and symptoms of uveitis. I. Anterior uveitis. *American Journal of Ophthalmology*, *47*(5), 155–170. doi:10.1016/S0002-9394(14)78239-X PMID:13649855

Jabs, D. A., Nussenblatt, R. B., & Rosenbaum, J. T. (2005). Standardization of uveitis nomenclature for reporting clinical data. Results of the first international workshop. *American Journal of Ophthalmology*, *140*(3), 509–516. doi:10.1016/j.ajo.2005.03.057 PMID:16196117

Jacobs, K., & Meire, F. M. (2000). Lenticonus. Department of Ophthalmology, Ghent University Hospital. *Bulletin de la Société Belge d'Ophtalmologie*, *277*, 65–70.

Pelegrín, L., De La Maza, M. S., Molins, B., Ríos, J., & Adán, A. (2015, July). Long-Term Evaluation Of Dexamethasone Intravitreal Implant In Vitrectomized And Non-Vitrectomized Eyes With Macular Edema Secondary To Non-Infectious Uveitis. *Eye (London, England)*, *29*(7), 943–950. doi:10.1038/eye.2015.73 PMID:25998942

Ramanan, A. V., Dick, A. D., Jones, A. P., McKay, A., Williamson, P. R., Compeyrot-Lacassagne, S., Hardwick, B., Hickey, H., Hughes, D., Woo, P., Benton, D., Edelsten, C., & Beresford, M. W. (2017). Adalimumab plus methotrexate for uveitis in juvenile idiopathic arthritis. *The New England Journal of Medicine*, *376*(17), 1637–1646. doi:10.1056/NEJMoa1614160 PMID:28445659

Rothova, A., La Hey, E., & Baarsma, G. S. (1994). Iris nodules in Fuchs' heterochromic uveitis. *American Journal of Ophthalmology*, *118*, 338–342.

Scheie, H. G., & Yanoff, M. (1975). Iris nevus (Cogan-Reese) syndrome. *Archives of Ophthalmology*, *93*, 963–970.

Shields, C. L., Shields, J. A., Materin, M., Gershenbaum, E., Singh, A. D., & Smith, A. (2001). Iris melanoma: Risk factors for metastasis in 169 consecutive patients. *Ophthalmology*, *108*(1), 172–178.

Sugita, S., Shimizu, N., Watanabe, K., Mizukami, M., Morio, T., Sugamoto, Y., & Mochizuki, M. (2008). Use of multiplex PCR and real-time PCR to detect human herpes virus genome in ocular fluids of patients with uveitis. *The British Journal of Ophthalmology*, *92*(7), 928–932. doi:10.1136/bjo.2007.133967 PMID:18408082

Vallet, H., Seve, P., Biard, L., Baptiste Fraison, J., Bielefeld, P., Perard, L., Bienvenu, B., Abad, S., Rigolet, A., Deroux, A., Sene, D., Perlat, A., Marie, I., Feurer, E., Hachulla, E., Fain, O., Clavel, G., Riviere, S., Bouche, P.-A., ... Saadoun, D. (2016). Infliximab versus adalimumab in the treatment of refractory inflammatory uveitis: A multicenter study from the French Uveitis network. *Arthritis & Rheumatology (Hoboken, N.J.)*, *68*(6), 1522–1530. doi:10.1002/art.39667 PMID:27015607

Van der Lelij, Ooijman, & Kijlstra. (2000). Anterior uveitis with sectoral iris atrophy in the absence of keratitis: A distinct clinical entity among herpetic eye diseases. *Ophthalmology*, *107*, 1164–1170.

Yanoff, M. (1979). Discussion of presentation by Dr. M Bruce Shields et al. *Trans Am Acad Ophthalmol.*, *86*, 1549–1550.

Yanoff, M. (1979). Iridocorneal endothelial syndrome: Unification of a disease spectrum. *Survey of Ophthalmology*, *24*, 1–2.

Yanoff, M., & Sassani, J. W. (2009). *Ocular Pathology* (6th ed.). Elsevier.

Chapter 11
Congenital Disorders

ABSTRACT

This chapter is devoted to specific diseases presenting usually in early infancy or childhood as a result of disruption in the normal development of the cornea and its associated structures. These disorders may develop due to one or a combination of various genetic, infectious, inflammatory, toxic, metabolic, traumatic, or mechanical processes and may occur at any time during tissue induction, differentiation, and maturation. Adjacent structures (anterior chamber angle, iris, and lens) can be impacted too. Congenital limbal stem cell deficiency is usually associated with aniridia and ectodermal dysplasia. Aniridia can occur in a sporadic or familial form. The familial inheritance pattern of aniridia is predominantly autosomal dominant. The aniridia phenotype varies depending on the mutation present. Interesting ocular congenital disorders associated with Neurofibromatosis, Axenfeld-Rieger syndrome, Icthyosis are shown in this chapter. It presents a rare case of porphyria-associated sclerocorneal melting with before and after treatment photos.

INTRODUCTION

Megalocornea refers to an enlarged cornea, which is defined as having a horizontal diameter greater than 13mm. It is a nonprogressive condition that is usually bilateral and symmetric. It is most frequently an isolated condition but may be associated with other ocular findings. Often, megalocornea is associated with congenital glaucoma (Fig 1) (Meire et al, 1994). In the presence of congenital glaucoma, the intraocular pressure is elevated; Haab striae are seen. Haab striae are tears in the Descemet membrane, more commonly localized horizontally and concentric to the limbus. No treatment is required in isolated anomaly. The treatment should be directed to associated diseases.

Microcornea refers to a cornea having a horizontal diameter less than or equal to 10mm in an otherwise normal-shaped globe. This condition is nonprogressive and may be unilateral and bilateral (Fig 2). Usually, microcornea is not isolated and can be associated with aniridia, autosomal dominant vitreoretinochoroidopathy, and Axenfeld syndrome (Salmon et al, 1988). No treatment is required in isolated anomaly. The treatment should be directed to associated diseases.

DOI: 10.4018/978-1-7998-6937-5.ch011

Figure 1. Megalocornea associated with congenital glaucoma. PK performed for bullous keratopathy due to chronic glaucoma. The diameter of the cornea is 15mm

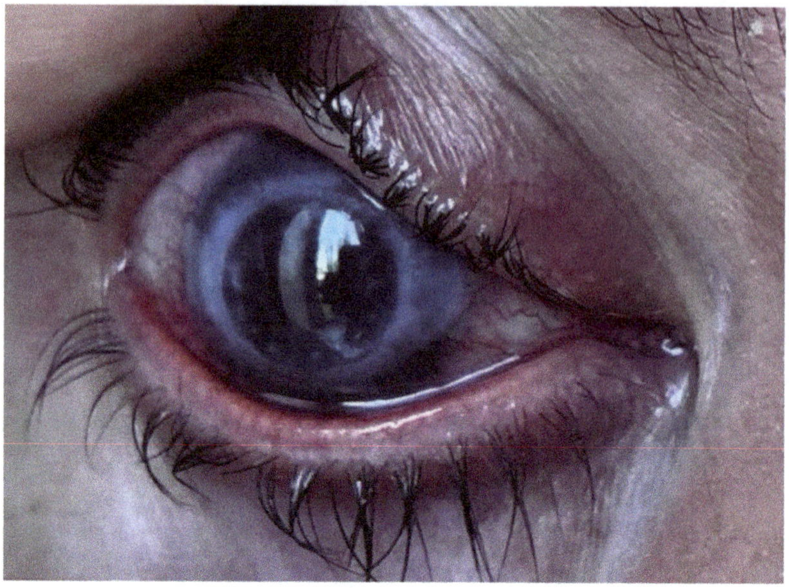

Figure 2. Microcornea, the diameter of the cornea is 9mm

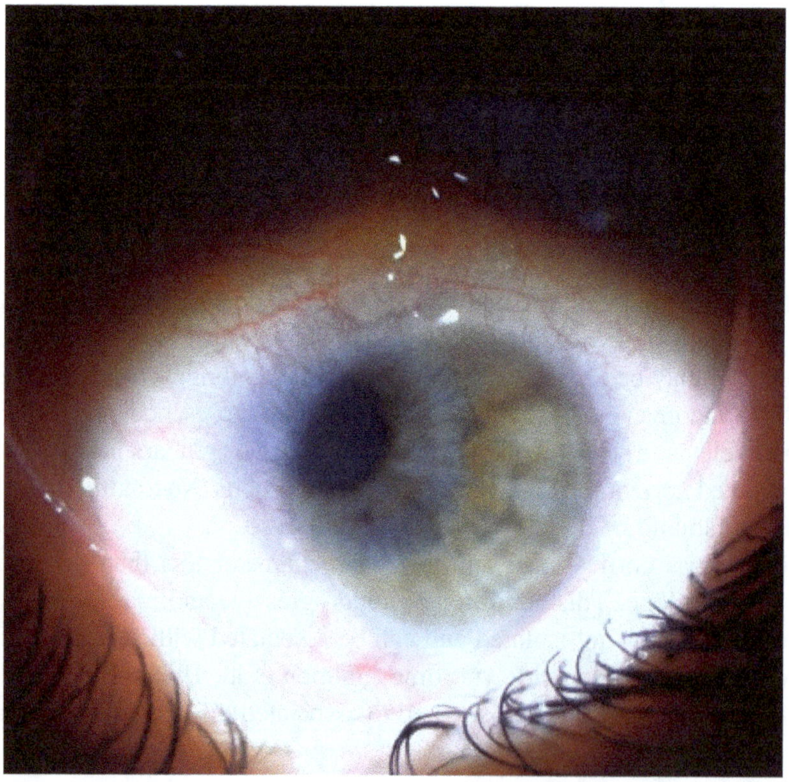

Sclerocornea is a congenital anomaly of the eye in which the cornea is scleralized. Sclerocornea is commonly bilateral and asymmetric rather than unilateral. Scleralization occurs in varying degrees and progresses from the periphery toward the center. Sleralization can be complete (total sclerocornea, Fig 5-8) and incomplete (Fig 3). Sclerocornea can be associated with Peters anomaly and cornea plana (Fig 4) (Sharkey et al, 1992; Kenyon et al, 1975). If the disorder is unilateral and the other eye has good visual acuity, the decision whether to operate becomes more difficult, and surgery can be performed only if other ocular structures are comparably normal. If the condition affects the central corneas bilaterally, inducing a substantial reduction in visual acuity, penetrating keratoplasty should be performed to attain useful vision.

Limbal stem cell deficiency is usually acquired but can be congenital as well. Aniridia, the most common cause of congenital limbal stem cell deficiency, is a bilateral, congenital disorder involving multiple ocular structures (Elsas et al, 1977). Affected individuals may have a different spectrum of iris anatomy, with the most severe being a total absence of the iris to the least severe being mild stromal hypoplasia with a normal-appearing pupil (Fig 9-12). The familial inheritance pattern of aniridia is predominantly autosomal dominant. The keratopathy manifests in the first decade of life and represents as a thickened irregular peripheral epithelium. This epitheliopathy, often followed by fine superficial neovascularization, advances and may involve the entire cornea. Subepithelial fibrosis and stromal scarring may develop. The most common approach to treatment is supportive therapy including lubricants, tarsorrhaphy, and bandage contact lenses for early disease stages. However, if the limbal stem cell deficiency is not treated early, the disease will often lead to stromal scarring. Although it is now understood that the etiology of aniridic keratopathy is a limbal stem cell deficiency, penetrating or lamellar keratoplasty is still often being performed to rehabilitate vision as much as possible. The published results for penetrating keratoplasty without limbal stem cell transplantation for aniridic keratopathy are dismal (Holland et al, 2003). In patients in whom the epithelial disease had progressed to the stromal scarring stage, penetrating keratoplasty was necessary after keratolimbal allograft for visual rehabilitation (Gomes et al, 1966).

Figure 3. Bilateral incomplete sclerocornea. The right and left eyes of the same patient. Scleralization looking like an American football ball is seen

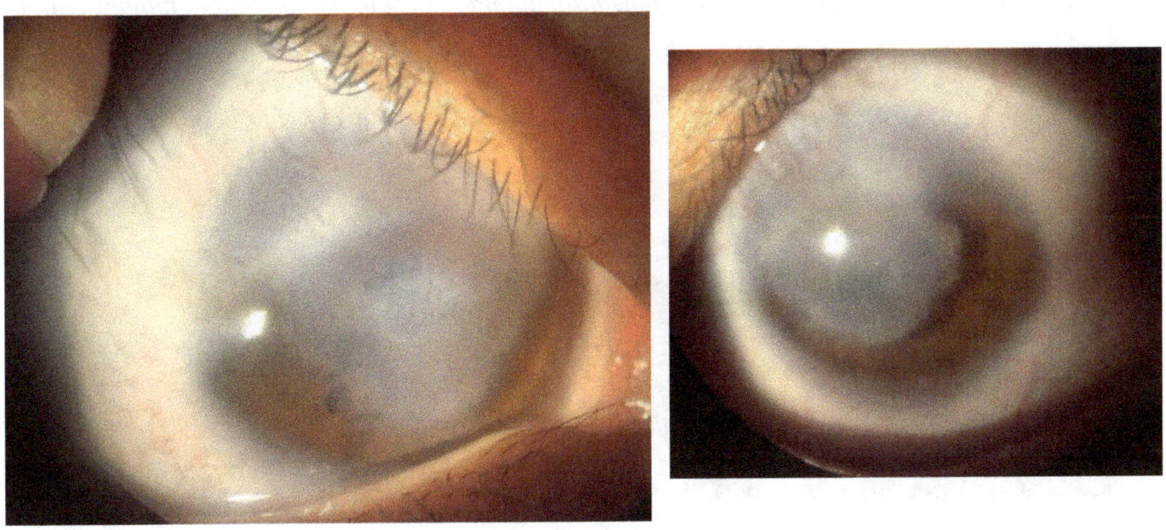

Figure 4. The sister of the previous patient. Incomplete sclerocornea associated with cornea plana (right photo). The scleralization of the cornea is seen superiorly

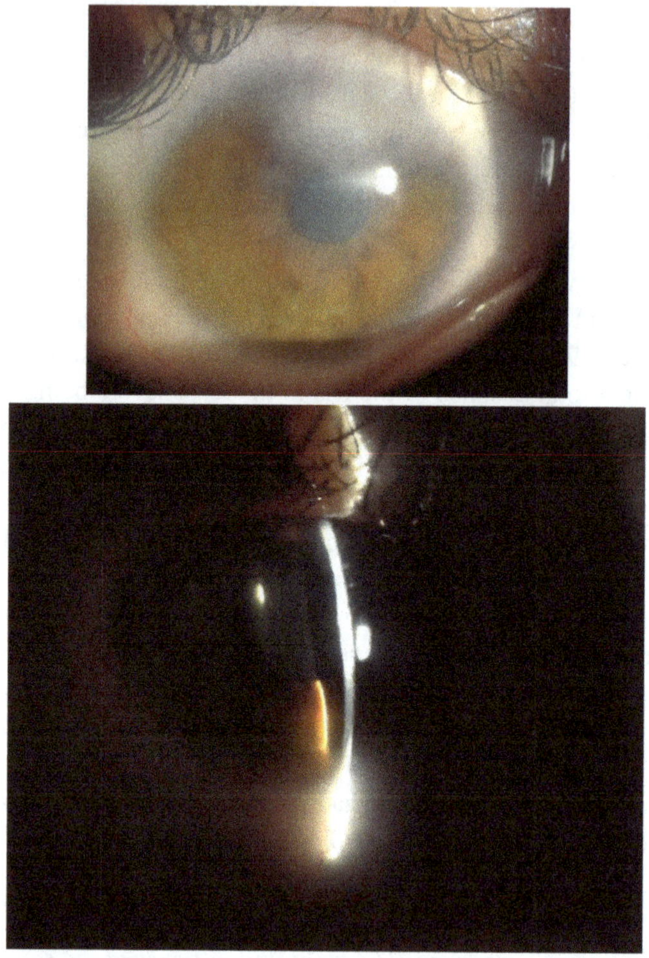

Figure 5. Total sclerocornea. The eye of the same patient under slit lamp and without magnification

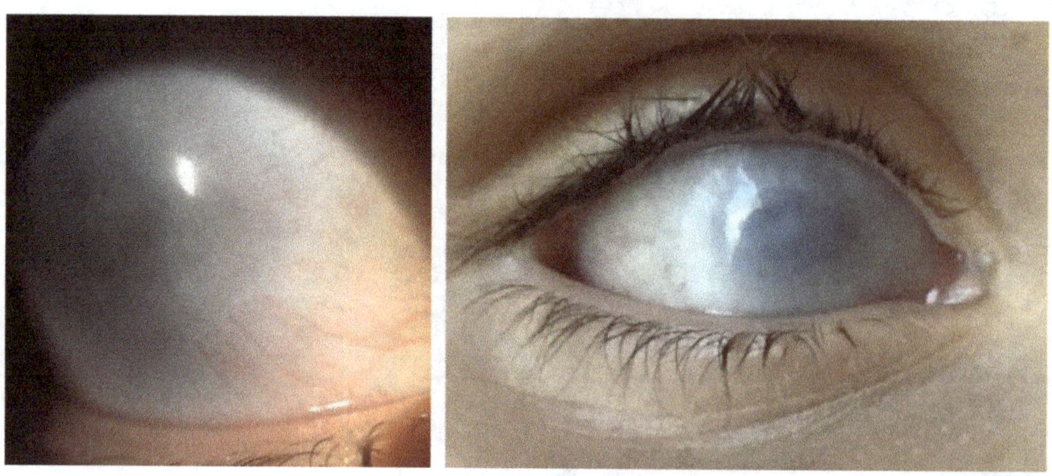

Figure 6. Bilateral total sclerocornea. Child is 26 months old

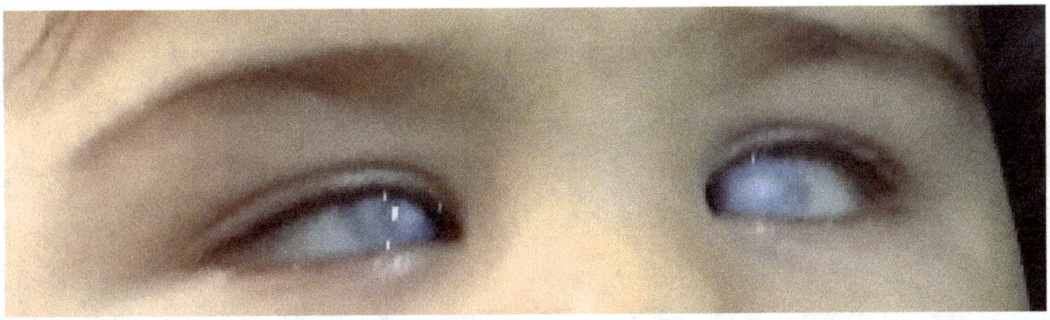

Figure 7. The same patient 2 years after PK in the right eye. Transplant remains clear. Child has 20/200 VA

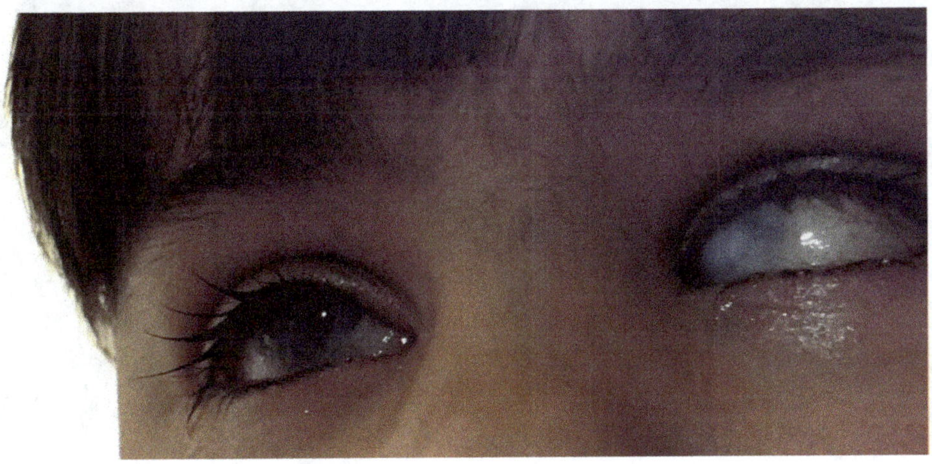

Figure 8. The same eye under a slit lamp

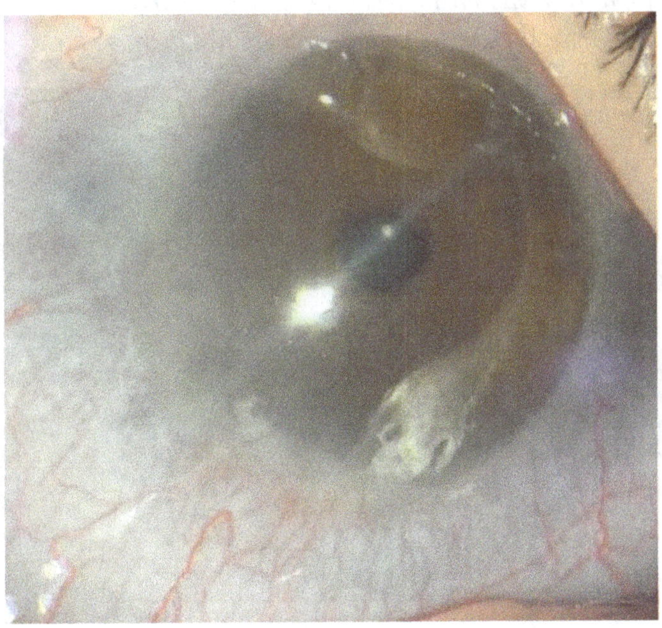

Figure 9. Aridic keratopathy. The hypoplastic iris is seen with 360 degrees of NV due to limbal stem cell deficiency

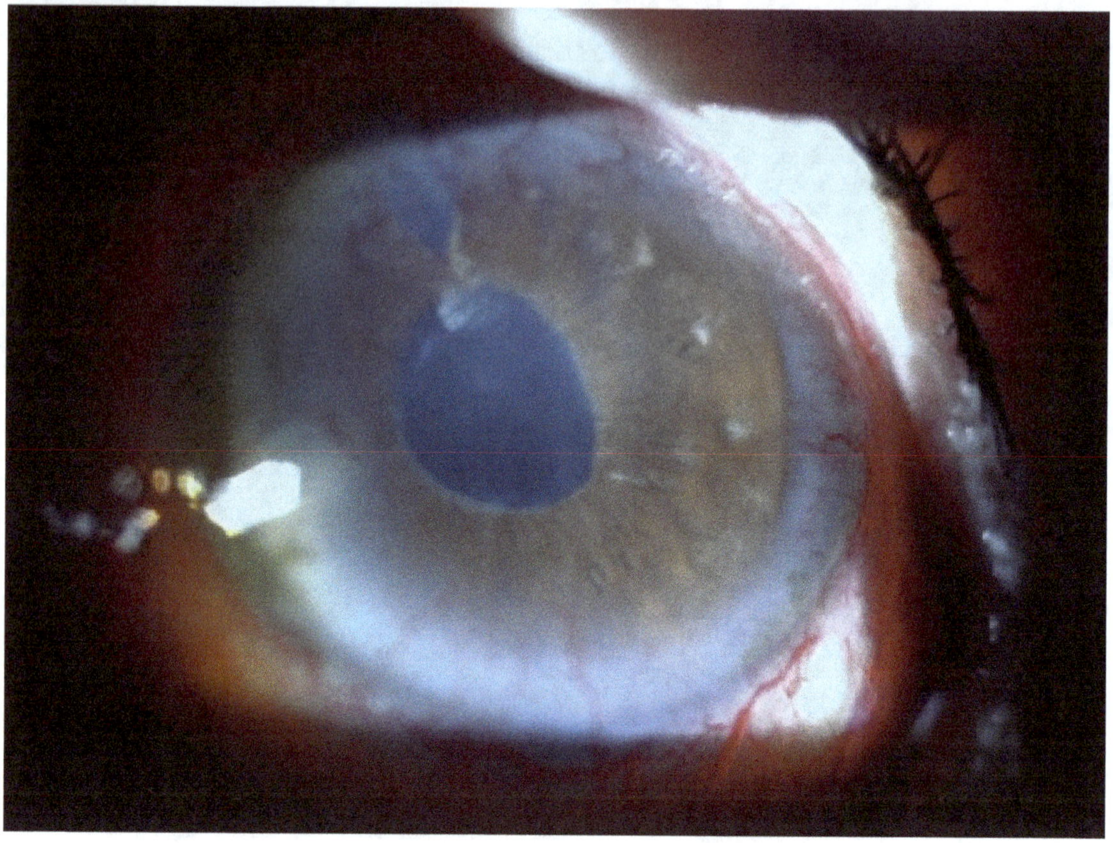

Figure 10. Aniridic keratopathy. Hypoplastic iris is noted with scarring and neovascularization in both eyes. Mother of the same patient. Both patients have severe nystagmus

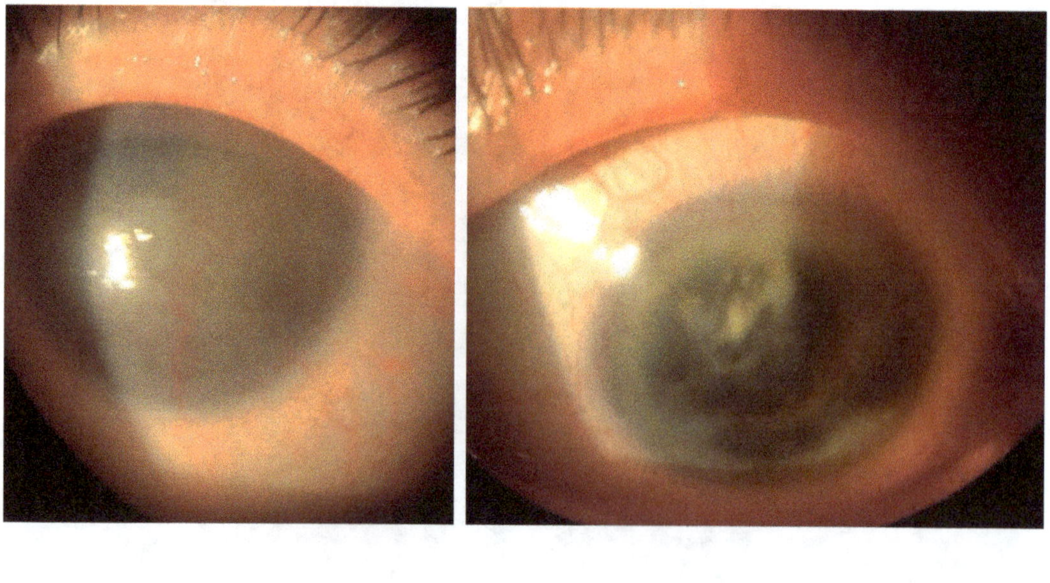

Figure 11. Aniridic keratopathy. Corneal scarring and neovascularization in seen (left photo) and the same eye under retroillumination showing the total absence of the iris

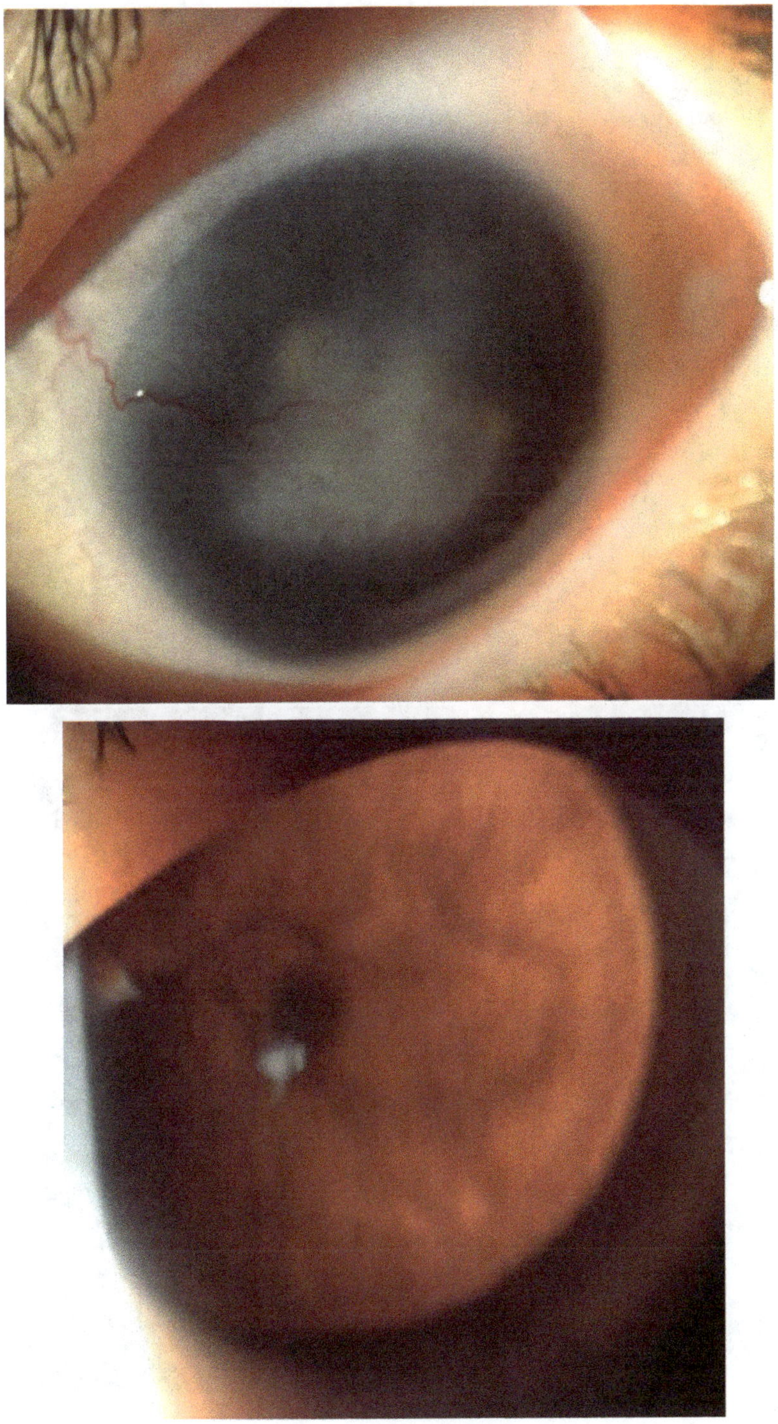

Figure 12. Aniridic keratopathy. The fellow eye of the same patient. The corneal scarring (left photo) with iris hypoplasia (right photo) is seen

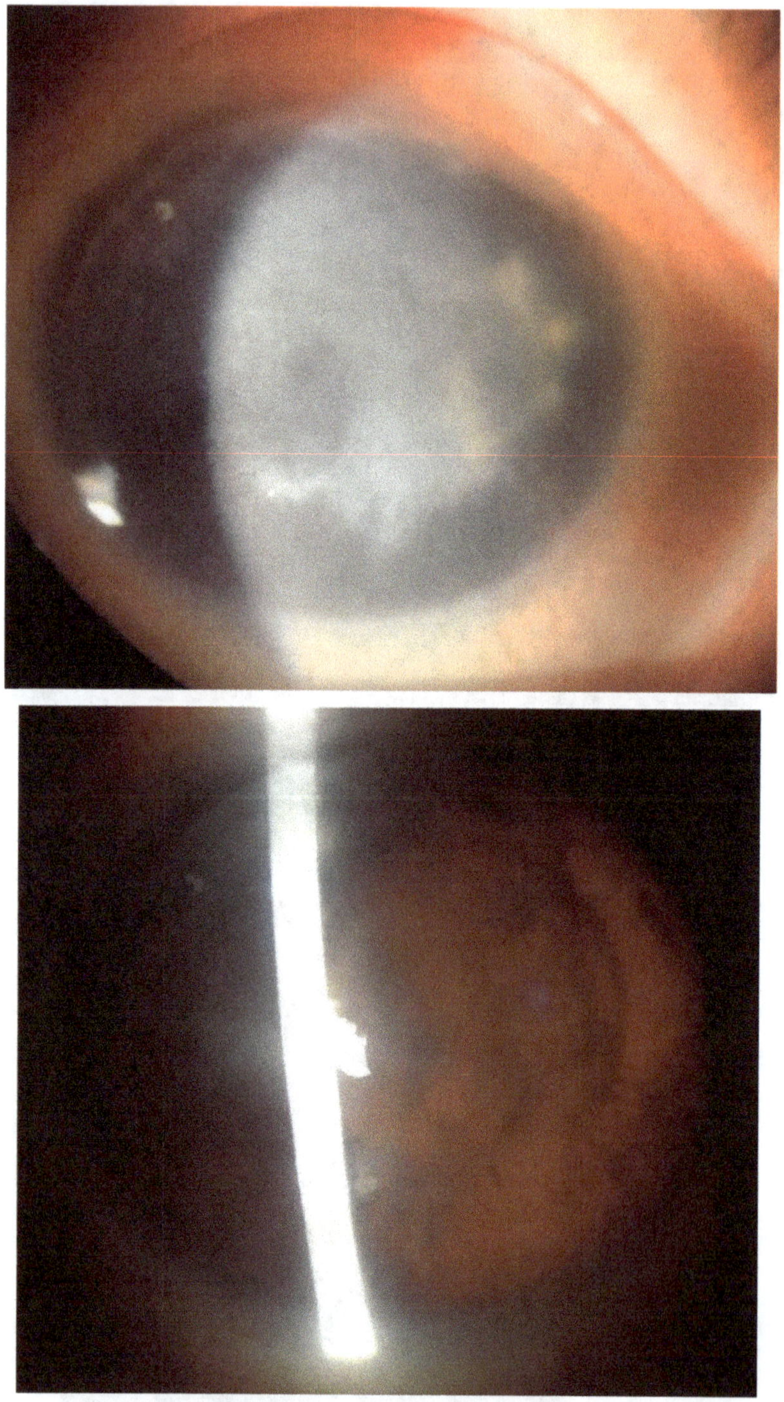

Axenfeld-Rieger syndrome is an autosomal dominant inherited disease characterized by bilateral anterior segment dysgenesis and systemic abnormalities (Murray et al, 1992). Common clinical findings are correctopia, polycoria, ectropion uveae, posterior embryotoxon, and increased intraocular pressure. These patients often have a characteristic slate-gray to chocolate-brown iris color (Fig 13, 14). Systemically, patients may have mild craniofacial dysmorphism, dental abnormalities, and redundant umbilical skin (Shields et al, 1985). The cornea rarely presents an issue in Axenfeld-Rieger syndrome. The goal of treatment is to control the glaucoma.

Figure 13. Axenfeld-Rieger syndrome. The right and left eyes of the same patient. Hypoplastic iris with a specific color is noted

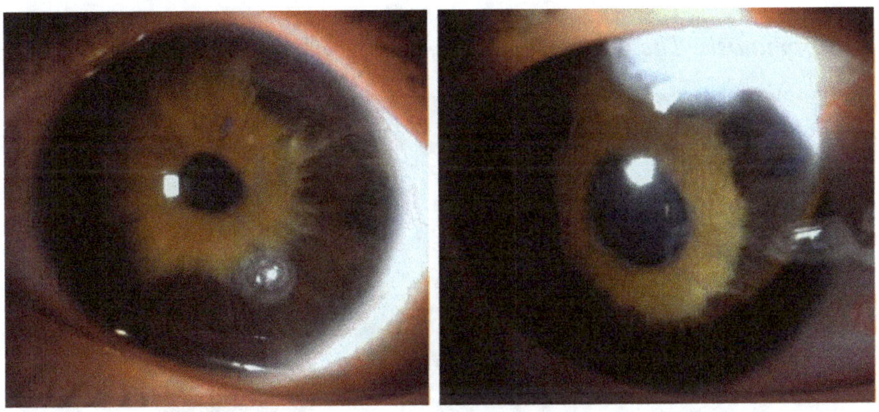

Figure 14. The same patient. The bleb after sinustrabeculectomy is seen

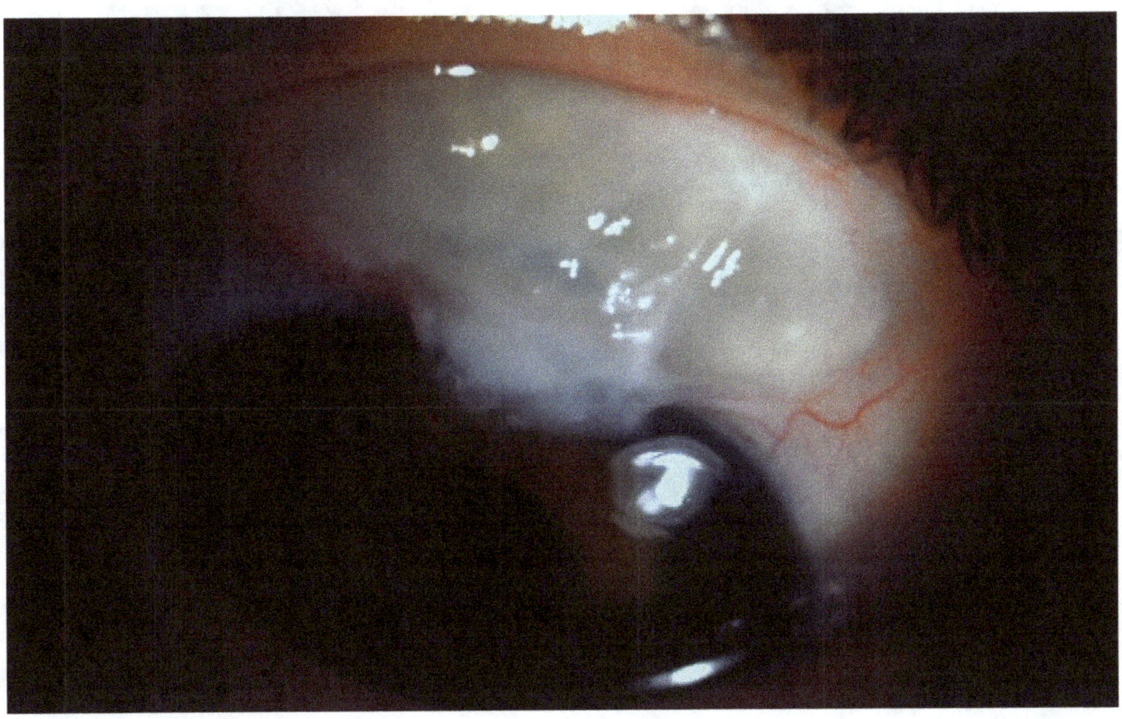

Neurofibromatosis (NF) type 1 (NF-1) is a disease characterized by the growth of noncancerous tumors called neurofibromas and has autosome dominant inheritance (Xu et al, 1990). Usually, these tumors are found on or just underneath the skin, as well as in the brain and peripheral nervous system. Ophthalmologic manifestations of NF-1 include iris Lisch nodules, plexiform neurofibromas, choroid hamartomas, retinal tumors, optic nerve gliomas, and prominent corneal nerves. Lisch nodules are the most common type of ocular involvement in NF-1. They are melanocytic hamartomas, usually clear yellow to brown, and dome-shaped elevations projecting from the iris's surface. Nowadays, no standardized treatments for NF1 and its complications are available. However, in recent years, increasing knowledge of the pathogenetic mechanisms has driven the scientific search behind biological agents that may affect the course of the disease.

Figure 15. Neurofibromatosis. The iris Lisch nodules are seen

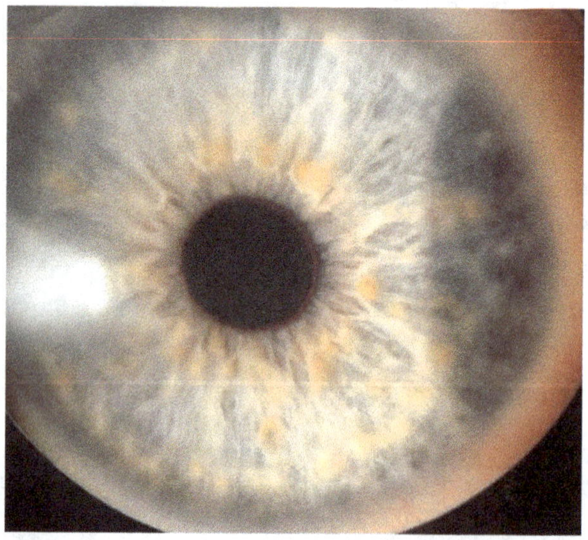

Figure 16. Multiple lesions on the lids and on the right eyebrow

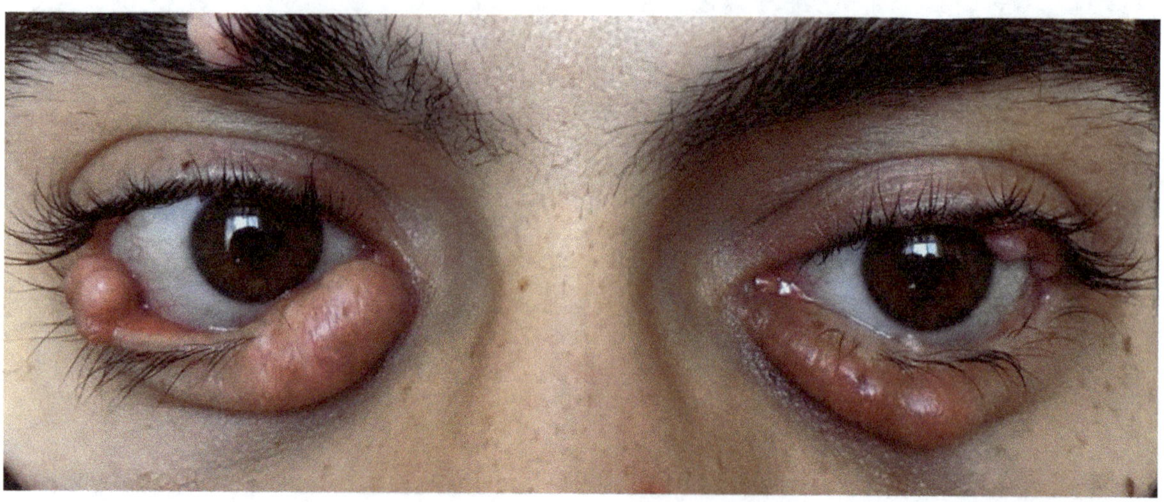

Ichthyosis refers to a relatively uncommon group of skin disorders characterized by excessive amounts of dry surface (Fig 17). Five distinct types of inherited ichthyosis are noted: ichthyosis vulgaris, lamellar ichthyosis, epidermolytic hyperkeratosis, congenital ichthyosiform erythroderma, and X-linked ichthyosis. In X-linked ichthyosis, generalized scaling is present at or shortly after birth (Shields et al, 1985). Irregular stromal corneal opacities located anterior to the Descemet membrane are found in 16-50% of male patients (Xu et al, 1990). This finding may be used to distinguish this form of ichthyosis from all other types. Ichthyosis doesn't have a known treatment, and the goal is to manage associated conditions. Lubricating drops and control of inflammation are required to relieve symptoms.

Figure 17. Ichthyosis. Corneal scarring is noted in the right eye

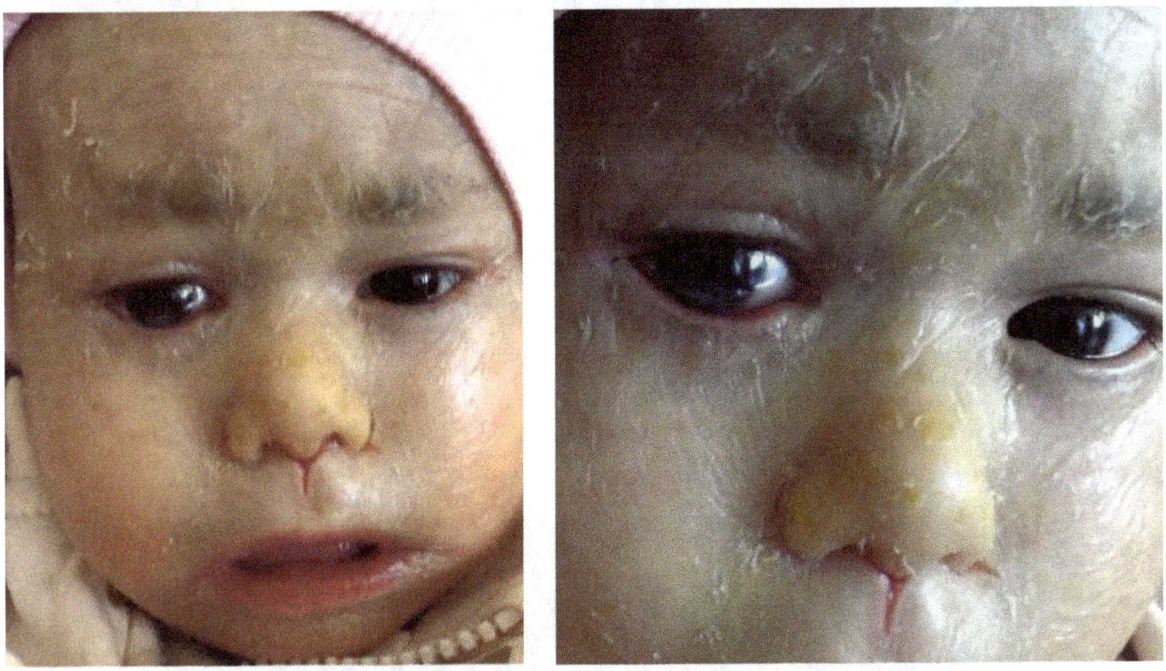

Porphyria (por-FEAR-e-uh) refers to a group of disorders that result from a buildup of natural chemicals that produce porphyrin in the body. There are two general categories of porphyria: acute, which mainly affects the nervous system, and cutaneous, which mainly affects the skin. Some types of porphyria have both nervous system symptoms and skin symptoms. Porphyria is usually inherited — one or both parents pass along an abnormal gene to their child. Eye involvement in porphyria is exceedingly rare and may manifest as a lid scarring, ectropion, pinguecula, pterygium, acute scleritis with scleral necrosis, corneal thinning, and corneal perforation (Fig 18 – 21). Treatment for acute porphyria involves intravenous (heme or glucose) infusions. For people diagnosed with cutaneous porphyria, avoiding sunlight is key to recovery.

Figure 18. Patient with porphyria. Facial characteristics and hands

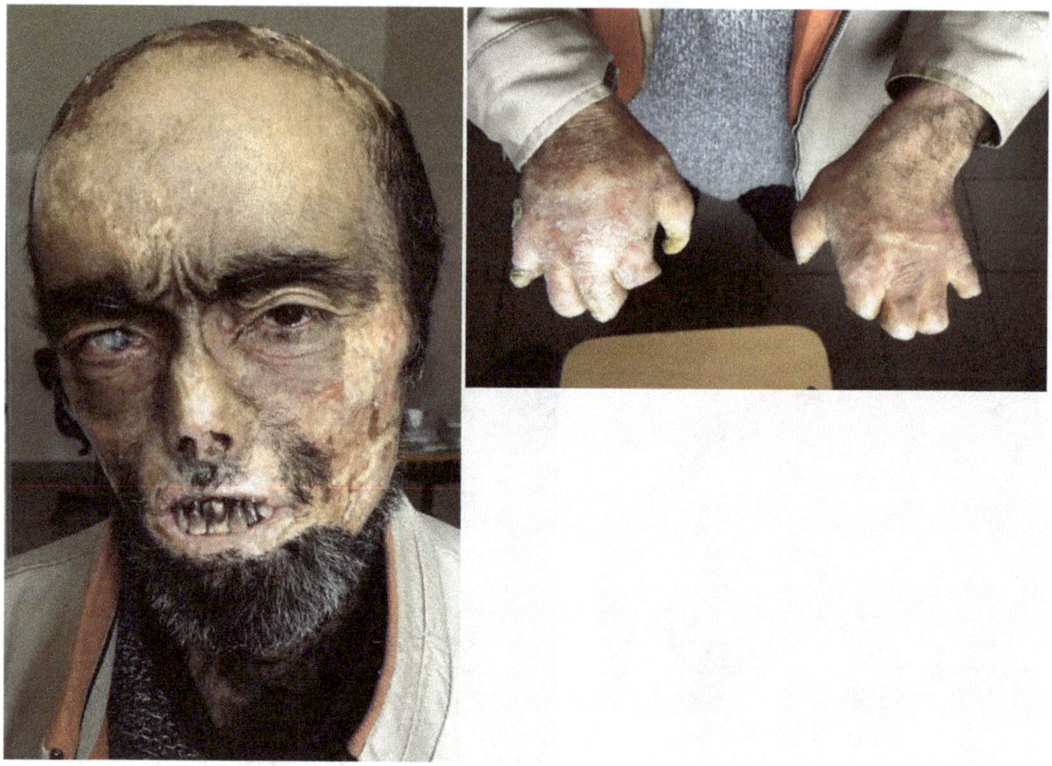

Figure 19. Same patient. Peripheral corneal thinning, scleral necrosis

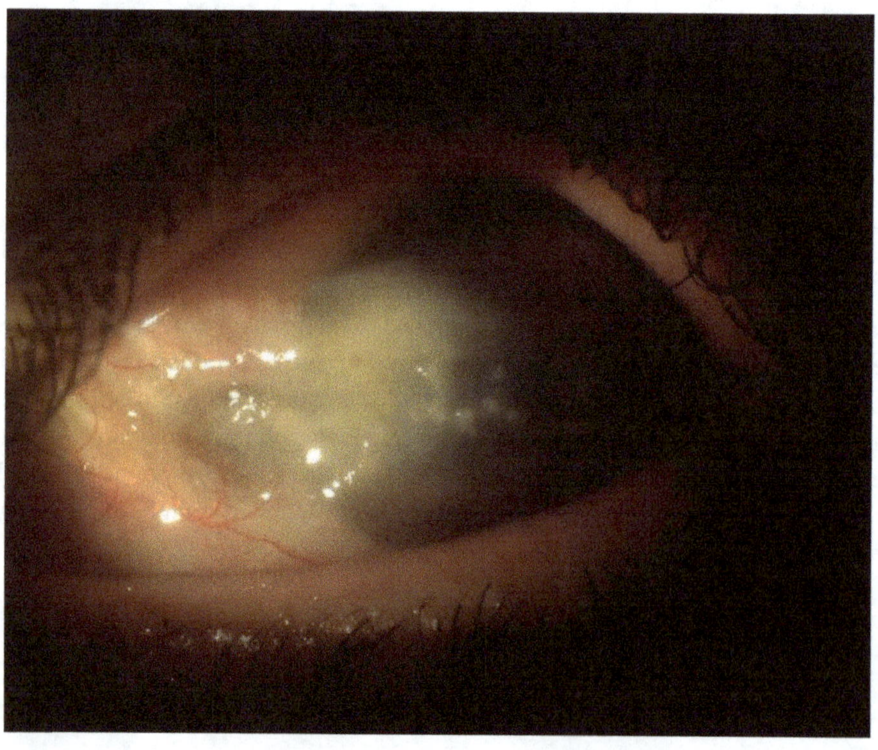

Figure 20. Amniotic membrane transplantation

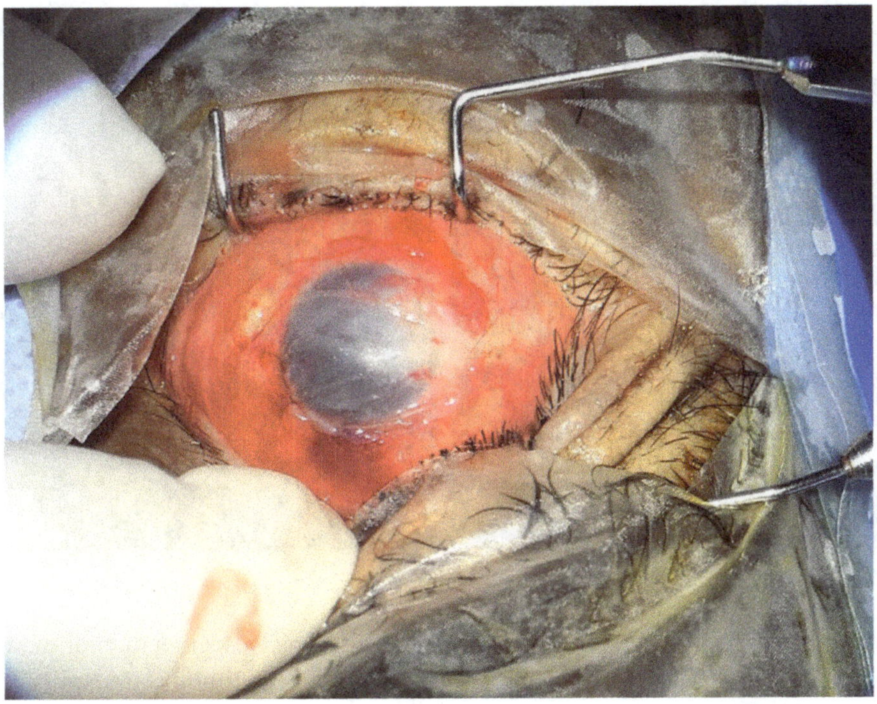

Figure 21. Appearance of the eye 1-month post-surgery and medical treatment involving oral Doxycycline, mild topical steroids (FML), cycloplegics, tears, and topical antibiotics for prophylaxis (Chloramphenicol)

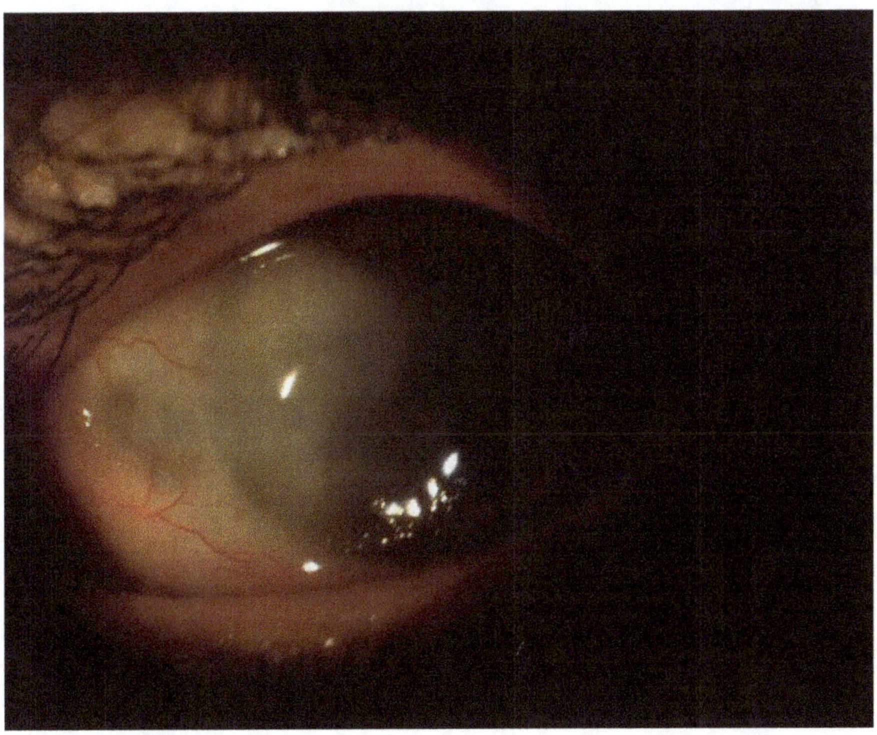

Figure 22. Haab Striae

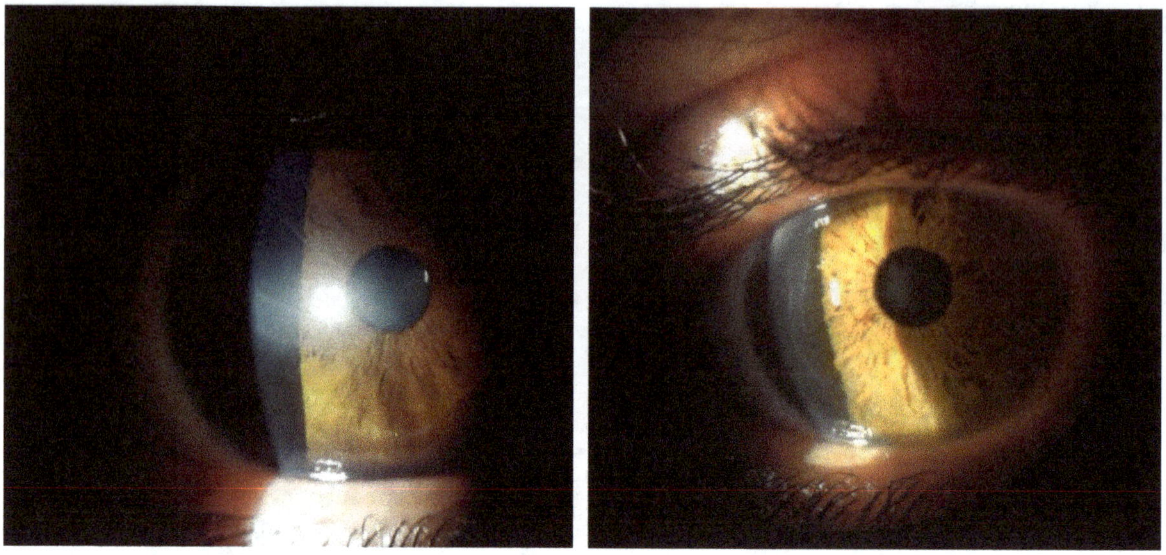

Haab's striae, or **Descemet's tears**, are horizontal breaks in the Descemet membrane associated with congenital glaucoma. Tears are usually peripheral, concentric to the limbus, and appear as lines with a double contour (Fig 22) (Turgut et al, 2009). Management of glaucoma is required.

REFERENCES

Costenbader, F. D., & Kwitko, M. L. (1967). Congenital glaucoma: An analysis of seventy-seven consecutive eyes. *Journal of Pediatric Ophthalmology*, *4*, 9.

Elsas, F. J., Maumenee, I. H., Kenyon, K. R., & Yoder, F. (1977). Familial aniridia with preserved ocular function. *American Journal of Ophthalmology*, *83*(5), 718–724. doi:10.1016/0002-9394(77)90139-8 PMID:868970

Gomes, J. A. P., Eagle, R. C. Jr, Gomes, A. K. G. D. P., Rapuano, C. J., Cohen, E. J., & Laibson, P. R. (1996). Recurrent keratopathy after penetrating keratoplasty for aniridia. *Cornea*, *15*(5), 457–462. doi:10.1097/00003226-199609000-00004 PMID:8862921

Holland, E. J., Djalilian, A. R., & Schwartz, G. S. (2003). Management of aniridic keratopathy with keratolimbal allograft: A limbal stem cell transplantation technique. *Ophthalmology*, *110*(1), 125–130. doi:10.1016/S0161-6420(02)01451-3 PMID:12511357

Kenyon, K. R. (1975). Mesenchymal dysgenesis in Peters' anomaly, sclerocornea and congenital endothelial dystrophy. *Experimental Eye Research*, *21*(2), 125–142. doi:10.1016/0014-4835(75)90077-9 PMID:1100415

Lee, H. J., & Colby, K. A. (2013). A review of the clinical and genetic aspects of aniridia. *Seminars in Ophthalmology*, *28*(5–6), 306–312. doi:10.3109/08820538.2013.825293 PMID:24138039

Meire, F. M. (1994). Megalocornea. Clinical and genetic aspects. *Documenta Ophthalmologica. Advances in Ophthalmology*, *87*(1), 1–121. doi:10.1007/BF01676641 PMID:7835180

Murray, J. C., Bennett, S. R., Kwitek, A. E., Small, K. W., Schinzel, A., Alward, W. L. M., Weber, J. L., Bell, G. I., & Buetow, K. H. (1992). Linkage of Rieger syndrome to the region of the epidermal growth factor gene on chromosome 4. *Nature Genetics*, *2*(1), 46–49. doi:10.1038/ng0992-46 PMID:1303248

Salmon, J., Wallis, C., & Murray, A. (1988). Variable expressivity of autosomal dominant microcornea with cataract. *Archives of Ophthalmology*, *106*(4), 505–510. doi:10.1001/archopht.1988.01060130551034 PMID:3355418

Sharkey, J. A., Kervick, G. N., Jackson, A. J., & Johnston, P. B. (1992). Cornea plana and sclerocornea in association with recessive epidermolysis bullosa dystrophica. *Cornea*, *11*(1), 83–85. doi:10.1097/00003226-199201000-00013 PMID:1559352

Shields, M. B., Buckley, E., Klintworth, G. K., & Thresher, R. (1985). Axenfeld-Rieger syndrome. A spectrum of developmental disorders. *Survey of Ophthalmology*, *29*(6), 387–409. doi:10.1016/0039-6257(85)90205-X PMID:3892740

Stein, P. E., Badminton, M. N., & Rees, D. C. (2017). Update review of the acute porphyrias. *British Journal of Haematology*, *176*(4), 527–538. doi:10.1111/bjh.14459 PMID:27982422

Turgut, B., Aydemir, O., Kaya, M., Turkcuoglu, P., Demir, T., & Clekir, U. (2009). Spontaneous corneal perforation in a patient with lamellar ichthyosis and dry eye. *Clinical Ophthalmology (Auckland, N.Z.)*, (3), 611–613. doi:10.2147/OPTH.S8407 PMID:19997563

Xu, G., O'Connell, P., Viskochil, D., Cawthon, R., Robertson, M., Culver, M., Dunn, D., Stevens, J., Gesteland, R., White, R., & Weiss, R. (1990). The neurofibromatosis type 1 gene encodes a protein related to GAP. *Cell*, *62*(3), 599–608. doi:10.1016/0092-8674(90)90024-9 PMID:2116237

Chapter 12
Corneal Trauma

ABSTRACT

Trauma is often the main cause of unilateral loss of vision in developing countries. Although corneal trauma can range from tiny corneal abrasions to sight-threatening and penetrating ocular injuries, even minor corneal trauma that breaches the epithelium has the potential to result in microbial keratitis and its associated complications, up until complete loss of vision. Even though ocular trauma is a global problem, blindness from eye injuries occurs mostly in developing countries, especially those where wars and civil conflicts bring around eye traumas from various weapons such as land mines, chemical substances, etc. Chemical injuries from both acids and alkalies are common causes of corneal injury due to their easy availability and soft regulations regarding their use. This chapter includes photos of trauma cases of the anterior segment, corneal and conjunctival foreign bodies, sequelae of blunt and penetrating trauma, chemical injuries, as well as a case of posttraumatic iris cyst.

INTRODUCTION

Foreign bodies should always be suspected when examining a patient with anterior segment trauma. Corneal foreign bodies are the second most common form of ophthalmic trauma after corneal abrasions. The source and composition of the foreign body determines the potential for ocular toxicity. Most corneal foreign bodies are easily seen by slit lamp examination, although the findings may be subtle. A metallic foreign body resulting from striking metal is usually sterile due to the heat generated by the striking force. Ferrous foreign bodies pose a special threat when embedded in the cornea, since they rust on contact with the tear film, forming rust rings. Plant and insect corneal foreign bodies shouldn't be underestimated since these types of materials can result in injuries with long-term corneal and ocular consequences. Foreign material of plant origin has a high incidence of microbial contamination. Thus, any patient with a plant-derived foreign body should be followed carefully for the development of a subsequent infection, and, in the events of infection developments, appropriate laboratory studies must be initiated, with special attention to fungal cultures (Fig 1-10). Foreign bodies located on the surface can be removed using different approaches. In most cases of superficial foreign bodies, a 27- or 30-gauge needle is an effective instrument for removal. After removing a foreign body, patients should be prescribed broad-spectrum topical ophthalmic antibiotics for one week or until the corneal surface is re-epithelialized. Short-acting topical cycloplegic drops can be used to mitigate discomfort (Murchison et al, 2017).

DOI: 10.4018/978-1-7998-6937-5.ch012

Figure 1. Multiple subconjunctival foreign bodies

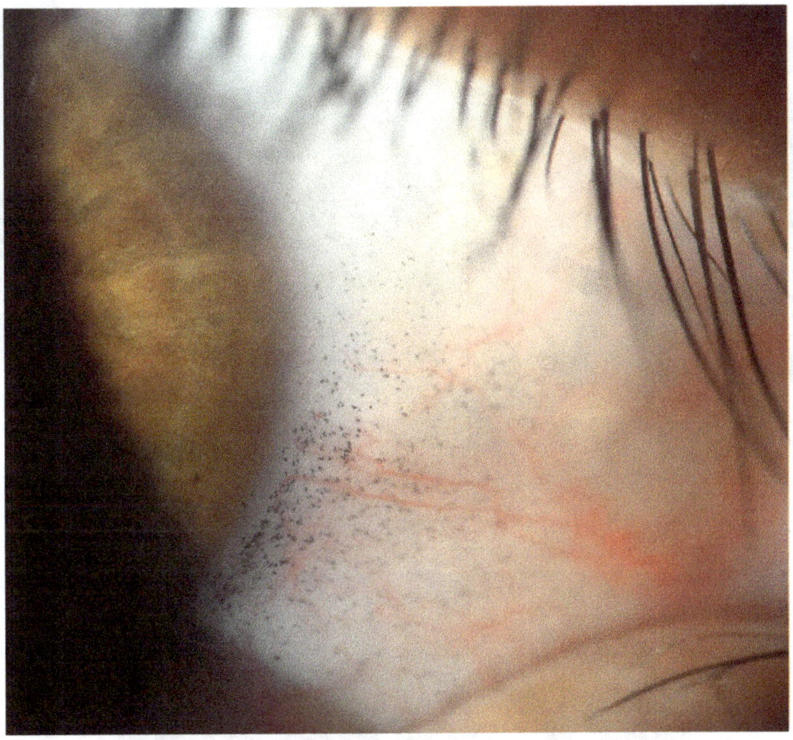

Figure 2. Cement in cul-de-sac

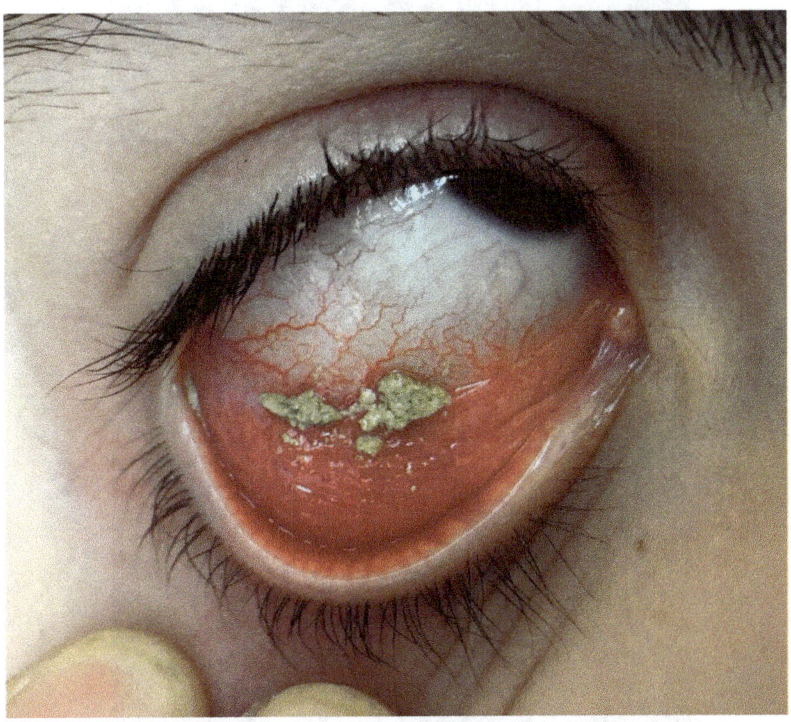

Figure 3. Intracorneal metallic foreign bodies

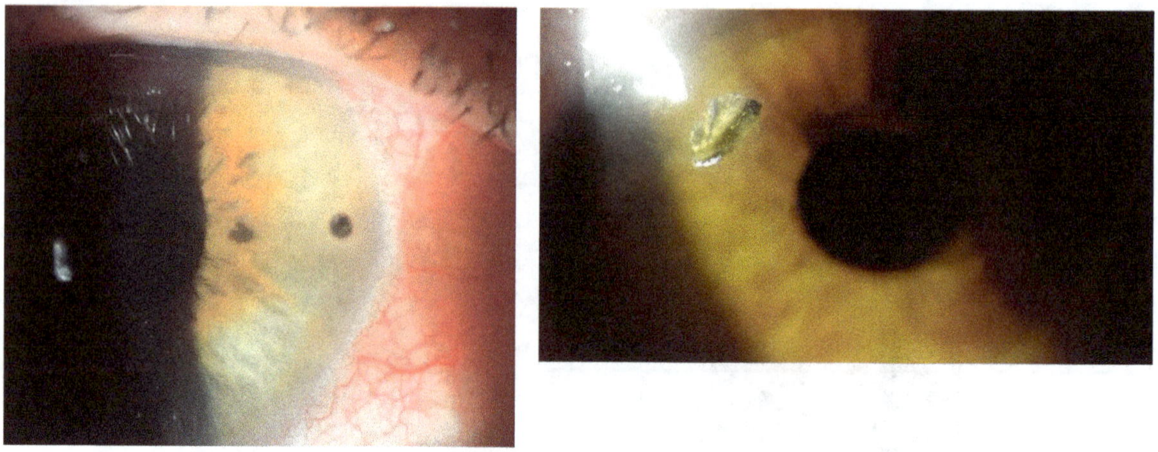

Figure 4. Intracorneal thorn bush shown by arrow

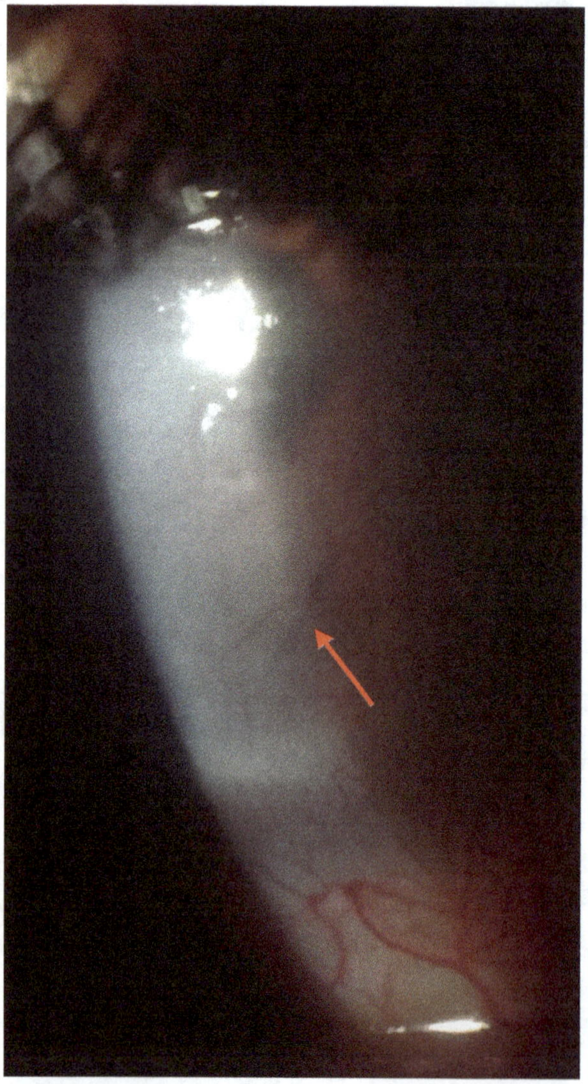

Figure 5. Wooden foreign body in anterior chamber penetrating the cornea (shown by arrow) associated with hypopyon

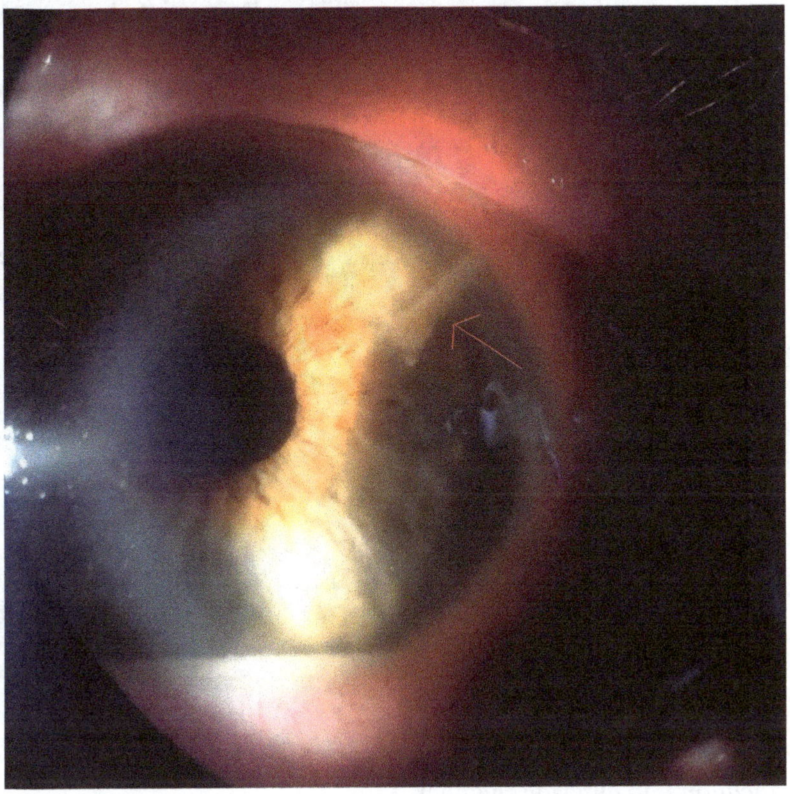

Figure 6. The same eye 4 weeks after foreign body removal and topical broad-spectrum antibiotic treatment with cycloplegic drops

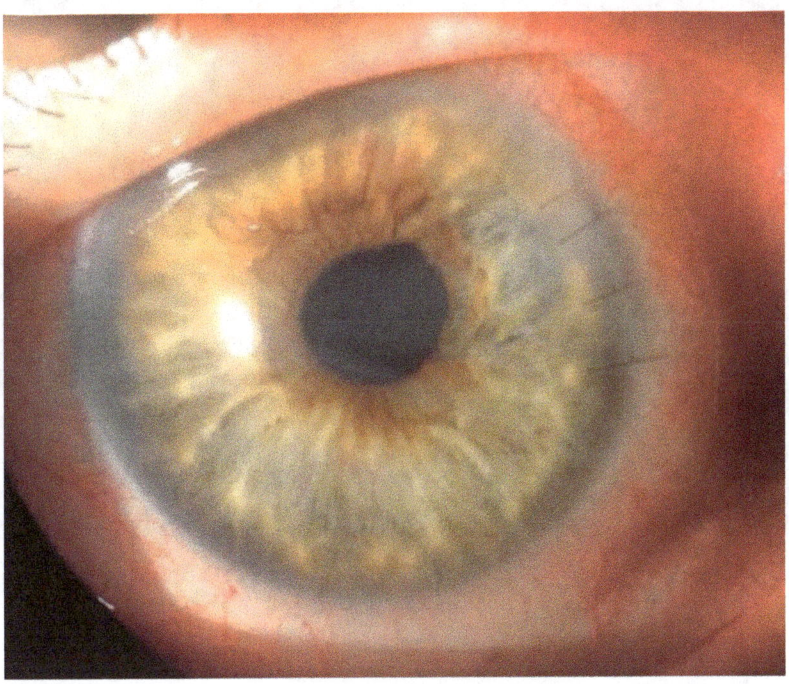

Figure 7. Anterior stromal scar after a penetrating trauma

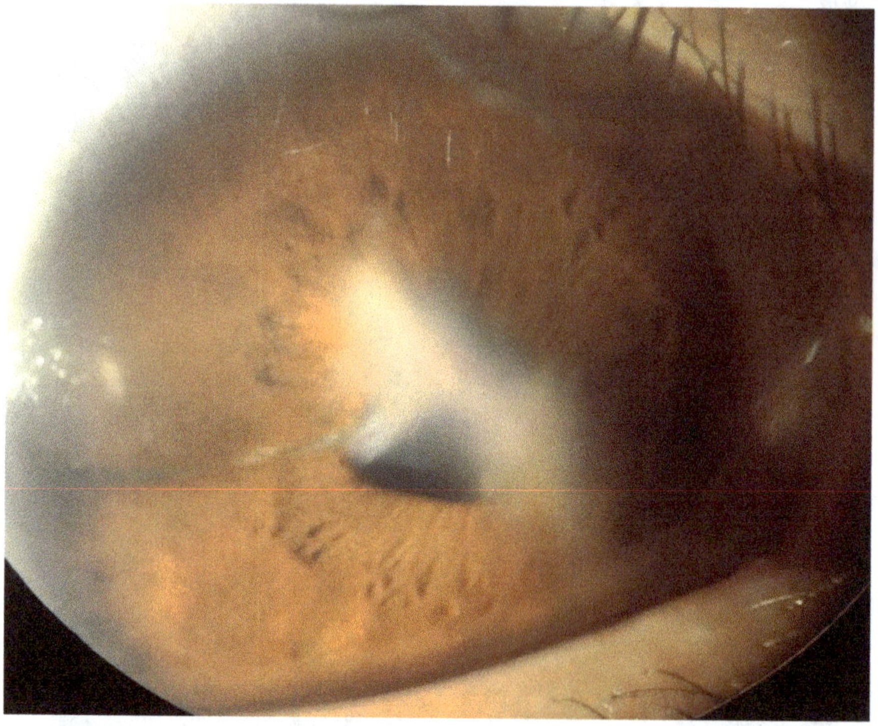

Figure 8. Penetrating trauma caused by exploded glass bottle. Picture taken after primary wound surgical repair. Lens dislocation into anterior chamber

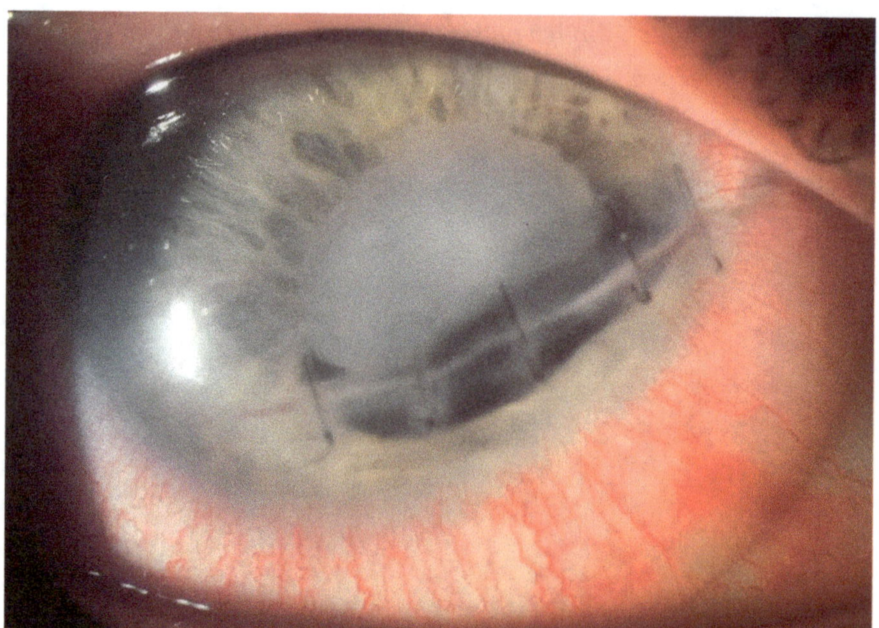

Figure 9. Corneoscleral laceration with prolapse of iris and choroid due to mine explosion

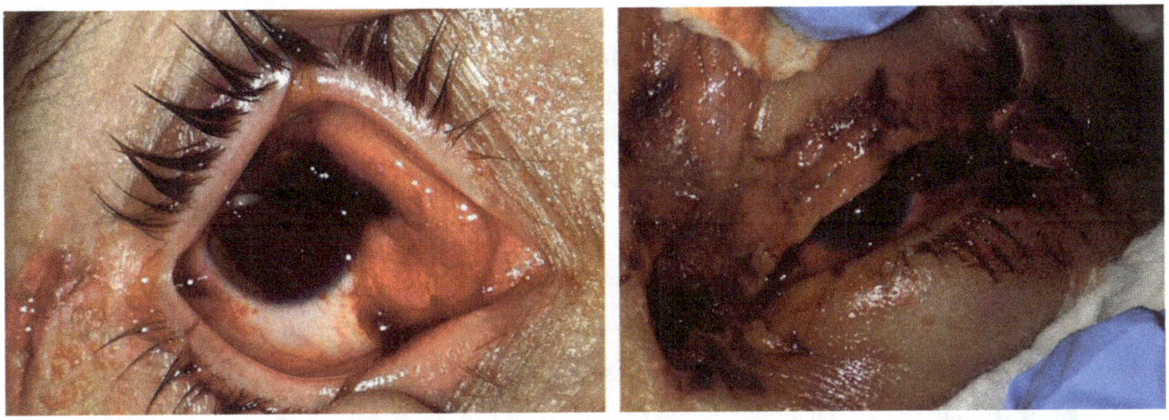

Figure 10. Nonleaking healed penetrating corneal trauma cause by knife

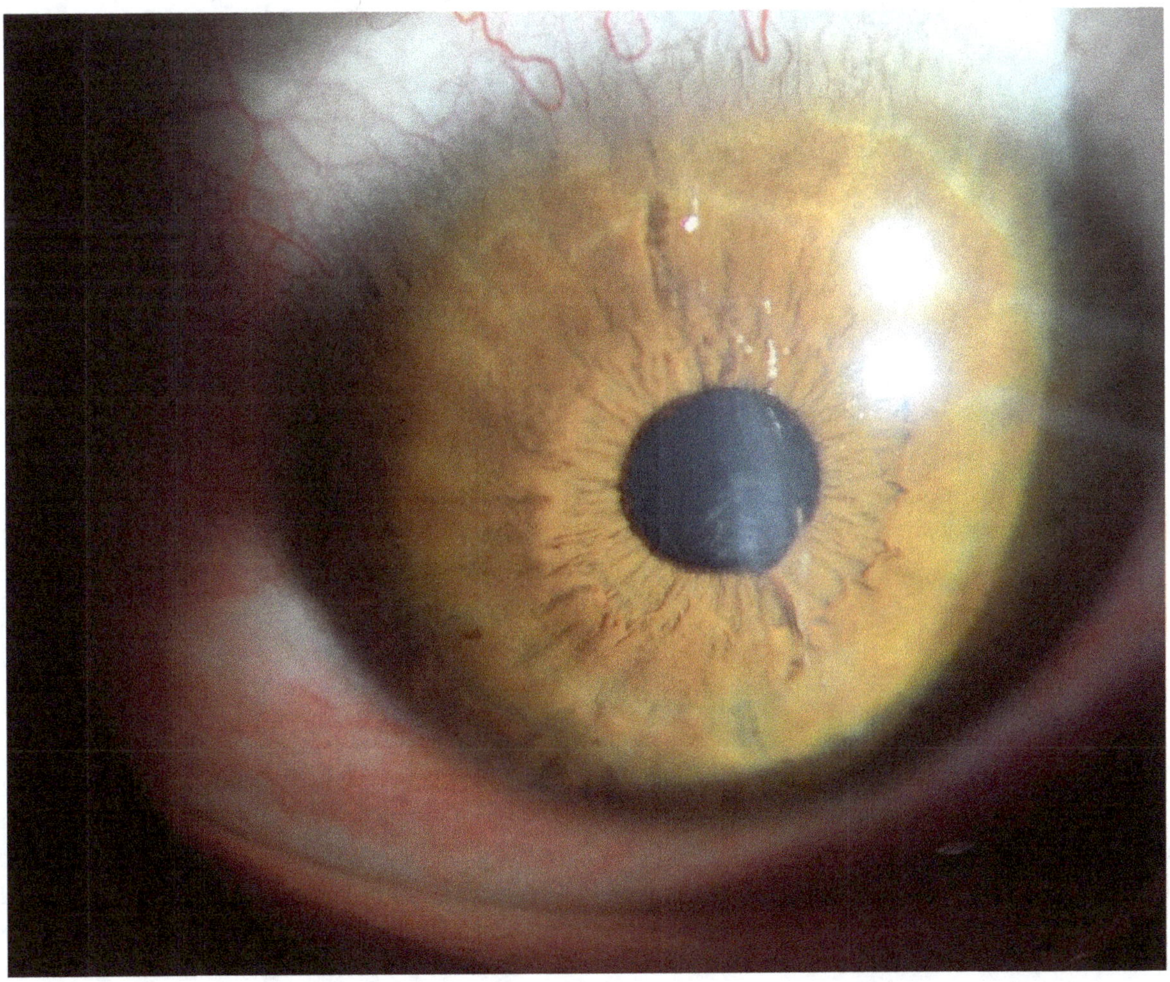

Blunt trauma refers to injuries that result from an impact with a noncutting instrument, in which the tissue damage is the result of a rapid transfer of compressive force. The most common patterns of iris injury after severe blunt trauma are sphincter tears which can be a reason of posttraumatic mydriasis and dialysis of the iris root. Traumatic iridodialysis can cause glare or diplopia (Fig 11) (Slingsby et al, 1981). Traumatic iridodialysis is repaired only when it is large enough to cause substantial, disabling glare or diplopia (Dağlioğlu et al, 2014).

Figure 11. Traumatic iridodialysis is seen

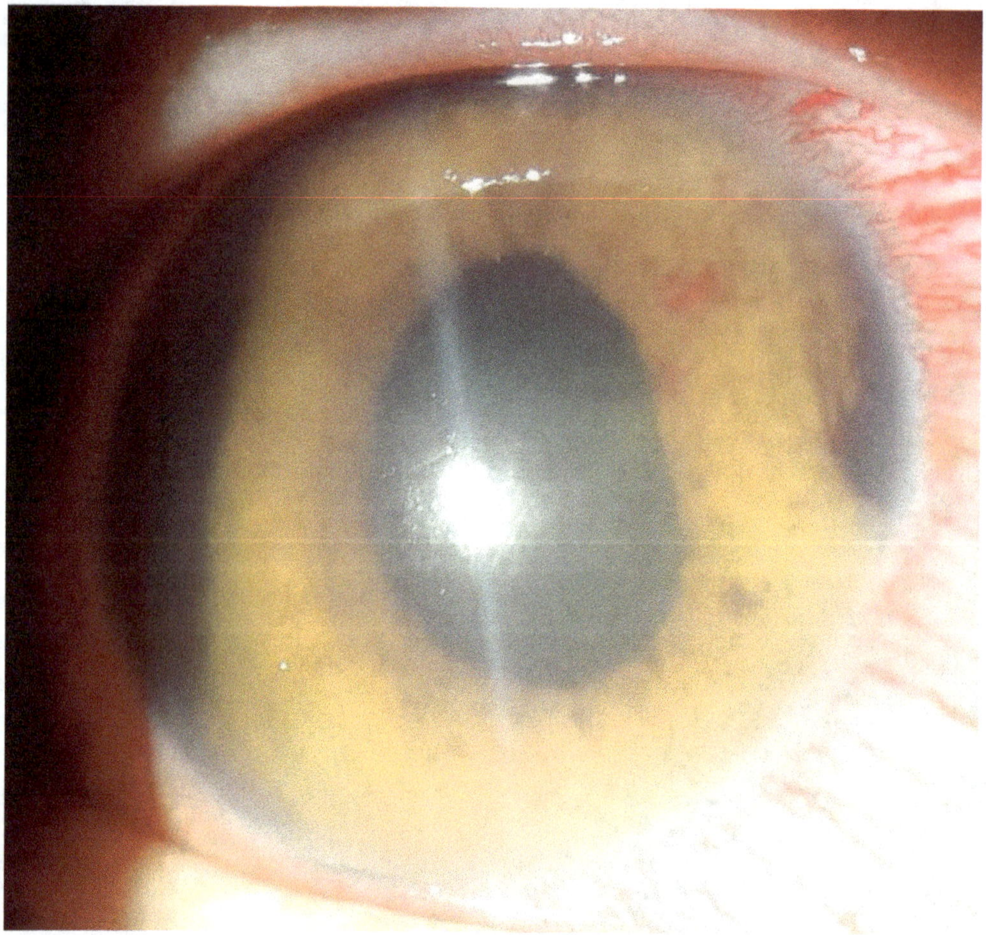

Lens injury with cataract formation frequently occurs in penetrating ocular trauma. Subluxation or dislocation of the lens is thought to be a result of equatorial expansion due to the shortening of the anterior to the posterior globe axis during blunt trauma (Fig 12-14) (Shah et al, 2014). Standard phacoemulsification may be achieved if the lens capsule is intact and there is sufficient zonular support. If anterior dislocation or extreme zonular instability are present, intracapsular cataract extraction may be required. Anterior dislocation of the lens into the anterior chamber is considered an emergency and requires immediate removal surgery due to possible pupillary block glaucoma development. Posterior capsulectomy and anterior vitrectomy improve visual outcomes (Walton et al, 2002).

Figure 12. Traumatic cataract after blunt trauma. The half opacified lens is seen

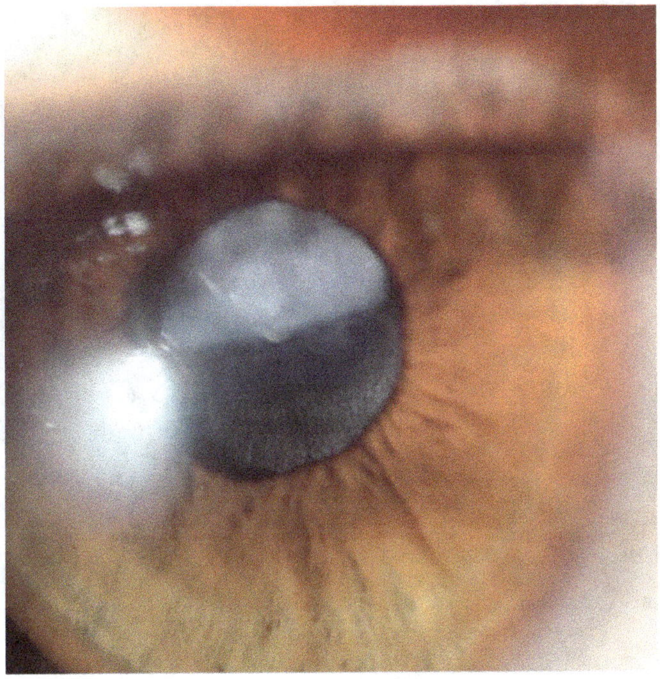

Figure 13. Dislocated lens after blunt trauma. Lens equator is seen through the pupil

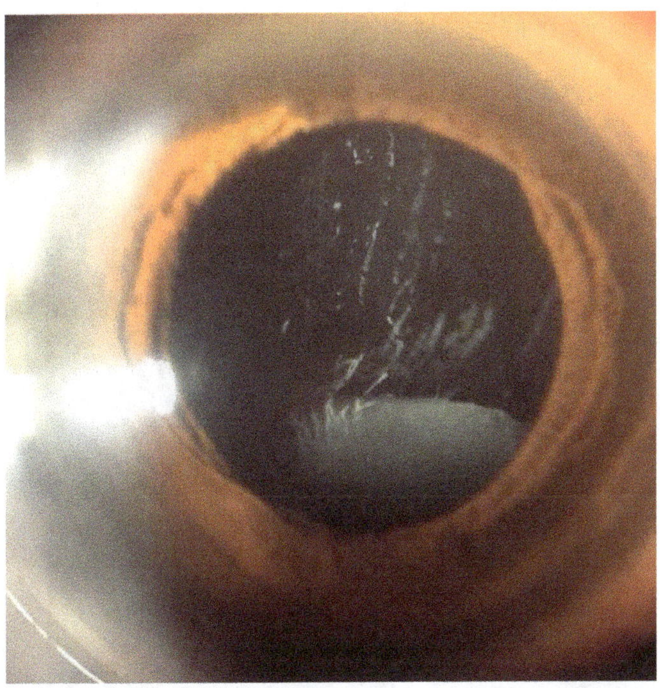

Figure 14. Lens dislocation into the anterior chamber after trauma

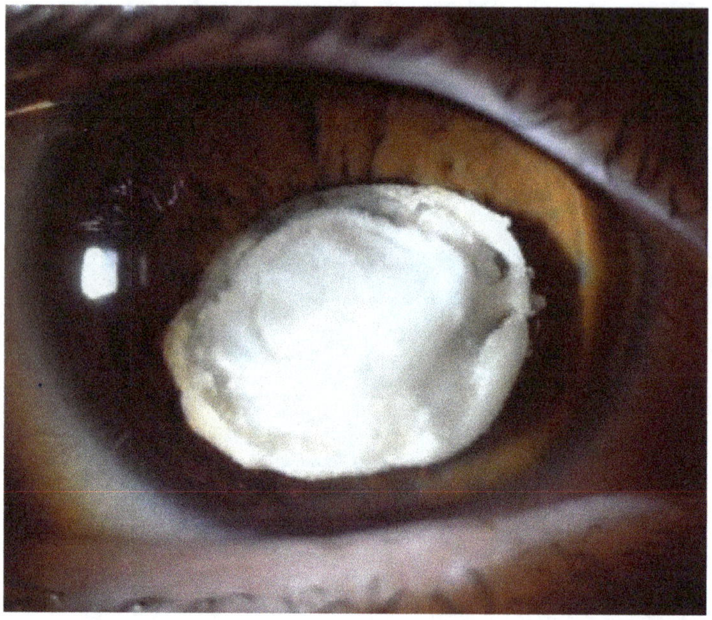

Hyphema is the accumulation of blood in the anterior chamber. The main cause of hyphema is blunt trauma; it can also be seen after intraocular surgeries as a complication (Fig 15) (Walton et al, 2008). Detailed evaluation is necessary as there is a risk of recurrent hemorrhage and glaucoma. In general, management includes restriction of physical activity and shielding the eye with the use of topical steroids (Nash et al, 2019).

Figure 15. Hyphema after a blunt trauma

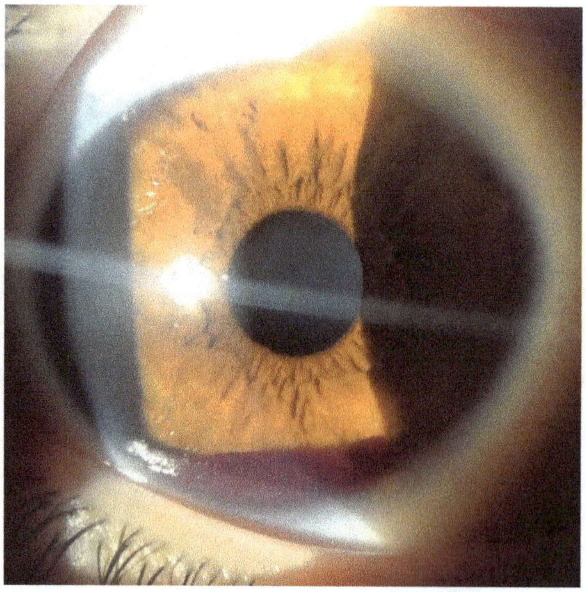

Ocular chemical injuries are true ophthalmic emergencies due to the potential for permanent corneal and intraocular damage leading to visual impairment or blindness. Acids and alkalis are the agents most commonly associated with significant chemical eye injuries. Common causes of alkali injury include cement, ammonia, lime, potassium hydroxide, and magnesium hydroxide. Acid injuries of the eye are associated with sulphuric, sulphuruous, hydrofluoric, acetic, chromic, and hydrochloric acids. Severe chemical injuries can cause perilimbal ischemia, corneal haze, and stromal collagenolytic processes, which may progress to ulceration and perforation (Fig 16-22) (Pfister et al, 1983; Wagoner et al, 1997). Immediate copious irrigation remains the single most important therapy for treating chemical injuries. Placement of a therapeutic bandage contact lens until the epithelium has regenerated can be helpful in some patients (Wagoner et al, 2000). Therapeutic treatment includes serum tears, topical antibiotics for prophylaxis, cycloplegics, lubricating drops, oral Doxycycline. Amniotic membrane transplant in eyes with acute ocular burns promotes faster healing of epithelial defects in patients with moderate grade burns (Clare et al, 2012). Controlling inflammation with topical steroids help halt the inflammatory cycle. Surgical treatment includes removal of inciting chemicals, and procedures as follows: limbal stem cell transplantion (Kawashima et al, 2007), either autologous from a fellow healthy eye or allograft from a living relative or cadaver, penetrating keratoplasty with or without cataract extraction (Tuft et al, 2009), keratoprosthesis. The surgeon decides on what procedure to implement depending on the nuances of the particular case.

Figure 16. Chemical (alkali) injury caused by cement. Hypopyon and total corneal edema is seen

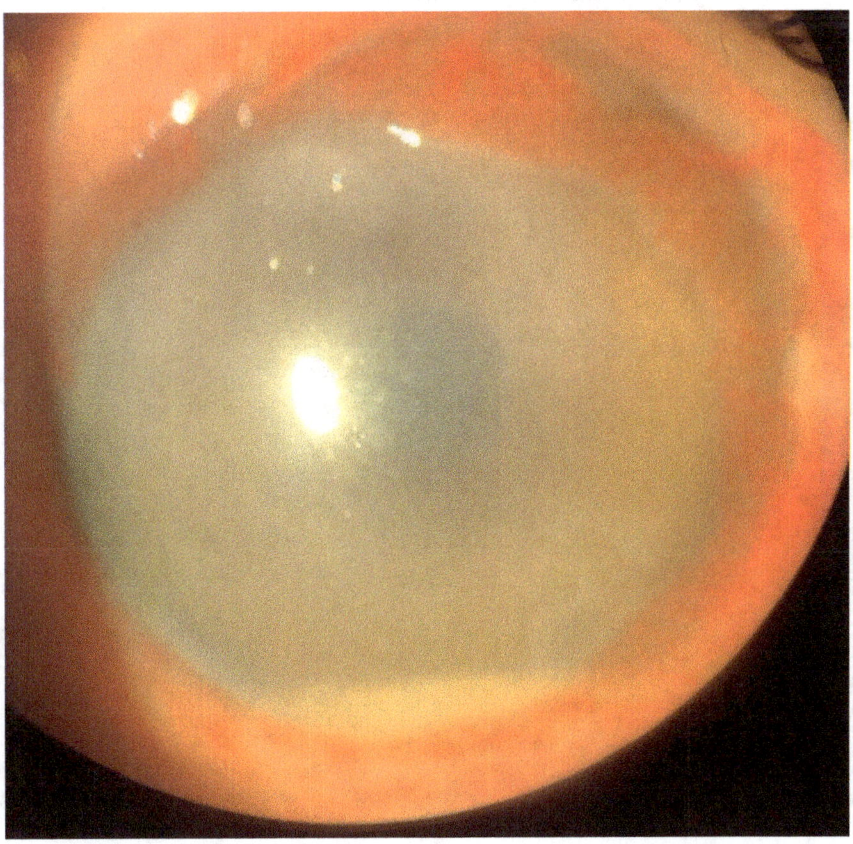

Figure 17. The same eye stained with fluorescein. Total epithelial defect is seen

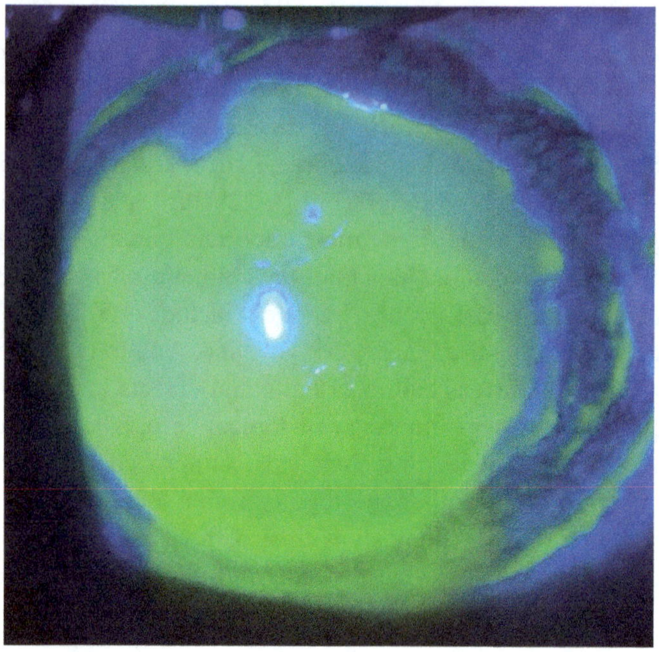

Figure 18. Chemical injury (alkali) caused by ammonia

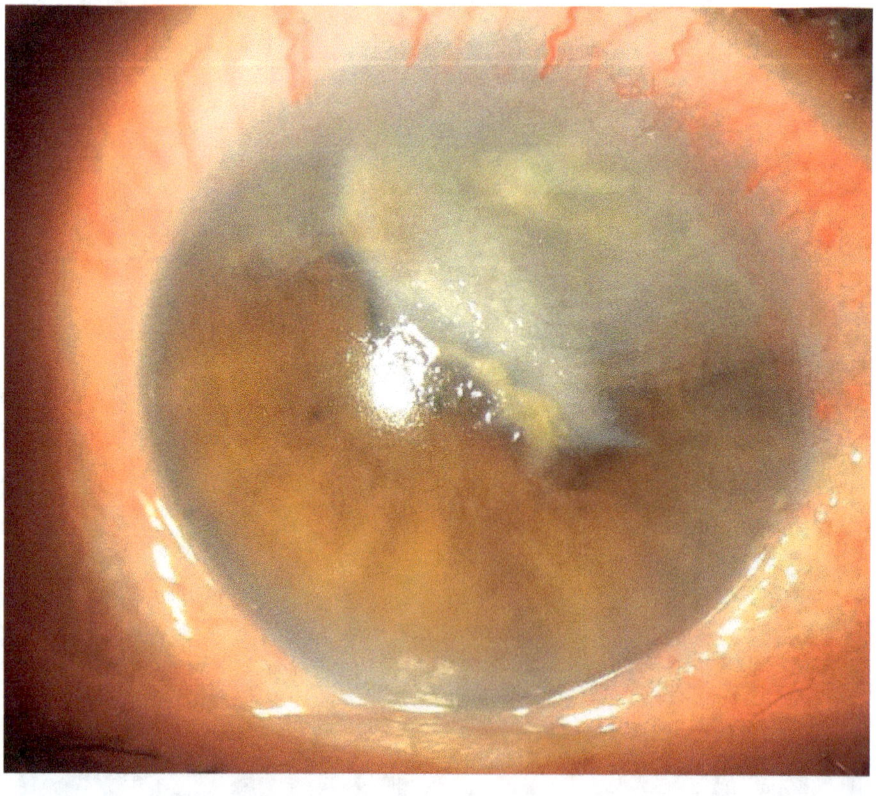

Figure 19. Acid Injury. Subtotal corneal epithelial and conjunctival defect (left photo). The same eye with chemical agent in the conjunctival cul-de-sac (right photo)

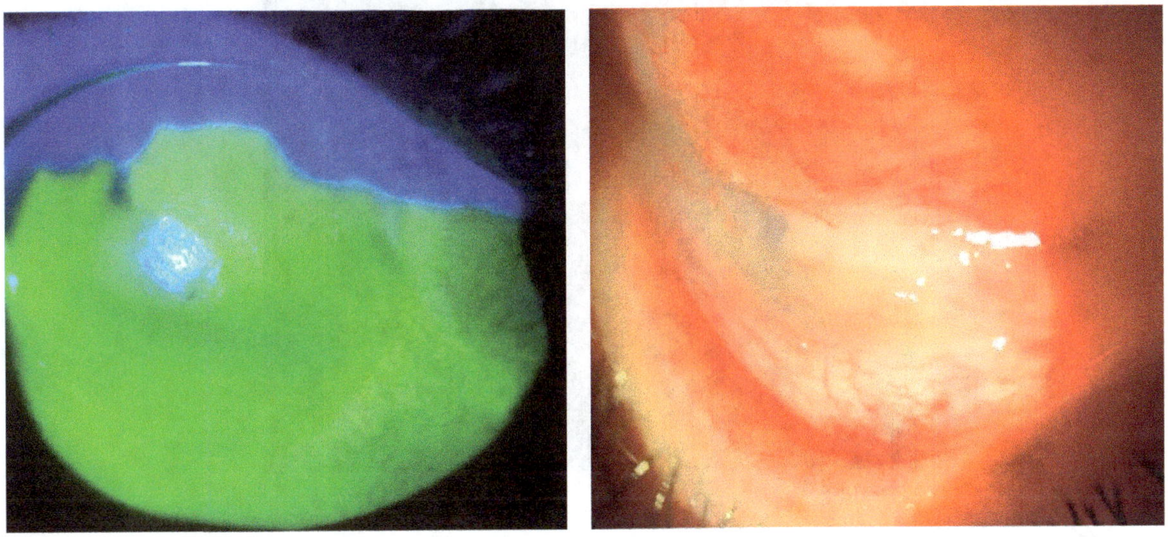

Figure 20. Chemical (acid) injury caused by hydrochloric acid; total conjunctivalization of the surface

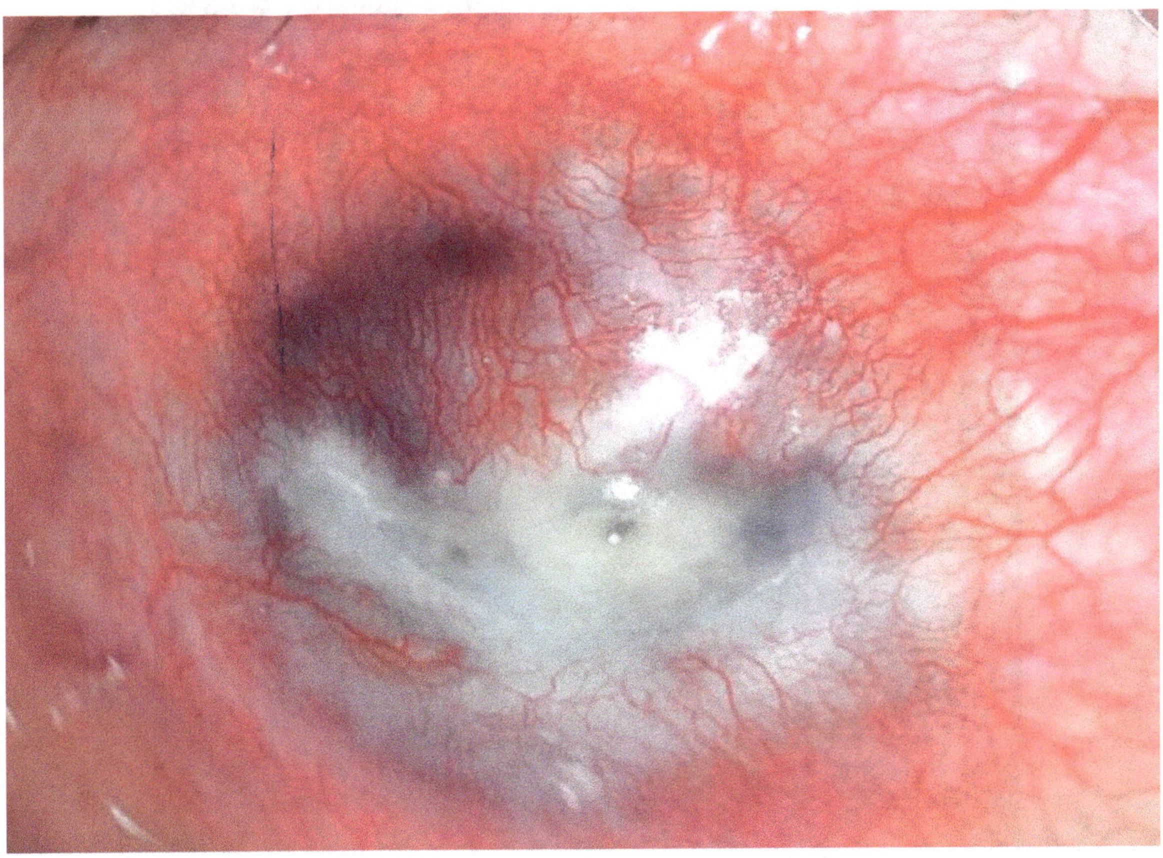

Figure 21. Chemical injury caused by cement. Thinning of cornea (pending perforation) is seen

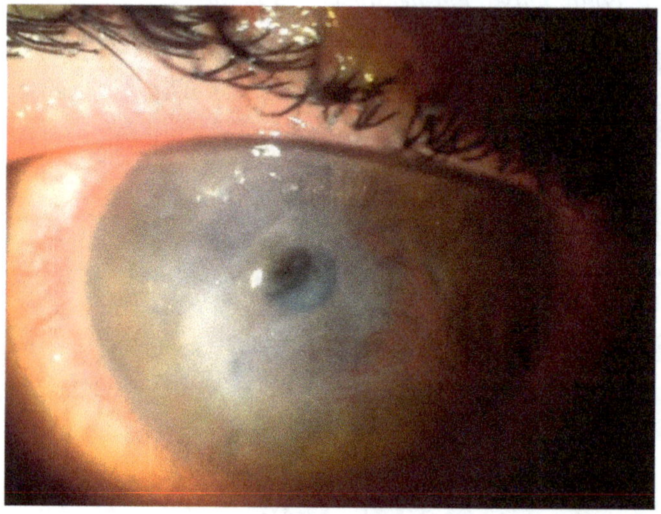

Figure 22. The same eye after 3 weeks of treatment with topical antibiotics, oral Doxycycline, mild steroids, cycloplegics, lubricants and serum tears. Anterior stromal scar is formed

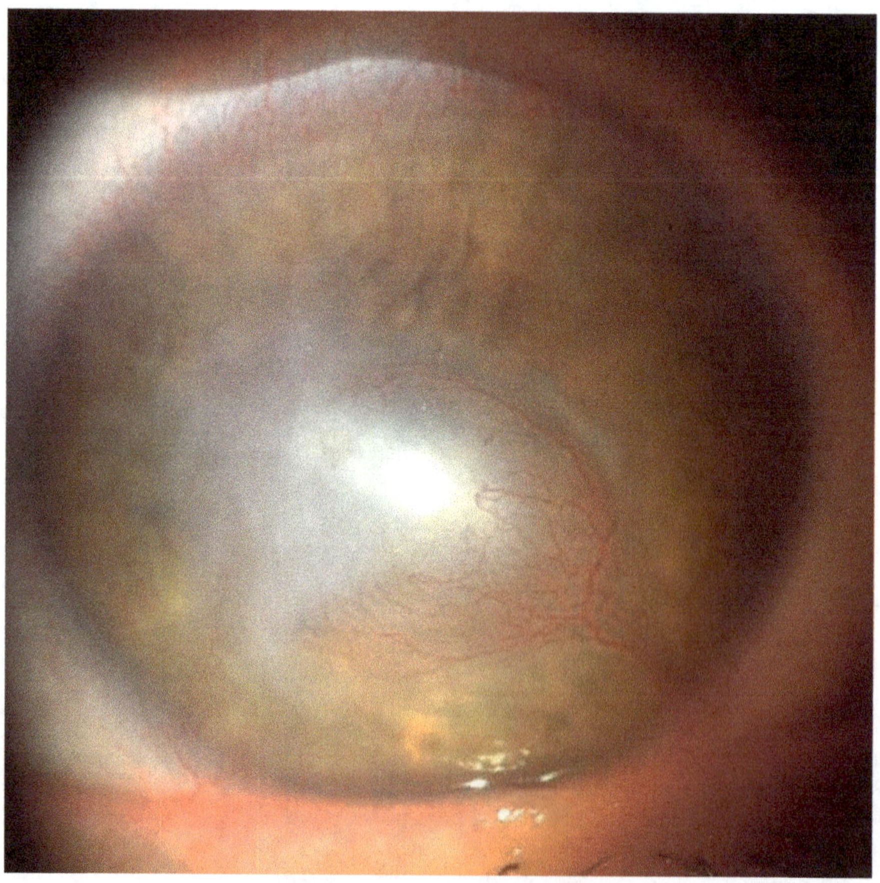

Injury of the cornea occurs from the placement of the forceps blade across the globe and the orbit during delivery, causing blunt trauma and rupture of the Descemet membrane (Cotran et al 1992). Left eyes seem to be affected more commonly than right eyes because neonates usually present in the left-occiput-anterior position. The Descemet tears in birth trauma are usually unilateral, central, and lines are seen in vertical or oblique patterns (Fig 23).

Figure 23. Birth trauma. Vertical Descemet tears are seen

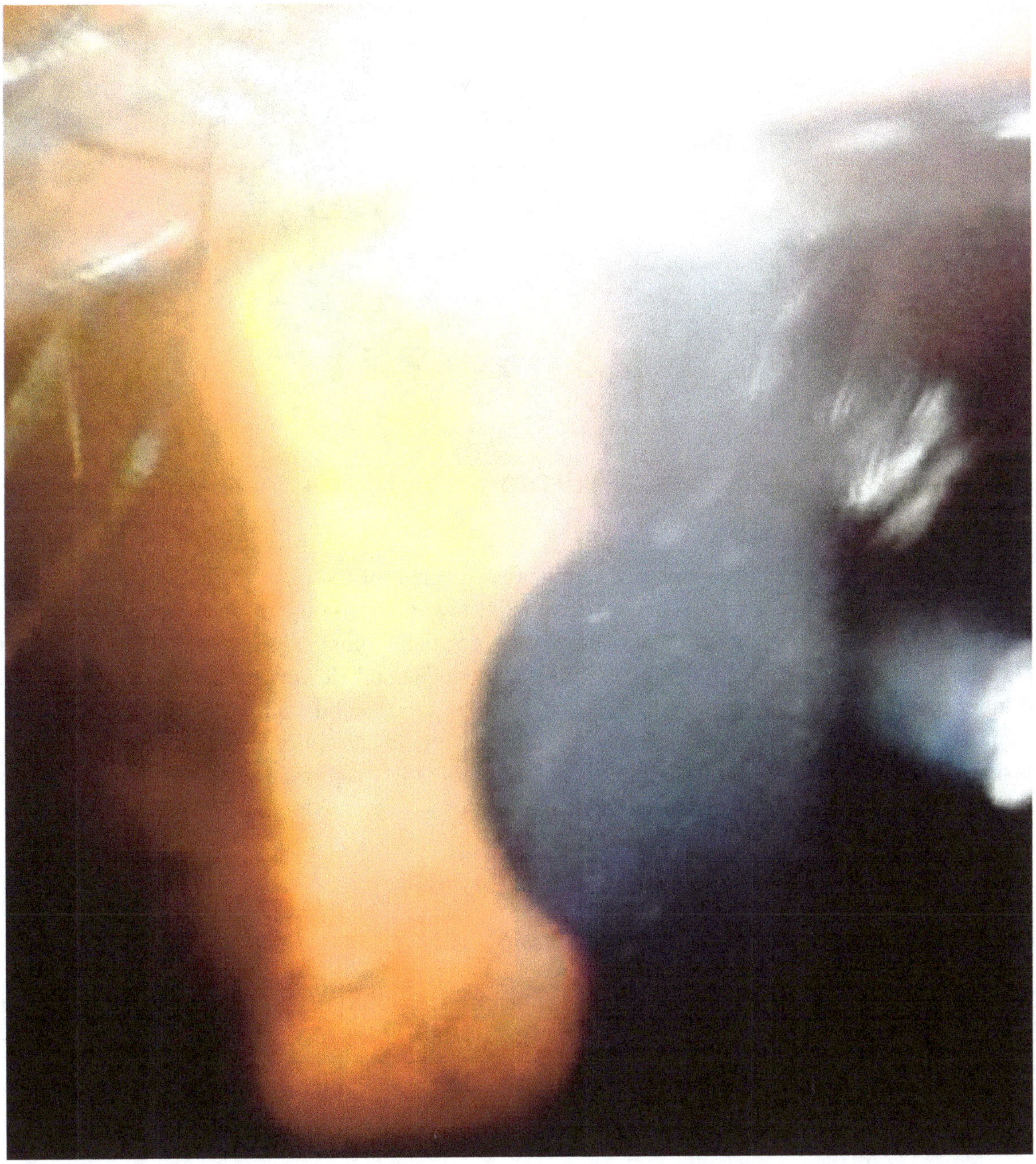

Figure 24. Iris cyst 6 months after a penetrating trauma

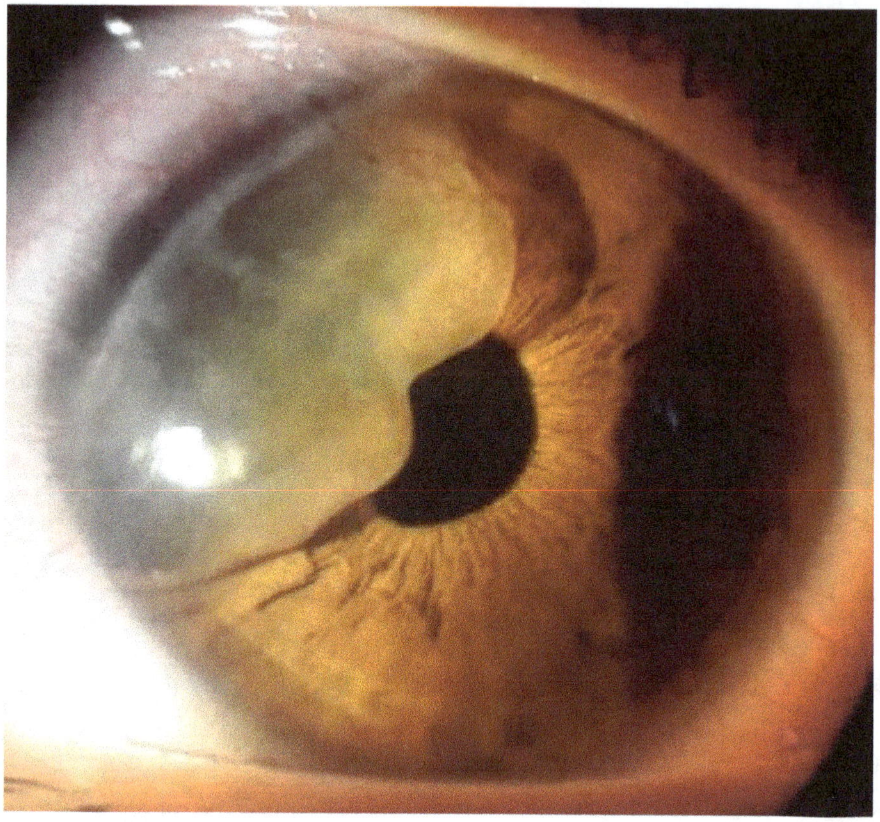

An **iris cyst** is an epithelial-lined space that involves a layer of the iris, which can be primary and secondary. Secondary iris cyst can occur due to epithelial downgrowth (surgical and non-surgical trauma, Fig 24), intraocular tumors, and medications (miotics, prostaglandins) (Shields et al, 1981). If the iris cyst is small and asymptomatic, close observation may be sufficient. However, larger iris cysts can grow and induce pupillary block and secondary glaucoma, uveitis, corneal decompensation, and ultimately, a painful, blind eye (Bruner et al, 1981). Many different treatment options, ranging from minimally invasive techniques such as aspiration of the cyst or laser therapy, to aggressive surgical procedures like block excision have been described for the management of iris cysts (Moreno-López et al, 2007; Xiao et al, 2006).

REFERENCES

Bruner, W. E., Michels, R. G., Stark, W. J., & Maumenee, A. E. (1981). Management of epithelial cysts of the anterior chamber. *Ophthalmic Surgery*, *12*(4), 279–285.

Chung, M. Y., Milly, K. M., & Weissman, B. A. (2009). Morcher iris reconstruction lens and rigid contact lens for traumatic aniridia. *Eye & Contact Lens*, *35*(2), 108–110. doi:10.1097/ICL.0b013e318199b00b PMID:19265334

Clare, G., Suleman, H., Bunce, C., & Dua, H. (2012, September 12). Amniotic membrane transplantation for acute ocular burns. *Cochrane Database of Systematic Reviews*, *9*, CD009379.

Cotran, P. R., & Bajart, A. M. (1992). Congenital corneal opacities. *International Ophthalmology Clinics*, *32*(1), 93–105.

Dağlioğlu, M. C., Coşkun, M., Ilhan, N., Ayintap, E., Tuzcu, E. A., İlhan, Ö., & Öksüz, H. (2014). Repair of iridodialysis using 8-0 polypropylene. *Seminars in Ophthalmology*, *29*(3), 159–162. doi:10.3109/08820538.2013.796395 PMID:23879224

Kawashima, M., Kawakita, T., Satake, Y., Higa, K., & Shimazaki, J. (2007, October). Phenotypic study after cultivated limbal epithelial transplantation for limbal stem cell deficiency. *Archives of Ophthalmology*, *125*(10), 1337–1344.

Moreno-López, M., Arruabarrena, C., Regueras, A., & Noval, S. (2007). Conservative surgical management of a post-traumatic iris cyst. *Archivos de la Sociedad Espanola de Oftalmologia*, *82*(7), 455–457.

Murchison. (2017). *Corneal Abrasions and Corneal Foreign Bodies*. Merck Manual.

Nash & Sheppard. (2019). *Hyphema*. Medscape Drugs & Diseases from WebMD.

Negrel, A. D., & Thylefors, B. (1998). The global impact of eye injuries. *Ophthalmic Epidemiology*, *5*(3), 143–169. doi:10.1076/opep.5.3.143.8364 PMID:9805347

Pfister, R. R. (1983). Chemical injuries of the eye. *Ophthalmology*, *90*, 1246–1253.

Shah, M. A., Shah, S. M., Patel, K. D., Shah, A. H., & Pandya, J. S. (2014, November). Maximizing the visual outcome in traumatic cataract cases: The value of a primary posterior capsulotomy and anterior vitrectomy. *Indian Journal of Ophthalmology*, *62*(11), 1077–1081. doi:10.4103/0301-4738.146757 PMID:25494250

Shields, J. A. (1981). Primary cysts of the iris. *Transactions of the American Ophthalmological Society*, *79*, 771–809.

Slingsby, J. G., & Forstot, S. L. (1981). Effect of blunt trauma on the corneal endothelium. *Archives of Ophthalmology*, *99*(6), 1041–1043. doi:10.1001/archopht.1981.03930011041011 PMID:7236101

Tuft, S. J., & Shortt, A. J. (2009, January 23). Surgical rehabilitation following severe ocular burns. *Eye (London, England)*.

Wagoner, M. D. (1997). Chemical injuries of the eye: Current concepts in pathophysiology and therapy. *Survey of Ophthalmology*, *41*, 275–313.

Wagoner, M. D., & Kenyon, K. R. (2000). Chemical injuries of the eye. Clinical Practice. Principles and Practice of Ophthalmology, 2, 943-59.

Walton, W., Von Hagen, S., Grigorian, R., & Zarbin, M. (2002). Management of traumatic hyphema. *Survey of Ophthalmology*, *47*(4), 297–334. doi:10.1016/S0039-6257(02)00317-X PMID:12161209

Xiao, Y., Wang, Y., Niu, G., & Li, K. (2006). Transpupillary argon laser photocoagulation and Nd:YAG laser cystotomy for peripheral iris pigment epithelium cyst. *American Journal of Ophthalmology*, *142*(4), 691–693. doi:10.1016/j.ajo.2006.04.050

Yuen, N. S., Hui, S. P., & Woo, D. C. (2006). New method of surgical repair for 360-degree cyclodialysis. *Journal of Cataract and Refractive Surgery*, *32*(1), 13–17. doi:10.1016/j.jcrs.2005.05.035 PMID:16516773

Chapter 13
Corneal Surgeries

ABSTRACT

This chapter includes corneal surgeries performed in the center such as corneal transplantation (PK, DALK, DSAEK, DMEK) with all possible complications: graft rejections, recurrence of previous diseases, reactivation of previous infection, and other rare complications. Photos of conjunctival limbal autotransplantation, Boston type 1 keratoprosthesis surgery, and corneal tattooing are included as well. Some interesting cases are discussed with management. Several possible complications after excimer laser procedures are also presented.

CORNEAL TRANSPLANT SURGERIES

Penetrating keratoplasty (PK) is a procedure through which a full-thickness host corneal tissue is replaced with a donor corneal tissue. The indications for PK are as follows: to establish a clear central cornea/visual axis, provide tectonic support, eliminate infections. It is also occasionally performed for cosmesis (Fig 1-4).

Deep anterior lamellar keratoplasty (DALK) is currently the preferred technique to restore corneal transparency and curvature in corneal stromal diseases with a healthy endothelium. The advantage of DALK is the elimination of the risk of endothelial allograft rejection. The visual outcome is much better compared to that of penetrating keratoplasty (PK). There are several techniques for separating a layer. Among the most popular DALK techniques, there is layer-by-layer manual dissection, hydrodissection, viscoelastic dissection, air big bubble (BB), and cannula BB (Fig 5, 6) (Melles et al, 1998; Terry et la, 2005; Gorovoy et al, 2006; Price et al, 2006; Anwar et al, 2002).

Endothelial keratoplasty (EK) has become the preferred choice for endothelial dysfunction, both for adult and pediatric patients. EK is not recommended for patients with significant anterior corneal scarring. There are several types of EK procedures: Descemet stripping (automated) endothelial keratoplasty (DSEK/DSAEK, Fig 7, 8), ultra-thin DSAEK (UT-DSAEK), and Descemet membrane (automated) endothelial keratoplasty (DMEK/DMAEK). The indication for endothelial keratoplasty is any cause of endothelial dysfunction, including endothelial dystrophies such as Fuchs endothelial dystrophy, posterior polymorphous dystrophy (PPMD) or congenital hereditary endothelial dystrophy (CHED), and

DOI: 10.4018/978-1-7998-6937-5.ch013

Figure 1. Postherpetic scar (left photo) and the same eye after PK in OR (right photo)

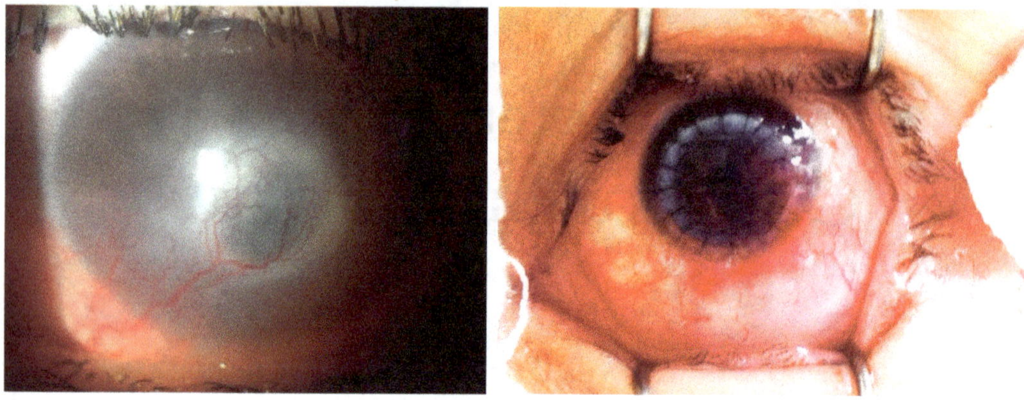

Figure 2. Total corneal scar and neovascularization after a chemical injury (left photo) and the same eye 2 weeks after PK (right photo) with the history of previous CLAU transplantation surgery from the fellow eye

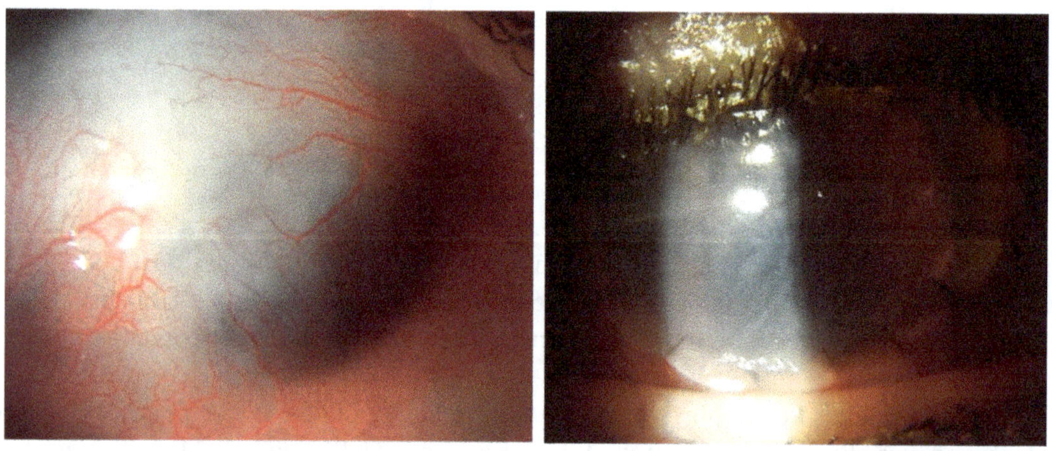

Figure 3. Fungal recurrence on the graft 3 months post initial surgery with loose sutures (left photo) and the same eye 10 days post PK (right photo)

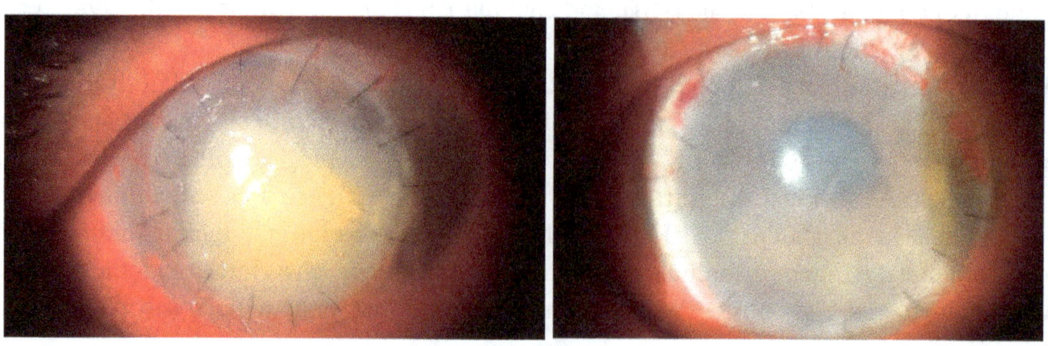

Figure 4. Keratoconus (left photo) and the same eye 1 week after PK (right photo)

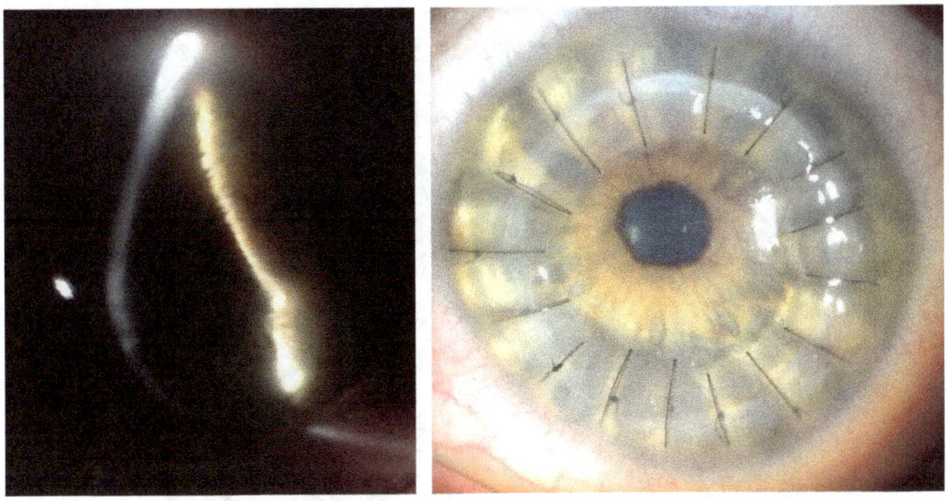

Figure 5. Keratoconus in OR (left photo). The same eye with big bubble (middle photo) and after visco-elastic dissection where only Descemet's membrane is left (right photo)

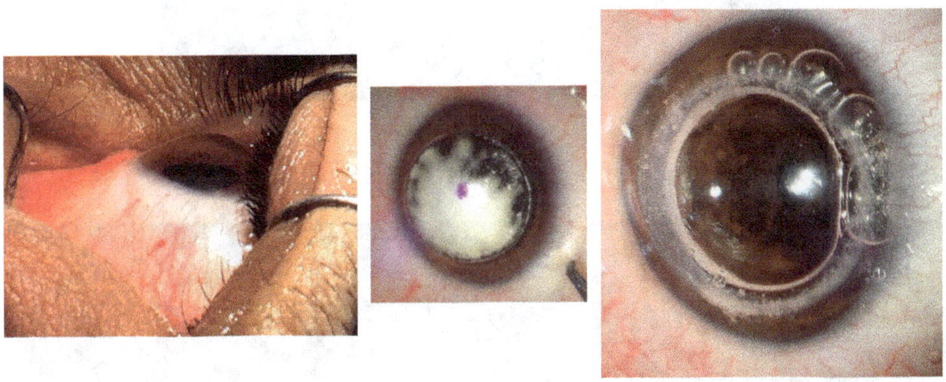

Figure 6. The same eye with 4 sutures (left photo) and at the end of the surgery (right photo)

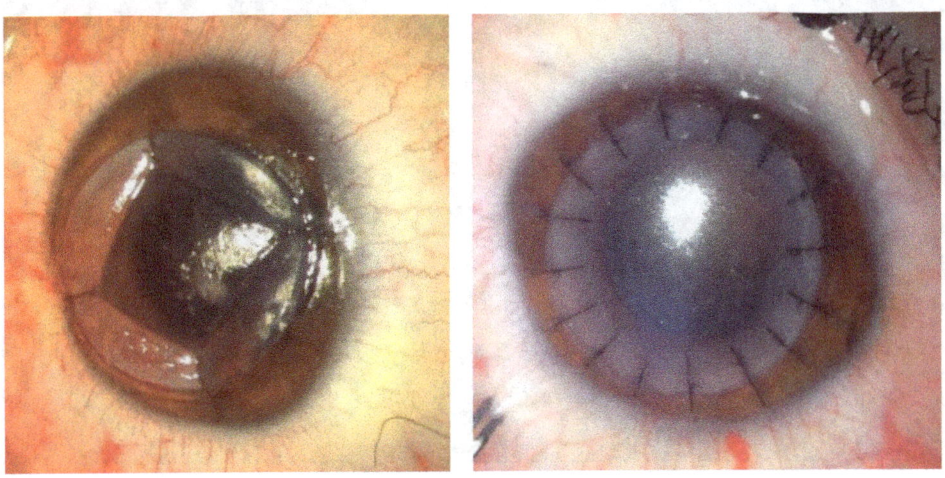

Figure 7. DSAEK performed for Fuchs endothelial dystrophy with a big air bubble in the anterior chamber in OR

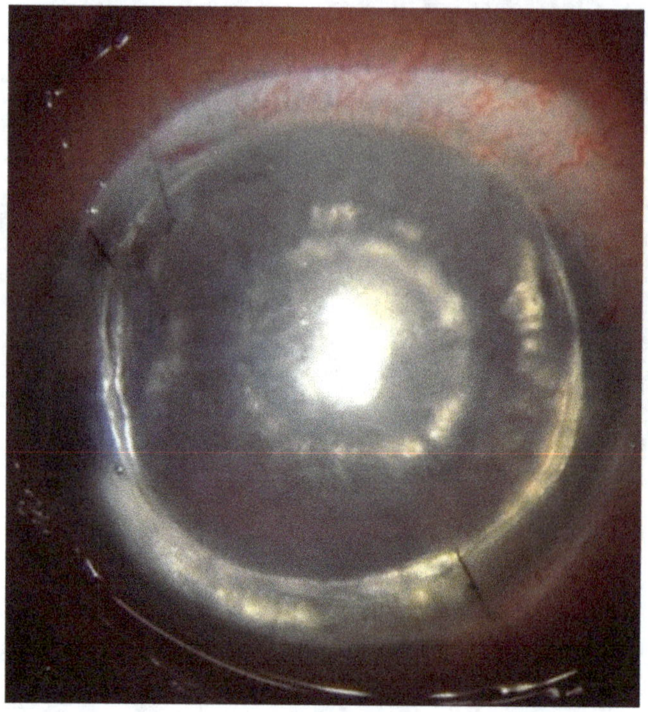

Figure 8. The same eye the next day with residual air and almost clear graft

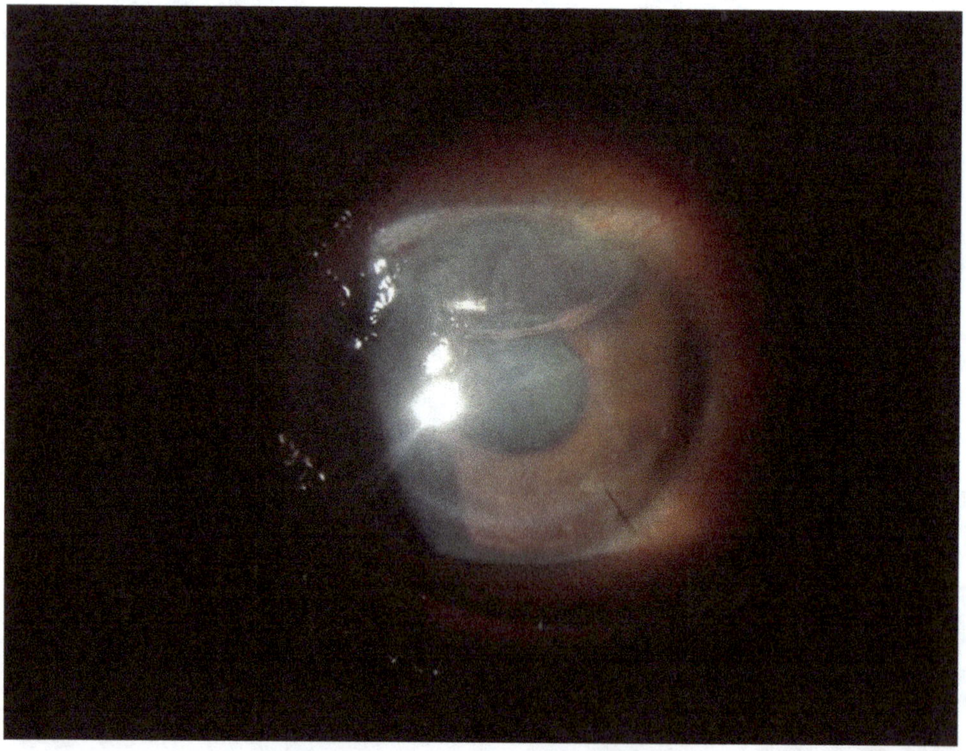

conditions like pseudophakic or aphakic bullous keratopathy, iridocorneal endothelial (ICE) syndrome, endothelial decompensation from trauma, etc (Melles et al, 1999; Giebel et al, 2008; Price et al, 2009; Chaurasia et al, 2014).

Complications of transplant surgery include graft rejections, suture abscesses, ICK and other infectious keratitis, recurrences of previous diseases, etc.

Kaye dots are white punctate epithelial opacities. They represent epithelial cells in various stages of degeneration. Kaye dots are not visually significant and do not bear any clinical significance either (Fig 9) (Lee et al, 2010).

Figure 9. Multiple Kaye dots located in the epithelium anterior to the suture line of a corneal graft

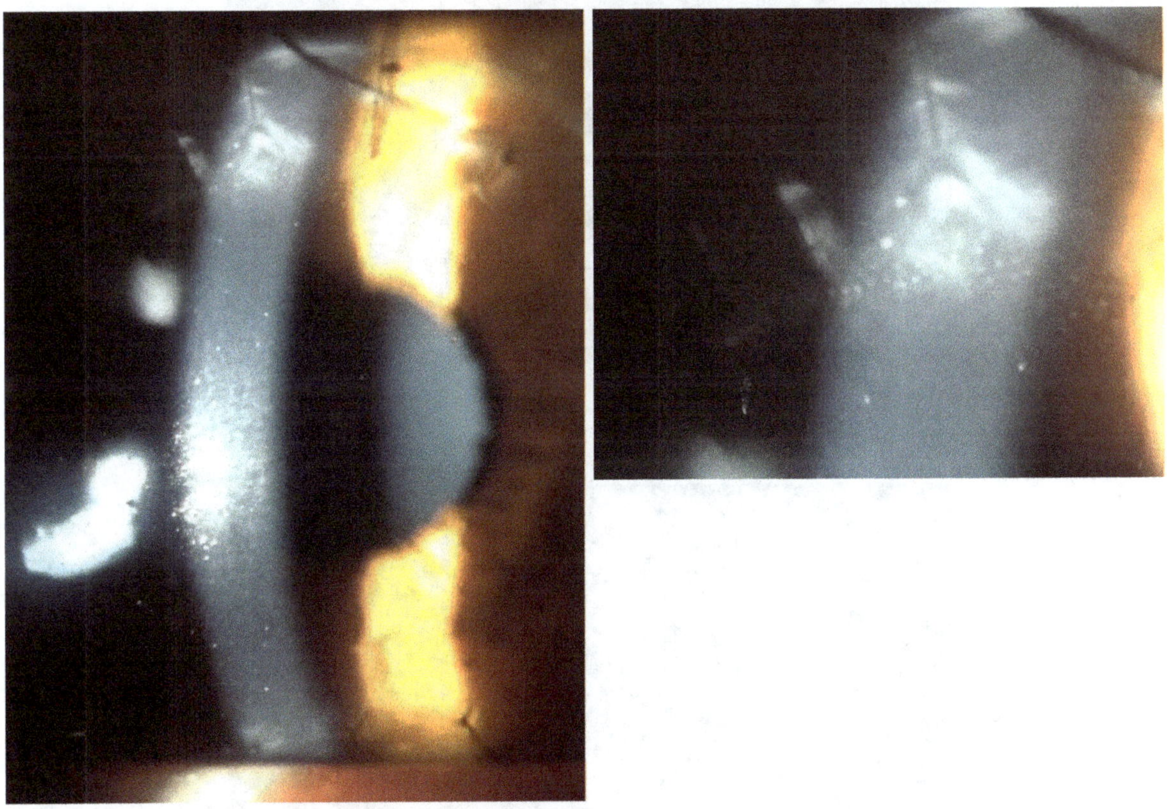

Superficial hypertrophic dendriform epitheliopathy is a relatively new entity that occurs after keratoplasty among the patients with preexisting chronic ocular inflammation (Fig 12).[11]

Epithelial downgrowth represents the entrance of epithelium through an incompletely healed wound, leading to the progressive epithelialization of the anterior chamber. The source of the invading could be the conjunctival and/or the corneal epithelial tissue. PK has a significantly lower incidence of epithelial downgrowth than cataract surgery (Sugar et al, 1977).

Corneal allograft rejection is still the leading cause of corneal graft failure. Young age, pre- or postoperative vascularization, and preoperative inflammation are considered risk factors for graft failure after penetrating keratoplasty. Most episodes of rejection are treatable with topical corticosteroids;

Figure 10. The broken suture is shown by an arrow

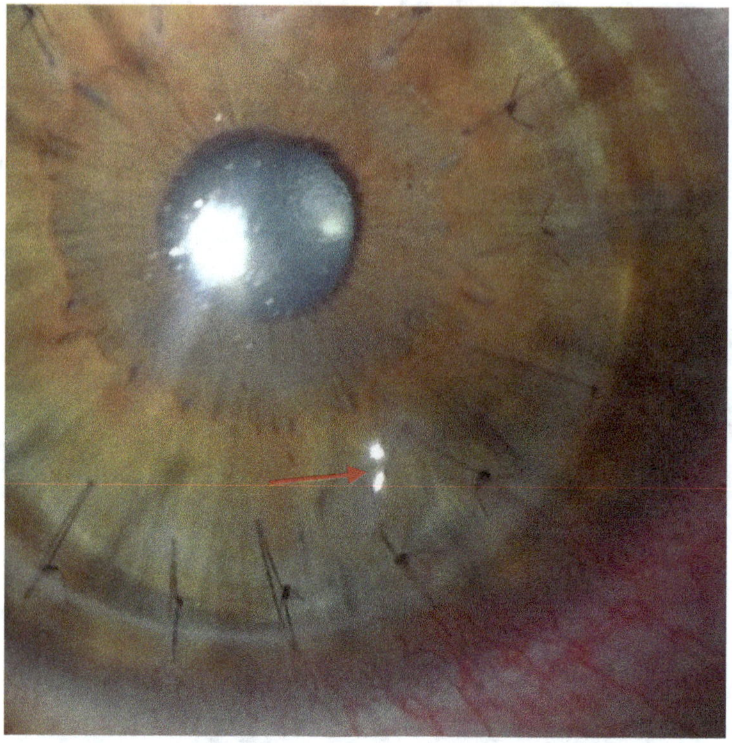

Figure 11. Loose sutures with surrounding epithelial and stromal edema

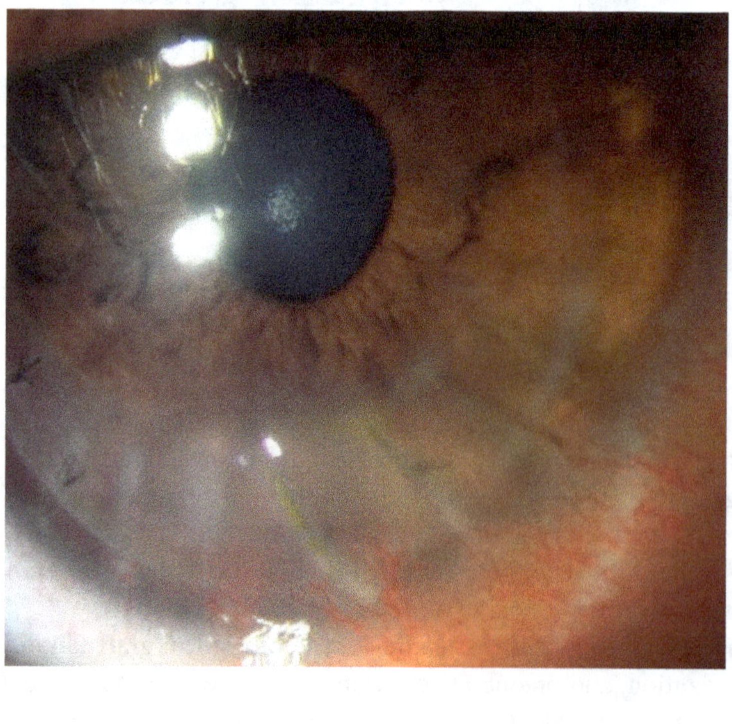

Figure 12. Superficial hypertrophic dendriform epitheliopathy on the graft

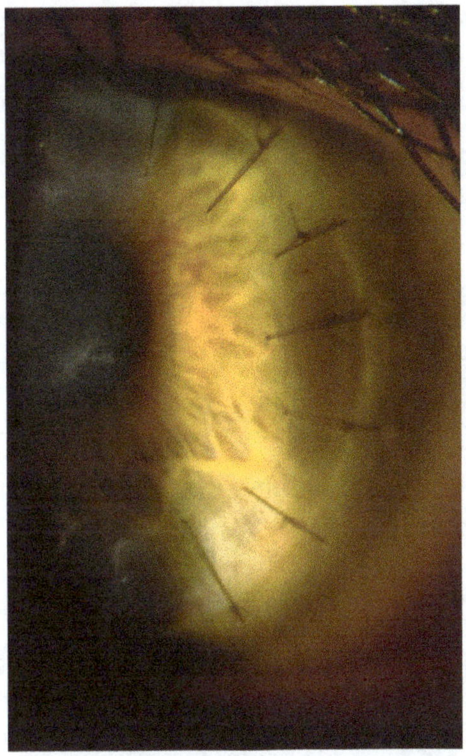

Figure 13. Mild epithelial downgrowth as thin vertical line is seen

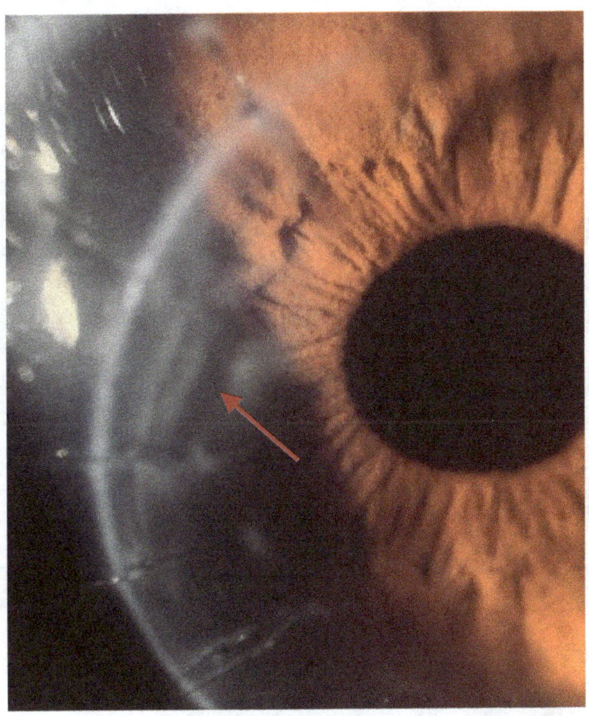

Figure 14. Epithelial rejection. Epithelial rejection line is seen as a wave consisting of cellular infiltrates

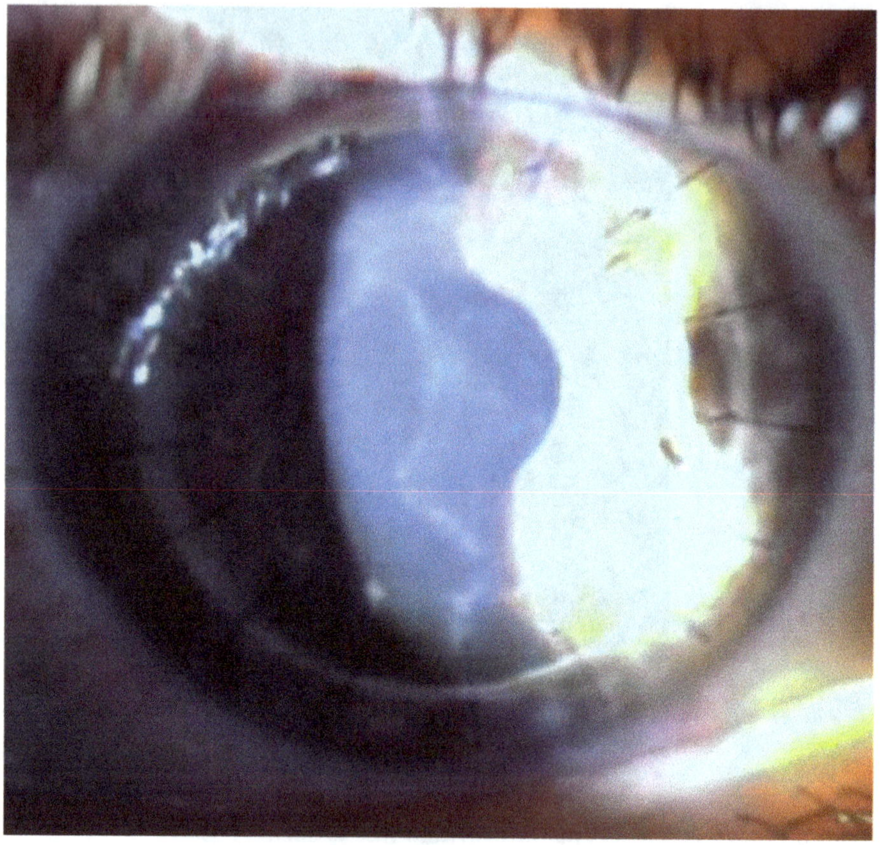

Figure 15. Epithelial rejection. Fine rejection line is seen

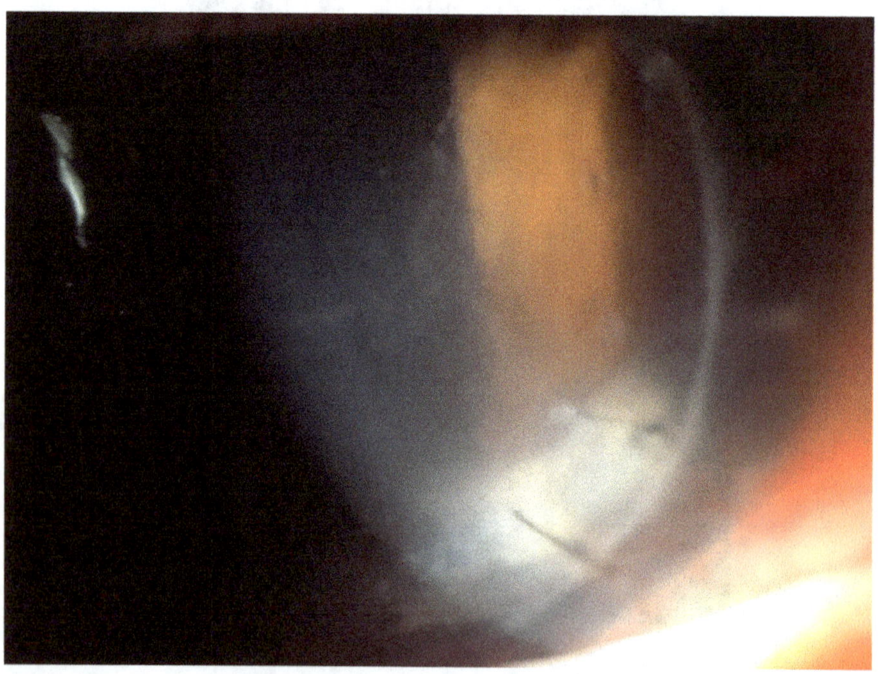

however, early recognition and intervention are crucial for success. Often, ciliary injection is the initial sign of rejection, and it can occur before the clinical appearance of cellular infiltrates in the cornea or the anterior chamber. Every layer of the cornea can be a target of rejection; thus epithelial, subepithelial, stromal, and endothelial rejections are observed (Alldredge et al, 1981).

Epithelial rejections are rare and usually can be seen earlier in the postoperative period (1 to 13 months) because the replacement of the epithelium obviates its rejection in patients with older grafts (Fig 14, 15) (Leahey et al, 1993).

Subepithelial rejection represents cellular infiltration of the cornea as discrete subepithelial infiltrates mimicking those seen in epidemic keratoconjunctivitis. They are usually scattered in the central cornea and occur exclusively in the donor tissue (Fig 16).

Figure 16. Subepithelial rejection. Small, round, subepithelial lesions are seen

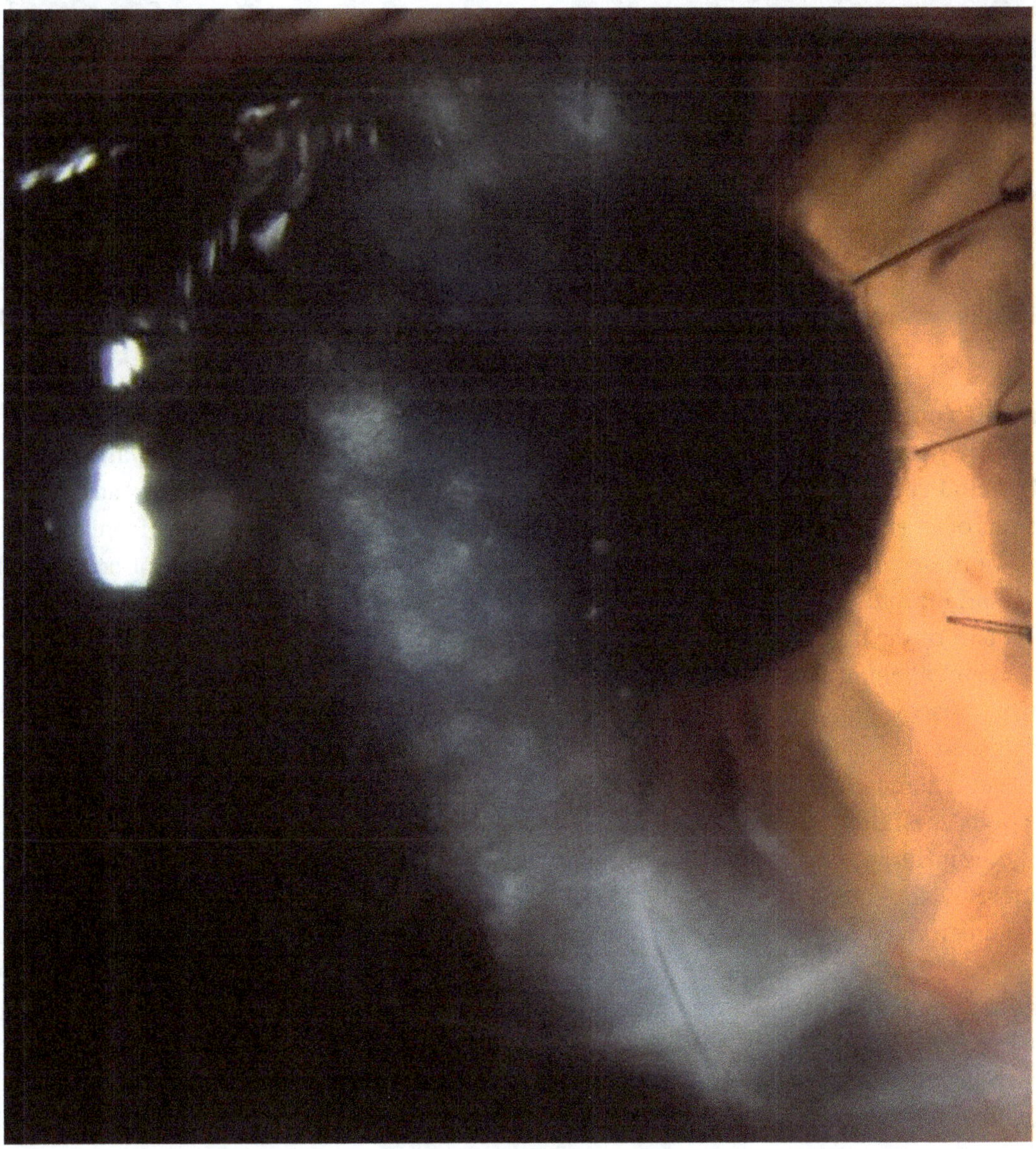

Figure 17. Severe stromal rejection. Marked neovascularization and stromal melt is seen

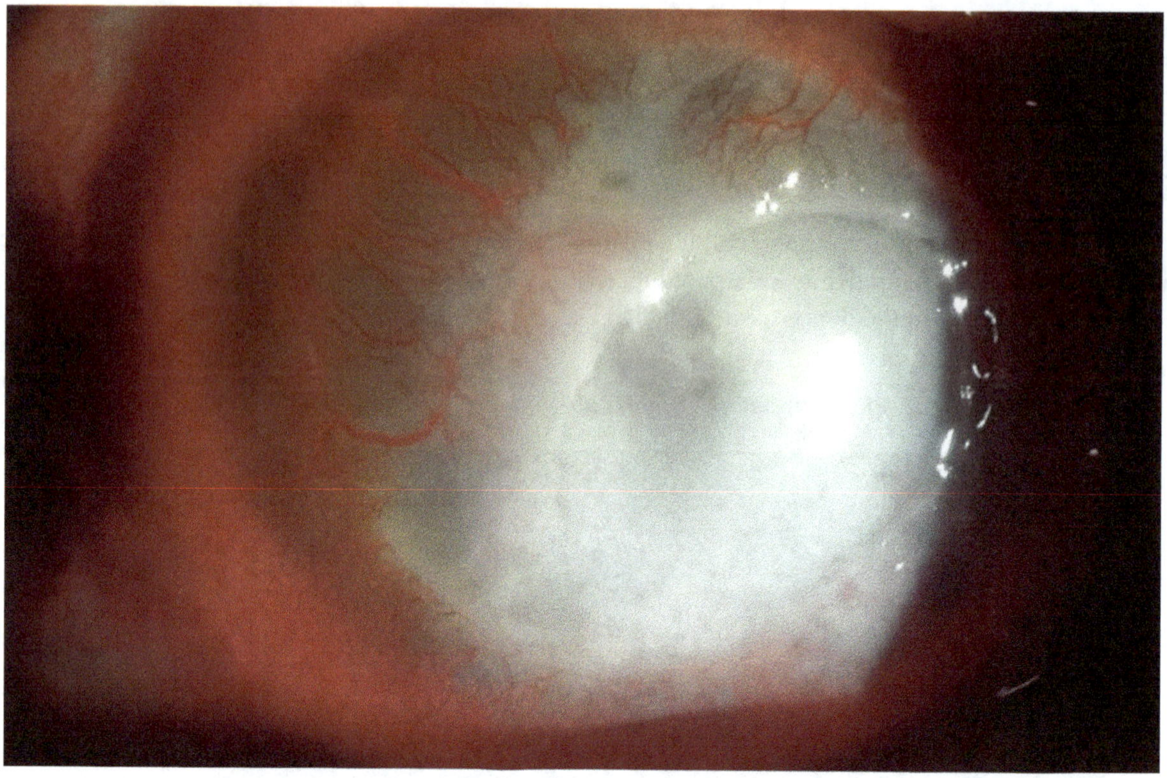

Isolated stromal rejection is uncommon but can be seen as stromal infiltrates and neovascularization. In severe graft rejection, the stroma can become necrotic (Fig 17) (Alldredge et al, 1981).

Endothelial rejection is the most common type. Endothelial keratic precipitates can occur as scattered lesions or as a linearly oriented wave (Khodadoust line) of leukocytes migrating from the peripheral cornea toward the center. The Khodadoust line has been considered the hallmark of corneal allograft rejection, and it represents a border between the edematous and clear cornea. Edema of the graft can occur as a part of the inflammatory reaction, but more commonly as a result of the stress or damage to the corneal endothelium (Fig 18-21) (Alldredge et al, 1981).

A **suture abscess** presents an infiltrate in either the donor or recipient cornea, which is in direct contact with, or close to, the suture material. The most common isolated organisms are S. epidermidis, S. pneumoniae, and S. aureus, although cases of Gram-negative infections can occur as well (Fig 22, 23).[14,15,16]

Infectious crystalline keratopathy (ICK) is an intrastromal bacterial colonization of a corneal graft. Clinically, the infiltrate is a gray-white, crystalline, needle-like branching opacities within the stroma close to the suture track. Although the most commonly reported causative organism in ICK is Streptococcus viridans, numerous pathogens have been implicated in causing ICK (Zabel et al, 1988). These organisms include S. pneumoniae, coagulase-negative Streptococcus, Peptostreptococcus species, Haemophilus aphrophilus, Haemophilus influenzae, Mycobacterium species, P. aeruginosa, Enterococcus species, Candida species, Serratia marcescens, etc (Matoba et al, 1994; Wilhelmus et al, 1991; Abry et al, 2010).

Herpetic recurrences on the graft are seen frequently after PK performed for postherpetic corneal opacification or severe melting/perforation cases unresponsive to medical treatment (Fig 25-29) (Pfister et al, 1972).

Figure 18. Endothelial rejection. The central marked edema is seen with underlying scattered KPs

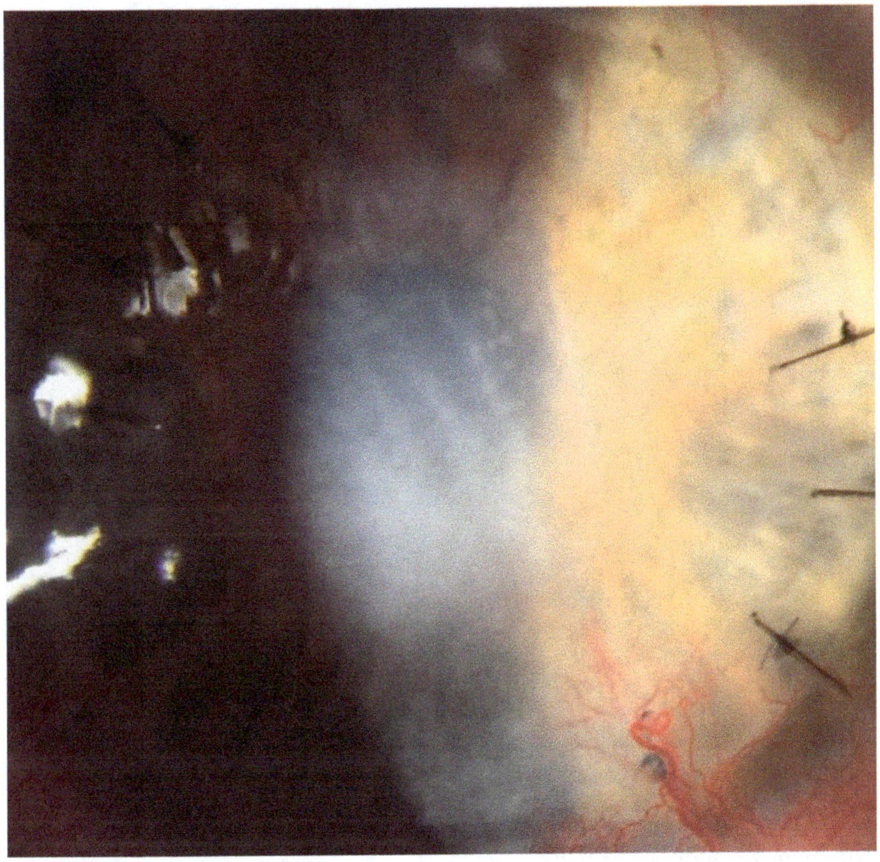

Figure 19. Endothelial rejection. Khodadust line is seen with edematous (above) and clear cornea (below)

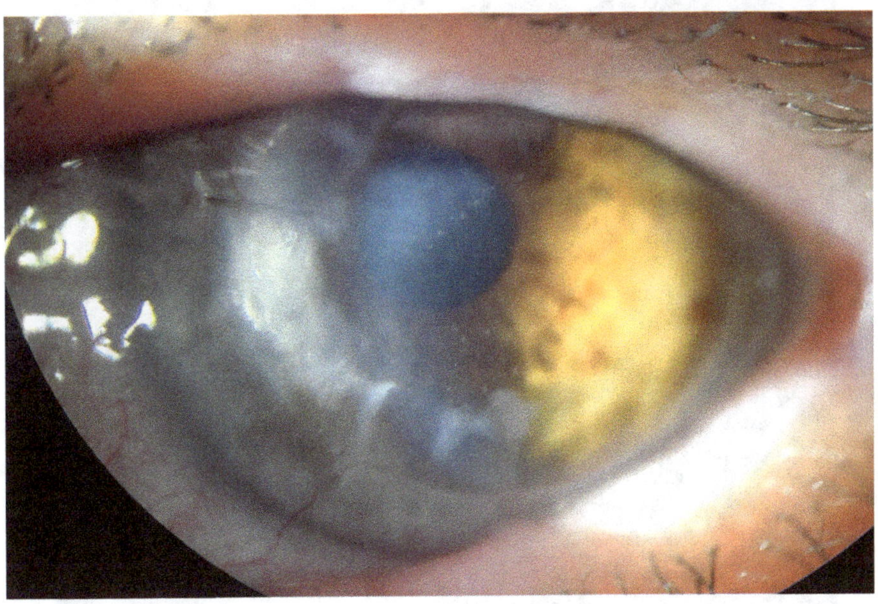

Figure 20. Khodadust line. Linear pigmented KPs are seen

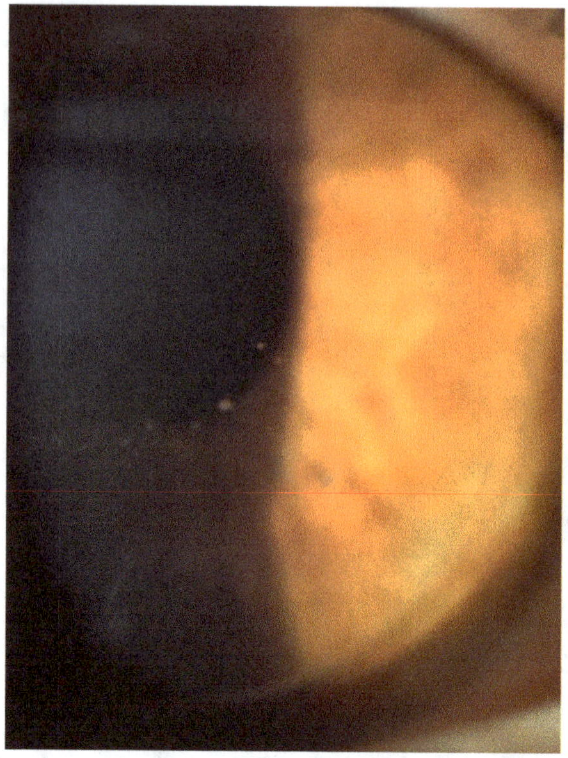

Figure 21. Mixed rejection. Khodadust line with KPs are seen between the edematous and clear cornea. Fine subepithelial lesions are noted as well

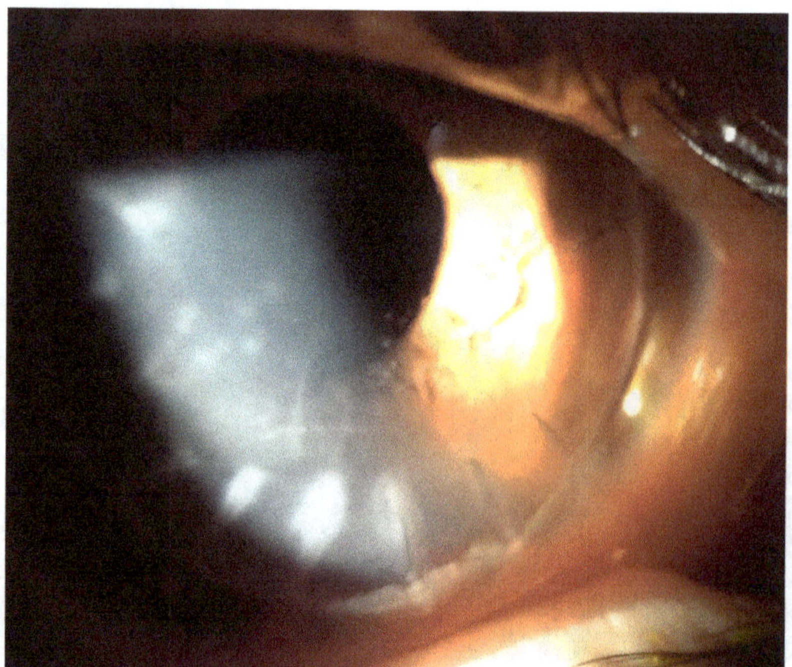

Figure 22. Suture abscess caused by S. Epidermidis. The infiltrate is located on 5 o'clock (left photo) and the same eye after 3 weeks of treatment with topical Moxifloxacin; mild corneal haze is seen (right photo)

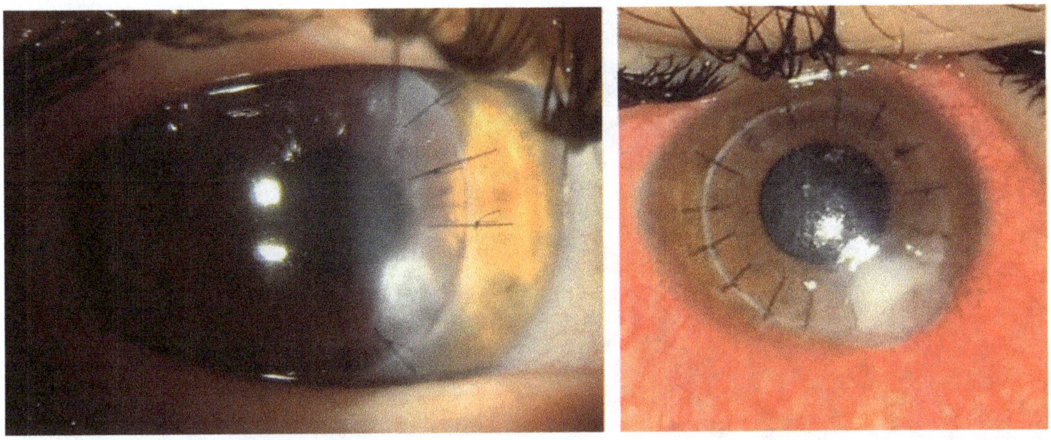

Figure 23. Suture abscess caused by S. aureus. The large infiltrate is seen involving donor cornea and interface (left photo), and the same eye 4 weeks after treatment (topical Moxifloxacin, Erythromycin ointment, cycloplegics and mild steroids) with mild anterior stromal scar (right photo)

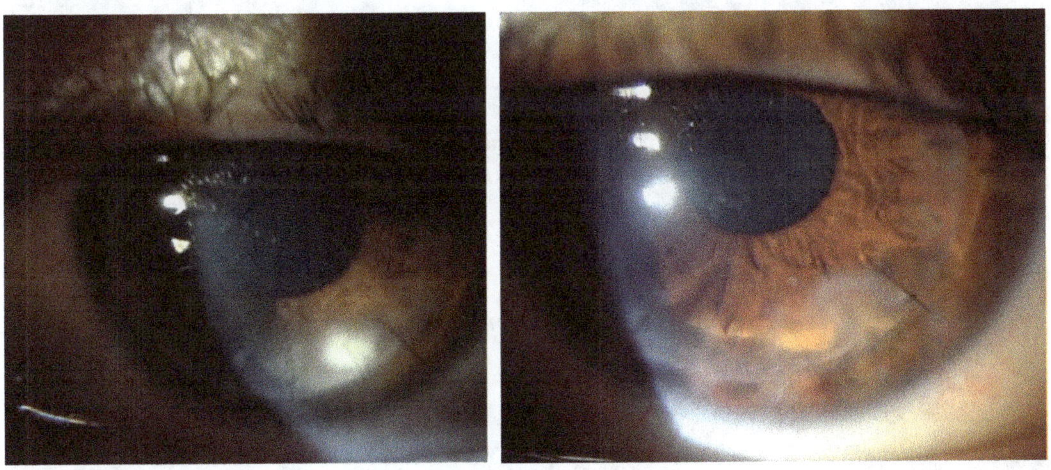

Figure 24. ICK, Crystalline-looking stromal infiltrate are seen

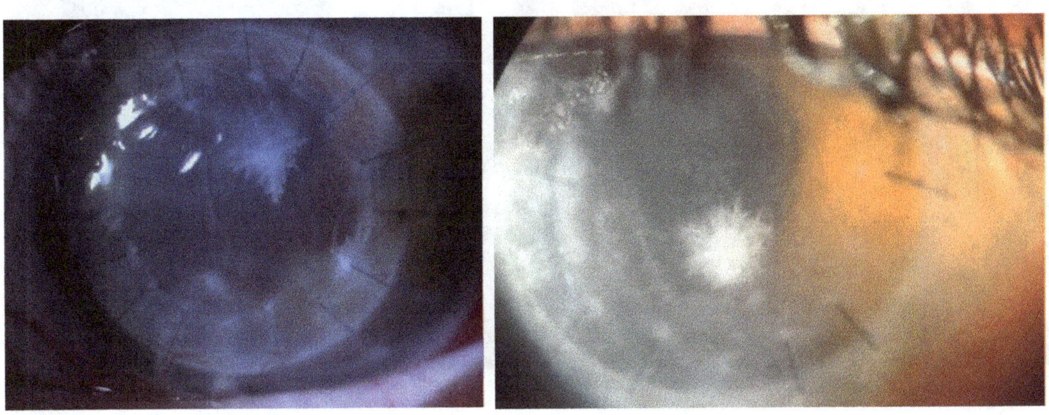

Figure 25. Dendritic and geographic herpetic ulcer recurrence on the graft. Involvement of host cornea is seen. The ulcers are stained with fluorescein. Photo is taken under cobalt-blue illumination

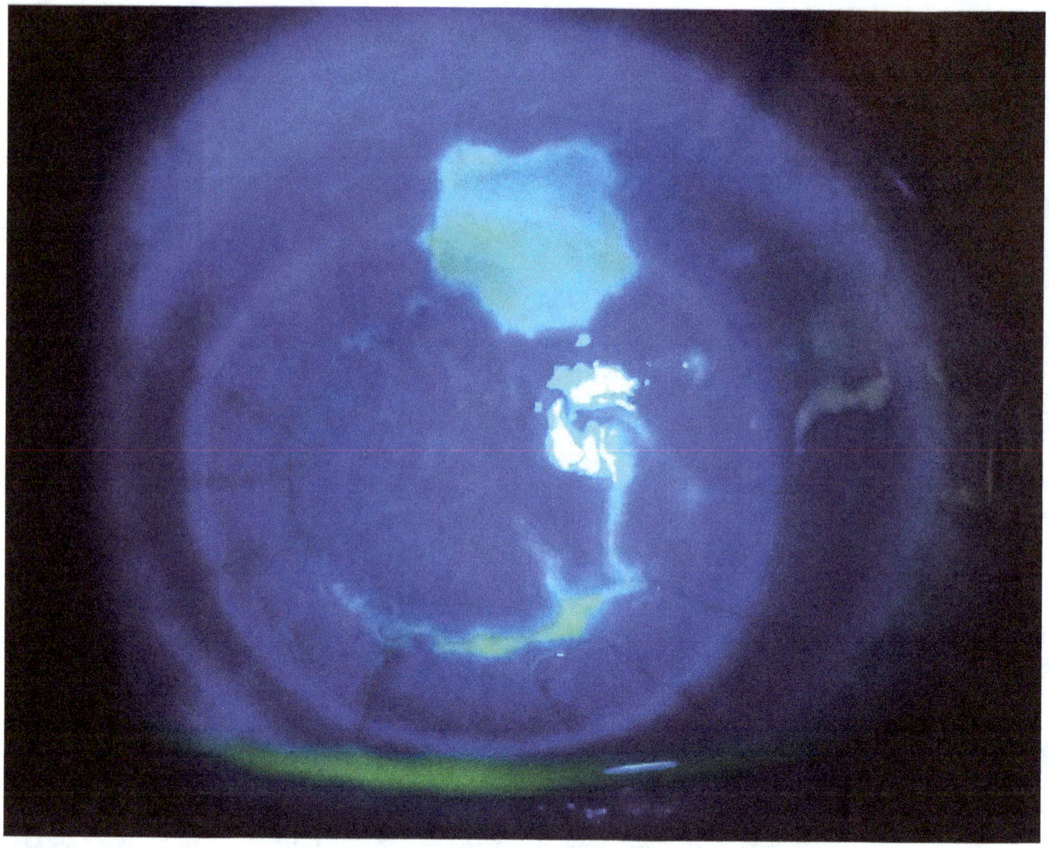

Figure 26. Herpetic geographic and dendritic ulcer on the graft with a loose suture (left photo). Geographic ulcer (right photo)

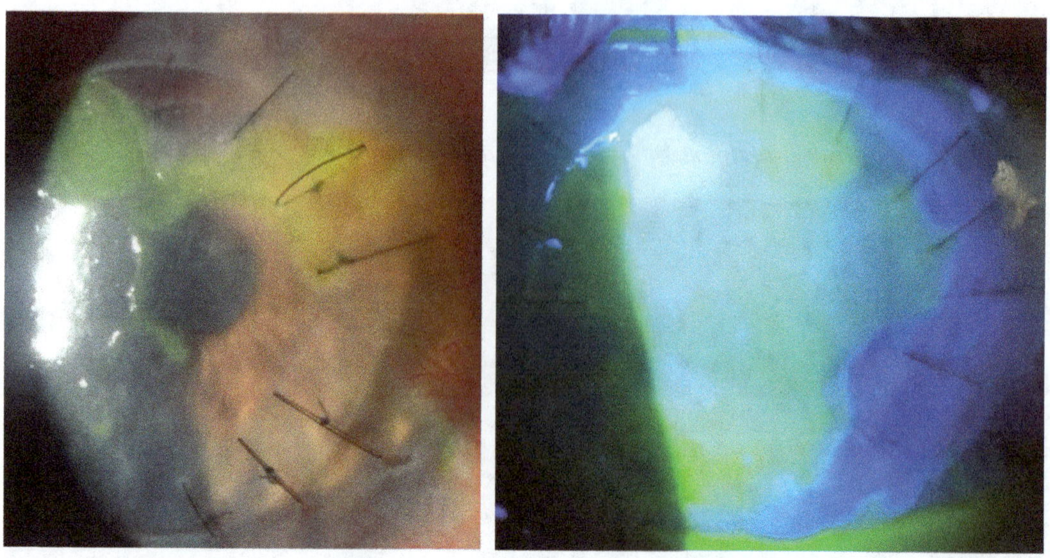

Figure 27. Severe herpetic geographic ulcer stained with fluorescein. The host cornea involvement is seen (left photo) and the same eye after 3 weeks of treatment with healed epithelium (right photo). Treatment included oral Acyclovir and topical Ganciclovir eye gel, cycloplegics and tears

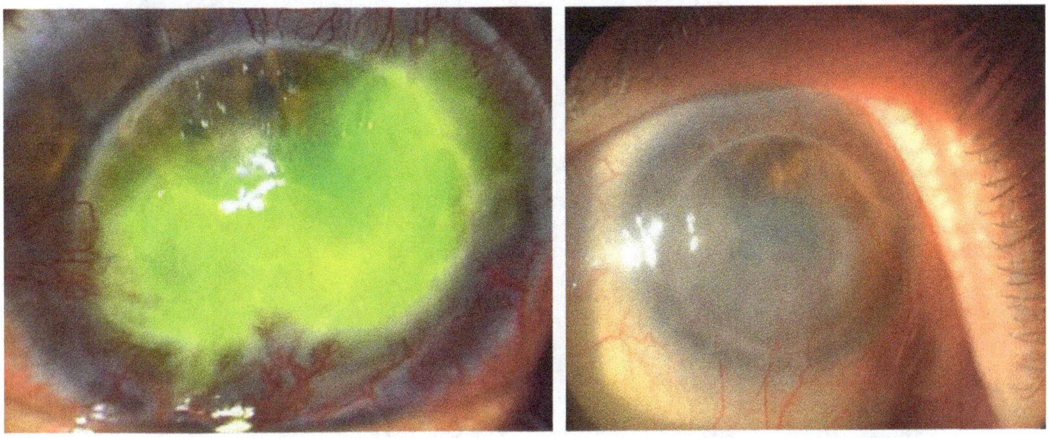

Figure 28. Postherpetic neurotrophic ulcer on the graft

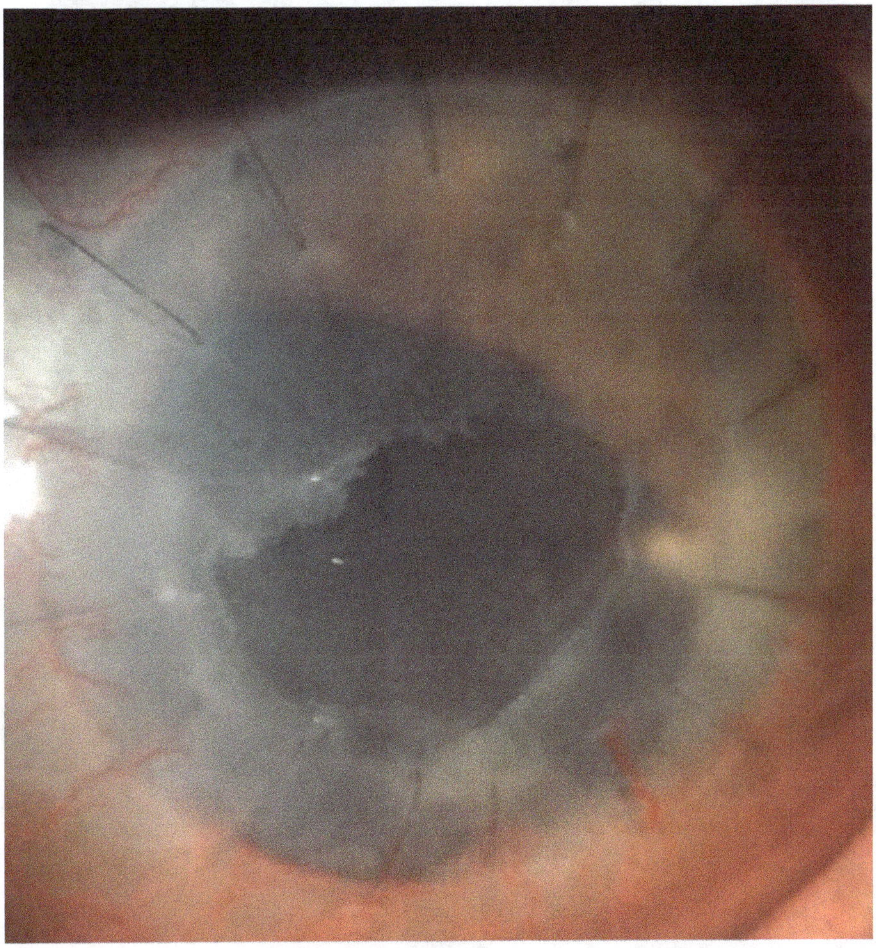

Figure 29. Necrotizing stromal herpetic keratitis on the graft. The large epithelial defect with underlying stromal infiltrate and hypopyon is seen

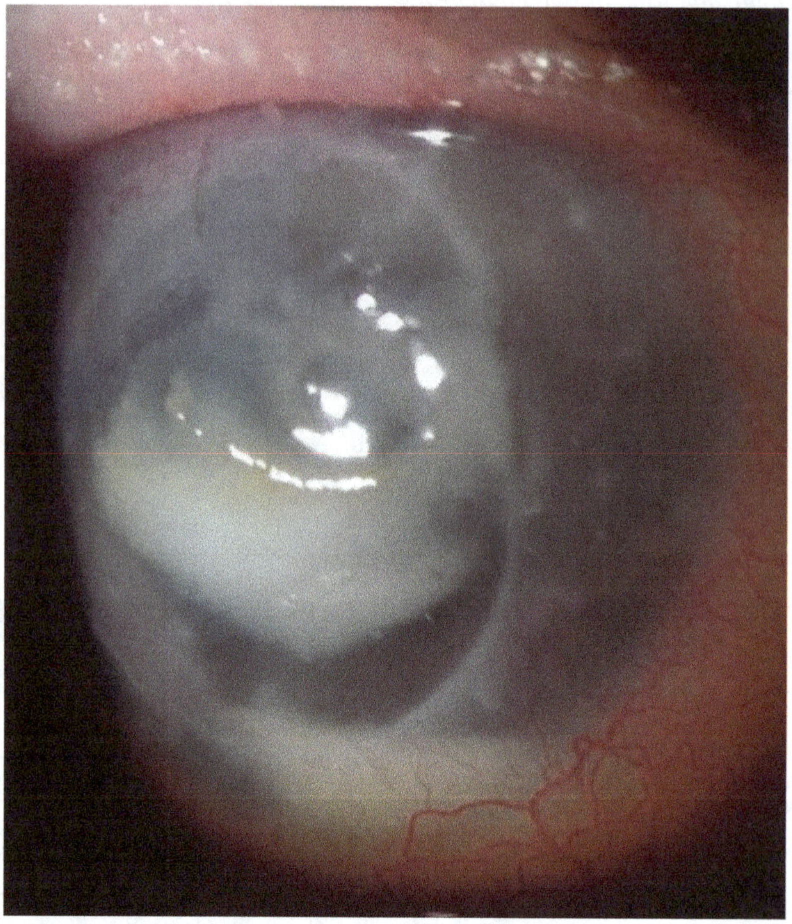

Figure 30. The recurrence of the granular dystrophy on the graft 4 years after surgery with remaining sutures (left photo) and the fellow eye of the same patient with granular dystrophy (right photo)

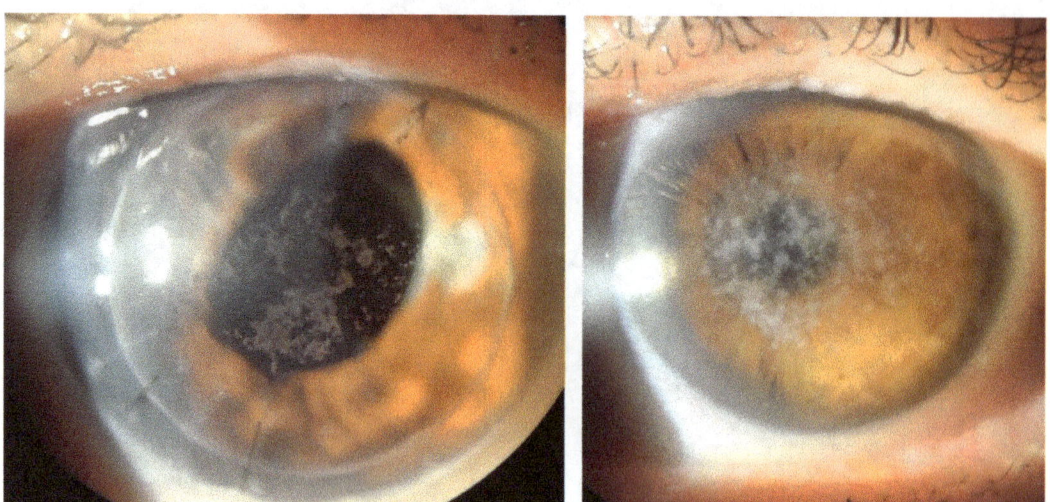

Figure 31. Recurrence of macular dystrophy on the graft 6 years after PK

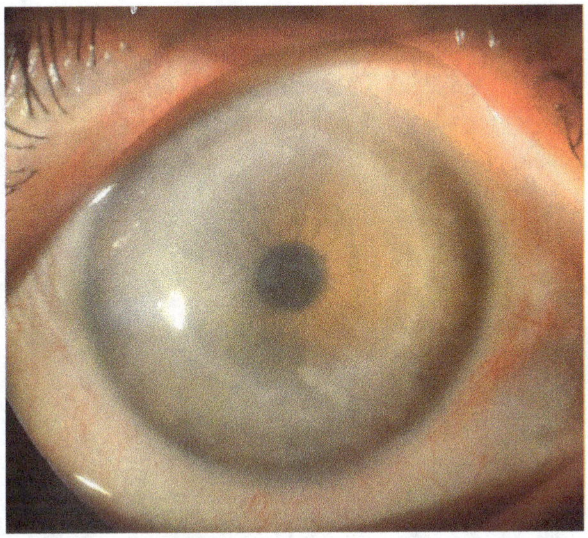

Figure 32. Double anterior chamber after DALK

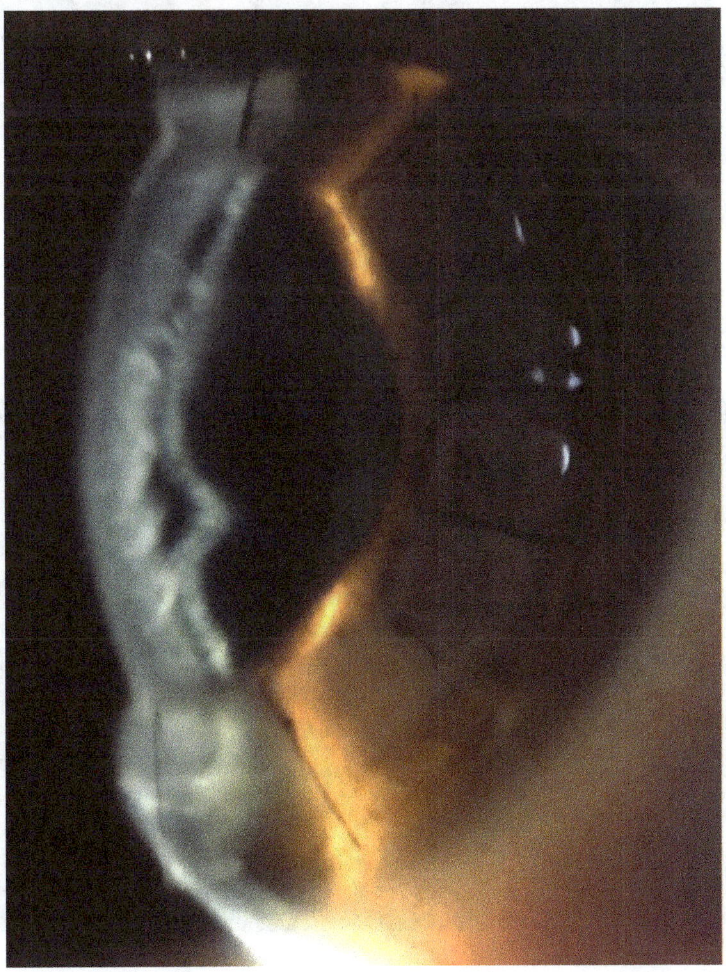

Figure 33. The same patient 3 weeks after air bubble injection into the anterior chamber

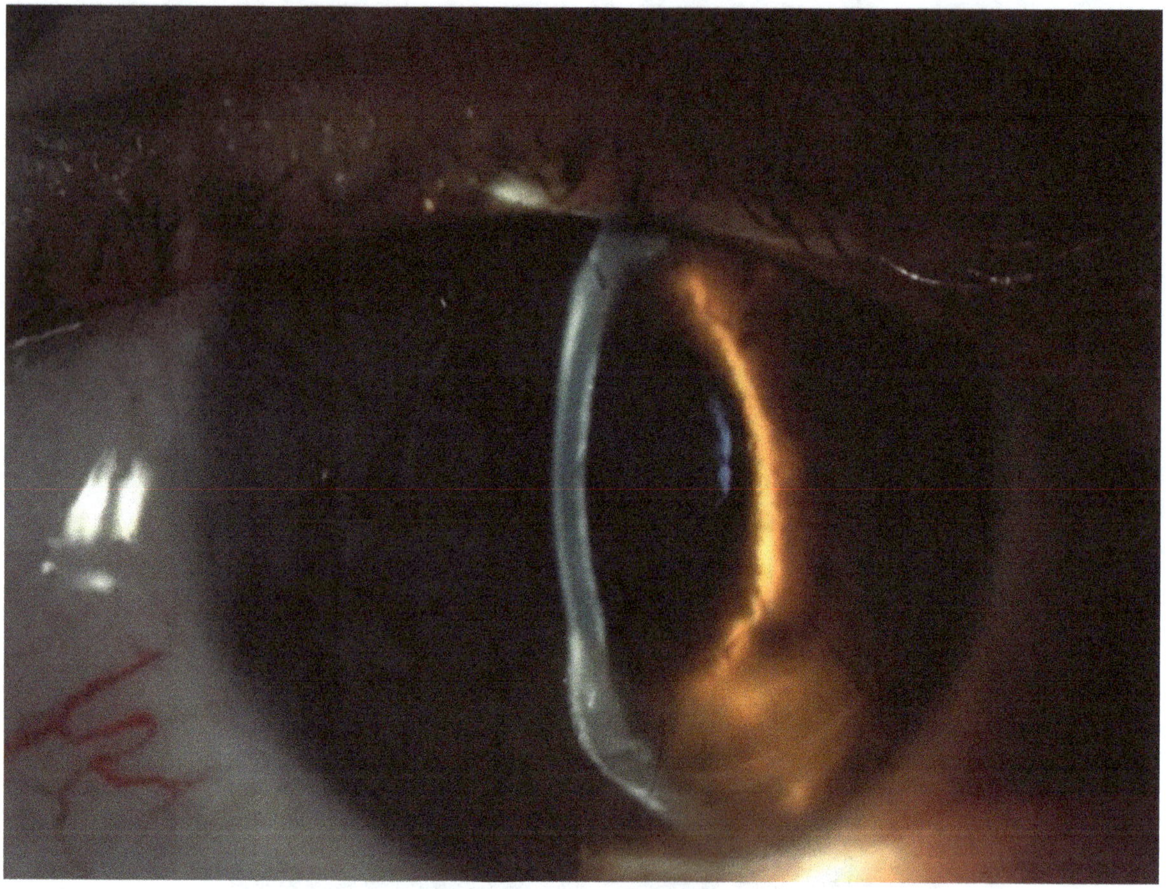

Figure 34. Anterior segment OCT. Endothelial detachment after DSAEK

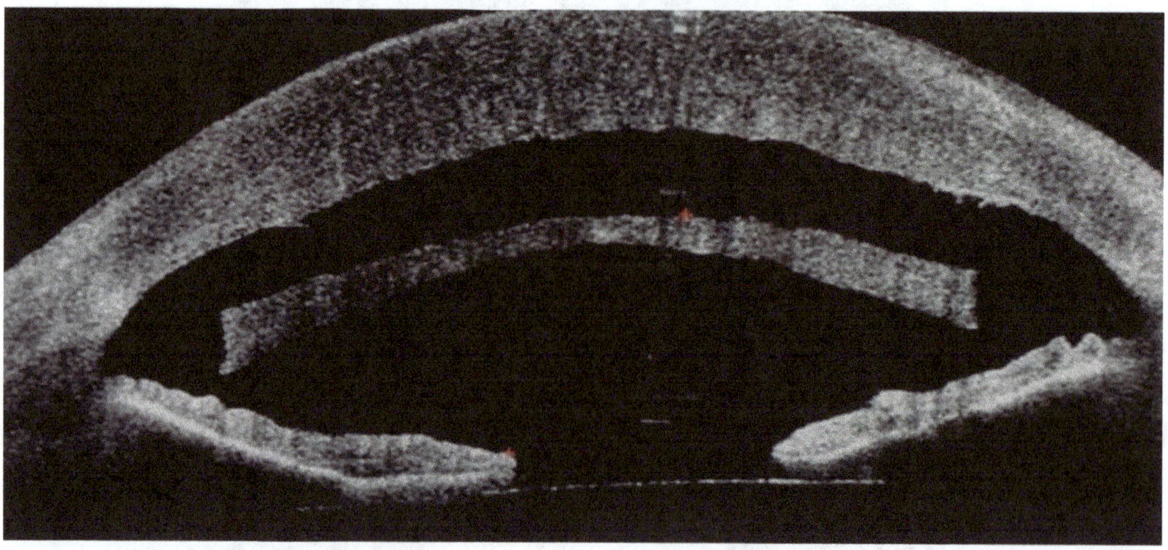

Figure 35. The same eye the next day with air bubble injection into the anterior chamber (left photo), and 1 month after treatment (right photo)

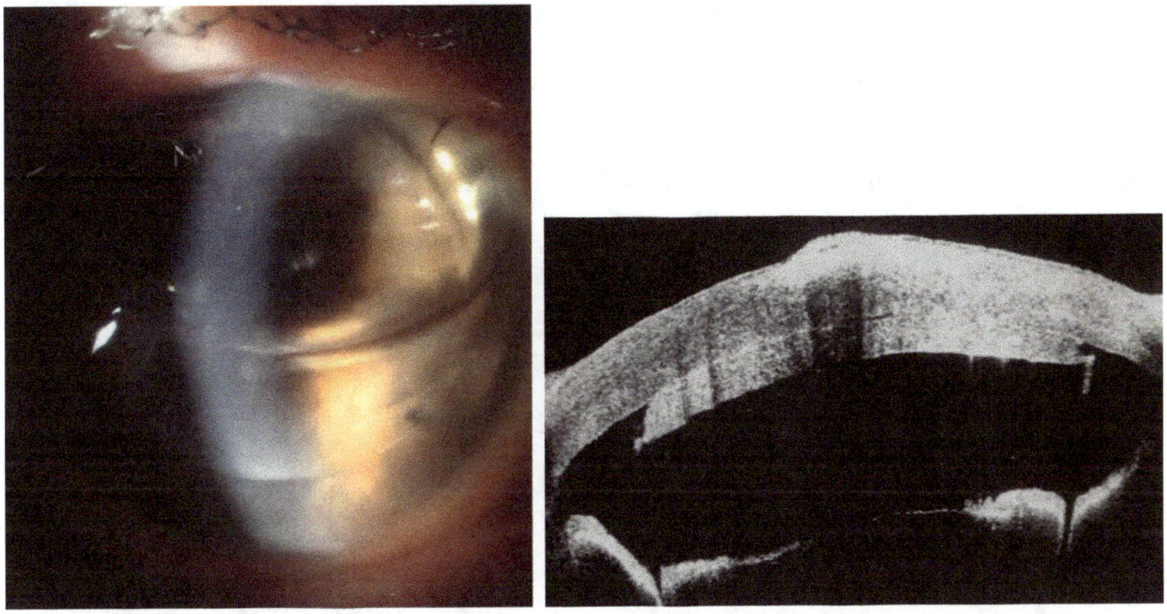

Recurrences of corneal dystrophies can always be seen after keratoplasty (Fig 20, 31)

Double anterior chamber formation is an uncommon complication of deep anterior lamellar keratoplasty (DALK) due to microperforation of the Descemet's membrane (Fig 31, 33).

Conjunctival Limbal Autografting

Conjunctival limbal autografting (CLAU) is a procedure in which the limbal tissue, together with adjacent conjunctival carrier, is transplanted from the healthy eye of a patient to the contralateral stem

Figure 36. Stem cell deficiency caused by chemical alkali injury. Total conjunctivalization of corneal surface is seen (OR photo)

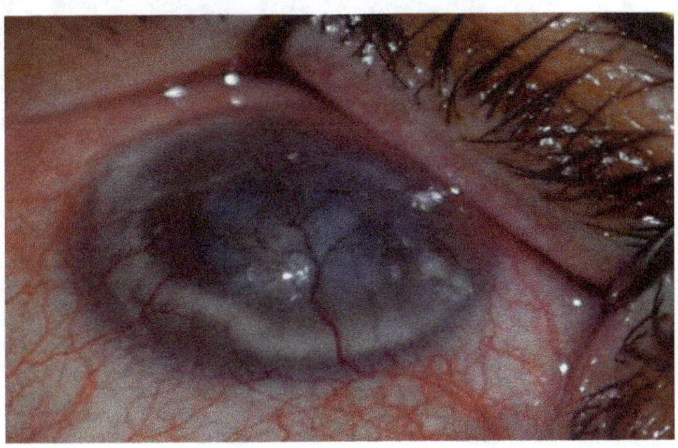

cell-deficient eye. It is the procedure of choice for unilateral cases of limbal stem cell deficiency. Its main advantage over other allograft procedures is that CLAU does not require immunosuppression. Limbal stem cells deficiency can be congenital (aniridia, ectodermic dysplasia, iatrogenic), traumatic (chemical and thermal injuries), contact lens wearing, and can also be associated with diseases (OCP, SJS, etc.) (Fig 36-45) (Tsubota et al, 1996; Holland et al, 1996; Sayegh et al, 2008).

Figure 37. Harvesting conjunctivolimbal autograft from the healthy eye

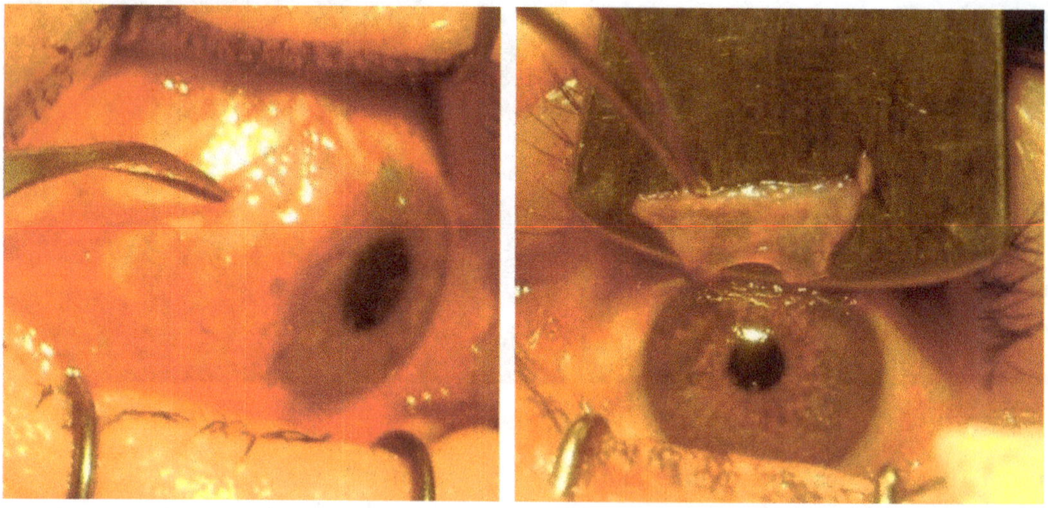

Figure 38. The same eye 2 months after the surgery. Healthy corneal smooth epithelial surface is noted

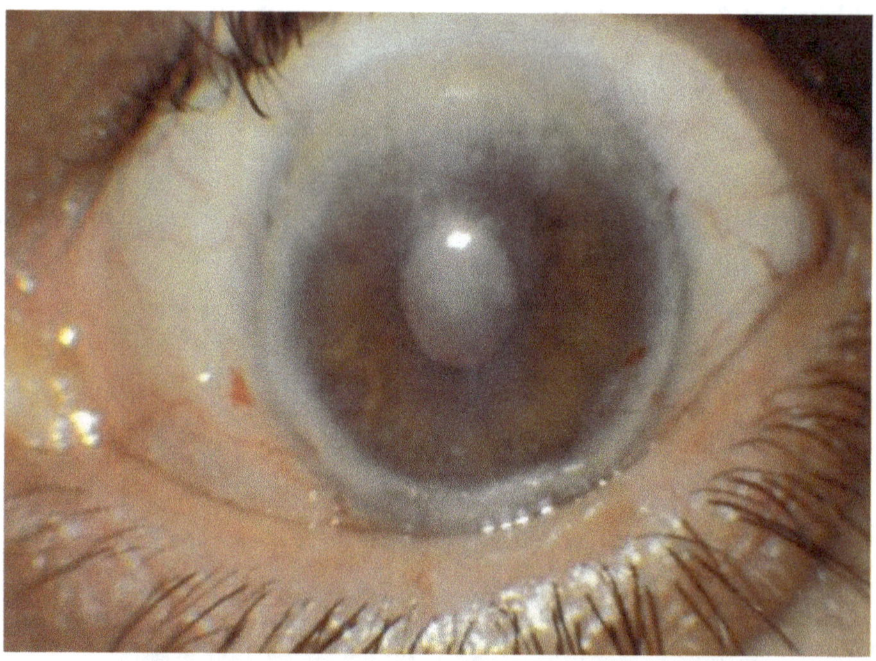

Figure 39. Stem cells deficiency after multiple surgeries with h/o 2 PKs

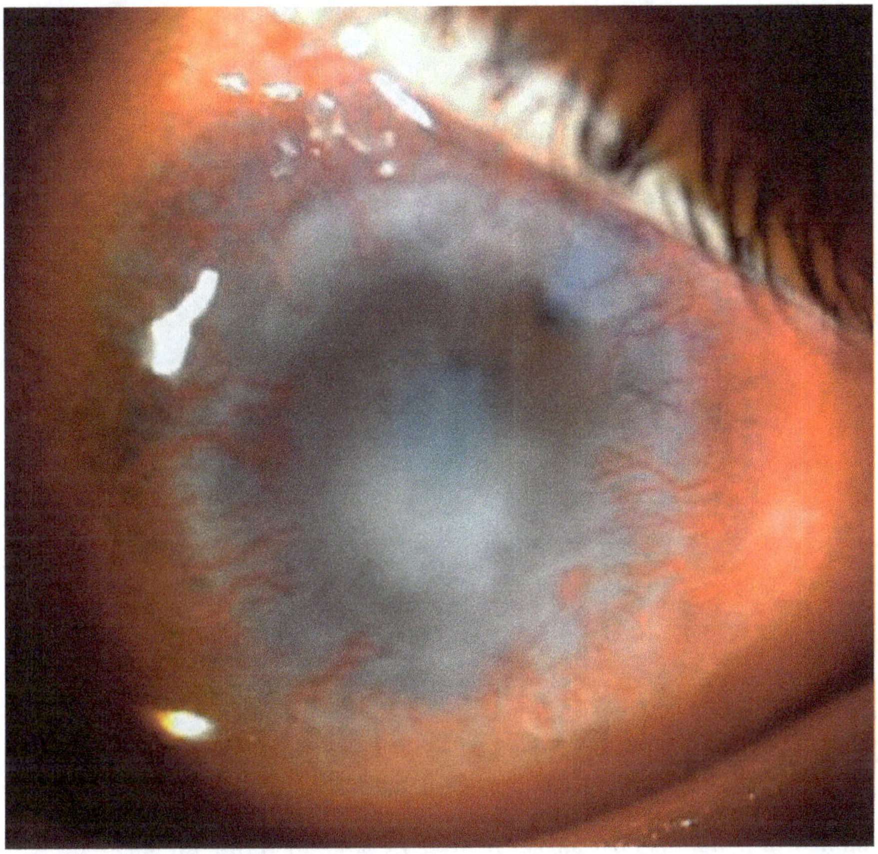

Figure 40. The same patient 2 years after the CLAU procedure and repeated PK subsequently

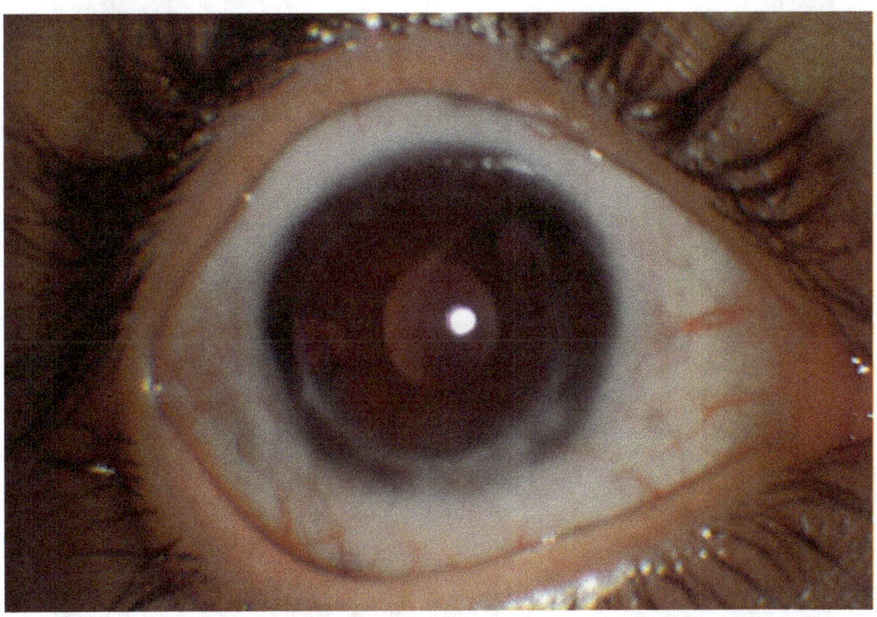

Figure 41. Stem cell deficiency secondary to chemical acid injury. The 360 degrees of neovascularization/pannus and total conjunctivalization of the surface is seen

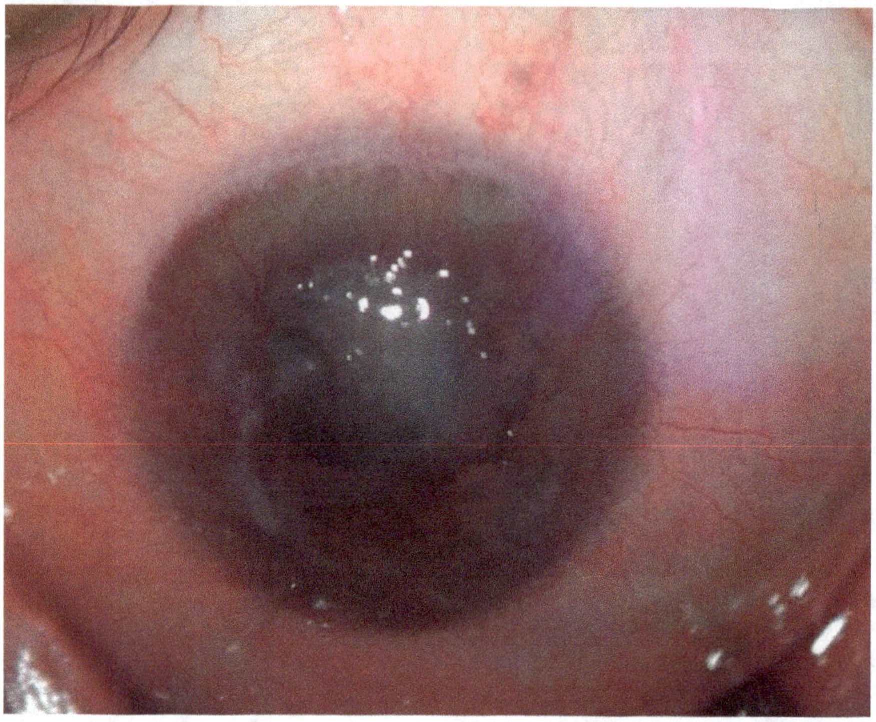

Figure 42. The same eye 2 months post-surgery. Note the smooth epithelial surface

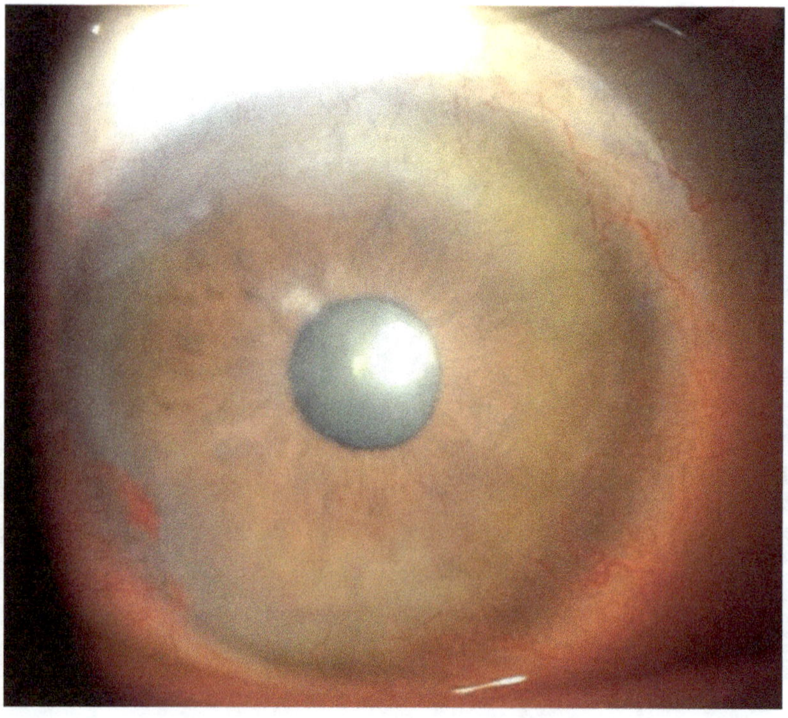

Figure 43. Stem cell deficiency after chemical injury. 280 degrees of conjucnctivalization of corneal surface is seen with paracentral stromal scarring

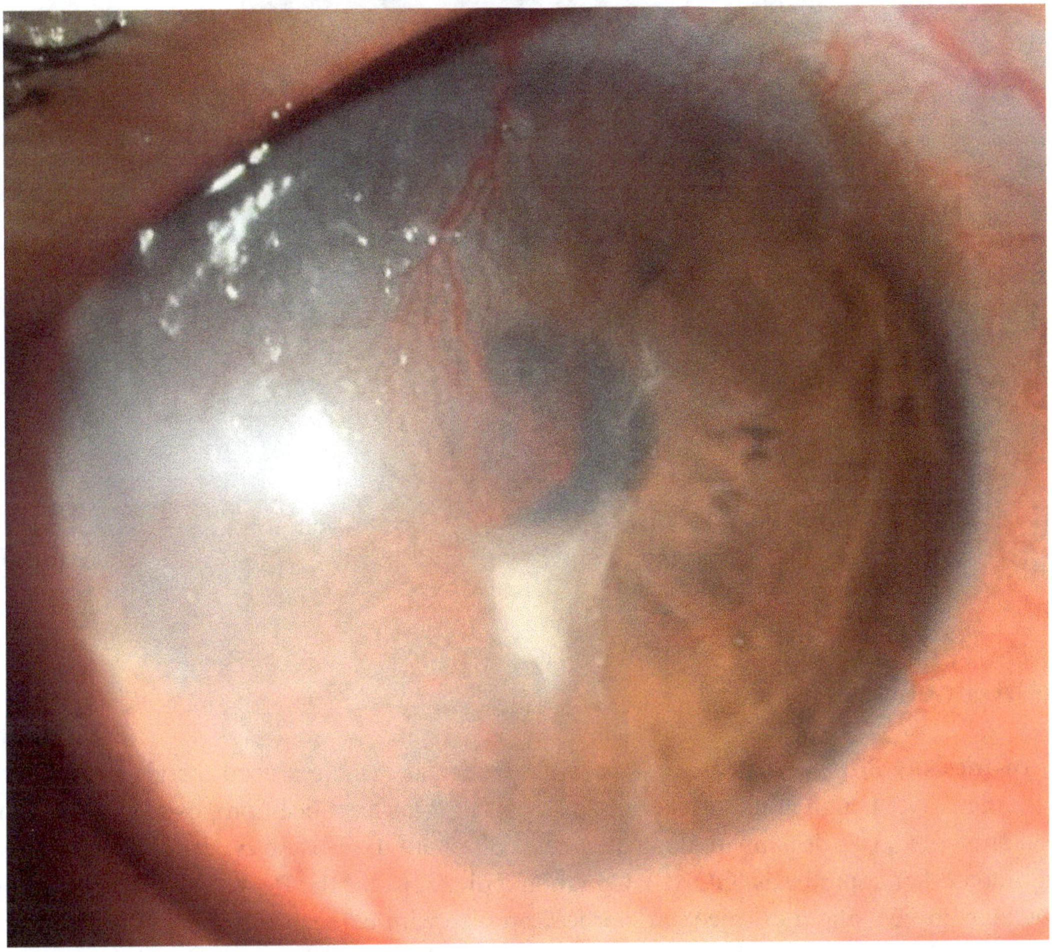

Figure 44. CLAU. Harvesting stem cells from the healthy eye (left photo) and the injured eye after autograft transplantation covered by amniotic membrane (right photo)

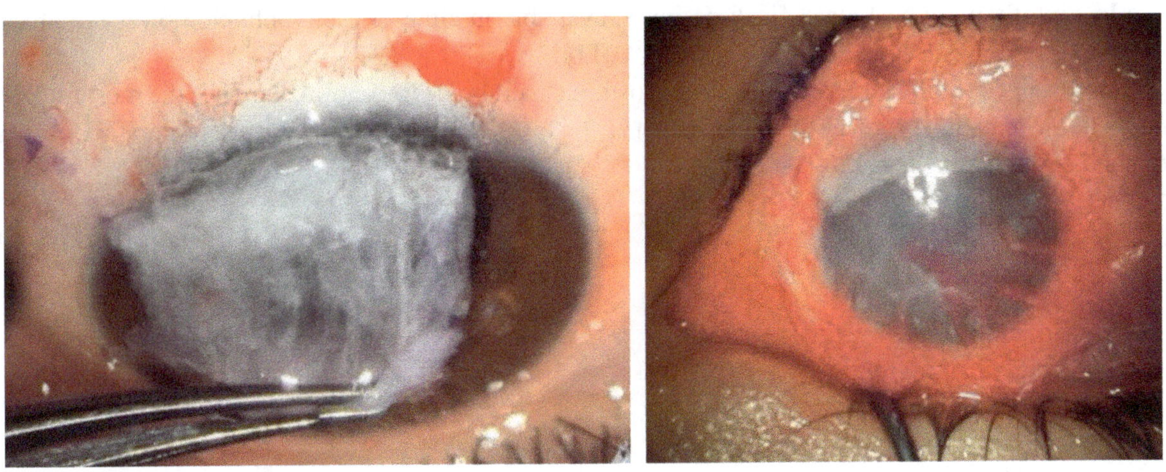

Figure 45. The same eye 1month after surgery

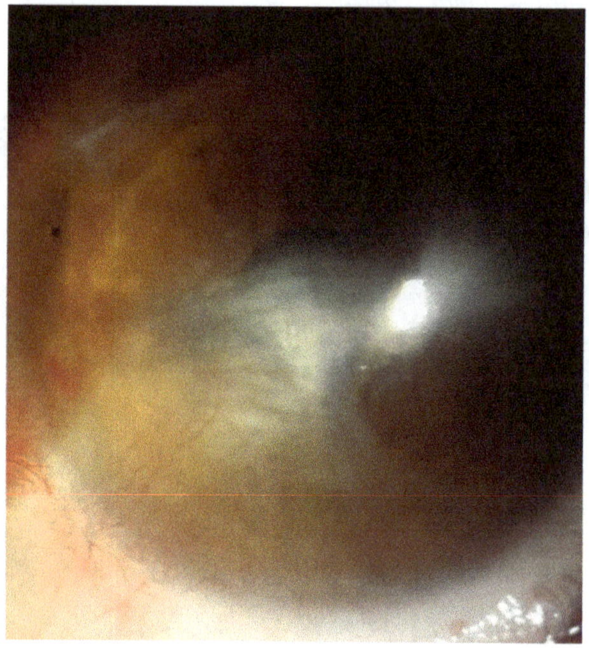

Keratoprosthesis

Keratoprosthesis (KPro) is an artificial corneal replacement, which is used for visual restoration of corneal blindness. Although numerous keratoprosthesis designs have been proposed and some of them have been attempted, two designs implemented most often are the Boston type 1 keratoprosthesis and the osteo-odonto-keratoprothesis (OOKP). Common indications for the Boston keratoprosthesis type 1 device include corneal allograft rejection, corneal opacity with extensive corneal neovascularization, limbal stem cell deficiency including aniridia, SJS, OCP, mild to moderate chemical injury, etc. Boston keratoprosthesis type 1 has an older snap-in design and a newer click-on design. The snap-in design consists of three components: a PMMA front plate with an optical stem, a PMMA or titanium backplate, and a titanium locking C-ring. The click-on design consists of only two parts, a PMMA front plate/stem, and a locking titanium backplate. Each design is available in either a pseudophakic power or aphakic power (46-57) (Sayegh et al, 2008; Pujari et al, 2011).

KPro surgery complications include: retroprosthetic membrane formation, which is the most frequent complication, glaucoma with the main long-term vision loss, endophthalmitis, infectious keratitis, corneal melt, and sterile keratolysis (58-63).[31-37]

Figure 46. Patient with h/o severe chemical alkali injury

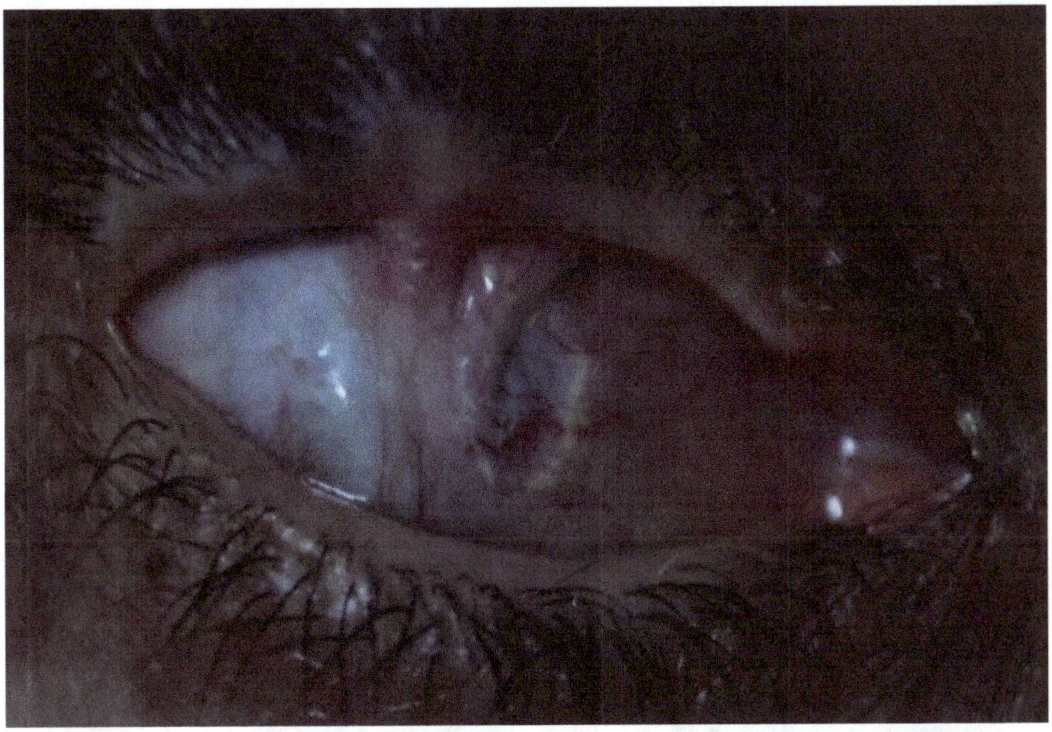

Figure 47. The same eye 6 months after Boston type 1 keratoprosthesis

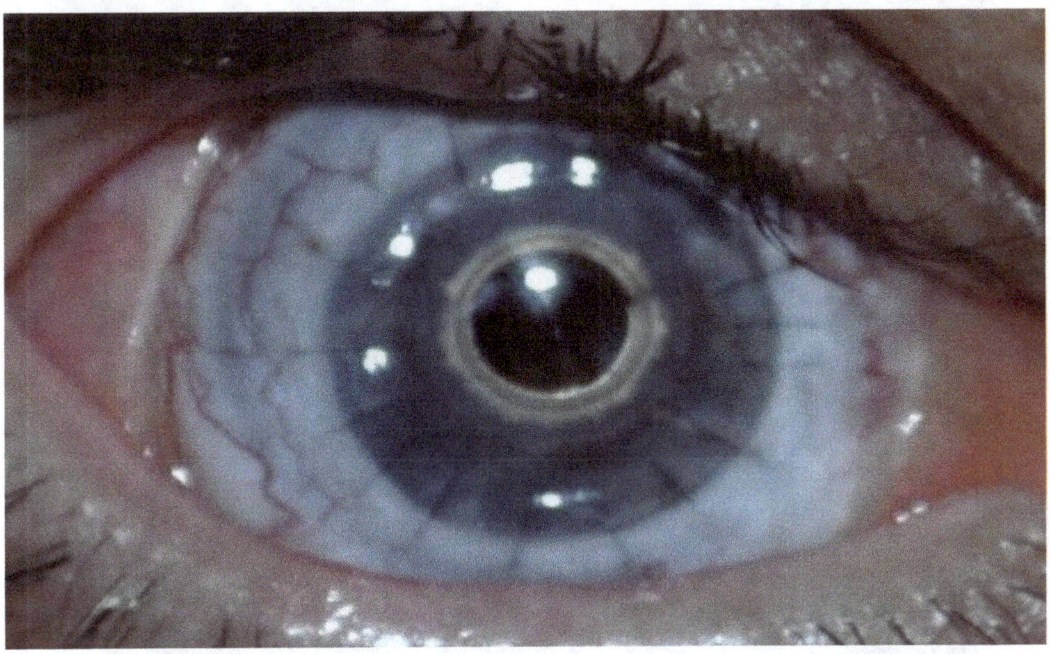

Figure 48. Severe chemical injury. Scarring and conjunctivalization is seen (left photo) and the same eye 2 weeks after surgery (right photo)

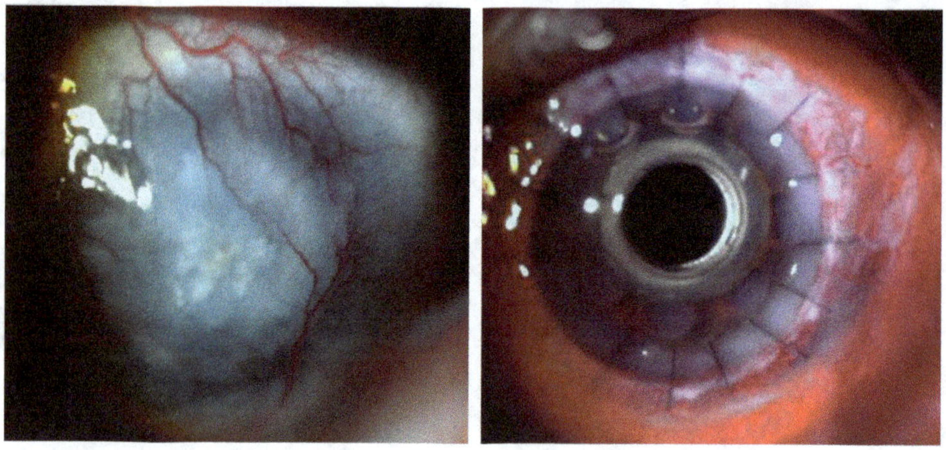

Figure 49. Postherpetic severe ectasia (left photo) and the same eye 6 months after Boston type 1 keratoprosthesis surgery (right photo)

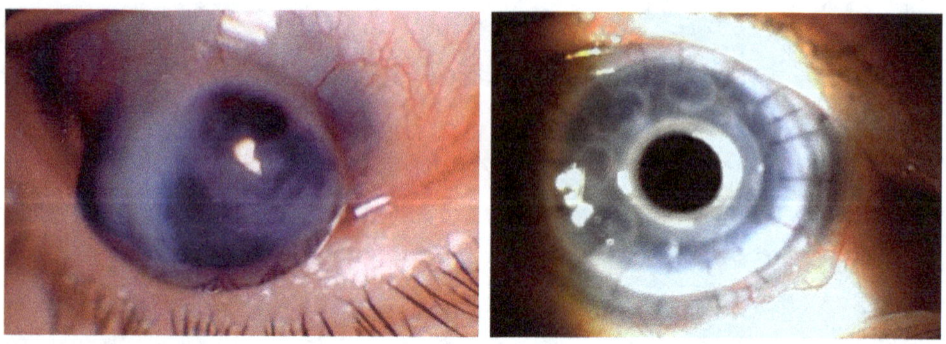

Figure 50. Vascularized cornea with h/o acid chemical injury and 2 failed PKs (left photo) and the same eye 2 weeks after Boston type 1 keratoprosthesis (right photo)

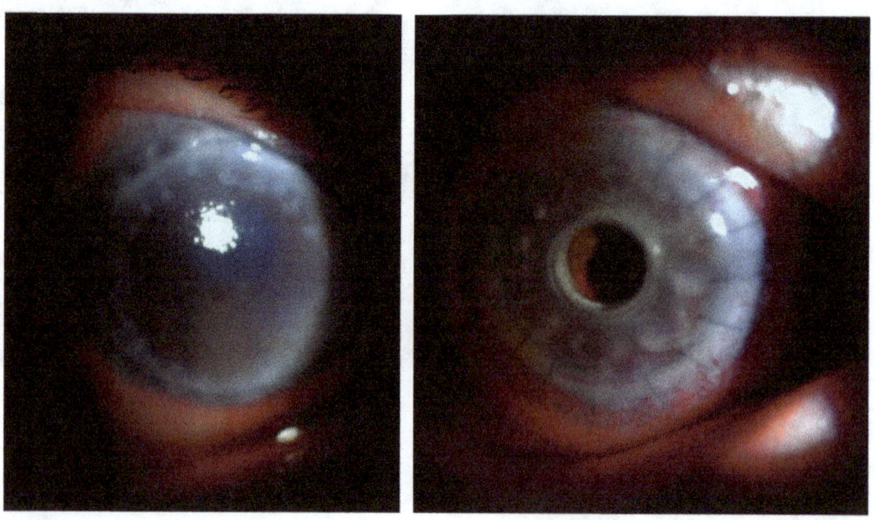

Figure 51. Ankyloblepharon due to OCP (left photo) and the same patient after eyelids reconstruction and further keratoprosthesis surgery 6 months later (right photo)

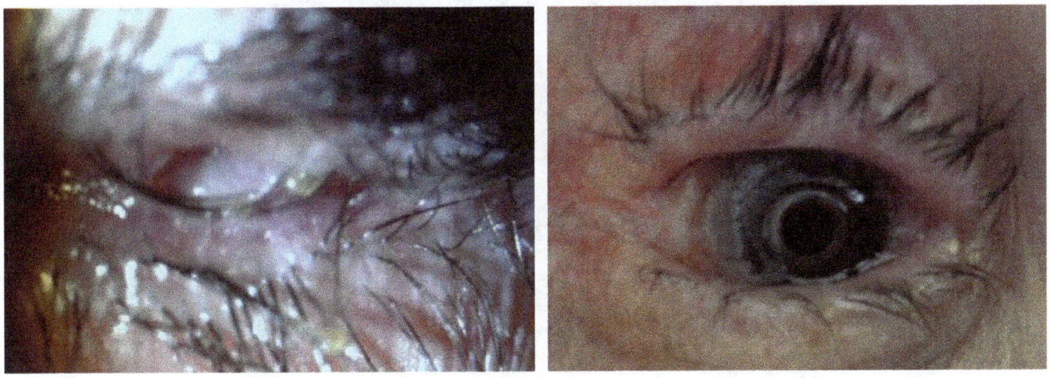

Figure 52. Corneal scaring and severe neovascularization caused by penetrating trauma with h/o multiple surgeries

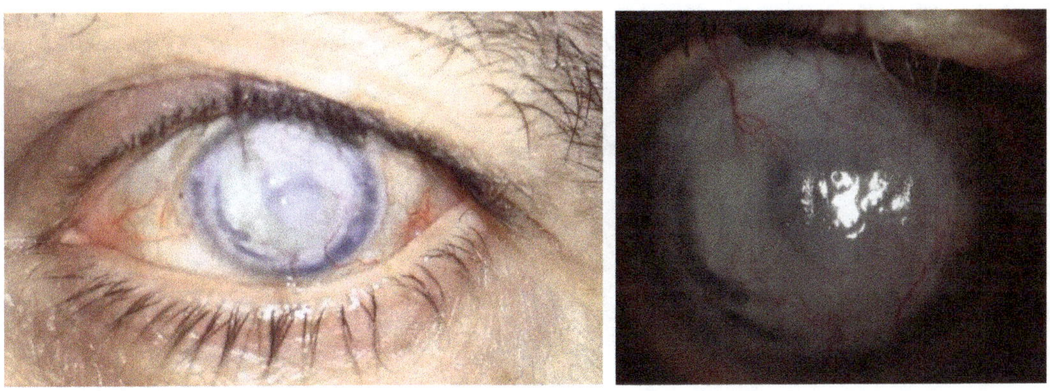

Figure 53. The same eye in OR. The artificial iris is seen

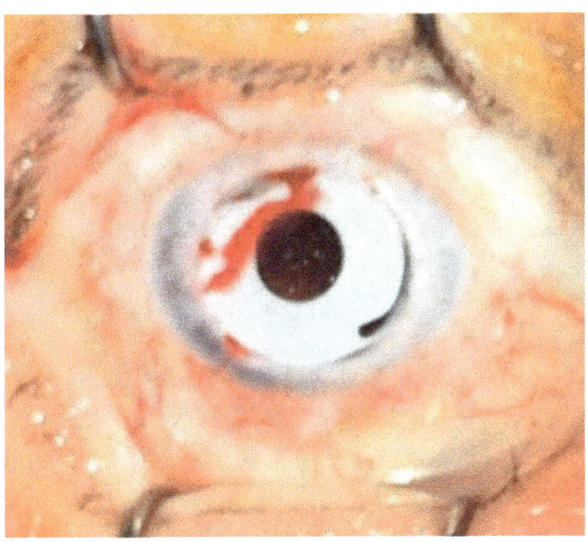

Figure 54. The same eye after KPro surgery in OR

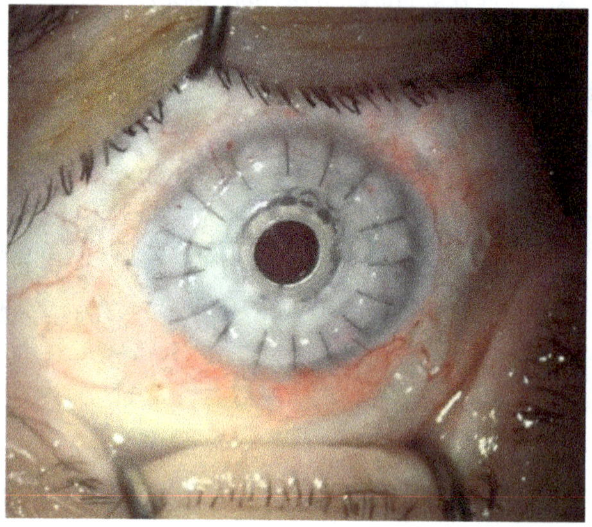

Figure 55. Bilateral keratoprosthesis. 14 years after surgery; h/o thermal injury (mine explosion)

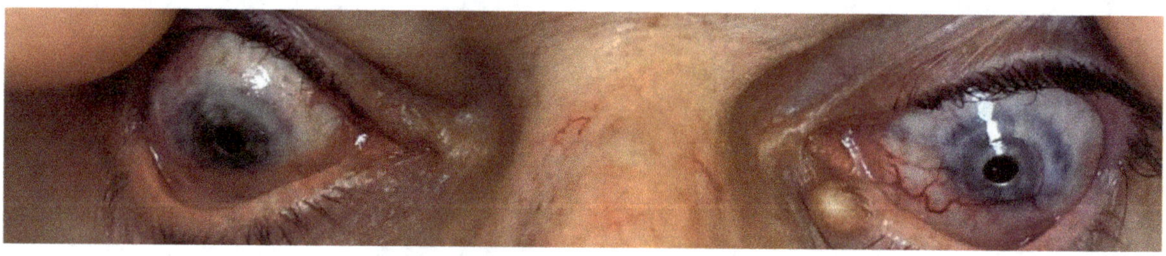

Figure 56. 6 y/o boy with h/o alkali chemical injury. Symblepharons and total conjunctivalization of external eye surface

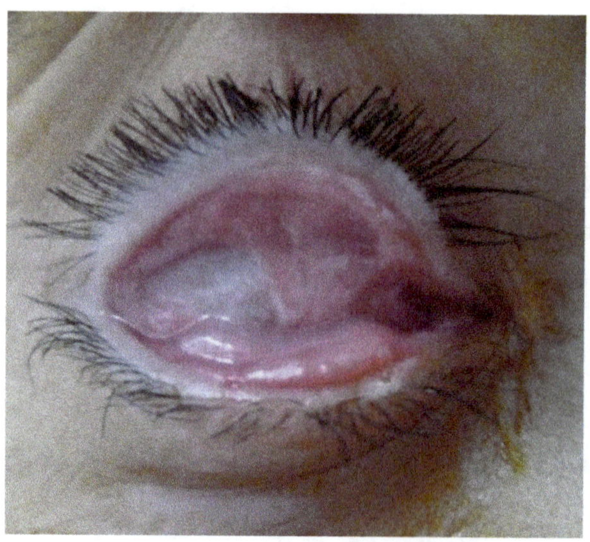

Figure 57. The same eye after surgery in OR (left photo) and 1 week later (right photo)

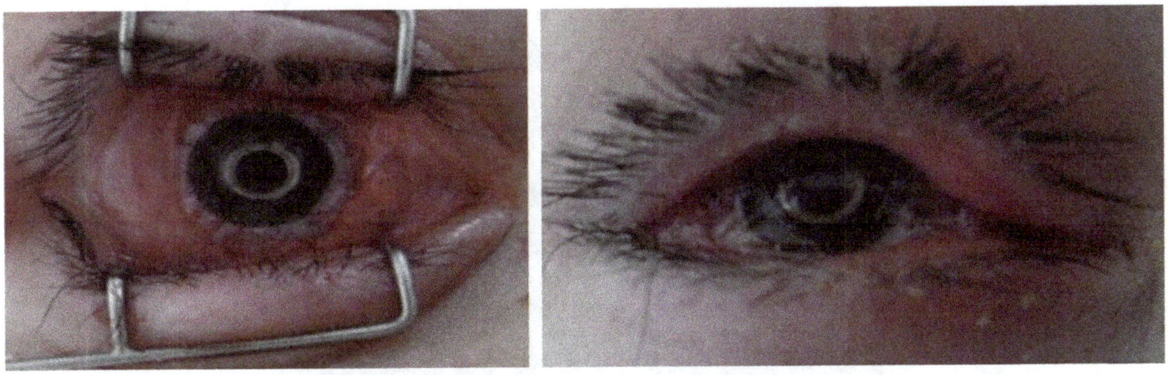

Figure 58. Retroprosthetic membrane is seen through the pupil

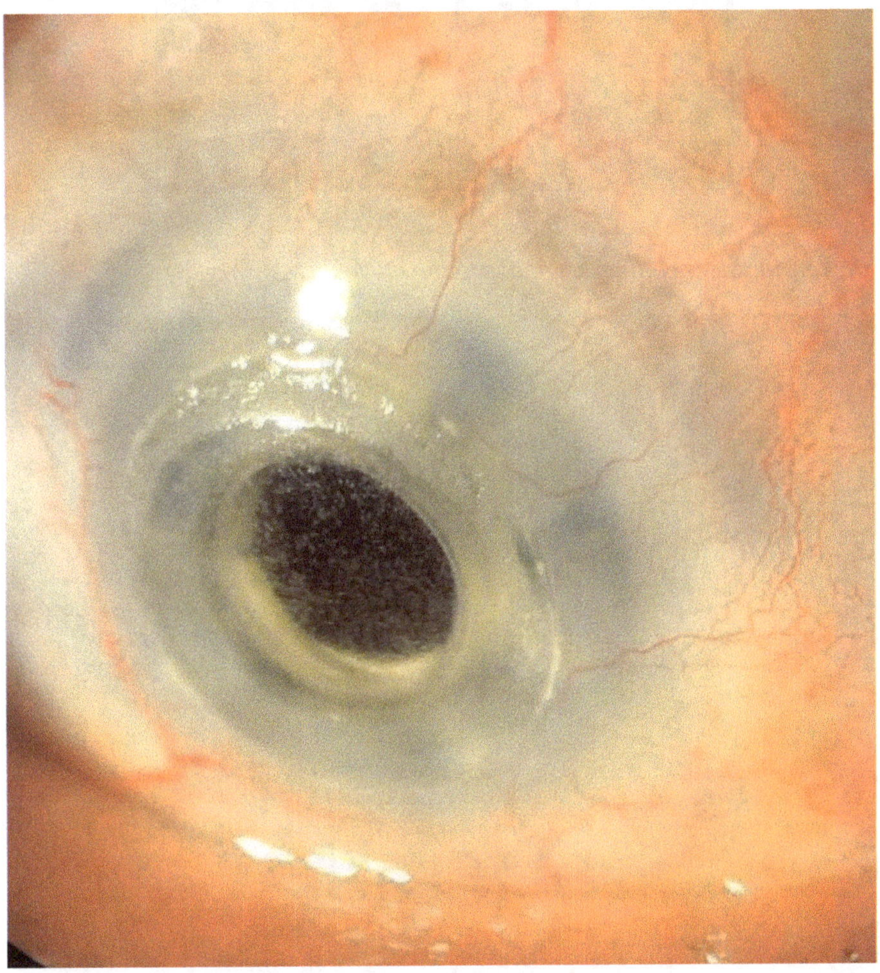

Figure 59. Donor cornea lysis 10 years after keratoprosthesis surgery

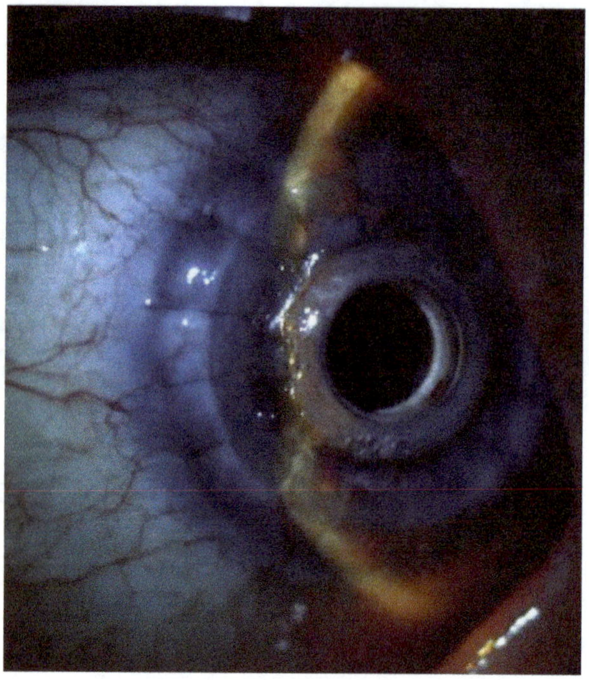

Figure 60. Sterile keratolysis, pending KPro extrusion, 1-year post surgery

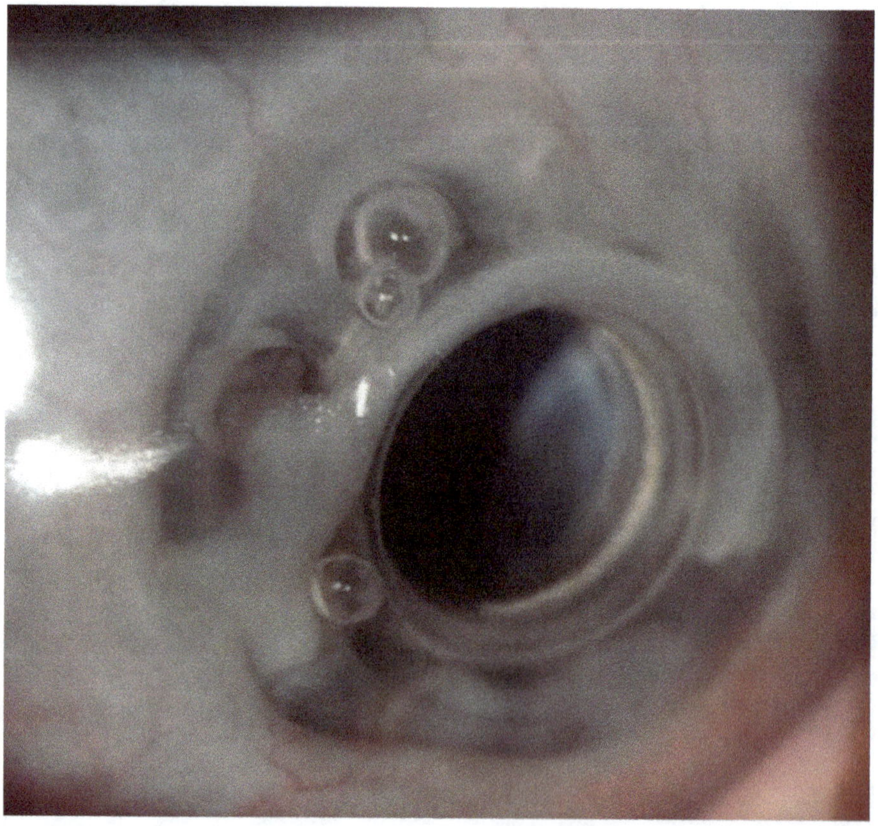

Figure 61. Endophthalmitis 8 years after keratoprosthesis surgery performed for corneal scarring due to chemical alkali injury

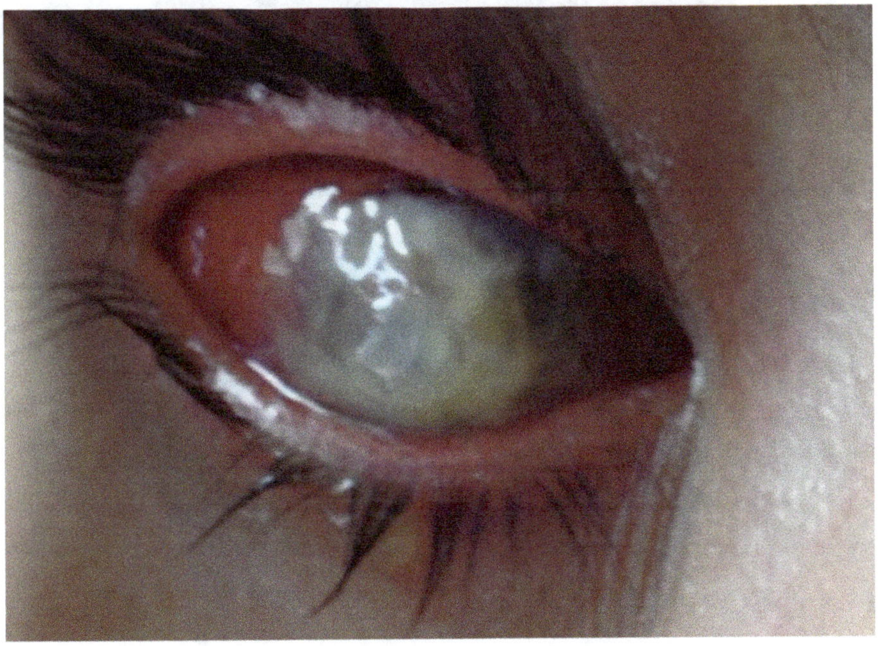

Figure 62. KPro extrusion

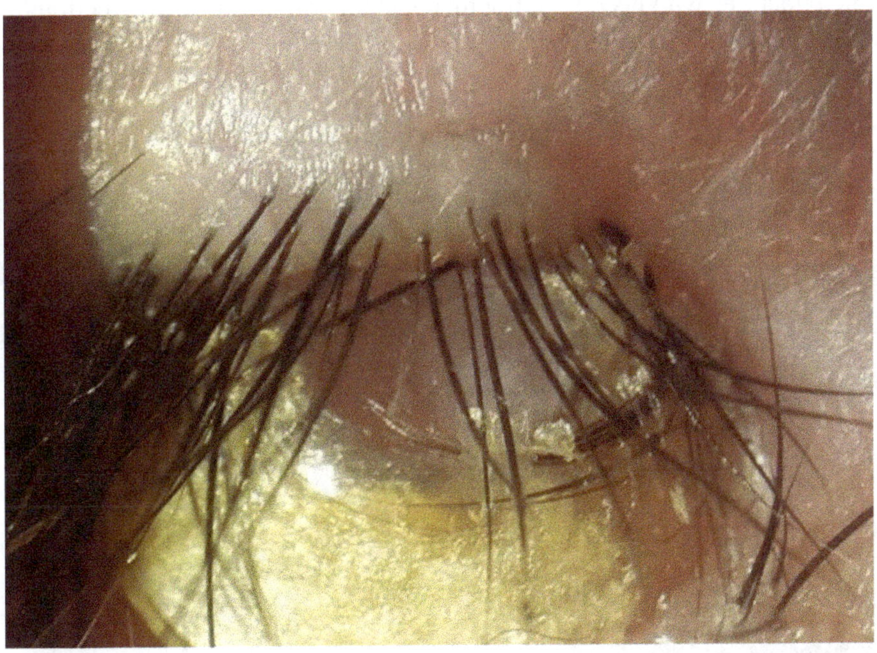

Figure 63. Total donor corneal melt, KPro extrusion

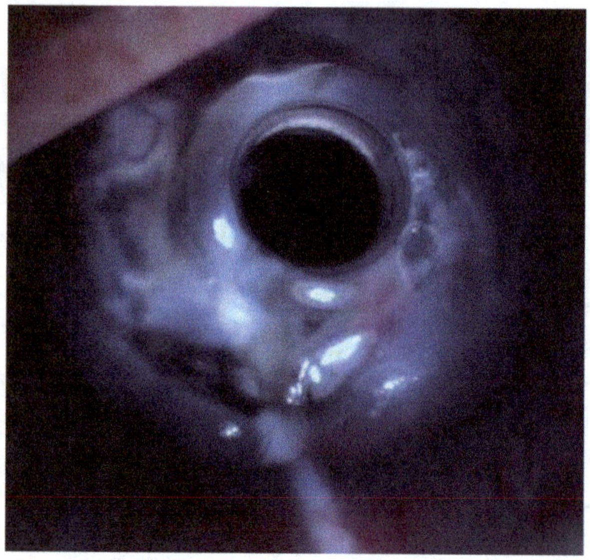

Corneal Tattooing Surgery

Corneal tattooing is mainly performed as a cosmetic surgery on blind patients with different types of corneal opacifications. Our technique includes deepithelization (superficial keartectomy), and application of ink via multiple punctures with needle to Bowman's membrane in oblique directions. The procedure usually takes 30 minutes.

Figure 64. Corneal opacification due to blind trauma before tattooing

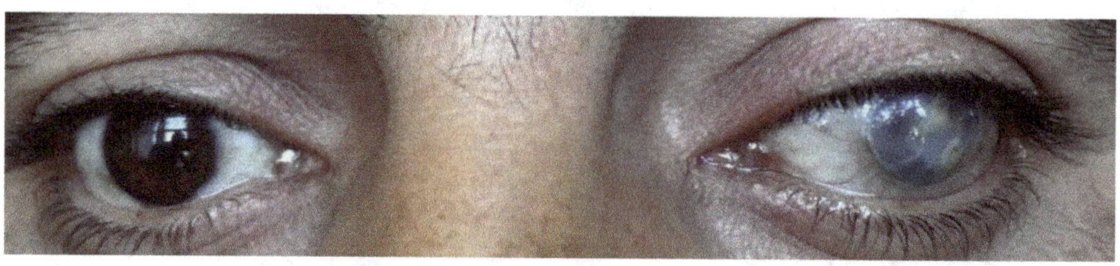

Figure 65. The same eye 2 weeks after tattooing

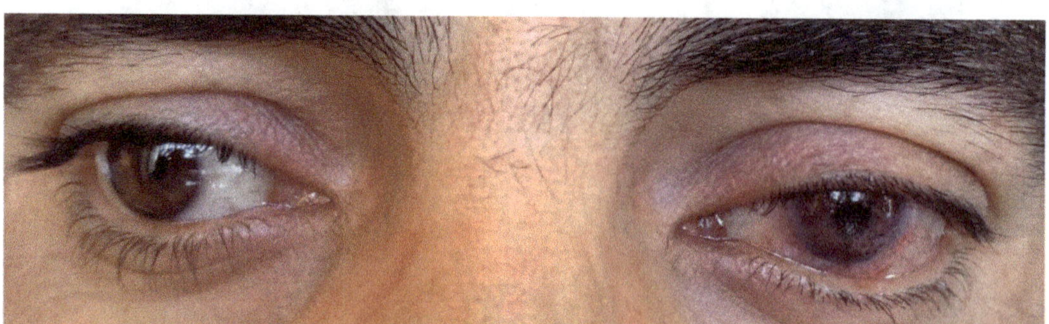

Figure 66. Mature cataract, old retinal detachment (left photo). The same eye after tattooing (right photo)

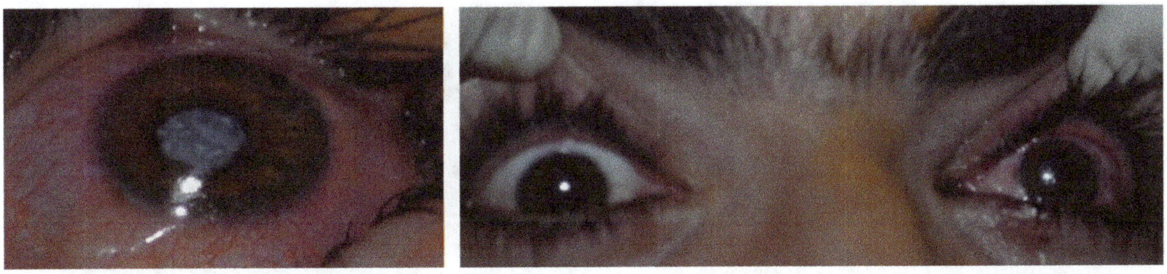

Figure 67. Corneal opacification due to blunt trauma

Figure 68. The same eye after tattooing, 2 months later

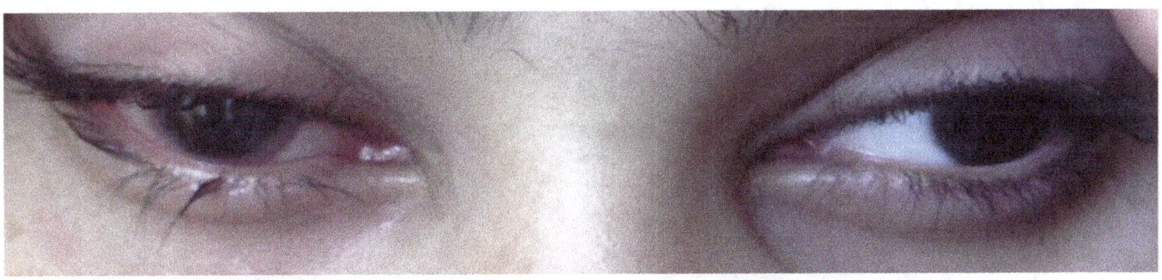

Figure 69. The same eye under a slit lamp

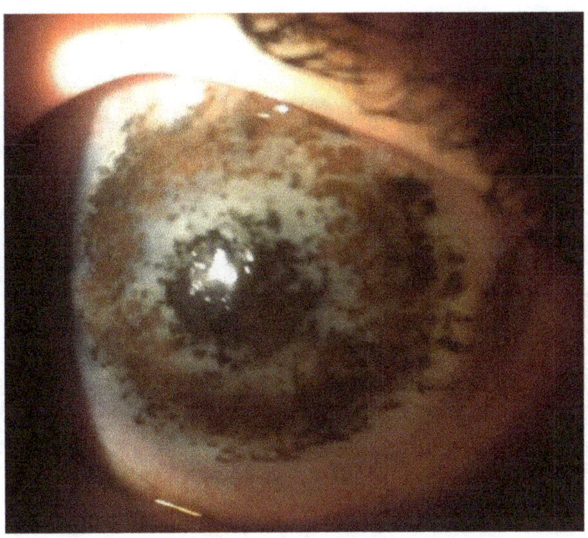

Figure 70. H/o penetrating trauma, corneal opacification

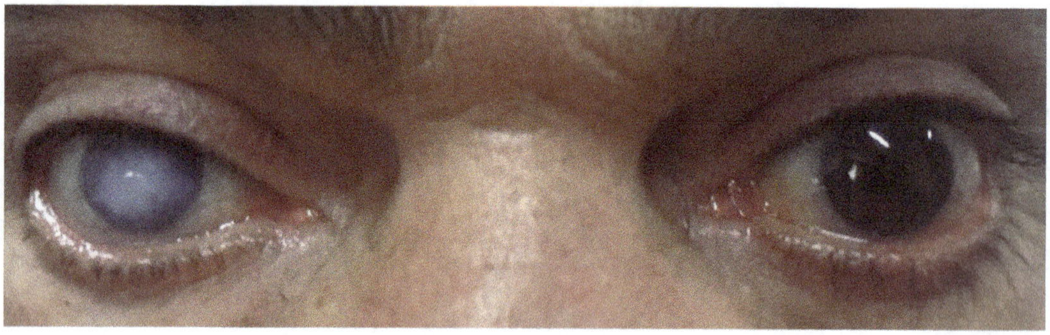

Figure 71. The same eye 1 week after the surgery

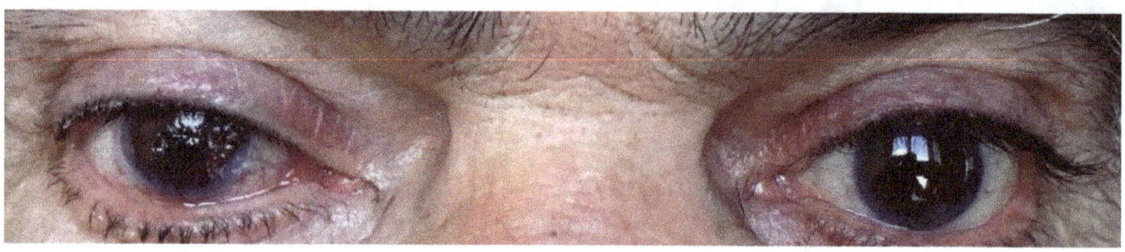

Figure 72. Half-opacified cornea due to penetrating trauma

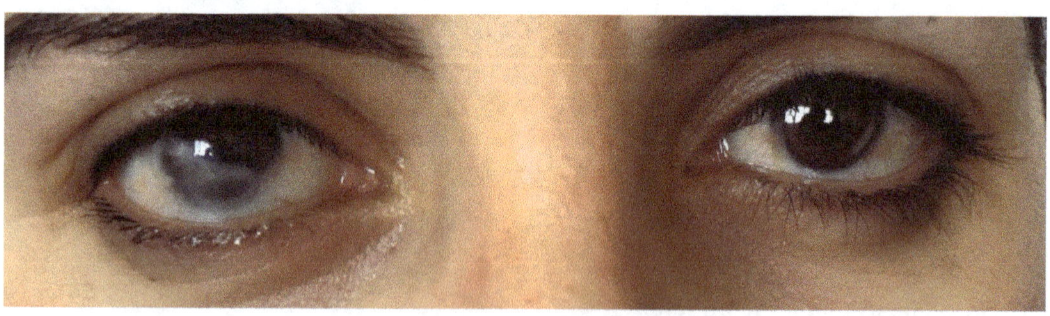

Figure 73. The same eye after tattooing in OR

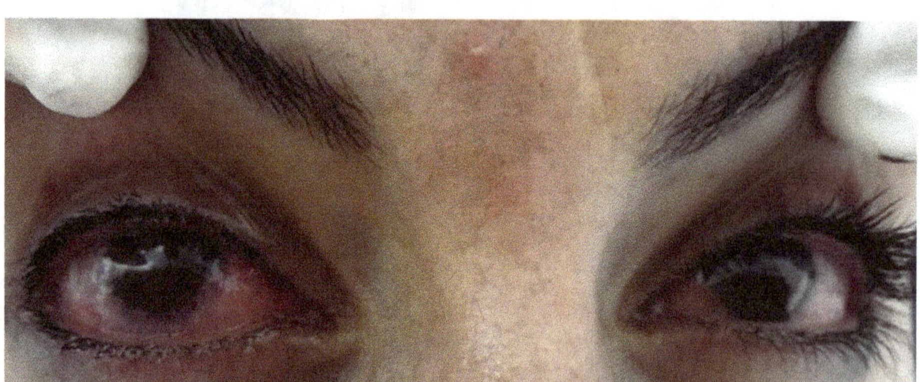

Figure 74. The opacified cornea due to old penetrating trauma

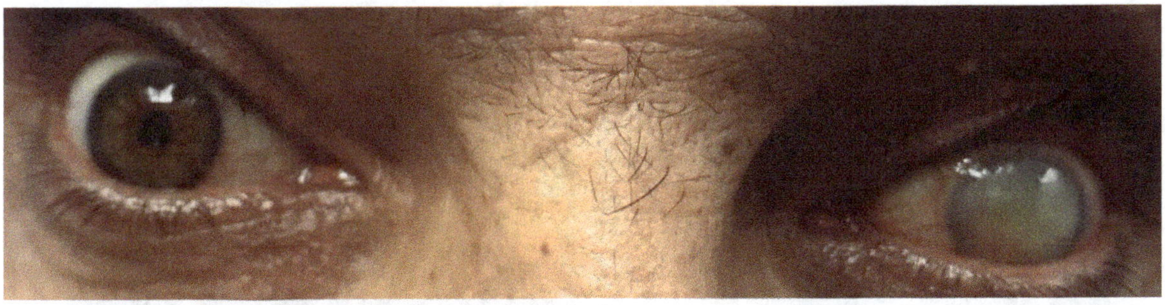

Figure 75. The same eye after tattooing in OR

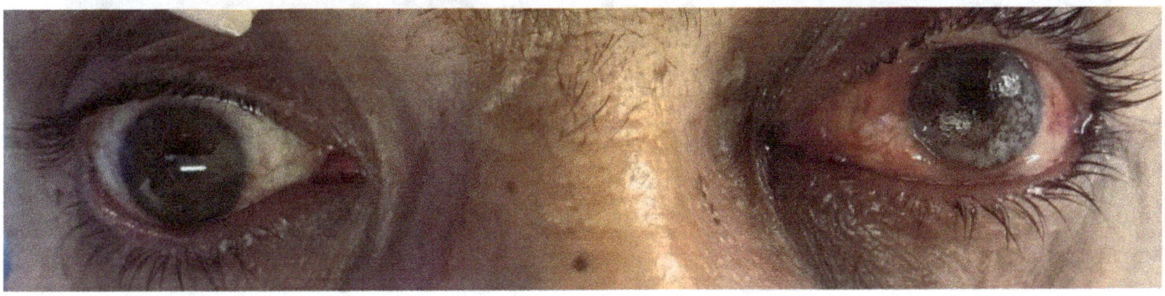

COMPLICATIONS

Rare Complications After Excimer Procedures, Cross-Linking and Other Intraocular Surgeries

Epithelial ingrowth occurs when the corneal epithelial cells grow within the lamellar interface beneath the LASIK flap.

Figure 76. Epithelial Ingrowth 3 months post LASIK

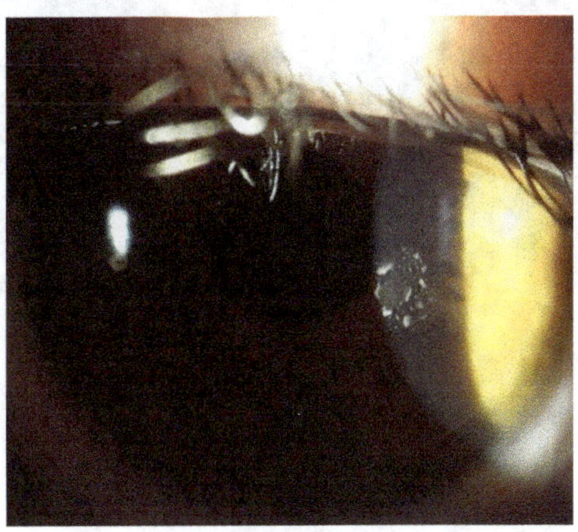

Figure 77. The right and left eyes of the patient. **Fibrosis** *after LASIK associated with severe dryness*

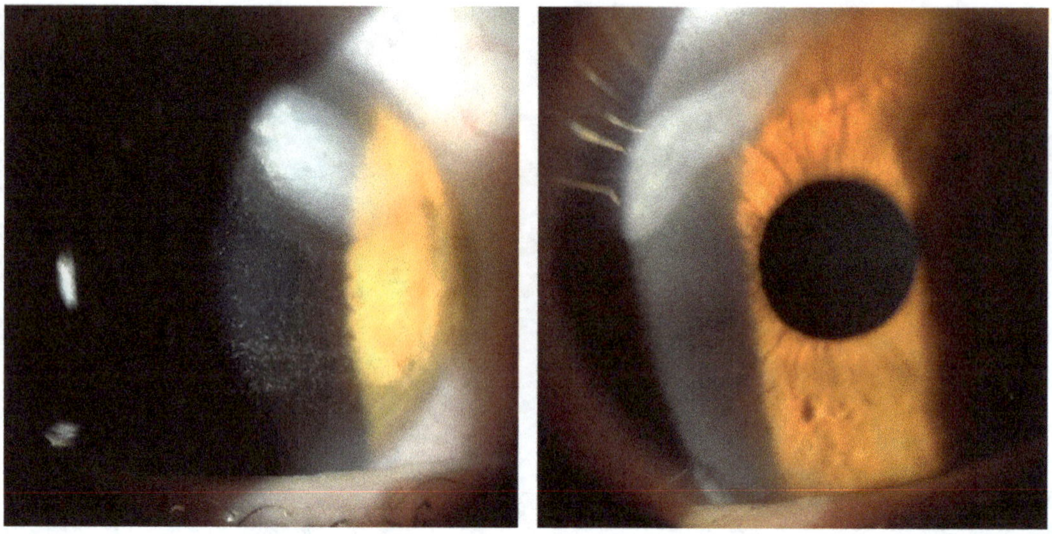

Diffuse lamellar keratitis (DLK) is a rare, noninfectious complication of refractive surgery characterized by inflammatory infiltrates beneath the corneal flap interface. The characteristic accumulation of fine white infiltrates manifests clinically as a grainy corneal opacification termed as "sands of Sahara syndrome."

Figure 78. DLK. The right and left eyes of the same patient after LASIK

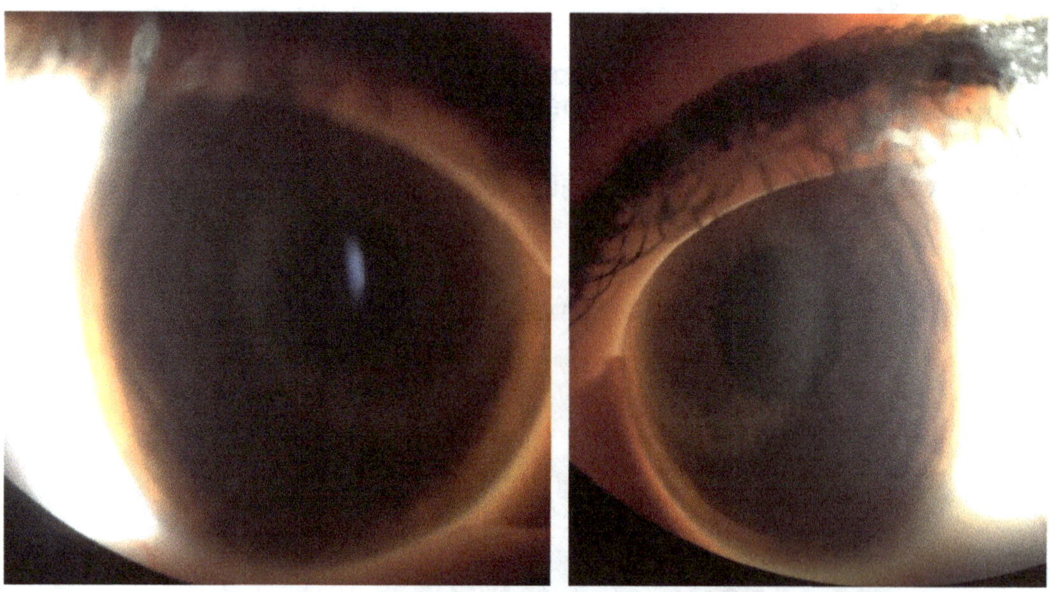

Figure 79. The same eye

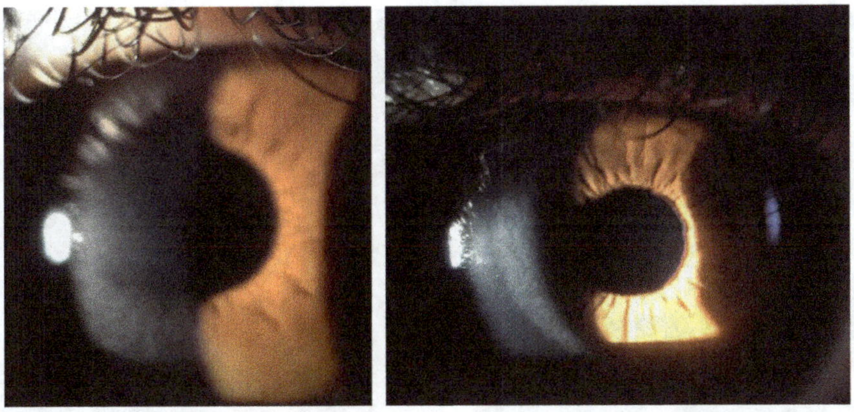

Sterile keratitis is a rare complication following corneal collagen crosslinking (CXL) treatment. The etiology remains unclear.

Figure 80. Sterile immune infiltrates/burns after cross-linking (left photo) and the same eye after 3 weeks of treatment with steroid drops, oral Vit. C, tears (right photo); edema has resolved, mild scarring is left

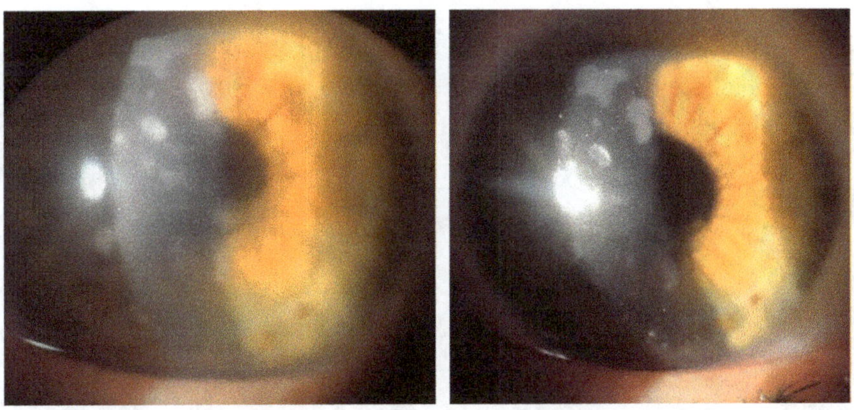

Figure 81. Post-LASIK infectious keratitis caused by Neisseria sicca

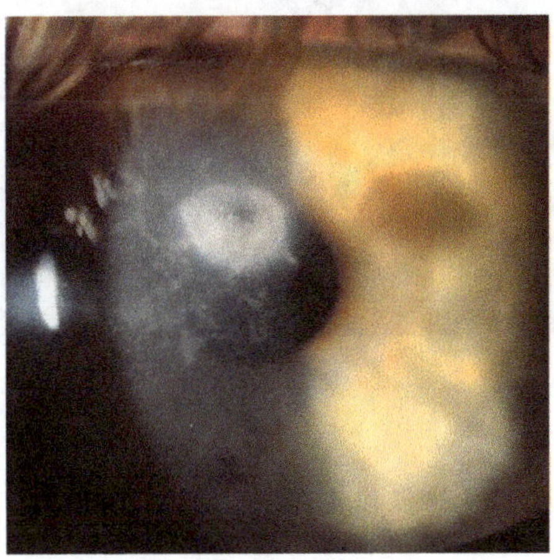

Figure 82. RK and AK cuts performed in Moscow, Russia in early 1980s

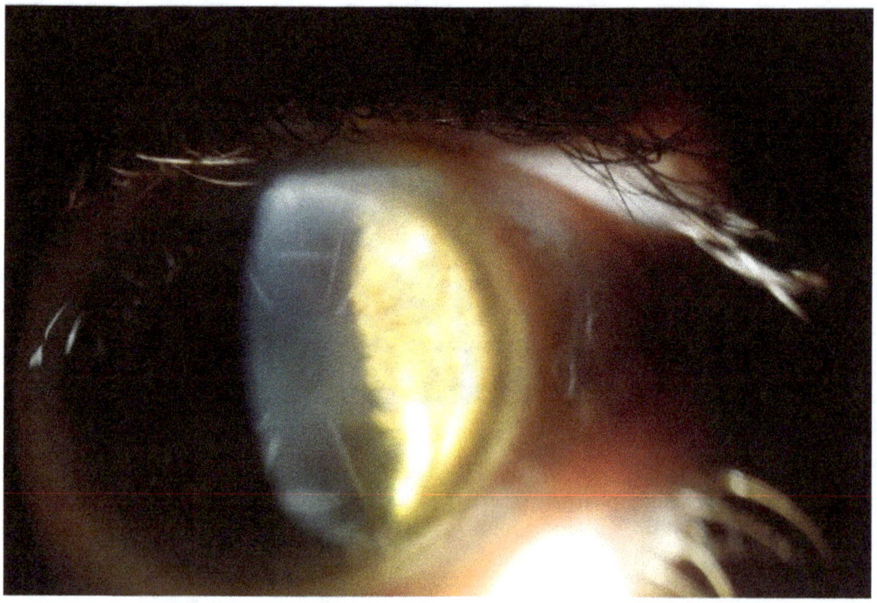

Figure 83. Conductive keratoplasty (CK) scars, performed for moderate hyperopia in Moscow, Russia

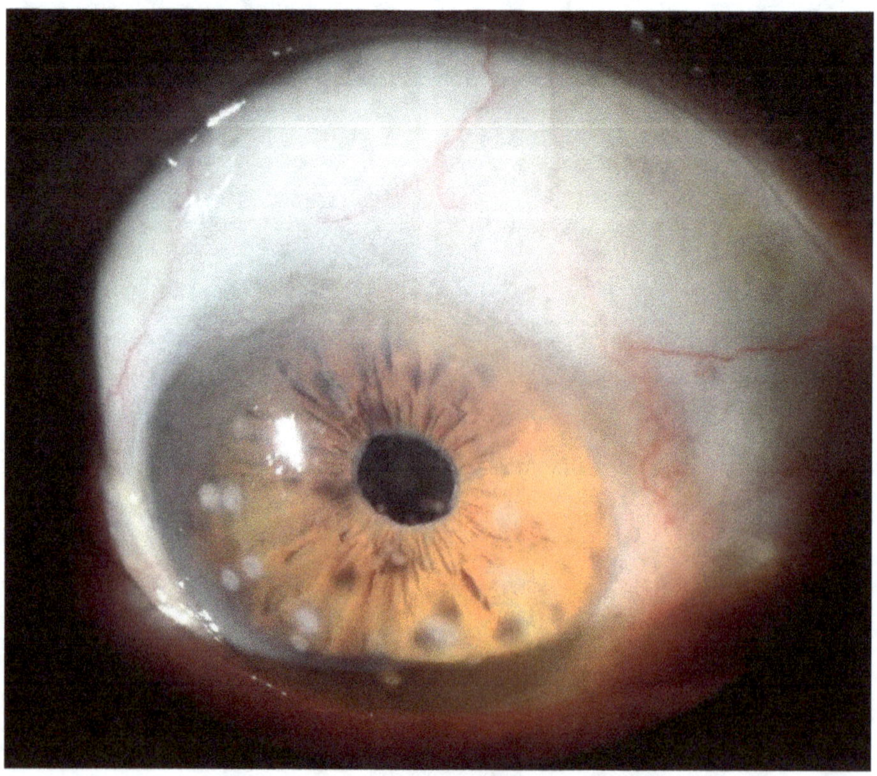

Figure 84. Fungal (Candida) keratitis with feathery borders after cross-linking, the hypopyon is seen in the right photo. Procedure performed for keratoconus

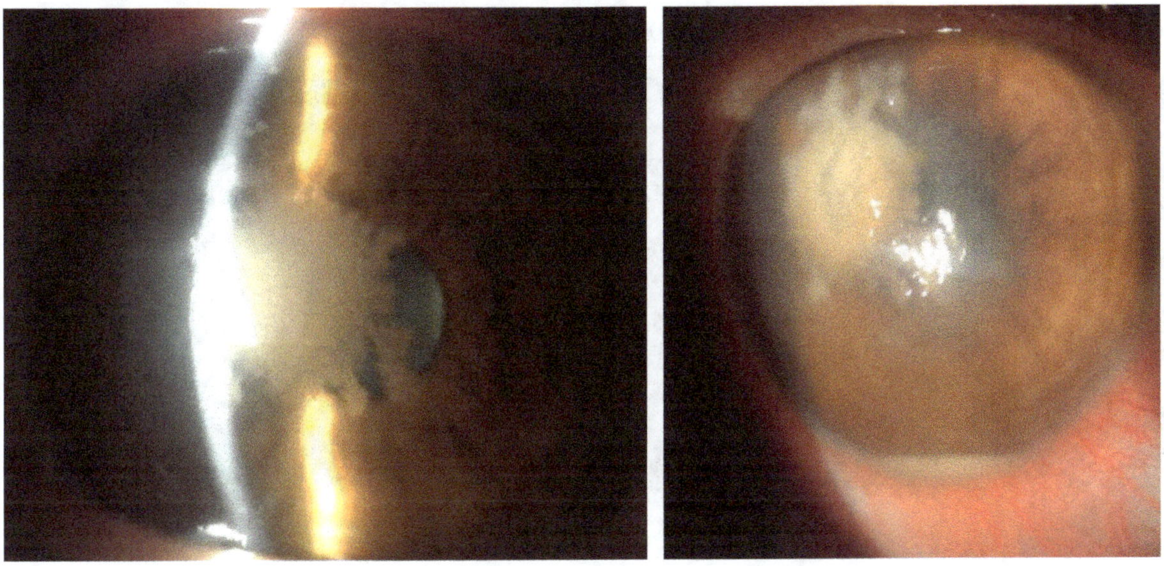

Figure 85. The same eye after 5 months of medical treatment with Amphotericin 0.15% eye drops, Fluconazole drops and subconjunctival injections; subepithelial haze formation is noted

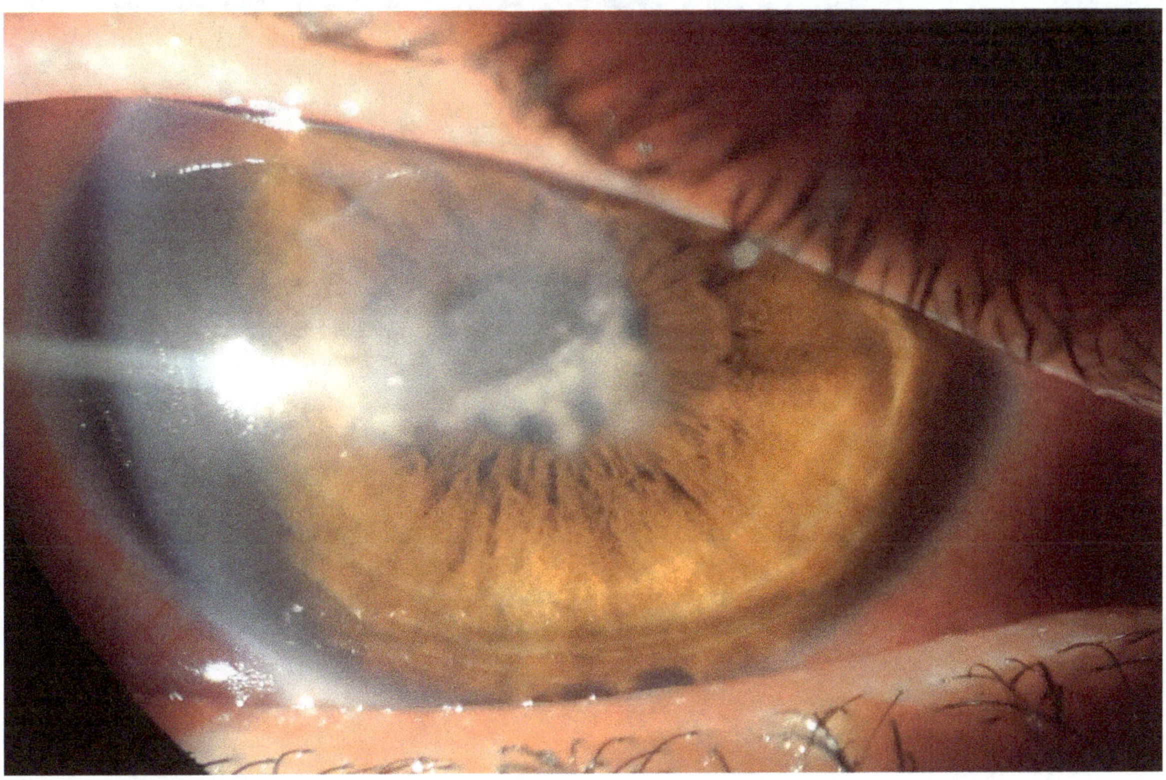

Descemet Membrane Detachment after Phacoemulsification Surgery

Figure 86. Descemet detachment noted the next day after cataract surgery. OCT image (right photo)

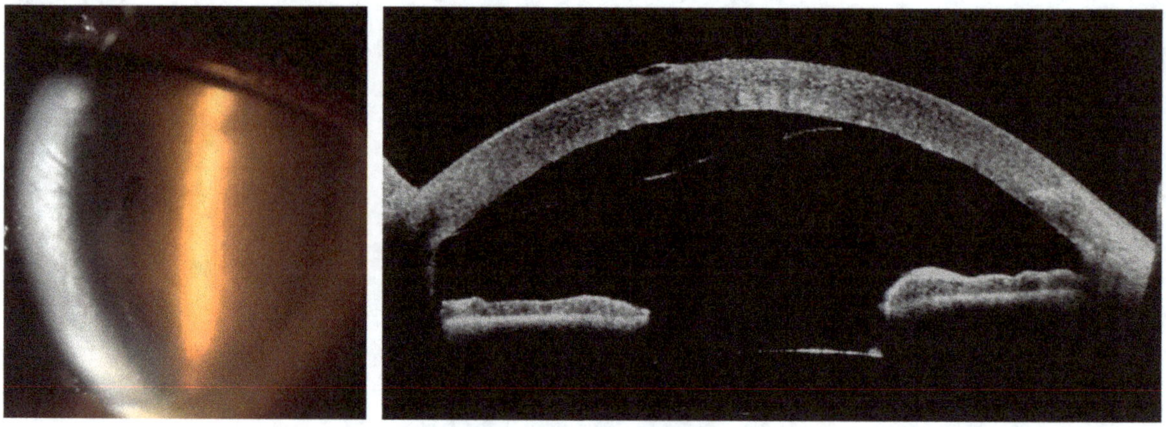

Figure 87. The same eye the next day after air injection with residual air seen in the anterior chamber (left photo). The same eye after 1 week of air injection. Descemet's membrane is attached (right photo)

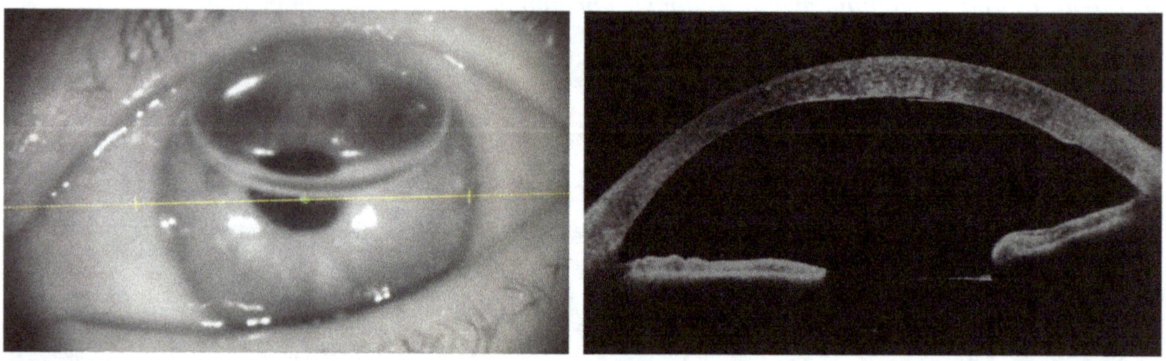

Bleb-Associated Endophthalmitis

Figure 88. Bleb-associated endophthalmitis with sectoral infectious scleritis caused by Pseudomonas aeruginosa

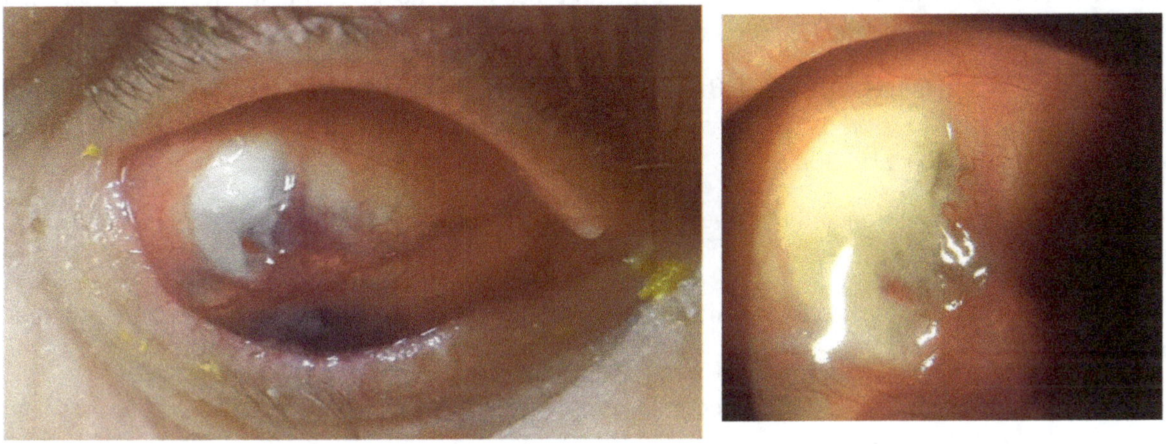

Figure 89. The same eye covered with a cosmetic contact lens 8 weeks after of treatment with I/v Ciprofloxacin, topical Ciprofloxacin, topical Tobramycin, Cycloplegics, Oral Doxycycline and tears

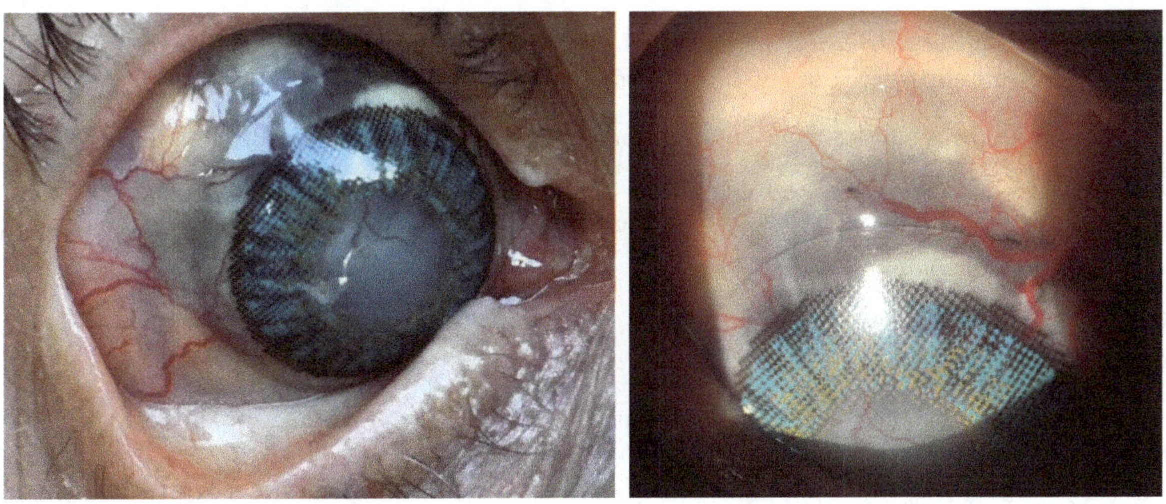

REFERENCES

Abry, Sauer, & Riegel. (2010). Infectious crystalline keratopathy caused by Streptococcus abiotrophia. *Cornea*, *29*, 934–936.

Alldredge, O. C., & Krachmer, J. H. (1981). Clinical types of corneal transplant rejection: Their manifestations, frequency, preoperative correlates and treatment. *Archives of Ophthalmology*, *99*, 599–604.

Anwar, M., & Teichmann, K. D. (2002). Big–bubble technique to bare Descemet's membrane in anterior lamellar keratoplasty. *Journal of Cataract and Refractive Surgery*, *28*(3), 398–403. doi:10.1016/S0886-3350(01)01181-6 PMID:11973083

Banitt, M. (2011). Evaluation and management of glaucoma after keratoprosthesis. *Current Opinion in Ophthalmology*, *22*, 133–136.

Chan, C. C., & Holland, E. J. (2012). Infectious endophthalmitis after Boston type 1 keratoprosthesis implantation. *Cornea*, *31*, 346–349.

Chan, C. C., & Holland, E. J. (2012). Infectious keratitis after Boston type 1 keratoprosthesis implantation. *Cornea*, *31*, 1128–1134.

Chaurasia, S., Price, F. W. Jr, & Gunderson, L. (2014). Descemet's membrane endothelial keratoplasty: Clinical results of single versus triple procedures (combined with cataract surgery). *Ophthalmology*, *121*, 454–458.

Christo, C. G., van Rooij, J., & Geerards, A. J. M. (2001). Suture-related complications following keratoplasty. A 5-year retrospective study. *Cornea*, *20*, 816–819.

Connell, M. (2006). A case of recurrent infectious crystalline keratopathy secondary to Haemophilus influenzae. *Eye*, *21*, 427–428.

Eiferman, R. A., Ogden, L. L., & Snyder, J. (1985). Anaerobic peptostreptococcal keratitis. *American Journal of Ophthalmology*, *100*, 335–336.

Giebel, A. W., & Price, F. W. (2008). *Air management of posterior grafts. FW Price MO Price DSEK: all you need to know about endothelial keratoplasty*. Slack Thorofare.

Gorovoy, M. S. (2006). Descemet-stripping automated endothelial keratoplasty. *Cornea*, *25*(8), 886–889. doi:10.1097/01.ico.0000214224.90743.01 PMID:17102661

Greiner, M. A., Li, J. Y., & Mannis, M. J. (2011). Longer-term vision outcomes and complications with the Boston Type 1 keratoprosthesis at the University of California, Davis. *Ophthalmology*, *118*, 1543–1550.

Groden, L. R., Pascucci, S. E., & Brinser, J. H. (1987). Haemophilus aphrophilus as a cause of crystalline keratopathy. *American Journal of Ophthalmology*, *104*, 89–90.

Holland, E. J., & Schwartz, G. S. (1996). The evolution of epithelial transplantation for severe ocular surface disease and a proposed classification system. *Cornea*, *15*, 549–556.

Hood, C. T., Lee, B. J., & Jeng, B. H. (2011). Incidence, occurrence rate, and characteristics of suture-related corneal infections after penetrating keratoplasty. *Cornea*, *30*, 624–628.

Hu, F. R. (1990). Infectious crystalline keratopathy caused by Mycobacterium fortuitum and Pseudomonas aeruginosa. *American Journal of Ophthalmology*, *109*, 738–739.

Kenyon & Tseng. (1989). Limbal autograft transplantation for ocular surface disorders. *Ophthalmology, 6*, 709-722.

Kim, M. J., Yu, F., & Aldave, A. J. (2013). Microbial keratitis after Boston type I keratoprosthesis implantation: Incidence, organisms, risk factors, and outcomes. *Ophthalmology*, *120*, 2209–2216.

Leahey, A. B., Avery, R. L., & Gottsch, J. D. (1993). Suture abscesses after penetrating keratoplasty. *Cornea*, *12*, 489–492.

Lee, J., & Sugar, J. (2008). Corneal graft rejection and Kaye's dots. *Survey of Ophthalmology*, *53*(1), 90–91.

Lee, W. B., Mannis, M. J., Mehra, N., & Garcia-Ferrer, F. (2006). Superficial hypertrophic dendriform epitheliopathy: A follow-up series. *Cornea*, *25*(3), 273–276.

Matoba, A. Y., O'Brien, T. P., & Wilhelmus, K. R. (1994). Infectious crystalline keratopathy due to Streptococcus pneumoniae: Possible association with serotype. *Ophthalmology*, *101*, 1000–1004.

Melles, G. R., Lander, F., Beekhuis, W. H., Remeijer, L., & Binder, P. S. (1999). Posterior lamellar keratoplasty for a case of pseudophakic bullous keratopathy. *American Journal of Ophthalmology*, *127*(3), 340–341. doi:10.1016/S0002-9394(98)00324-9 PMID:10088746

Melles, G. R. J., Eggink, F. A. G. J., Lander, F., Pels, E., Rietveld, F. J. R., Beekhuis, W. H., & Binder, P. S. (1998). A surgical technique for posterior lamellar keratoplasty. *Cornea*, *17*(6), 618–626. doi:10.1097/00003226-199811000-00010 PMID:9820943

Pfister, R. R., Richards, J. S. F., & Dohlman, C. H. (1972). Recurrence of herpetic keratitis in corneal grafts. *American Journal of Ophthalmology*, *73*, 192–196.

Price, F. W. Jr, & Price, M. O. (2006). Descemet's stripping with endothelial keratoplasty in 200 eyes. Early challenges and techniques to enhance donor adherence. *Journal of Cataract and Refractive Surgery*, *32*(3), 411–418. doi:10.1016/j.jcrs.2005.12.078 PMID:16631048

Price, M. O., Giebel, A. W., & Fairchild, K. M. (2009). Descemet's membrane endothelial keratoplasty: Prospective multicenter study of visual and refractive outcomes and endothelial survival. *Ophthalmology*, *116*, 2361–2368.

Pujari, S., Siddique, S. S., & Dohlman, C. H. (2011). The Boston keratoprosthesis type 2: The Massachusetts Eye and Ear Infirmary experience. *Cornea*, *30*(12), 1298–1303.

Robert, M. C., & Dohlman, C. H. (2014). A Review of corneal melting after Boston Keratoprosthesis. *Seminars in Ophthalmology*, *29*, 349–357.

Rudnisky, C. J., Belin, M. W., & Todani, A. (2012). Risk factors for the development of retroprosthetic membranes with Boston Keratoprosthesis Type 1 Multicenter Study Results. *Ophthalmology*, *119*, 951–955.

Sayegh, R. R., Ang, L. P., & Foster, C. S. (2008). The Boston keratoprosthesis in Stevens–Johnson syndrome. *American Journal of Ophthalmology*, *145*(3), 438–444.

Sugar, A., Meyer, R. F., & Hood, I. (1977). Epithelial downgrowth following penetrating keratoplasty in the aphake. *Archives of Ophthalmology*, *95*, 464.

Terry, M. A., & Ousley, P. J. (2005). Deep lamellar endothelial keratoplasty visual acuity, astigmatism, and endothelial survival in a large prospective series. *Ophthalmology*, *112*(9), 1541–1548. doi:10.1016/j.ophtha.2005.03.026 PMID:16005975

Tsubota, K., Toda, I., & Saito, H. (1995). Reconstruction of the corneal epithelium by limbal allograft transplantation for severe ocular surface disorders. *Ophthalmology*, *102*, 1486–1496.

Wilhelmus, K. R., & Robinson, N. M. (1991). Infectious crystalline keratopathy caused by Candida albicans. *American Journal of Ophthalmology*, *112*, 322–325.

Zabel, R. W., Mintsioulis, G., & MacDonald, I. (1988). Infectious crystalline keratopathy. *Canadian Journal of Ophthalmology*, *23*, 311–314.

About the Author

Anna Hovakimyan, MD, PhD, is a practicing ophthalmologist and the head of the Cornea-Uveitis department at the S.V. Malayan Eye Center in Yerevan, Armenia. She also holds professorship at the Yerevan State Medical University and is a coauthor of a hundred journal and conference publications. Her education outside her country includes two fellowships at the UCSF, Proctor Foundation, 2000-2001, and at the Cincinnati Eye Institute, 2004-2005, among many others. Her work has been recognized by numerous awards in Armenia, including a Silver Medal from AECP for 25 years of service, Avetis Aharonyan second degree silver award by "1.5mln+1 Armenia-Diaspora cultural bridge", award of Meria of Yerevan as a doctor with high sense of responsibility, and many others. She is married and has three children.

Index

F

G

H

I

K

L

M

N

O

P

S

T

V

W

X

www.ingramcontent.com/pod-product-compliance
Lightning Source LLC
LaVergne TN
LVHW080535300926
849162LV00007B/1611